Sleep, Health, and Society

Sleep, Health, and Society
From Aetiology to Public Health

Edited by

Francesco P. Cappuccio

Michelle A. Miller

Steven W. Lockley

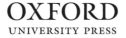

OXFORD
UNIVERSITY PRESS

OXFORD

UNIVERSITY PRESS

Great Clarendon Street, Oxford OX2 6DP

Oxford University Press is a department of the University of Oxford.
It furthers the University's objective of excellence in research, scholarship,
and education by publishing worldwide in

Oxford New York

Auckland Cape Town Dar es Salaam Hong Kong Karachi
Kuala Lumpur Madrid Melbourne Mexico City Nairobi
New Delhi Shanghai Taipei Toronto

With offices in

Argentina Austria Brazil Chile Czech Republic France Greece
Guatemala Hungary Italy Japan Poland Portugal Singapore
South Korea Switzerland Thailand Turkey Ukraine Vietnam

Oxford is a registered trade mark of Oxford University Press
in the UK and in certain other countries

Published in the United States
by Oxford University Press Inc., New York

© Oxford University Press 2010

British Library Cataloguing in Publication Data
Data available

Library of Congress Cataloging in Publication Data
Data available

Typeset in Minion by Glyph International, Bangalore, India
Printed in Great Britain
on acid-free paper by
CPI Antony Rowe, Chippenham, Wiltshire

ISBN 978–0–19–956659–4

10 9 8 7 6 5 4 3 2 1

Foreword

Macbeth does murder sleep, the innocent sleep,
Sleep that knits up the ravell'd sleeve of care,
The death of each day's life, sore labour's bath,
Balm of hurt minds, great nature's second course,
Chief nourisher in life's feast.

W. Shakespeare, *Macbeth*, Act 2 Scene 2

Is sleep a cause, a consequence, or a symptom? Shakespeare says it rather well: all three. Lack of sleep is a **cause** of distress and ill health. If we miss sleep we miss the balm of hurt minds, the chief nourisher in life's feast. Second, Macbeth's actions and his distress murder sleep. Sleep disturbance is a **consequence** of the circumstances of people's lives. Macbeth thinks he will sleep no more because he has just murdered King Duncan. More prosaically, shift work, overtime, and poor living conditions can all affect sleep with the likely ill-effects that causes. Third, Lady Macbeth's heart is sorely charged and her sleep is disturbed. Sleep disturbance is a **symptom** of depression and perhaps other illness.

These three – cause, consequence, and symptom – can all interact. Too much sleep, too little, or poor quality sleep can be the result of other problems but can, in their turn, cause other problems. Although the possibility of interaction must be always considered, it is important to sort out which of the three is operating, as interventions might be quite different. Sleep research has mostly been the subject of specialized small scale studies. This volume builds on and brings together epidemiological studies of sleep. It is greatly to be welcomed. Shakespeare knew sleep to be important and we know sleep to be important, but with what consequences and what we can do about it, has been unclear.

The first issue, of course, is the difficulty of measurement. It is said that for anyone who has had a baby or been a junior doctor on call, or both, the concept of a "normal" night's sleep is forever changed. Epidemiological studies described here rely for the most part on self-report. People are inaccurate enough in reporting what they do when they are awake, let alone when consciousness is doubtful or absent. That said, measurement error is a challenge to be overcome not a counsel of despair. People can report how long they slept and if they have disturbed nights. The results are extraordinarily interesting. Short sleep, overly long sleep, and sleep disturbance all seem to play a role in disease.

Second, it is not at all surprising that sleep should be intimately bound up with hormonal and metabolic changes and that these will have effects on health and disease. The surprise is that we should not have given sleep, this fundamental part of life, all the attention it deserves. The link between short sleep and obesity via an effect of short duration on leptin and ghrelin and hence on appetite regulation is an elegant example. As the book makes clear we now need much more work to explore both the nature of the link between aspects of sleep and chronic disease and the mechanisms by which they occur.

This leads to the third big issue. If, as seems likely, the evidence firms up that sleep quality and duration are important, what is to be done? As an example, we know that shift work and overtime work with their impact on sleep, have deleterious health effects. There will be other features of the circumstances in which people live and work with impacts on sleep. How should they be addressed?

One in particular relates to children. As this book makes clear sleep in childhood is likely to be important. Yet data from Britain show that the likelihood of a regular bed time for children diminishes the lower the socioeconomic position of their parents. This was highlighted by the Review we conducted of Health Inequalities in England. We emphasized the likely consequences on child development and hence on health inequalities in adult life.

The big achievement of this volume is to bring together research on the health consequences of sleep and put sleep on the agenda for research in epidemiology and public health. It is timely indeed.

Professor Sir Michael Marmot MBBS, MPH, PhD, FRCP, FFPHM
Director, University College London International Institute for Society and Health
Head of the University College London Department of Epidemiology and Public Health
Chairman, Commission on Social Determinants of Health
President, British Medical Association

Foreword

There are currently 6.85 billion people on Earth, and every one of them is subject to the biological imperative of daily sleep. Our genetic code instantiates this imperative in a circadian rhythm of sleep and waking, which reflects evolutionary adaptation that extends back to the oldest complex animals. Modern societies often question the need to sleep each day, and many social factors (e.g., television viewing, commute time to/from work) result in reduction of time for sleep in exchange for time spent in work, leisure, and other more socially and economically valued pursuits. However, this modern view of sleep as a low-value, nonessential activity is increasingly contradicted by a steady flow of scientific evidence on the physiological and neurobehavioural effects of sleep deprivation, suggesting that sleep serves critical biological needs. However, experimental evidence such as this has not stemmed the tide of political, social, and economic pressure to have more people awake for more amount of time, especially in nonstop industrialized societies with their heavy reliance on electronic technologies and machine automation.

What has begun to give pause to the view that sleep is merely an archaic arbitrary activity that has no meaningful relation to health and lifespan is the recent explosion of population science on sleep health, sleep duration, and sleep timing, relative to obesity, disease, and mortality. While epidemiological studies of self-reported sleep time and health status began to appear more than 40 years ago, many of the hundreds of published population studies on sleep in relation to public health have appeared in the past 15 years, and have come from all over the globe, as population science and sleep science have matured in parallel in academic institutions, and as obesity has increased around the world, as time has become more valuable, and as stress and psychological uncertainty have become normative for many humans. Collectively, these post-Cold War global changes have caused concern that public health may require attention to factors other than the traditional focus on sanitation and clean water, vaccinations, management of toxins, etc. As a result of widespread evidence that sleep duration in particular has an association with obesity, serious common diseases, and mortality, sleep and sleep disorders have become visible as possible significant contributors to the health of both children and adults.

What has been missing in the scientific and policy debates about whether adequate sleep is important for public health is a thoughtful integration of the rapidly expanding epidemiological literature on sleep. Fortunately, this marvelously comprehensive book, *Sleep, Health, and Society: From Aetiology to Public Health*, edited by Cappuccio, Miller, and Lockley, is a much-needed integration of the burgeoning data on sleep need and public health. It is the first systematic review of this literature by content experts in their fields, and it provides an overdue and essential critical evaluation of the strengths and weaknesses of the data, the conclusions that can be drawn from the available evidence, the limitations of arguments used pro and con relative to sleep need in relation to obesity, health, accidents, and mortality, and the need for specific types of studies going forward.

The extensive evidence reviewed in the well-written chapters of this text reveals that sleeping 7–8 hours per night may be optimal for health for a great many people, but the authors conclude that, in many cases, this general statement cannot be asserted as factual causality until prospective studies, mechanistic studies, and intervention studies confirm it. On the other hand, public health policy does not always have to wait for conclusive evidence of causality, especially if an epidemic is moving rapidly and in vulnerable populations, as is the case with obesity in children. There is ample evidence that reduced sleep duration and obesity are associated in children. As reviewed by Gozal and Spruyt in Chapter 10, chronic inadequate sleep may contribute not only to obesity in children but also to neurobehavioural problems, which appear to be increasing in frequency. Whether there is a direct or indirect causal relationship between sleep duration and obesity in children, it would seem unwise to avoid doing the needed prospective interventional studies with objective measures of sleep and obesity.

It is well established that inadequate sleep – whether voluntary or from disorders that disrupt sleep continuity or duration – often leads to significant risk of accidents relative to driving and other safety-sensitive activities. As a result, public policies continue to evolve in many countries regarding treatment of sleep disorders, fatigue management in the work place, and improved schedules for those who work nights, rotating shifts, and prolonged and irregular duty periods. The public health and policy response to inadequate sleep and increased risk to safety is by no means sufficient, however, as the last seven chapters of this text reveal. Nevertheless, these policy responses are further along than the as-yet-nonexistent public policies regarding the need for healthy adequate sleep duration. This text highlights the importance of public health research mobilized around objective measures of sleep and health, using study designs superior to extensive cross-sectional research conducted to date.

Surprisingly, it is often argued that large-scale population-based intervention trials to evaluate the benefits of extending sleep time are too costly or infeasible. This perspective is somewhat needlessly pessimistic and reminds one of reasoning used to avoid studying women and myocardial infarcts, minorities in health-related outcome studies, and interventions for weight loss. Yet, in all of these cases, when public health research was properly conducted, the resulting science provided definitive answers regarding actual risks and benefits. Why should assessing the benefits of improving sleep quality or extending sleep time be any different than evaluating diets, or exercise, or other interventions? As many of the authors argue in chapters throughout the book, we must push the science beyond reliance on self-report measures of sleep and cross-sectional designs. Even if prospective intervention studies demonstrate that cost-benefits argue in favour of allowing sleep to be curtailed (likely) for economic reasons, public health understanding of the scope of the problems posed by sleep loss for the most vulnerable populations will be enriched, and public awareness may affect behavioural changes.

Sleep, Health, and Society presents a comprehensive and critical look at the remarkable accumulation of data on the association between sleep and public health risks. It points out the most promising paths to follow scientifically to determine why these associations continue to be found globally. What is needed now is the public policy will and resources to resolve these important and promising opportunities for improving public health by understanding how alterations in sleep quality and quantity affect weight gain, cardiovascular and respiratory health, metabolism, neurological status, and mortality. The text offers the first comprehensive public health focus on what we know about sleep and its potential criticality for healthy populations. It points to the path that enlightened societies should take relative to one of nature's oldest and most important biological imperatives.

David F. Dinges, PhD
Professor, Director, Unit for Experimental Psychiatry
Chief, Division of Sleep and Chronobiology
Vice Chair for Faculty Affairs and Professional Development
Department of Psychiatry
University of Pennsylvania School of Medicine
Philadelphia, USA

Acknowledgements

We are delighted to see the publication of this book which represents one of the first comprehensive textbooks of Sleep Epidemiology. The seeds were laid in late 2005 with the establishment of the *Sleep, Health, & Society Programme* at the University of Warwick in close collaboration with the Division of Sleep Medicine at Brigham and Women's Hospital and Harvard Medical School. The ambition was to close important gaps in medical teaching and research in the area of sleep medicine and to expand our knowledge of the population implications of sleep disturbances and sleep disorders. It is extraordinary to reflect on the speed with which this discipline has developed and gained momentum in just a few years. It goes without saying that this book would not have been possible without the scholarly and highly professional contributions of many authors who gave time, expertise, and enthusiasm to the project. Our gratitude and appreciation go to them primarily.

Such an achievement, however, would not have been reached without the aid of many others. The *Sleep, Health, & Society Programme* has been supported by a multidisciplinary team of researchers and we wish to thank, in particular, Anne Bakewell, Lanfranco D'Elia, Richard Donahue, Joan Dorn, Mair Edmunds, Chen Ji, N-B Kandala, Pasquale Strazzullo, Jason Sullivan, Frances Taggart, Maurizio Trevisan, and Geraldine Ward for their fundamental role in the development of the *Sleep, Health, & Society* research programme.

First and foremost, our particular thanks go to Yvonne Carter, founding Dean of Warwick Medical School, who provided encouragement and support to us: sadly she is no longer with us to enjoy this book. We also thank Ed Peile, who had the foresight to develop the first formal medical school training course in Sleep Medicine nationwide in 2004. Over 60 medical students have now completed the Special Study Module in Sleep Medicine, initiating a new generation of physicians to the importance of getting good sleep for keeping good health. We are grateful for their positive feedback and the participation that makes our teaching module a continuing success. Each year we have had students who have developed a keener interest in research aspects of the discipline. In particular, we wish to thank Daniel Cooper, Andrew Currie, and Alex Lowe who have participated more actively in several research projects in their own time with commendable commitment and professionalism.

A special note of gratitude also goes to Paul Blake for his initial vision, significant support, and tireless encouragement, and for allowing total independence on the direction of travel.

We express our thanks to the staff at Oxford University Press, in particular to Georgia Pinteau, who guided us through the early stages of our proposal giving time, expertise, and encouragement, Eloise Moir-Ford and Jenny Wright, and more recently Nic Wilson, whose expert knowledge of the editorial process coupled with a profound understanding of the academic domains contributed to the completion of the book. Finally, we owe much gratitude to Patricia McCabe for her unreserved administrative support to the project, her long hours devoted to it, the sense of commitment and diplomacy in dealing with publisher, editors, and authors, and her resilience. For all these reasons, and for much more, we are grateful!

Francesco P. Cappuccio
Michelle A. Miller
Steven W. Lockley
February 2010

Contents

Abbreviations

%SEI	Sleep efficiency index in %
95% CI	95% confidence interval
A	Actigraphy
AASM	American Academy of Sleep Medicine
ABMS	American Board of Medical Specialities
ACGME	Accreditation Council for Graduate Medical Education
ACQ	Asthma Control Questionnaire
ACTH	Adrenocorticotropic hormone
AD	Alzheimer's disease
ADHD	Attention-deficit hyperactivity disorder
AEE	Activity-related energy expenditure
AF	Atrial fibrillation
AHI	Apnoea-hypopnoea index
AIDS	Auto immuno-deficiency syndrome
AIRG	Acute insulin response to glucose
AMI	Acute myocardial infarction
aMT6s	6-Sulphatoxymelatonin
ApoE4	Apolipoprotein E4
AQOL	Asthma quality of life
ASDA	American Sleep Disorders Association
ASPS	Advanced sleep phase syndrome
BMA	British Medical Association
BMI	Body mass index
BT	Bedtime
CAC	Coronary artery calcification
CAD	Coronary artery disease
CAR	Cortisol awakening response
CARDIA	Coronary artery risk development in young adults
CBT	Core body temperature
CDC	Centres for Disease Control
cGMP	Cyclic guanosine monophosphate
CHD	Coronary heart disease
CI	Confidence interval
CMS	Centers for Medicare and Medicaid Services
CNS	Central nervous system
CO_2	Carbon dioxide
COPD	Chronic obstructive pulmonary disease

COR	Chain of responsibility
Cox-2	Cyclooxygenase-2
CPAP	Continuous positive airways pressure
CPSI	American Cancer Society's Cancer Prevention Study I (baseline 1959–60)
CPSII	American Cancer Society's Cancer Prevention Study II (baseline 1982)
CR	Constant routine
CRH	Corticotropin-releasing hormone
CRSD	Circadian rhythm sleep disorders
CRY	Crytochrome
CSA	Central sleep apnoea
CSF	Cerebrospinal fluid
CSHQ	Children's Sleep Habits Questionnaire
CVD	Cardiovascular disease
DI	Disposition index
DIMS	Difficulties of initiating and maintaining sleep
DLB	Dementia with Lewy bodies
DSM	Diagnostic and statistical manual of mental disorders
DSPD	Delayed sleep phase disorder
DSPS	Delayed sleep phase syndrome
ED	Excessive sleepiness
EDS	Excessive daytime sleepiness
EEG	Electroencephalogram or Electroencephalography
EMG	Electromyogram or electromyography
EOG	Electrooculogram or electrooculography
ER	Emergency room
ERV	Expiratory reserve volume
ESS	Epworth Sleepiness Scale
EU	European Union
EWTD	European Working Time Directive
FAI	Fatigue assessment instrument
FDA	Federal Drugs Authority
$FEV_1\%$	Forced expiratory volume in one second as % of predicted value
FFI	Fatal familial insomnia
fMRI	functional magnetic resonance imaging

FMSCA	Federal Motor Carrier Safety Administration		LVEF	Left ventricular ejection fraction
FRC	Functional residual capacity		m	Metre
FVC%	Forced vital capacity as % of predicted value		M	Method
			MetS	Metabolic syndrome
GERD	Gastroesophageal reflux disease		MG	Myasthenia gravis
GH	Growth hormone		MI	Myocardial infarction
GHRH	Growth hormone releasing hormone		MRE	Mortality risk estimates
GME	Graduate Medical Education		MS	Multiple sclerosis
GWS	Genome wide scan		MSA	Multiple system atrophy
H@N	Hospital at Night		MSLT	Multiple sleep latency test
HbA1c	Haemoglobin A1c		MVA	Motor vehicle accidents
HDL	High-density lipoprotein		MVV	Maximum minute ventilation
HIV	Human immunodeficiency virus		MWT	Maintenance of wakefulness test
HLA	Human leukocyte antigen		N1	Stage 1 sleep
HOMA-IR	Homeostasis model assessment-estimated insulin resistance		N2	Stage 2 sleep
			N3	Stage 3 sleep
HOS	Hours of service		NADPH	Nicotinamide adenine dinucleotide phosphate
HPA axis	Hypothalamic-pituitary-adrenal axis		NAEPP	National Asthma Education and Prevention Program
HR	Hazard ratio			
HRT	Hormone replacement therapy		NCSDR	National Commission of Sleep Disorders Research
hs-CRP	C-reactive protein (high-sensitivity)			
HVDF	Heavy vehicle driver fatigue		NDD	Neurodevelopmental disorders
ICAM-1	Intracellular adhesion molecule-1		NFLE	Nocturnal frontal lobe epilepsy
ICS	Inhaled corticosteroid		NF- B	Nuclear factor-Kappa B
ICSD-2	International Classification of Sleep Disorders, 2nd Edition		ng/mL	Nanograms per millilitre
			NHANES	National Health and Nutrition Examination Survey (USA)
ICU	Intensive care unit			
IFN-γ	Interferon-gamma		NHLBI	National Heart, Lung and Blood Institute
IH	Intermittent hypoxia			
IL-1	Interleukin-1		NHS	National Health Service
ILD	Interstitial lung disease		NMD	Neuromuscular disorders
ILO	International Labour Organization		NO	Nitric oxide
IMT	Intima-media thickness		NOS	Nitric oxide synthase
IOM	Institute of Medicine		NREM	Non-rapid eye movement
ISR	Insulin secretory rate		NSF	National Sleep Foundation
ivGTT	Intravenous glucose tolerance test		NTSB	National Transport Safety Board
JACC	Japan Collaborative Cohort study		O_2	Oxygen
Kcal	Kilocalorie		OAD	Obstructive airway disease
KDT	Karolinska drowsiness test		OCP	Oral contraceptive pill
kg	Kilogram		ODI	Oxygen desaturation index
KLS	Kleine-Levin syndrome		OHS	Obesity hyperventilation syndrome
KSS	Karolinska Sleepiness Scale		OR	Odds ratio
LDL	Low-density lipoprotein		OSA	Obstructive sleep apnoea
LPL	Lipoprotein lipase		OSAS	Obstructive sleep apnoea syndrome
LPS	Lipopolysaccharide		$PaCO_2$	Arterial CO_2 pressure

PAI-1	Plasminogen activator inhibitor		SD	Standard deviation
PaO$_2$	Arterial O$_2$ pressure		SDB	Sleep-disordered breathing
PCI	Percutaneous coronary intervention		SES	Social economic status
PCOD	Polycystic ovary disease		SEWS	Standardized early warning score
PEF	Peak expiratory flow		SF-36	Short form of medical outcomes study questionnaire (36 questions)
PEFR	Peak expiratory flow rate			
Per	Period gene		SGRQ	St. George's Respiratory Questionnaire
Pes	Esophageal pressure (measured on esophageal manometry)		SHHS	Sleep Heart Health Study
PET	Positron emission tomography		SI	Insulin sensitivity
PFT	Pulmonary function test		SOL	Sleep onset latency
PGO	Ponto-geniculo-occipital		SpO$_2$	Oxyhaemoglobin saturation
PH	Pulmonary hypertension		SpRs	Specialist Registrars
PKG	Protein kinase G		SPT	sleep period time
PLMD	Periodic limb movement disorder (nocturnal myoclonus)		SRS	Sleep regulatory substance
			SSM	Special Study Module
PLMS	Periodic limb movements of sleep		SSRI	Structured sleep-related interview
PNE	Primary nocturnal enuresis		SSRIs	Selective serotonin re-uptake inhibitors
PRC	Phase response curve			
PSG	Polysomnography		SSS	Stanford Sleepiness Scale
PSQI	Pittsburgh Sleep Quality Index		SWS	Slow wave sleep
PTSD	Post-traumatic stress disorder		SWSD	Shift-work sleep disorders
PVT	Psychomotor vigilance test		T2DM	Type 2 diabetes mellitus
PYY	Peptide YY		TD	Time-diary
Q	Questionnaire		TEE	Total energy expenditure
QOL	Quality of life		TEM	Thermic effect of meals
RA	Rheumatoid arthritis		TI	Telephone interview
RBD	REM sleep behaviour disorder		TIB	Time in bed
RCP	Royal College of Physicians		TLC%	Total lung capacity as % of predicted value
RDI	Respiratory disturbance index			
REM	Rapid eye movement		TLRs	Toll-like receptors
RHT	Retinohypothalamic tract		Tmin	Temperature minimum
R$_L$	Total airway resistance		TNF-α	Tissue necrosis factor-alpha
R$_{LL}$	Lower airway resistance		TSH	Thyroid-stimulating hormone
RLS	Restless legs syndrome		TST	Total sleep time
RMR	Resting metabolic rate		TST$_{SaO2<90\%}$	Total sleep time with oxyhaemoglobin saturation<90%
RNA	Ribonucleic acid			
ROS	Reactive oxygen species		TV	Tidal volume
RR	Relative risk		U.S.	United States
R$_{UAW}$	Upper airway resistance		U.K.	United Kingdom
RV	Residual volume		UAW	Upper airway
S	Survey		UK	United Kingdom
SAH	Sleep apnoea-hypopnoea		UPPP	Uvulopharyngopalatoplasty
SCI	Spinal cord injury		US	Unites States
SCN	Suprachiasmatic nucleus/nuclei		UTR	Untranslated region
			V/Q	Ventilation/perfusion ratio

VCAM-1	Vascular cell adhesion molecule-1	WASE	Wakefulness after sleep end
V_E	Minute ventilation	WGBH	A Boston-based public broadcasting station
VEGF	Vascular endothelial growth factor		
VNTR	Variable number tandem repeat	WHO	World Health Organization
V_T	Tidal volume	WHR	Waist-hip ratio
		WU	Wake-up time

Contributors

Torbjörn Åkerstedt, PhD
Professor of Behavioural Physiology,
Director of the Stress Research Institute
Stockholm University,
Clinical Neuroscience,
Karolinska Institutet,
Stockholm, Sweden

Sara Arber, PhD, AcSS, FBA
Professor of Sociology,
Co-Director, Centre for Research
on Ageing and Gender (CRAG)
Department of Sociology,
University of Surrey, Guildford,
Surrey, UK

John Axelsson, PhD
Associate Professor,
Osher Center for Integrative Medicine and
the section for Psychology
Department for Clinical Neuroscience,
Karolinska Institutet,
Stockholm, Sweden

Josiane Broussard, B.S.
PhD candidate,
Department of Medicine,
University of Chicago,
Chicago, USA

Francesco P. Cappuccio,
MD, MSc, FRCP, FFPH, FAHA
Cephalon Professor of Cardiovascular
Medicine & Epidemiology,
Honorary Consultant Cardiovascular
Physician;
Head, World Health Organization
Collaborating Centre for Nutrition;
Director, European Centre of Excellence in
Hypertension and Cardio-Metabolic Research,
University of Warwick Medical School &
University Hospitals Coventry &
Warwickshire NHS Trust,
Coventry, UK

Daniel A. Cohen, MD, MMSc
Instructor in Neurology,
Harvard Medical School,
Cognitive Neurology and Sleep Medicine,
Department of Neurology,
Beth Israel Deaconess Medical Center;
Associate Physician,
Division of Sleep Medicine,
Department of Medicine,
Brigham and Women's Hospital,
Boston, USA

Charles A. Czeisler, PhD, MD, FRCP
Baldino Professor of Sleep Medicine,
Harvard Medical School;
Director, Division of Sleep Medicine,
Harvard Medical School;
Chief, Division of Sleep Medicine,
Brigham and Women's Hospital
Senior Physician,
Division of Sleep Medicine,
Department of Medicine,
Brigham and Women's Hospital
Affiliated Faculty,
Department of Neurobiology,
Harvard Medical School,
Boston, USA

Jane E. Ferrie, PhD
Senior Research Fellow;
Department of Epidemiology and
Public Health,
University College London Medical School,
London, UK

David Gozal, MD
Herbert T. Abelson Professor of Pediatrics,
Chair, Department of Pediatrics and
Comer Children's Hospital,
Pritzker School of Medicine,
University of Chicago,
Chicago, USA

Laura Herpel, MD
Assistant Professor of Medicine,
Division of Pulmonary, Critical Care,
Allergy & Sleep Medicine,
Medical University of South Carolina,
Charleston, South Carolina, USA

Christopher B. Jones, LLB, PhD
School of Psychology,
Psychiatry and Psychological Medicine,
Monash University,
Victoria, Australia

Rahul Kakkar, MD, FCCP, FAASM
Sleep Specialist,
North Florida-South Georgia VA
Health System,
St Augustine, Florida, USA

Göran Kecklund, PhD
Associate Professor,
Stress Research Institute,
Stockholm University,
Stockholm, Sweden

Mika Kivimäki, PhD
Professor of Social Epidemiology,
Department of Epidemiology and
Public Health,
University College London Medical School,
London, UK

Kristen Knutson, PhD
Assistant Professor of Medicine,
Department of Medicine,
University of Chicago,
Chicago, Ohio, USA

Vidya Krishnan, MD
Associate Director of Center for Sleep
Medicine, MHMC
Assistant Professor of Medicine,
Division of Pulmonary,
Critical Care and Sleep Medicine
Case Western Reserve University,
Cleveland, Ohio, USA

Christopher P. Landrigan, MD, MPH
Assistant Professor of Pediatrics and Medicine,
Harvard Medical School;
Director,
Sleep and Patient Safety Program,
Division of Sleep Medicine,
Department of Medicine,
Brigham and Women's Hospital;
Research and Fellowship Director,
Inpatient Pediatrics Service,
Division of General Pediatrics,
Department of Medicine,
Children's Hospital Boston,
Boston, USA

Clark J. Lee, JD
Member,
Maryland and District of Columbia Bars
Law and Policy Analyst,
Center for Health and Homeland Security,
University of Maryland
Baltimore, USA

Steven W. Lockley, PhD
Assistant Professor of Medicine,
Harvard Medical School
Associate Neuroscientist,
Division of Sleep Medicine,
Department of Medicine,
Brigham and Women's Hospital,
Boston, USA
Honorary Associate Professor in Sleep Medicine,
Warwick Medical School, UK
Adjunct Associate Professor,
School of Psychology and Psychiatry,
Monash University, Australia

Nathaniel S. Marshall, PhD
Research Fellow and Clinical Senior Lecturer
NHMRC Centre for Integrated Research and
Understanding of Sleep (CIRUS),
Woolcock Institute of Medical Research,
Sydney Medical School, The University of
Sydney, Australia

Robert Meadows, LLB, MA, PhD
Lecturer in Sociology,
Department of Sociology,
University of Surrey,
Guildford, UK

Michelle A. Miller, PhD
Associate Professor (Reader) in
Biochemical Medicine,
University of Warwick Medical School,
Coventry, UK

Ed Peile, MB, BS, EdD, FRCP, FRCGP, FRCPCH, LFHEA, FAcadMed
Emeritus Professor of Medical Education,
University of Warwick Medical School,
Coventry, UK

Shantha M.W. Rajaratnam, LLB, PhD
Associate Professor,
School of Psychology and Psychiatry,
Monash University, Victoria, Australia
Lecturer in Medicine,
Division of Sleep Medicine,
Brigham and Women's Hospital and
Harvard Medical School,
Boston, USA

Asim Roy, MD, FAASM
Assistant Clinical Professor of Neurology,
University of Pittsburgh Medical Center,
Pittsburgh, USA

Mikael Sallinen, PhD
Team Leader,
Brain and Work Research Centre,
Finnish Institute of Occupational Health,
Helsinki, Finland
Research Professor,
Agroa Center,
University of Jyväskylä, Jyväskylä, Finland

Martin Shipley, PhD
Senior Lecturer in Medical Statistics,
Department of Epidemiology and
Public Health, University College London
Medical School, London, UK

Karen Spruyt, PhD
Assistant Professor of Pediatrics,
Section of Pediatric Sleep Medicine
Department of Pediatrics,
Pritzker School of Medicine,
Division of Biological Science
University of Chicago,
Chicago, USA

Gregory Stores, MD, MA, DPM, FRCPsych, FRCP
Emeritus Professor of Developmental
Neuropsychiatry,
University of Oxford,
Oxford, UK

Saverio Stranges, MD, PhD, FFPH
Associate Clinical Professor of
Cardiovascular Epidemiology,
University of Warwick Medical School,
Coventry, UK

Mihai C. Teodorescu, MD
Assistant Clinical Professor of Medicine,
Section of Geriatrics and Gerontology,
Center for Sleep Medicine and Sleep Research,
University of Wisconsin School of Medicine
and Public Health, William S. Middleton
Memorial VA Hospital, Madison,
Wisconsin, USA

Mihaela Teodorescu, MD
Assistant Professor of Medicine,
Section of Allergy, Pulmonary and
Critical Care Medicine, Center for
Sleep Medicine and Sleep Research,
University of Wisconsin School of
Medicine and Public Health,
William S. Middleton Memorial VA Hospital,
Madison, Wisconsin, USA

Scott Weich, MSc, MD, FRCPsych
Professor of Psychiatry,
University of Warwick Medical School
Honorary Consultant Psychiatrist,
Coventry and Warwickshire Partnership Trust
Coventry, UK

Simon Williams, BA, MSc, PhD
Professor in Sociology,
Department of Sociology,
University of Warwick,
Coventry, UK

Ailiang Xie, MD, PhD
Senior Scientist,
Section of Allergy, Pulmonary and
Critical Care Medicine,
University of Wisconsin School of
Medicine and Public Health,
Madison, Wisconsin, USA

Chapter 1

Sleep, health, and society: the contribution of epidemiology

F.P. Cappuccio, M.A. Miller, and S.W. Lockley

Introduction

Sleep disturbances and sleep deprivation are common in modern society. Most studies show that since the beginning of the century, populations have been subjected to a steady constant decline in the number of hours devoted to sleep, due to changes in a variety of environmental and social conditions (e.g. less dependence on daylight for most activities, extended shift work, 24/7 round-the-clock activities). The potential detrimental effects to health of sustained sleep deprivation and disruption were first acknowledged by industry (like airlines, long-distance driving, shift-work manufacturing industry, and emergency services). Only recently, however, has the wider implication for the population at large been unveiled. Through the application of epidemiological methods of investigation, sleep deprivation has been shown to be associated with a variety of chronic conditions and poor health outcomes, detectable across the entire lifespan, from childhood to adulthood to older age. This book is designed to summarize for the first time the epidemiological evidence linking disturbances of sleep quantity and quality to several chronic conditions, to assess the epidemiological evidence for causality, and to explore the public health implications with a view to inform a discourse on possible preventive strategies.

Textbooks of Sleep Medicine have traditionally focused predominantly on the physiology and pathophysiology of sleep (Kryger et al., 2005) with a view to help diagnose and treat a variety of sleep-related conditions. Mainly directed to physiologists, sleep technicians, respiratory physicians, psychiatrists, and paediatricians, these textbooks almost invariably glance at the growing epidemiology of sleep and at the implications for public health. The scope of the present book is to fill a significant gap in the population-based approach to the problem of sleep-related disease risk.

The role of epidemiology

Epidemiology differs from clinical medicine in that the unit of interest is the population, not the individual. Clinical investigations are conducted on sick people, the results relate to patients, and decisions are related to treatment of individuals. Epidemiological research studies the sick and the well, results relate to populations, and decisions are related to public health (Rose, 1985). Epidemiology may be defined as the *quantitative study of the distribution, frequency, determinants, and control of health problems and disease in populations* (Fig. 1.1).

The purpose of epidemiology is to obtain, interpret, and use health information to promote health and reduce disease. Using this definition, it is clear that epidemiology is concerned with populations, not only death, illness, and disability in populations, but also with more positive health states and with the means to improve health.

Quantitative	=	how much there is of a particular health problem or disease or hazard
Distribution	=	variation of disease in the population by time, place and person
Determinants	=	causes of disease
Control	=	what to do about the problem, planning and setting priorities evaluating the risk and benefits of intervention
Disease or health problem	=	what it is and what is its natural history
Populations	=	the methods of study and the findings relate to populations

Fig. 1.1 Definition of epidemiology.

Epidemiology is a crucial discipline for the promotion of public health. It provides a set of skills, approaches, and a philosophy which allows causes of health problems to be detected, the association between ill-health and a variety of risk factors to be quantified, treatments and public health interventions to be tested, and changes in states of health over time to be monitored. It is a discipline which allows the distribution of health and ill-health in a population to be described (e.g. *what* is the problem and its frequency? *who* is affected? *where* and *when* does this health problem manifest in the population?). It also provides the tools to compare the health characteristics of populations. Epidemiology may play a role in identifying the *cause* of a health problem (e.g. a genetic trait, an infectious agent, a particular behaviour, an environmental exposure). The epidemiological approach provides a framework within which 'causation' can be hypothesized and tested. The primary objective in epidemiology is to judge whether an association between exposure and disease or health problem is, in fact, causal. A *causal association* is one in which a change in the frequency or quality of an exposure or characteristic results in a corresponding change in the frequency of a disease or outcome of interest. *Causality* is more likely if an association between exposure and disease can satisfy most of the following criteria: *strength, consistency, specificity, right time sequence, dose relationship, reversibility, biological plausibility, coherence* (Hill, 1965). Making judgements about causality would require an assessment of the *validity* of the findings and of the *likelihood of alternative explanations* for the results. It would then require the assessment of the role of *chance*, the role of *bias*, and the role of *confounding*.

Once the disease occurs, epidemiology provides a means for monitoring the course and outcome (*natural history*) of the condition. It also allows us to answer questions regarding the *effectiveness of interventions* and therapies and their impact on populations (i.e. how effective are particular interventions for controlling disease in communities? is intervention A more effective than intervention B? what are the outcomes of these two lines of intervention?). Of course, such information needs to be placed alongside other data before a choice of interventions is made (e.g. what are the side effects of the treatments? what are the views of consumers and patients about the procedure? how much does the intervention cost?). Such data may help determine where best to direct resources. Identifying health states in the population may facilitate establishing the *need for services* and the *determination of priorities*. Given limited resources, public health practitioners are always under pressure to use resources optimally and to produce the greatest return, in the form of health gain, for a given investment of time, money, materials, and personnel. Epidemiology cannot do this alone: it needs to interact with health services research, health economics, and other social sciences if wise public health decisions are to be made and health promoted on a population level.

Epidemiology thus has many applications and is an essential tool in providing useful information about public health problems, their magnitude and distribution, causation, prevention, prognosis, and treatment, and likely impact of interventions. If epidemiological data are to be of use in policy-making, they need to address questions for which policy-makers require answers, and need to do so in a convincing and compelling way. Yet still, epidemiology is just one contribution to the policy debate. Increasing our understanding of health problems and their determinants and possible solutions places us in a better position to make appropriate policy.

The book

The book is structured in 21 chapters. Chapter 1 is an introduction that builds on the basic science and clinical knowledge of the physiology of sleep and the clinical manifestations of sleep disturbances and explains how the development of this discipline is now in need of an epidemiological approach to fill the gap in knowledge to assess the population and public health implications of sleep disturbances. Chapter 2 is an introduction to the principles of sleep physiology that will allow the reader to grasp the key factors without going too deeply into the subject, extensively covered by existing literature. Chapter 3 describes the epidemiology of sleep deprivation and disruption, their risk factors and markers, and discusses the concept of causality in an epidemiological framework. Chapters 4 to 10 pay attention mostly to new areas of population-based research addressing the relevance of sleep disturbances as potential determinants of ill-health and mortality, cardiovascular, metabolic, and respiratory diseases, and the interplay with depression and neurological conditions, with special attention to manifestations in children. Chapters 11 and 12 focus mainly on new biochemical and genetic mechanisms that might underpin the role of sleep as a determinant, or risk marker, of ill-health. Chapter 13 is new in that it addresses the sociological dimensions of sleep and the personal and societal implications. Chapter 14 is an extensive perusal of the psychosocial and medical consequences of misinterpreting sleep disturbances and, with Chapter 19, makes a plea for improving education and training in sleep medicine and sleep-related disorders not only amongst medical students and doctors but also among health professionals at large. Chapters 15–21 enter into the sphere of public health through an extensive review of the perils associated with shift-work, not only in industrial settings, but also in the medical profession, to both individuals who work in shifts and to those who would benefit from the activities of shift-workers (e.g. the patients served by junior doctors working shifts). The societal and medico-legal implications are also covered, with an overview of the implications in different legal systems worldwide.

The brief to authors was to take a population perspective, and to consider the extent to which their particular area of expertise translates into the population and public health arena. To maximize the take-home messages on the population and public health perspective, most chapters end with a Box summarizing the main points for easy reference.

The intended primary readership of this book is epidemiologists and public health professionals as well as medical students and those of allied professions. We hope our book will also appeal to psychologists, cardiologists, and cardiovascular physicians, specialists in metabolic or respiratory diseases, neurologists, psychiatrists, policy-makers, specialists in medical education, professionals involved in shift-work, occupational health professionals, regulatory bodies and voluntary organizations, as well as patients' groups.

Brief historical note

As clearly highlighted by William Dement (Dement, 2005), 'Interest in sleep and dreams has existed since the dawn of history' and there is a wealth of scholarly work that highlights the interests, concerns, beliefs, and roles of sleep and associated activities (e.g. dreams, nightmares) over the centuries, from prehistoric ages to our modern society (Thorpy, 1991). Until very recently, sleep had been considered a passive state. In MacNish's definition of 1834 (MacNish, 1834), '*Sleep is the intermediate state between wakefulness and death: wakefulness being regarded as the active state of all the animal and intellectual functions, and death as that of their total suspension*'. It was not until the end of the nineteenth century and well into the twentieth century that the concept that sleep could be an active and dynamic state gained credence and some scientific support through early experiments in animals (Legendre and Pieron, 1910) and humans (Kleitman, 1939). The discovery that the electrical activity and rhythms of the human brain, using an electroencephalogram (EEG), vary significantly and constantly during wakefulness and sleep (Berger, 1930) sparked an increased interest in unravelling the scientific basis of sleep. The work of Sigmund Freud and his interpretation of dreams arguably contributed to creating an interest in sleep among health professionals.

In the latter half of the twentieth century we witness the start of animal experimentation on sleep, leading to the understanding of some of the deep brain mechanisms underpinning sleep and wakefulness, the modern neuroscience.

At a similar pace it developed the understanding of the pathology of sleep, from insomnia, narcolepsy with cataplexy, and, much later, obstructive sleep apnoea syndrome, firstly described in 1836 by Charles Dickens in the Young Dropsy, a young obese, always sleepy, boy who snored (referred to as Pickwickian syndrome). Similarly the discipline now known as 'chronobiology', which for centuries had described the 24-hour rhythmic cycles governing the biological activities of the plant and animal kingdoms, began being applied to the sleep-wake cycles of animals and humans (see also Chapter 2).

Scientific output, measured by the number of publications in the field of sleep research since 1945, provides a crude indication of the exponential growth of knowledge and highlights some milestone discoveries (Fig. 1.2).

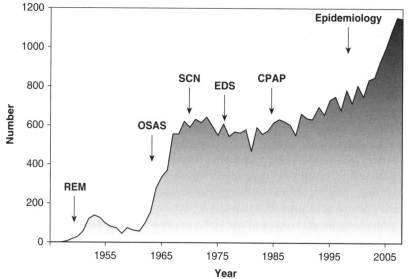

Fig. 1.2 Publication trends in the field of sleep research.
Source: Medline search 1945–2008 for sleep.

The first description that rapid eye movements (REMs) occur in sleep (de Toni, 1933) precedes the landmark study that suggested that REMs represented a 'lightening' of sleep and might indicate dreaming, due to the close association with irregular respiration and an increase in heart rate (Aserinsky and Kleitman, 1953). A second spark in the research progress in sleep medicine was the discovery of sleep apnoea in 1965 (Gastaut et al., 1965; Jung and Kuhlo, 1965). In the early 1970s, the internal biological clock regulating the sleep-wake cycle and many other rhythmic biological activities (the suprachiasmatic nucleus or SCN) was described (Moore and Eichler, 1972; Stephan and Zucker, 1972) (see also Chapter 2). This autonomous circadian pacemaker has since been intensively studied (Weaver, 1998) and, more recently, its genetic regulation (e.g. *Clock* genes) has been detailed (see also Chapter 12). The 1980s and 1990s were dominated by studies of the importance of excessive daytime sleepiness (EDS; see also Chapters 15–18) and the discovery and applications of the continuous positive airways pressure (CPAP) for the management of obstructive sleep apnoea syndrome and its complications (see also Chapter 7). Finally, at the end of the twentieth century and at the dawn of the twenty-first century, there was a very sharp increase in the scientific output of sleep research, with a disproportionate representation of population studies on the effect of sleep on health risks and a debate on the public health issues associated with declining trends in the quantity and quality of sleep in the modern society as potential contributing factors to, or risk markers for, ill-health and reduced safety (see also Chapters 4–6, 13, and 15–21).

Sleep, health, and society

Throughout our life we spend approximately a third of our time asleep. We spend more time asleep as babies and children and then settle for a pattern that is of approximately 7- to 8-hour per night. Although subjective sleep duration remains fairly constant with age, sleep patterns, however, directly measured with polysomnography seem to indicate that, with age, total sleeping time, sleep efficiency, and slow wave sleep decline and waking after sleep onset increases (Bixler, 2009). Sufficient sleep is necessary for optimal daytime performance and well-being, yet there is a large difference in how much sleep people report, ranging from <6 hours to >9 hours per night. The epidemiology of sleep duration indicates that a good night's sleep equates to at least 6 hours and ideally 8 hours of continuous sleep, with changes in sleep duration or continuity being associated with negative impacts on health outcomes. In one study in Britain, the average duration of sleep in an adult population was 7.04 hours per night (standard deviation, SD 1.55 hours) (Groeger et al., 2004). Approximately three-quarters of men and women slept between 6 hours and 8 hours per night. However, another quarter reported sleep time either <5 hours per night (approximately 5% with <4 hours per night) or >9 hours (more than 5% with >11 hours per night), indicating large inter-individual variation within the same population. Adult women report sleeping consistently less than men up to the age of 50–55 years, then the pattern reverses (see also Chapter 13). There are also geographical variations in average sleeping time (whether due to environmental, genetic, or socioeconomic factors). In a study of 18- to 30-year-old university students from countries around the world, the majority reported sleeping between 7 hours and 8 hours per night (Steptoe et al., 2006). Exceptions were students in East Asian countries (Japan, Korea, Taiwan, and Thailand) who slept on average <6 hours per night, and those of some European countries (Spain and Romania) with >8 hours per night. This variation was associated, in short sleepers, with increased self-reported ill-health. Both short and long sleep have been associated with increased all-cause mortality (Cappuccio et al., 2010) and other outcomes from chronic disease (see also Chapters 4 and 5). Many have speculated that the secular increase in chronic diseases, like cardiovascular disease, diabetes, and obesity, have been paralleled by a steady deterioration in sleeping patterns, with an increase in the proportion on short sleepers, and that these two phenomena might be related. A recent analysis of self-reported sleep hours in the United States between 1975 and 2006 did not detect any significant increase in the odds of short sleep (<6 hours per night) over the 31-year period (Knutson et al., 2010). However, when the analysis was carried out by employment status, a significant increase in the odds (odds ratio, OR = 1.19) was detected amongst full-time workers, with the excess time awake being spent predominantly in working activities. Working overtime and working shifts is associated with negative health outcomes and with reduced performance posing risk to others (see also Chapters 15–18). Lack of sleep should be considered as a potential mediator of these effects since trends in shorter sleep is associated with longer working hours (Knutson et al., 2010). Finally, there is evidence to suggest that reducing the amount of time we spend asleep strongly predicts cardiovascular outcomes (Ferrie et al., 2007) and risk of some types of cancer. On the other hand, increasing sleeping hours over time may be a marker of general ill-health predicting non-cardiovascular mortality (Ferrie et al., 2007).

Sleep education and awareness

As the world population increases and individuals become larger, the number of individuals suffering from sleep disorders will increase. In the United States, it is estimated that over the next 20 years, the number of Americans suffering from sleep disorders will double. However, the public awareness of the need for adequate sleep both for adults and children and the awareness of sleep-related conditions are poor. Moreover, the physicians who treat them receive minimal training in sleep disorders medicine (Stores and Crawford, 1998) (see also Chapter 14). In fact, they themselves are forced to endure excessive work schedules during their internship and residency training, which desensitizes them to sleep as a fundamental biological necessity, degrades their ability to provide quality patient care and to benefit fully from their training experience, and places them at increased risk of ill-health, injuries, and sleep-related motor vehicle accidents during their training (Landrigan et al., 2004; Barger et al., 2005) (see also Chapters 17 and 18). These difficult, and often conflicting, interests need to be addressed so that the medical field can provide an optimal platform for learning and patient care (Buysse et al., 2003).

In 1993, a national survey of 126 accredited medical schools in the United States indicated that less than 2 hours of total teaching time was allocated to sleep and sleep disorders, on average, with 37 schools reporting no structured teaching time whatever in this area (Rosen et al., 1993). Furthermore, it was reported that only 8% of medical students are trained in the use of sleep laboratory procedures, and 11% have participated in the clinical evaluation of sleep-disordered patients. Over two-thirds of the survey respondents reported that they believed that the provision of teaching time for sleep medicine was inadequate and that more time should be provided. Thus, it would appear that although there is increasing evidence to support the idea that sleep is a fundamental requirement for patient health and well-being, the provision of medical education in this area is currently inadequate.

There has been an increasing awareness of the widening gap between scientific research and clinical teaching in sleep and sleep disorders. The survey of the Taskforce 2000 established by the American Sleep Disorders Association (ASDA) to address the deficiencies in current medical education in sleep (Rosen et al., 1998) (see also Chapter 19) indicated that the majority of respondents (65.2%) are currently involved in teaching sleep to medical students or postgraduate trainees. The average amount of teaching time for sleep reported for undergraduates was only 2.1 hours and that for graduates was 4.8 hours. The results from the survey also indicated that the teaching of sleep laboratory procedures and clinical evaluation of sleep-disordered patients is limited at either an undergraduate or postgraduate level.

A similar situation, with regards to lack of sleep education, exists in Medical Schools in the United Kingdom (Stores and Crawford, 1998). The provision of any medical education on sleep and its disorders varied widely from 6% to 80%. However, the median time reported for such teaching was restricted to 15 minutes for preclinical teaching and zero in clinical teaching. The study concluded that in the United Kingdom, undergraduate medical teaching does not provide an adequate training basis for the development of competence in diagnosing and treating sleep disorders. It was recommended that changes in medical education were required to address this issue. Some examples of dramatic increase in teaching and research in the area of sleep medicine have become available recently (see also Chapter 19 for Warwick Medical School).

The public awareness of the importance of sleep, the need for good sleep hygiene and awareness of sleep disorders in general is poor in both adults and children. Various professional bodies worldwide are attempting to redress the balance, but there is much to do. In the U.K. education system, for example, children are taught about the importance of diet and exercise but sleep education is rarely addressed. Poor sleep habits in early life may have long-term consequences for health (see also Chapters 5, 6, and 10).

Conclusion

Taken together, these issues bring the results of the epidemiology of sleep outside the clinical setting and well within the domain of public health. One of the main questions still to answer is whether in these circumstances, sleep disturbances are the consequence of ill-health, are intermediate markers in the pathways of disease causation, or whether changes in sleep patterns can be causal in the determination of chronic disease and, more generally, ill-health. The bi-directional relationships between sleep duration and disease and their non-linear associations remain important research challenges to overcome towards aetiological answers. A long-term intervention trial of sleep manipulation would be necessary to test the effect of sleep duration on chronic disease outcome. However, this is an unlikely scenario, since such a study would be impractical, large, long, and expensive. This leaves the burden of proof on observational epidemiology to inform potential changes in public health policies. At the same time, the deleterious effects of shift work on several outcomes, like risk of self-harm and harm to others (e.g. medical errors, road accidents, attentional failures in high risk occupations) (Landrigan et al., 2004; Lockley et al., 2004; Barger et al., 2005) (see also Chapters 15–18), which are by and large mediated by excessive sleepiness and fatigue caused by sleep debt, have recently benefited from stronger evidence from randomized clinical trials and are now informing policy changes.

References

Aserinsky, E. & Kleitman, N. (1953). Regularly occurring periods of eye motility, and concomitant phenomena, during sleep. *Science*, **118**, 273–274.

Barger, L.K., Cade, B.E., Ayas, N.T., et al. (2005). Extended work shifts and the risk of motor vehicle crashes among interns. *N Engl J Med*, **352**, 125–134.

Berger, H. (1930). Über das Elektroenkephalogramm des Menschen. *J Psychol Neurol*, **40**, 160–179.

Bixler, E. (2009). Sleep and society: an epidemiological perspective. *Sleep Med*, **10**, S3–S6.

Buysse, D.J., Barzansky, B., Dinges, D., et al. (2003). Sleep, fatigue, and medical training: setting an agenda for optimal learning and patient care. *Sleep*, **26**(2), 218–225.

Cappuccio, F.P., D'Elia, L., Strazzullo, P. & Miller, M.A. (2010). Sleep duration and all-cause mortality: a systematic review and meta-analysis of prospective studies. *Sleep*, **33**(5): 585–592.

Dement, W.C. (2005). History of sleep physiology and medicine. In: Kryger, M.H., Roth, T. & Dement, W.C. (eds.), *Principles and Practice of Sleep Medicine*. Fourth edition. The Netherlands: Elsevier, pp. 1–12.

de Toni, G. (1933). I movimenti pendolari dei bulbi oculari dei bambini durante il sonno fisiologico, ed in alcuni stati morbosi. *Pediatria*, **41**, 489–498.

Ferrie, J.E., Shipley, M.J., Cappuccio, F.P., et al. (2007). A prospective study of change in sleep duration: associations with mortality in the Whitehall II cohort. *Sleep*, **30**, 1659–1666.

Gastaut, H., Tassinari, C. & Duron, B. (1965). Etude polygraphique des manifestations épisodiques (hypniques et respiratoires) du syndrome de Pickwick. *Rev Neurol*, **112**, 568–579.

Groeger, J.A., Zijlstra, F.R. & Dijk, D.J. (2004). Sleep quantity, sleep difficulties and their perceived consequences in a representative sample of some 2000 British adults. *J Sleep Res*, **13**, 359–371.

Hill, A.B. (1965). The environment and disease: association or causation? *J Royal Soc Med*, 58, 295–300.

Jung, R. & Kuhlo, W. (1965). Neurophysiological studies of abnormal night sleep and the pickwickian syndrome. *Prog Brain Res*, **18**, 140–159.

Kleitman, N. (1939). *Sleep and Wakefulness*. Chicago, IL: University of Chicago Press.

Knutson, K.L., Van Cauter, E., Rathouz, P.J., DeLeire, T. & Lauderdale, D.S. (2010). Trends in the prevalence of short sleepers in the USA: 1975–2006. *Sleep*, **33**, 37–45.

Kryger, M.H., Roth, T. & Dement, W.C. (2005). *Principles and Practice of Sleep Medicine*. Fourth edition. The Netherlands: Elsevier.

Landrigan, C.P., Rothschild, J.M., Cronin, J.W., et al. (2004). Effect of reducing interns' work hours on serious medical errors in intensive care units. *N Engl J Med*, **351**, 1838–1848.

Legendre, R. & Pieron, H. (1910). Le problème des facteurs du sommeil: resultats d'injections vasculaires et intracerebrales de liquids insomniques. *C R Soc Biol* (Paris), **68**, 1077–1079.

Lockley, S.W., Cronin, J.W., Evans, E.E., et al. (2004). Effect of reducing interns' weekly work hours on sleep and attentional failures. *N Engl J Med*, **351**, 1829–1837.

MacNish, R. (1834). *The Philosophy of Sleep*. New York, NY: D. Appleton and Company.

Moore, R.Y. & Eichler, V.B. (1972). Loss of a circadian adrenal corticosterone rhythm following suprachiasmatic lesions in the rat. *Brain Res*, **42**, 201–206.

Rose, G. (1985). Sick individuals and sick populations. *Int J Epidemiol*, **14**, 32–38.

Rosen, R.C., Rosekind, M., Rosevear, C., Cole, W.E. & Dement, W.C. (1993). Physician education in sleep and sleep disorders: a national survey of U.S. medical schools. *Sleep*, **16**(3), 249–254.

Rosen, R., Mahowald, M., Chesson, A., et al. (1998). The Taskforce 2000 survey on medical education in sleep and sleep disorders. *Sleep*, **21**(3), 235–238.

Stephan, F.K. & Zucker, I. (1972). Circadian rhythms in drinking and locomotor activity of rats are eliminated by hypothalamic lesions. *Proc Natl Acad Sci U S A*, **69**, 1583–1586.

Steptoe, A., Peacey, V. & Wardle, J. (2006). Sleep duration and health in young adults. *Arch Intern Med*, **166**, 1689–1692.

Stores, G. & Crawford, C. (1998). Medical student education in sleep and its disorders. *J R Coll Physicians Lond*, **32**(2), 149–153.

Thorpy, M. (1991). History of sleep and man. In: Thorpy, M. & Yager, J. (eds.), *The Encyclopaedia of Sleep and Sleep Disorders*. New York, NY: Facts on File.

Weaver, D.R. (1998). The suprachiasmatic nucleus: a 25-year retrospective. *J Biol Rhythms*, **13**, 100–112.

Chapter 2

Principles of sleep-wake regulation

S.W. Lockley

Introduction

Given the expanding number of associations emerging between sleep behaviour and health, measurement of sleep will become increasingly important, if not obligatory, in population-based public health research. The goal of this chapter is to provide the epidemiologist with a basic understanding of the physiological principles underlying sleep-wake regulation and how they might be considered when measuring sleep in epidemiological studies, in addition to highlighting possible confounders that might be considered when interpreting sleep data. The chapter is not intended to provide detailed basic knowledge about sleep, as that information is readily available in specialized texts for the interested reader (Kryger et al., 2005).

It is important to remember that sleep is an essential behaviour, as important as food in terms of survival (Everson et al., 1989) and is increasingly considered one of the pillars of good health, along with diet and exercise. The general exclusion of sleep from past public health research likely reflects the dismissive attitudes towards sleep of society in general, and the success of those lobbying on behalf of diet and exercise as public health issues. Although the societal attitudes towards sleep are changing only slowly, if at all, some in the epidemiological field have started to embrace sleep. These researchers are finding powerful associations between sleep and disease, and between sleep disorders and health, that often dwarf other more established risk factors. Indeed, determining sleep behaviour may be more important than some traditional markers in establishing health risk and in future, it is likely that sleep behaviour will become a core component of all public health research, as important as knowledge about smoking, alcohol, diet, and exercise. Epidemiology without sleep assessments will be missing essential information in establishing health risks, just as those who eat well and exercise regularly are missing an essential component of good health if they do not sleep well too.

Sleep-wake regulation

Basic sleep behaviour and physiology

Sleep has traditionally been described by the changes in behaviour that occur during a sleep state and, while brain electrophysiology and physiology have advanced our understanding of what happens to humans (and other animals) during sleep, measurement of the basic sleep behaviours will form the core tools in epidemiological sleep assessments. Sleep is a behavioural state characterized by minimal behaviour and a particular posture during which it is more difficult, but not impossible, to stimulate the individual. Sleep is therefore a state of relative, but not complete, disengagement with the environment while also being rapidly reversible, unlike coma or hibernation. The reasons for why we sleep are unclear but a number of hypotheses have been proposed including energy conservation, tissue repair, memory consolidation, and brain thermoregulation (Siegel, 2005).

Rodents will die of sleep deprivation at a rate on par with starvation and the multiple system failures that occur during sleep deprivation may reflect the universal importance of sleep for the recovery and repair of all body systems (Rechtschaffen et al., 1989).

In humans and many other mammals, sleep has been most carefully characterized by changes in brain electrophysiology. Discernible sleep 'stages' were first reported in the human electroencephalogram (EEG) during sleep in the 1930s and were formally defined by Rechtschaffen and Kales in 1968 (Rechtschaffen and Kales, 1968). This system still forms the main basis for classifying sleep stages, notwithstanding recent revisions (Iber et al., 2007).

When determined polysomnographically, there are two distinct types of sleep—rapid eye movement (REM) and non-rapid eye movement (NREM) sleep—which alternate every ~45 minutes to form a NREM-REM sleep cycle approximately every 90–100 minutes. Depending on the sleep episode duration, there are usually 4–5 sleep cycles per night. The proportion of NREM and REM sleep in each cycle changes throughout the night with a higher proportion of REM sleep in each cycle in the latter half of the night. NREM is generally associated with more stable physiology—regular breathing patterns, lower heart rate, lower temperature—whereas REM is a more active state with a more variable but generally higher breathing rate, heart rate, blood pressure, brain temperature, and brain blood flow (but lower core temperature). On average, about 25% of the sleep episode will consist of REM sleep. By definition, REM is usually associated with REMs detected in the electrooculogram (EOG) and inhibition of the skeletal muscles, measured using an electromyogram (EMG) from the muscles under the chin. Brain activity, as measured by EEG, is very active during REM sleep, exhibiting irregular, low amplitude, high frequency waves very similar to those seen during wakefulness. During NREM sleep the EEG activity is more synchronous, with higher amplitude, lower frequency ('slow') waves that gradually predominate with increasing 'depth' of sleep. NREM sleep is further divided into three sleep stages—N1, N2, and N3—which reflect increasing synchrony in the EEG and increasing thresholds for arousal. Stage N3 (formerly known as Stage 3–4 sleep), has the highest proportion of 'slow wave' sleep (SWS) and the amount of time spent in this stage is correlated with the duration of prior sleep deprivation, as discussed in the next section.

Two-process model of sleep-wake regulation

The two-process model of sleep regulation, first formally proposed by Alexander Borbély in 1982, remains the cornerstone on which our understanding of sleep-wake timing and structure is built (Borbély, 1982; Daan et al., 1984). The model proposes that two oscillatory processes, an hourglass-like homeostat and the endogenous 24-hour circadian pacemaker, interact to determine the timing, duration, and structure of sleep and the time course of daytime sleepiness and cognitive functioning. This model has withstood the test of time under most experimental conditions and has underpinned many advances in understanding sleep and sleep-like behaviour in both vertebrates and non-vertebrates, the role of medications and other substances on sleep and wake, and the impact of disruption in these homeostatic and circadian phase relationships on sleep and wake function.

It is well understood that it is generally easier to fall asleep at 1 o'clock in the morning compared to 1 o'clock in the afternoon. This 24-hour rhythm in sleep propensity is determined by an endogenous near-24-hour pacemaker in the suprachiasmatic nuclei (SCN) of the hypothalamus. The circadian ('about a day') pacemaker controls the timing of many rhythmic behavioural, physiological, and metabolic functions, including sleep propensity, sleep structure, temperature regulation, hormone production such as melatonin and cortisol, cardiac and lung function, glucose and insulin rhythms, and many more (Dijk and Czeisler, 1995; Cajochen et al., 1999; Czeisler and Klerman, 1999;

Hilton et al., 2000; Spengler et al., 2000; Shea et al., 2005). The circadian pacemaker determines the 24-hour patterns of sleepiness in the two-process model—defined as *Process C*—which predicts maximum sleep propensity at ~6:00 a.m., close to habitual waketime and minimum sleep propensity at ~9:00 p.m., prior to habitual bedtime and just before the onset of melatonin production (the Wake Maintenance Zone; see section 'Daytime functioning') (Fig. 2.1).

It is also intuitively understood that it is easier to fall asleep the longer one has been awake, and easier to wake up the longer one has been asleep. This homeostatic determinant of sleep propensity is defined as *Process S* in the model and is best represented physiologically by the amount of slow wave activity during sleep (SWS or Stage N3) or measured in the EEG during wake (delta activity, 0.5–5.0 Hz) (Dijk, 2009). Process S predicts maximum sleep propensity at the end of the waking day just before habitual bedtime, and minimal propensity for sleep just before waketime.

Under normal circumstances, these two processes oscillate in opposition in order to maintain a long bout of consolidated wakefulness during the day and a long bout of consolidated sleep at night (Dijk and Czeisler, 1994). The gradual increase in the circadian alerting signal through the day is counteracted by the increasing homeostatic pressure for sleep with longer time awake, permitting a prolonged consolidated wake episode. Conversely, the increasing circadian drive for sleep through the night is opposed by the reduction in homeostatic drive for sleep that decreases during the sleep episode, the sleep effectively 'releasing' the sleep pressure built up during the day, permitting a prolonged sleep episode.

Under normal conditions, distinguishing the relative contribution of these processes on sleep is not possible, as sleep always occurs at a particular part of the circadian cycle and generally after the same number of hours awake (Lockley et al., 2008). Experimentally, these processes can be forcibly desynchronized in order to quantify their relative impact on sleep (Dijk and Czeisler, 1995). The 'forced desynchrony' protocol schedules the sleep-wake cycle to a day-length that is outside the range of entrainment for the circadian pacemaker, forcibly desynchronizing the sleep-wake and dark-light cycle from the circadian clock, permitting the circadian pacemaker to revert to its endogenous period (Czeisler et al., 1999). Over a several-week study, the sleep-wake cycle will be scheduled to occur across all circadian phases, thereby allowing an examination of the effect of circadian phase on sleep structure. 'Day'-lengths employed range from 11 hours to 42.85 hours, but most commonly 20- or 28-hour 'days'.

Under these circumstances, the role of the circadian clock on sleep is revealed. It is clear that sleep duration depends on the circadian timing of sleep (Czeisler et al., 1980)—there is only a narrow window of time where sleep can continue for a long duration and remain uninterrupted (Fig. 2.1). Sleeping outside this circadian 'window' causes difficulties with falling asleep if sleep occurs too early, or difficulties staying asleep if the sleep opportunity is too late. The latter problem accounts for why shift-workers have trouble sleeping during the day—the circadian drive for alertness wakes them up. Regarding sleep structure, REM sleep is highly controlled by the circadian system with a distinct rhythm peaking in the early morning (Fig. 2.2). Sleeping at the wrong circadian phase will therefore reduce the amount of REM sleep. NREM sleep, particularly SWS, is much less under the control of the circadian system but is more influenced by the homeostatic Process S, and exhibits a strong sleep-dependent decline with increasing time asleep (Fig. 2.2) (Dijk, 2009). These processes also interact such that the circadian influence on sleep structure increases with increasing time asleep; as the homeostatic sleep pressure is reduced, the relative influence of the circadian system increases (Dijk and Czeisler, 1995).

Ageing

The circadian window for sleep changes in older age, further narrowing the time over which good sleep can be achieved (Fig. 2.1). This reduction in biological sleep opportunity is reflected in the

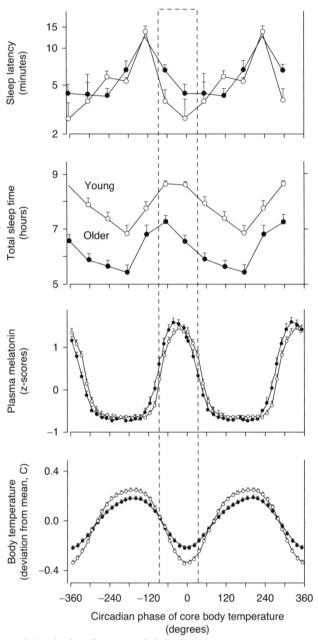

Fig. 2.1 Circadian variation in sleep latency and sleep duration.

Figure 2.1 shows the variation in sleep latency (top panel) and total sleep time (second panel) as a function of circadian phase in a group of 11 young men (21–30 years) and 13 older adults (64–74 years, 9 men). Subjects in these studies lived on a scheduled 28-hour 'day' (18:40 hours wake: 9:20 hours sleep) for several weeks in order to schedule sleep and wake uniformly across all circadian phases. Circadian phase is expressed in degrees (one circadian cycle = 360°) and was measured experimentally using core body temperature (CBT minimum = 0°) and plasma melatonin. Data are double-plotted to aid visualization of the rhythms. The open bar represents the timing of a normal

Fig. 2.1 (contd) 8-hour sleep period (~0:00–8:00 hours), if CBT minimum occurs at ~6:00 hours. Sleep latency is the duration of time taken to fall asleep at the start of each sleep opportunity and total sleep time is the duration spent asleep in each 9:20 hours scheduled sleep opportunity.

There is a distinct circadian rhythm in the propensity to fall asleep (sleep latency) with shortest sleep latencies during the biological night when melatonin is produced (top panel). Total sleep time also shows a distinct rhythm with the highest sleep duration obtained during the usual night in both young (o) and older (●) subjects, although overall sleep duration is lower in the older adults at all circadian phase (second panel). The 'window' of time when sleep duration is maximal differs between the groups and is narrower for the older subjects; sleep duration declines at an earlier circadian phase in the older (0°) as compared to the younger (60°) subjects (middle panel). Sleep latencies are also longer at this time in older subjects (top panel). The longest sleep latencies and shortest sleep durations in both groups are observed several hours before the onset of melatonin production, and illustrate the 'wake maintenance zone' or 'forbidden' zone for sleep which occurs prior to habitual bedtime (see text for details).

Source: Adapted with permission from Dijk, D.-J., Duffy, J.F. & Czeisler, C.A. (2000). Contribution of circadian physiology and sleep homeostasis to age-related changes in human sleep. *Chronobiol Int*, **17**(3), 285–311.

maximum sleep that older adults can obtain. In studies where young and old subjects are given long opportunities to sleep (either 14–16 hours a night for 9–28 nights or 12 hours per night plus a 4-hour nap for 3–7 days), sleep duration asymptotes at ~8.5 in young adults (Wehr et al., 1993; Rajaratnam et al., 2004; Klerman and Dijk, 2008) and about an hour less (7.4 hours) in older adults (Klerman and Dijk, 2008). It is not clear whether these sleep durations represent sleep 'need' in adults in terms of what is biologically required to maintain optimal function, but does represent at least their biological capacity to sleep. Failure to achieve these totals on a daily basis—termed chronic partial sleep deprivation—will result in a progressive decline in alertness and performance with time (Van Dongen et al., 2003; Belenky et al., 2003; Cohen et al., 2010).

Age-independent disruptions in the relative timing or 'phase relationship' of these two processes can also cause problems with both sleep and daytime function. As outlined in sections 'Diurnal preference' and 'Daytime functioning', there are inter-individual differences in the exact phase relationship of these two processes that determine individual differences in sleep timing, diurnal preference, and patterns of daytime alertness and performance. If these processes become completely desynchronized, as happens in shift-workers or following transmeridian travel ('jet lag'), symptoms of insomnia and excessive daytime sleepiness can reach clinical severity.

Diurnal preference

Diurnal preference, sometimes referred to as 'morningness-eveningness', or whether someone is a 'lark' or an 'owl', describes an individual's behavioural preference for sleep timing and for optimal daytime functioning. Questionnaires used to measure diurnal preference (Horne and Östberg, 1976; Roenneberg et al., 2003) ask about when one prefers to go to bed, or when one prefers to complete tasks requiring attention and concentration, or simply if one rates oneself an extreme or moderate morning or evening type.

Diurnal preference has been used in epidemiological studies to examine, for example, the relationship between clock genes polymorphisms and circadian timing, or between sleep timing and diurnal preference (e.g. Archer et al., 2003; Roenneberg et al., 2007). Self-reported diurnal preference is not a simple measure of circadian phase, however, but rather a reflection of the phase relationship—the 'phase angle of entrainment'—between the circadian and homeostatic processes.

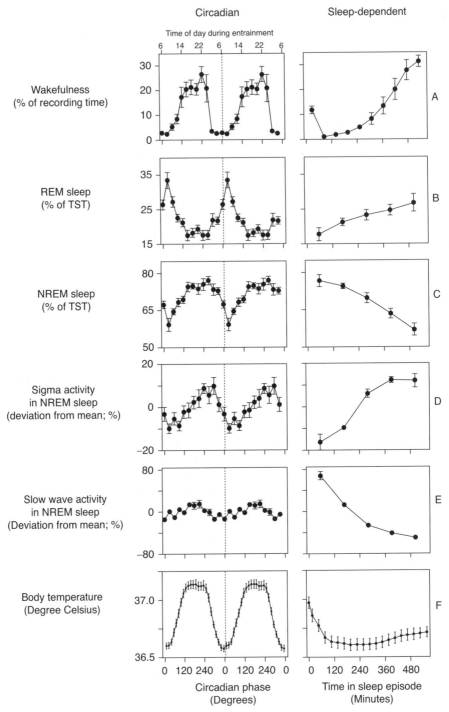

Fig. 2.2 Circadian and sleep-dependent changes in sleep structure.

Figure 2.2 shows the variation in sleep structure with respect to circadian phase (left column) and time asleep (right column) in subjects studied under a 28-hour day forced desynchrony protocol (see Fig. 2.1 legend).

Fig. 2.2 (contd) There are distinct circadian rhythms (left column) in wakefulness within sleep (A), REM sleep (B), and sigma ('sleep spindle') activity within NREM sleep (D). (The NREM rhythm in (C) is a function of REM sleep rhythmicity in the fixed sleep episode.) Slow wave activity in NREM (E) is marginally rhythmic but has a very clear sleep-dependent decline with increasing time asleep (E, right column) which is also apparent in NREM sleep overall (C). Wakefulness within sleep increases with increasing time asleep (A, right column) as does sleep spindle activity (D).

Source: Reproduced with permission from Dijk, D.-J. & Czeisler, C.A. (1995). Contribution of the circadian pacemaker and the sleep homeostat to sleep propensity, sleep structure, electroencephalographic slow waves, and sleep spindle activity in humans. *J Neurosci*, **15**, 3526–3538.

Imagine an experiment where a group of people are kept on the same light-dark schedule (16 hours light:8 hours dark) for several weeks; some people would go to bed and wake early, some would go to sleep late and lie-in, some would sleep for only 7 hours, some for 9 hours, and so on. Each person would find their own natural timing within the day, that is, their diurnal preference, and their natural sleep duration. Across a population, there is a range of diurnal preferences and a range of sleep durations (Roenneberg et al., 2003; Groeger et al., 2004). These behaviours reflect the interaction between the circadian and homeostatic processes—not either exclusively—and therefore the diurnal preference and sleep timing phenotypes are determined by multiple factors. For example, those people who tend to sleep and wake early ('larks') may either have a circadian clock that cycles faster than those who tend to sleep and wake later ('owls') (Duffy and Czeisler, 2002; Duffy et al., 2001; Wright Jr. et al., 2005), and/or may have a greater propensity to sleep early due to a quicker build up of homeostatic sleep pressure (Mongrain et al., 2008) or to wake early due to a quicker dissipation of homeostatic sleep pressure (Mongrain et al., 2005, 2006). Similarly, inter-individual differences in sleep duration may reflect differences in homeostatic dynamics during sleep (Aeschbach et al., 1996) and wake (Aeschbach et al., 2001) in addition to circadian timing.

The non-trait like properties of diurnal preference are further illustrated when examining the relationship of diurnal preference with age. In cross-sectional studies, there is a trend for older people to rate themselves as more morning-type compared to young people (Duffy et al., 1999; Robilliard et al., 2002; Roenneberg et al., 2007). When measured experimentally, older adults do indeed have an earlier circadian phase than younger adults and do wake at an earlier clock time (Duffy et al., 1998, 1999, 2002) (Fig. 2.3). Their phase angle of entrainment is different compared to young people, with wake time occurring at a relatively earlier circadian phase (Duffy et al., 1998, 1999, 2002) (Fig. 2.3). When young morning types are compared to young evening types, the opposite is the case: young morning types, although having an earlier circadian phase and clock time than young evening types, wake at a relatively later circadian phase than young evening types, and exhibit a very different phase angle of entrainment (Duffy et al., 1999; Dijk and Lockley, 2002) (Fig. 2.3). The self-reported diurnal preference is therefore not specific to a particular underlying phase relationship and may be misleading if used to estimate circadian timing (see section 'Using sleep and circadian rhythms as biomarkers').

Daytime functioning

The two-process model also describes the general time course of sleepiness and performance through the day, with a general increase in sleepiness with longer time awake, and a strong circadian rhythm in sleepiness, mood, and performance (Johnson et al., 1992; Boivin et al., 1997;

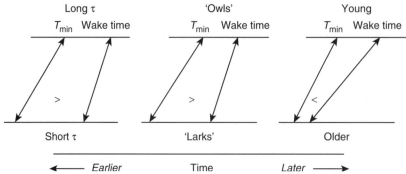

Fig. 2.3 Schematic representation of sleep and circadian rhythm timing differences due to diurnal preference, ageing, and circadian period.

Figure 2.3 shows the relative differences in the timing of circadian phase (as indicated by core body temperature minimum, T_{min}) and wake time in three different comparative groups. As might be predicted, young morning types ('Larks') have an earlier circadian phase and earlier wake time than young evening types ('Owls') (middle panel). The phase relationship between sleep timing and circadian phase is not the same, that is, the lines are not parallel. The time between T_{min} and wake time is longer (>) in morning as compared to evening types, indicating that morning types wake at a relatively later phase of their circadian cycle. These differences could theoretically be driven by differences in endogenous circadian period between these groups (left panel).

This internal phase relationship changes with ageing (right panel). Older adults, who usually tend to be more morning type, do indeed have an earlier circadian phase and earlier wake time than young subjects. Unlike young morning types, older subject wake at a relatively earlier circadian phase (<), closer to their T_{min} than young subjects.

Source: Reproduced from Dijk, D.-J. & Lockley, S.W. (2002). Integration of human sleep-wake regulation and circadian rhythmicity. *J Appl Physiol*, **92**, 852–862. Used with permission from the Am Physiol Soc.

Wyatt et al., 1999, 2004; Cajochen et al., 2002). Under normal sleep-wake conditions, daytime functioning is relatively stable during the day before exhibiting a wake-dependent decline towards the end of day. A third process is required to explain the sub-maximal alertness experienced upon awakening, as the two-process model would predict lowest sleep pressure at the end of the sleep episode and therefore maximal alertness upon waking. It takes some time to reach maximal alertness after waking up, however—up to 2 hours under laboratory conditions (Jewett et al., 1999; Wertz et al., 2006)—and the time course of this sleep inertia has been termed Process W (Folkard and Åkerstedt, 1987; Åkerstedt et al., 2008). Sleep inertia interacts with both Process C and Process S, exhibiting a greater severity and duration when waking from an adverse circadian phase or deeper sleep (Cavallero and Versace, 2003; Scheer et al., 2008).

Although alertness generally declines during the day, there is a window just before the habitual sleep episode where sleep is difficult to initiate and performance is maintained (Fig. 2.1). As explained above, this 'Wake Maintenance Zone' occurs due to the circadian rhythm in alertness, which is high towards the end of the day, not being fully counteracted by the wake-dependent decline in alertness. The end of the Wake Maintenance or 'forbidden' zone coincides with the onset of pineal melatonin production (see section 'Role of melatonin in sleep-wake regulation'), sometimes referred to as the opening of the 'sleep gate' (Lavie, 1986, 1997). There in a rapid increase in sleepiness and sleep propensity at this time (Fig. 2.1).

There is a non-linear interaction between the homeostatic and circadian processes that can cause a dramatic deterioration in alertness under certain circumstances and has potential safety implications.

As outlined above, the circadian sleep propensity rhythm is highest in the early morning and anyone awake at this time is inherently sleepy regardless of how long they have been awake. The severity of this sleepiness is amplified in a non-linear manner, depending on how long one has been awake at this time. For example, a night shift-worker is not only awake at 4:00–5:00 a.m., the sleepiest time according to their circadian rhythm, but often has also been awake for 12 hours or more by that time, exacerbating the circadian sleepiness with an additional wake-dependent decline (Fig. 2.4). This is a particularly vulnerable time for sleepiness-related accidents and injuries

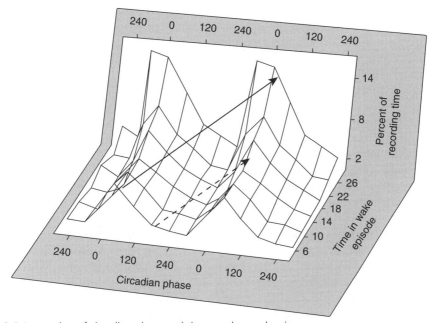

Fig. 2.4 Interaction of circadian phase and time awake on sleepiness.

Figure 2.4 shows the rate of slow-rolling eye movements, a reliable marker of sleepiness, measured during a forced desynchrony study (see Fig. 2.1 legend). Circadian phase (and relative time of day; 0° ≅ 6:00 a.m., 120° ≅ 2:00 p.m., 240° ≅ 10:00 p.m.) is plotted on the x-axis, increasing time awake on the y-axis and the percent of EOG recording time with slow eye movements plotted on the z-axis. There is a clear circadian rhythm in the rate of slow eye movements, with maximal sleepiness in the early morning (Process C). There is also an increase in sleepiness with increasing time awake (Process S). The non-linear interaction between these two processes is indicated by the two example time courses illustrated. The solid arrow indicates the evolution of sleepiness for an individual waking at 6:00 a.m. and then working a 24-hour shift (e.g. medical resident or firefighter). Sleepiness remains fairly stable for the first ~16 hours (0–240°) after which it rapidly increases as increased time awake coincides with the endogenous circadian rhythm in sleep propensity. The dotted arrow shows the sleepiness trajectory for someone working overnight having had a sleep prior to starting the night shift, thereby reducing their homeostatic build-up of sleep pressure. Although sleepiness also increases with increased time awake, the later time of day at which the wake episode starts reduces the cumulative interaction between time awake and adverse circadian phase; even if the individuals remain awake all night, they never reach as high a level of fatigue during the early hours as the resident on duty continuously.

Source: Adapted from Czeisler, C.A., Buxton, O.M. & Khalsa, S.B.S. (2005). The human circadian timing system and sleep-wake regulation. In: Kryger, M.H., Roth, T. & Dement, W.C. (eds.), *Principles and Practices of Sleep Medicine*. Fourth edition. Philadelphia, PA: W.B. Saunders, pp. 375–394, with permission from Elsevier.

(Folkard and Lombardi, 2006). In professions that require workers to be on duty round-the-clock continuously, for example physicians and firefighters, their circadian nadir can coincide with ~24 hours of prior wakefulness, increasing the risk of sleepiness on duty (Cajochen et al., 1999; Lockley et al., 2004; Elliott and Kuehl, 2007) (Fig. 2.4) and the rate of drowsy driving crashes on the drive home after work (Barger et al., 2005). These interactions are dramatically exacerbated when examined on a background of chronic partial sleep deprivation, the dynamics of which are only just starting to be understood (Cohen et al., 2010).

Although the contribution of these fundamental processes on waking function have been defined primarily in the laboratory, they are also readily apparent under real world conditions. As outlined above, there are differences in the phase angle of entrainment between morning and evening types such that morning types wake at a later circadian phase than evening types, even though they wake at an earlier actual clock time (Fig. 2.3). These differences in phase angle of entrainment are reflected in the different time course of sleepiness and performance exhibited by morning and evening types through the day (Horne et al., 1980; Kerkhof and Van Dongen, 1996; Kerkhof, 1998). Morning types, waking later in their circadian cycle, have high alertness and per-formance in the morning and then decline rapidly through the day, whereas evening types, waking earlier in their circadian cycle, are more sleepy and poorer performers in the morning but do not decline as much as morning types by the end of the day. The behavioural differences reported by morning and evening types, that is, that morning types feel more alert in the morning and prefer to perform critical tasks at this time, whereas evening types feel better and perform better later in the day, is therefore explained by the circadian phase at which they wake (Duffy et al., 1999; Baehr et al., 2000; Mongrain et al., 2004; Lockley et al., 2008). In totally blind people who have non-24-hour circadian rhythms (Lockley et al., 2007), the time course of their daytime alertness changes back and forth between the morning-type or evening-type profile depending on whether they are in a relatively advanced or delayed phase of their circadian cycle, respectively (Lockley et al., 2008), illustrating the primary role of phase angle in determining alertness, mood, and per-formance patterns. In adolescents, who generally report a tendency to eveningness, circadian rhythms are phase delayed, altering the phase relationship between the homeostatic and circadian processes (Carskadon et al., 2004). Consequently, sleep and wake occur at a relatively early circa-dian phase, compromising the ability of teens to remain awake and perform during the day. There are also marked changes in the dynamics of homeostatic sleep pressure during both wake and sleep during development that, in combination with the circadian system, increase sleepiness during the day, particularly in the mid-afternoon (Carskadon et al., 2004).

Factors affecting sleep-wake regulation

Role of light in sleep-wake regulation

An important consideration in sleep-wake regulation is the role of light, exposure to which can affect both circadian timing (Process C) and sleepiness and performance directly (Process S) (for reviews see: Czeisler and Gooley, 2007; Lockley, 2007; Cajochen, 2007; Brainard and Hanifin, 2005). Light has a number of 'non-visual' effects on human physiology separate and apart from vision, including resetting the circadian pacemaker, suppressing pineal melatonin production, increasing nighttime heart rate and core temperature levels, and acutely improving subjective and objective measures of alertness. These effects may have important consequences for health and well-being and have been an important consideration in a number of epidemio-logical findings.

As described above, the SCN controls 24-hour rhythms in many aspects of human physiology, metabolism, and behaviour. The endogenous period of this circadian pacemaker clock is near to, but not exactly, 24 hours and in order to ensure that these rhythms are timed appropriately to anticipate future environmental events (e.g. food availability), environmental time cues must reset this internal clock. The 24-hour light-dark cycle is the primary environmental time signal ('*zeitgeber*') and this light information is captured exclusively by the eyes primarily using specialized short-wavelength (blue) light sensitive retinal ganglion cells and transduced directly to the SCN via a dedicated neural pathway, the retinohypothalamic tract (RHT) (Gooley et al., 2003; Peirson and Foster, 2006). Each day the light-dark cycle resets the internal clock, which in turn synchronizes the physiology, metabolism, and behaviour controlled by the clock. Failure to receive this light-dark information, as experienced by many totally blind individuals, causes the circadian pacemaker to revert to its endogenous non-24-hour period and become desynchronized from the 24-hour light-dark cycle. Consequently, the majority of totally blind subjects suffer from non-24-hour sleep-wake disorder as their sleep-wake cycle, alertness, and performance patterns and other rhythms becomes desynchronized from the 24-hour social pattern (Lockley et al., 2007). Similar results were observed in early experiments of sighted subjects conducted in caves or underground bunkers without access to a natural light-dark cycle (Kleitman, 1963; Mills, 1964; Wever, 1979). Circadian misalignment also occurs in sighted subjects who are not exposed to a stable 24-hour light-dark cycle, for example in night shift-workers or after a rapid change in light-dark patterns following transmerdian travel ('jet lag'). Exposure to a stable 24-hour light-dark cycle is therefore required to maintain normal circadian entrainment, including entrainment of the sleep-wake cycle and sleep propensity rhythms described by Process C.

Light also has a direct effect on Process S in that light exposure can acutely enhance alertness and performance during both the day and the night (Phipps-Nelson et al., 2003; Rüger et al., 2006; Cajochen, 2007) and reduces homeostatic sleep pressure (SWS) in nighttime sleep following light exposure (Munch et al., 2006). Light is not required to generate or maintain the phase relationships between Process C and Process S, as these relationships persist in totally blind subjects whose circadian systems cannot detect light (Klein et al., 1993; Lockley et al., 1999).

The separate functional and anatomical distinction between the non-visual and visual photoreception systems gives rise to some differences in the dynamics of how light affects the two systems. The circadian resetting and alerting effects of light are determined by a range of light properties including the timing, intensity, duration, pattern, wavelength, and history of exposure and these factors may be important when interpreting light exposure 'risk'. Each of these is separately reviewed briefly below but under real-world conditions many of these factors will apply simultaneously to the net effects of light. A detailed review of these differences is provided in the Light and Health Committee Technical Report of the Illuminating and Engineering Society of North America (Figueiro et al., 2008).

An important factor in determining the circadian effect of light is the timing of the light exposure. Light can either phase advance (shift to an earlier time) or phase delay (shift to a later time) the circadian system depending on the timing of exposure. Under normal conditions, light in the late day/early night (~18:00–6:00 hours) causes a phase delay of the pacemaker whereas light exposure in the late night/early day (~6:00–18:00 hours) will phase advance the clock. The relationship between the timing of a stimulus and the direction and magnitude of the resultant shift is described in a phase response curve (PRC) (Honma and Honma, 1988; Czeisler et al., 1989; Khalsa et al., 2003) and is a vital tool when interpreting the effects of light. There are also non-linear relationships between the intensity or duration of light and its non-visual effects. For example, exposure to relatively dim indoor room light (~100 lux) for 6.5 hours at night can stimulate 50% of the maximum effect of an equal-duration exposure with 10- to 100-fold greater illuminance (Zeitzer et al., 2000a; Cajochen et al., 2000). An intermittent exposure will also induce a disproportionally greater response compared to continuous exposure (Rimmer et al., 2000;

Gronfier et al., 2004). The effect of a light stimulus is also dependent on light history. The circadian photoreception system exhibits adaptation to prior light exposure in determining the response to a current stimulus such that prior exposure to brighter light over previous hours or days reduces the impact of subsequent light exposure. Similarly, subjects routinely exposed to more bright light during the day over a week may have a reduced melatonin suppression response than following exposure to dimmer light, consistent with reports that seasonal light exposure changes the sensitivity to melatonin-suppressing effects of light (Hébert et al., 2002; Smith et al., 2004; Higuchi et al., 2007).

The wavelength sensitivity of the circadian and alerting effects of light is blue-shifted relative to the photopic (cone vision) and scotopic (rod vision) photoreceptor systems. The specialized retinal ganglion cells that detect light for circadian and alerting responses contain the novel photopigment melanopsin (Provencio et al., 2000), which is most sensitive to short-wavelength (blue) light ~480 nm (Berson et al., 2002; Hattar et al., 2002; Dacey et al., 2005). Blue light is a powerful stimulant of circadian and alerting responses to light in humans and has a similar peak spectral sensitivity to melanopsin (Brainard et al., 2001; Thapan et al., 2001; Hankins and Lucas, 2002; Zaidi et al., 2007).

Role of melatonin in sleep-wake regulation

The major biochemical correlate of the light-dark cycle is provided by the pineal melatonin rhythm. Under normal light-dark conditions, melatonin is produced only during the night and provides an internal representation of the environmental photoperiod, specifically night-length (scotoperiod), which has become an important proxy for sleep in epidemiology (see section 'Using sleep and circadian rhythms as biomarkers'). The synthesis and timing of melatonin production requires an intact afferent signal from the SCN to the pineal and ablation of this pathway, as occurs in some people due to spinal damage at the upper cervical level, completely abolishes melatonin production although other circadian rhythms not requiring this projection remain intact (Kneisley et al., 1978; Zeitzer et al., 2000b). Ocular light exposure during the night inhibits melatonin production acutely and provides an indirect assessment of light input to the SCN via the RHT. Given the close temporal relationship between the SCN and melatonin production, the melatonin rhythm is often used as a marker of circadian phase and the melatonin suppression response as a proxy for RHT-SCN integrity and sensitivity. The specific nighttime production of melatonin and its exquisite sensitivity to light also makes it a potential biomarker for assessing light exposure during the night, as outlined below.

The melatonin rhythm is also closely associated with sleep in diurnal animals such as humans but may not have a direct effect on sleep *in vivo*. Nocturnal animals such as rats and hamsters also produce melatonin at night during their active episode. As described previously, the human circadian sleep propensity rhythm is closely correlated with the melatonin profile and the opening of the sleep gate occurs simultaneously with the onset of melatonin (Nakagawa et al., 1992; Lavie, 1997; Lockley et al., 1997) (Fig. 2.1). These events may simply be contemporaneous, as individuals who do not produce melatonin (e.g. tetraplegic individuals, many people taking beta-blockers, pinealectomized patients) still exhibit circadian sleep-wake rhythms and have only minor changes in sleep timing and structure (Macchi and Bruce, 2004; Scheer et al., 2006). Similarly, if plasma melatonin is suppressed by light exposure at night, alertness levels simultaneously improve, suggesting that melatonin and sleepiness are directly related. Light exposure in the daytime will also improve alertness, at a time when melatonin is not produced, however suggesting that either melatonin is not a direct mediator of alertness and/or separate mechanisms exist during the day and night for enhancement of alertness by light (Lockley and Gooley, 2006; Cajochen, 2007). The presumed association between melatonin and sleep arises from the effects of exogenous melatonin treatment which does induce sleepiness and, when taken at a time when endogenous melatonin is not produced, can improve sleep (Dijk and Cajochen, 1997; Wyatt et al., 2006). These pharmacological effects are not necessarily an indication of endogenous melatonin function.

Sleep and circadian influences on endocrinology and metabolism

The effects of sleep disruption and clinical sleep disorders on health and disease, and potential mechanisms underlying these findings, are reviewed in detail in this book (see also Chapters 4–12). There are direct effects of sleep and circadian rhythms on a number of common hormonal and metabolic biomarkers that epidemiologists may need to take into account when developing protocols and interpreting findings, and these are reviewed briefly below (Czeisler and Klerman, 1999; Knutson et al., 2007).

Understanding the role of sleep and circadian phase on physiology and metabolism requires controlled experiments that attempt to isolate the effects of each. A simple approach to examine the direct effect of sleep is to compare the level and rhythms of biomarkers under normal sleep-wake (baseline) conditions with a sleep deprivation condition. Isolating circadian effects is more complicated and requires the elimination or equal distribution of factors that affect the endogenous circadian pacemaker, including light, sleep, activity, posture, meal timing, social interaction, knowledge of clock time, and so on. The constant routine (CR) protocol, first developed by Mills and colleagues in the 1970s (Mills et al., 1978), encompasses both approaches and has been used to examine both the role of sleep and circadian phase on physiology and metabolism. Subjects are studied under baseline conditions (usually 16 hours wake in room light and 8 hours sleep in darkness) and then undergo a CR procedure consisting of ~30–50 hours of constant wakefulness in dim light while maintaining a semi-recumbent posture. Subjects are not permitted access to time cues (e.g. TV, radio, Internet, clocks, etc.) and are provided with identical hourly snacks to control the effects of food on circadian rhythms (Duffy and Dijk, 2002). These controls either abolish or mitigate the effects of environmental time cues on the circadian pacemaker, revealing the endogenous phase and amplitude of the rhythm.

These studies have demonstrated that many hormones and peptides are influenced by the circadian system, sleep, or a combination of both. Some hormones have a strongly endogenous circadian rhythm that is minimally influenced by sleep. Pineal melatonin, which has a nighttime peak (~2:00 a.m.) under normal conditions, is virtually unaffected by sleep (Fig. 2.5), although it is strongly suppressed directly by exposure to light at night. Cortisol, which rises during sleep to a maximum shortly before habitual waketime, is also relatively unchanged during sleep or wake conditions, although waking from sleep causes a small direct elevation (Fig. 2.5). Conversely, some hormones, for example growth hormone (GH), are very strongly sleep-dependent with little influence of the circadian system. GH is secreted primarily during SWS and has lower levels under conditions of sleep deprivation. Sleep deprivation, therefore, could dramatically reduce GH secretion. Other outcomes are influenced by both. For example, thyroid-stimulating hormone (TSH) appears to be under minimal circadian control with only a small peak close to sleep onset under normal conditions. When assessed under CR conditions, a very different pattern emerges; TSH has a strong circadian rhythm with a nighttime peak that is suppressed by sleep at night under normal conditions (Fig. 2.5). Similar careful consideration is needed when examining insulin and glucose levels; although they are clearly influenced by meals, when hourly snacks are provided to spread out nutrient intake equally over 24 hours, an underlying circadian rhythm is revealed with minimal levels during the biological night and a morning peak, particularly for insulin (Shea et al., 2005). The effects of partial chronic sleep deprivation (Spiegel et al., 1999, 2004) and circadian desynchrony (Morgan et al., 1998; Scheer et al., 2009) on metabolic biomarkers have also been examined, with dramatic results: in a very short space of time—a matter of days—chronic sleep deprivation or circadian desynchrony can induce glucose levels on par with a pre-diabetic or even diabetic state in initially healthy young adults (Knutson et al., 2006; Scheer et al., 2009).

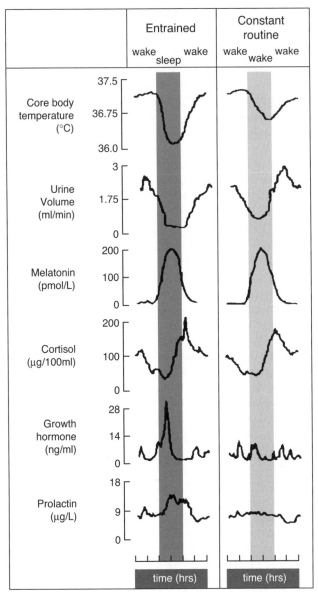

Fig. 2.5 Sleep and circadian-dependent influences on endocrine function.

Figure 2.5 shows the relative profiles of temperature, urine volume and a number of common endocrine markers under normal baseline 16 h wake - 8h sleep -16 h wake (W-S-W) conditions (left panels, sleep shown by dark shaded area) and under Constant Routine (CR) conditions where subjects remain awake in a time-free environment, under dim light and in a semi-recumbent posture with hourly snacks for 30 hours or more (see text for details).

Melatonin (third panel) and cortisol (fourth panel) profiles are relatively unchanged by sleep, except that there is a small wake-dependent rise in cortisol in the morning not seen during CR condition.

Fig. 2.5 (contd) Controlled dim light exposure is necessary to maintain melatonin levels under CR conditions, however, as light directly suppresses melatonin (see text). There is a large sleep-dependent increase in the amplitude of Core Body Temperature (top panel) and a lowering of the temperature minimum reached due to the direct hypothermic effect of sleep in addition to the circadian decline in temperature at night. Growth Hormone (fifth panel) and to a lesser extent, Prolactin (bottom panel) have a sleep-dependent increase in levels such that production of these hormones is greatly reduced if sleep is absent (right panels).

These examples serve to underscore the importance of understanding the time of day and sleep status of subjects being sampled to avoid possible systematic confounds when measuring biomarkers (see text).

Source: Adapted with permission from Figure 1 in Maywood, E.S., O'Neill, J.S., Chesham, J.E. & Hastings, M.H. (2007). Minireview: The circadian clockwork of the suprachiasmatic nuclei–analysis of a cellular oscillator that drives endocrine rhythms. *Endocrinol*, **148**, 5624–5634.

Considerations in epidemiology

Sleep and circadian confounds

The practice of using single time-point biomarkers or measurements in epidemiology brings potential confounds with respect to circadian and sleep influences. For example, a high cortisol level would be normal for a morning blood draw but abnormal for an evening draw (Fig. 2.5, part C). Accounting for time of day in analyses, or maintaining a fixed time of day for data collection, is therefore a minimum requirement for being able to interpret markers that have any circadian component to their variation. This is a compromise position, of course, as it assumes that all individuals have the same timing of their circadian rhythms. This is not the case and there is at least a 5-hour range in circadian phase across the population, even in normally phased healthy subjects (Wright Jr. et al., 2005). Systematic changes in circadian timing, for example those that occur in adolescence or old age, may be possible to account for on average but again, inter-individual variability in circadian phase will mean that these assumptions are potentially flawed.

The confound becomes more severe when dealing with a population who may have a greater degree of circadian disruption, for example in shift-workers or in pilots and flight attendants who are desynchronized due to jet lag, as the direction and magnitude of circadian misalignment is unpredictable (Arendt and Deacon, 1996; Dumont et al., 2001). For example, the melatonin metabolite 6-sulphatoxymelatonin (aMT6s) concentration in a morning void urine sample may reliably correlate with overall 24-hour production in non-shift-workers with normal circadian rhythms (Schernhammer and Hankinson, 2005) but has little predictive value in shift-workers who may be advanced or delayed relative to normal; a morning void aMT6s level might occur before the peak melatonin output if the circadian rhythm is delayed but may occur many hours after the melatonin peak if the rhythm was advanced. Similar confounds may exist in relation to sleep. As outlined above, the sleep duration in the night or nights prior to sampling may affect some biomarkers directly and therefore knowledge of at least the previous night's sleep may be an important covariate. These factors are particularly problematic if interpreting single time-point alertness or performance measures; as discussed earlier, the current vigilance level is highly dependent on the number of hours awake and circadian phase.

Understanding the differential effects of these factors on multiple biomarkers is also key when examining relationships and ratios; if one parameter has a circadian rhythm and one does not, then their ratio will be rhythmic and the ratio may be high or low depending on the time at which the sample is taken. If one biomarker is dependent on sleep and one is not, again their ratio may change depending on prior sleep duration. The limitations of circadian- or sleep-dependent biomarkers that are only sampled once or are sampled in populations with potential circadian misalignment should be acknowledged and results may be misleading, even in very large cohorts, if these confounds cannot be accounted for.

Using sleep and circadian rhythms as biomarkers

A number of sleep and circadian biomarkers have been used directly and as proxy markers in recent epidemiological studies, with variable success. A number of examples are outlined below as case examples of how sleep might be used as a biomarker to illustrate the advantages and disadvantages of such approaches.

An area where both indirect and direct estimations of circadian desynchrony and sleep have been relatively successful has been the examination of shift-work, sleep duration, and nighttime light exposure on breast cancer risk (Stevens et al., 2007). It has been shown in animal and *in vitro* that suppression of melatonin via pinealectomy or constant light exposure can increase the rate of mammary tumour growth, and that exposure to darkness or increasing melatonin levels can slow tumour growth down (Blask et al., 2002; Reiter et al., 2007). Inducing chronic circadian desynchrony by simulating continuous jet lag, even in species that do not produce melatonin, also increases tumour growth and mortality rates compared to animals kept on a stable light-dark cycle (Filipski et al., 2005; Sahar and Sassone-Corsi, 2009).

Measuring circadian desynchrony, light exposure at night or melatonin levels directly in order to test the hypothesis that light exposure at night may contribute to the increase in breast cancer risk observed in industrialized nations (Stevens, 2005) is difficult in large-scale epidemiological studies. Displacement of sleep by shift-work or jet lag has multiple consequences including circadian desynchrony, light exposure at night, and possible suppression of melatonin. Regular exposure to shift-work or jet lag has therefore been used to test the hypothesis that shift-working women would be at a greater risk of breast cancer than non-shift-workers in these epidemiological studies. A number (but not all) of epidemiological studies have reported a ~60% increased risk of breast cancer in shift-working women who worked overnight chronically (Davis et al., 2001; Schernhammer et al., 2001; Megdal et al., 2005) or routinely travelled across time zones (Rafnsson et al., 2001), prompting the World Health Organization to designate 'shift-work that involves circadian disruption' as a probable carcinogen (Group 2A) (Straif et al., 2007) placing it in the same category as UV light and diesel engine exhausts.

Epidemiologist have also considered what other proxy outcomes could be used to estimate exposure to light at night. As discussed previously, some totally blind subjects are unable to detect light for circadian entrainment and melatonin suppression and therefore a prediction of the 'light-at-night' hypothesis is that totally blind women, the majority of whom cannot detect light or have their melatonin suppressed by light (Czeisler et al., 1995), would have a reduced cancer risk compared to visually impaired or sighted women. This association has indeed been confirmed in a number of (but again not all) cross-sectional studies with totally blind women exhibiting about a 50% reduction in breast cancer risk (Hahn, 1991; Feychting et al., 1998; Flynn-Evans et al., 2009b) and increasing risk with increasing visual acuity (Pukkala et al., 2006; Flynn-Evans et al., 2009b). These findings do not appear to be due to differences in reproductive function (Flynn-Evans et al., 2009a).

Although measuring sleep and sleep disruption is of interest in its own right (see section 'Sleep-wake regulation'), it is important to remember that sleep also gates ocular light exposure for circadian entrainment and melatonin suppression (Dijk and Lockley, 2002). The sleep-wake pattern determines the light-dark exposure pattern, or photoperiod, as wake is associated with light exposure and sleep occurs with eyes closed, shutting off virtually all light input. Changes in sleep-wake patterns therefore also mean changes in light-dark exposure, which can have substantial effects on circadian rhythms (Czeisler et al., 1999). This reciprocal relationship has consequently been used to estimate light exposure at night from assessments of sleep duration (Verkasalo et al., 2005). Consistent with the results for shift-workers (who are an example of extremely 'short'—i.e. zero—sleepers during the night), women who reported sleeping most (≥9 hours per night) had the lowest breast cancer risk as compared to women who slept 7–8 or ≤6 hours per night (Verkasalo et al., 2005). A separate study showed that satellite-derived estimates of the intensity of light pollution at night were correlated with breast but not lung cancer risk (Kloog et al., 2008). Sleep duration may therefore be an important proxy biomarker for other outcomes, including light exposure at night and sleep- or light-affected hormones such as melatonin, cortisol, GH, and TSH.

Using similar assumptions, lack of sleep has been estimated indirectly from work hour records (Rothschild et al., 2009). A retrospective review of complications following surgery or labour used the recorded times of procedures to estimate the sleep opportunity available overnight to individual physicians. Analysis of the complications by sleep opportunity showed that complication rates were higher in those who had less than 6 hours sleep opportunity before the surgery as compared to those who had more than 6 hours sleep opportunity. Although sleep opportunity does not equal sleep duration, and some of those who had the opportunity to sleep may not have done so, this method allowed for identification of the maximum amount of sleep obtained before an event.

Measuring circadian rhythms themselves requires experimental control that is not usually available for epidemiological studies. A number of proxy markers have been used to estimate circadian phase including sleep timing, diurnal preference, and morning urinary melatonin levels. As outlined above, sleep timing and diurnal preference have some shortcomings when used to estimate circadian phase as there is at least a 5-hour range in the phase relationship between sleep and circadian phase for a given circadian phase even in normal sleepers (Wright Jr. et al., 2005). This range is likely to be broader in the general population meaning that the sleep time may misestimate circadian phase by many hours. Sleep may also bear no relationship at all with circadian phase under extreme cases, for example in shift-workers: if only sleep data were measured without knowledge of the work pattern, then the sleep timing would clearly not be an accurate measure of circadian phase in shift-workers.

Similar shortcomings exist for diurnal preference given that it is estimated largely on the basis of sleep preferences. Diurnal preference, and components therein, have been used as a proxy for circadian phase most notably in studies examining the effects of alterations in circadian clock genes (Von Schantz, 2008; Ellis et al., 2009). Although diurnal preference and entrained phase angle do correlate with circadian period (Duffy and Czeisler, 2002; Wright Jr. et al., 2005; Gronfier et al., 2007), the inconsistency in the studies comparing circadian clock gene polymorphisms and diurnal preference suggests that the diurnal preference phenotype may be determined by several possible mechanisms in addition to circadian phase, as described previously. For example, Katzenburg and colleagues (Katzenberg et al., 1998) reported an association between prevalence of the 3111C allele in the 3'-untranslated region (3'-UTR) of the circadian gene Clock and an evening-type preference that was not replicated in later studies (Robilliard et al., 2002; Johansson et al., 2003; Pedrazzoli et al., 2007) nor in DSPD (delayed sleep phase disorder) patients (Robilliard et al., 2002; Iwase et al., 2002). A variable number tandem repeat (VNTR) polymorphism of the circadian gene Period 3 (Per3) has also been reported to be associated with evening-type diurnal preference (Ebisawa et al., 2001; Archer et al., 2003; Pereira et al., 2005) and DSPD (Ebisawa et al., 2001; Archer et al., 2003), although not consistently (Pereira et al., 2005). The potential confounding effects of age on diurnal preference described above are illustrated here in that the association between Per3 and eveningness is dependent on age, and is much stronger in young people (Jones et al., 2007). Despite multiple demonstrations of the association between diurnal preference and the Per3 VNTR in population-based studies, the Per3 polymorphism was surprisingly not associated with any differences in circadian rhythms or sleep in a small population studied in detail following genetic selection for the Per3 polymorphism (Viola et al., 2007). The latter study showed a strong association between the Per3 polymorphism and overnight performance during a 40-hour CR, suggesting that Per3 may regulate the homeostatic, rather than the circadian control of sleepiness and performance (Viola et al., 2007; Groeger et al., 2008). As outlined earlier, different diurnal preference phenotypes may also be expressed due to differences in homeostatic sleep pressure and not necessarily changes in circadian phase. Diurnal preference may also be subject to sociological differences that affect reporting by different ethnic groups (Barbosa et al., 2010).

Other genetic polymorphisms associated with morning diurnal preference, for example in the Per1 (Carpen et al., 2006) or Per2 (Carpen et al., 2005) genes, have yet to be independently confirmed although the latter has been associated with advanced sleep phase disorder (Satoh et al., 2003). Some additional intriguing associations have also been reported, linking circadian clock gene polymorphisms with disorders in which circadian desynchrony or sleep problems are a factor; for example breast cancer (Zhu et al., 2005, 2008) and prostate cancer (Chu et al., 2008) risk and onset of bipolar disorder (Benedetti et al., 2008). Similarly, a strong association has been reported between a polymorphism in the melatonin receptor 1B gene and glucose and insulin metabolism and type 2 diabetes risk (Prokopenko et al., 2009; Lyssenko et al., 2009; Bouatia-Naji et al., 2009).

Given the wide-ranging impact of circadian rhythms and sleep on physiology, behaviour, and metabolism, it may not be surprising that alterations in clock- and sleep-related genes, and their subsequent effects on light exposure, hormone patterns, sleep and metabolism, are associated with disease risk. Similarly, systematic alterations in behaviour, whether genetically driven or societally induced, will also impact sleep and circadian organization with potentially important effects on medical and mental health. Epidemiology has an important role to play in understanding the contribution of sleep and circadian rhythms on the aetiology of poor health and disease and in distinguishing between the genetic or behavioural basis to disease. Epidemiologists must therefore understand how to measure sleep and circadian rhythms as accurately as possible and to understand how sleep, circadian phase, or light may affect the measurement, analysis, or interpretation of other outcomes. As stated at the start of the chapter, measuring sleep will become a core component of all health research and failure to include sleep will exclude a third of our entire lives.

Summary box

- Sleep is an essential behaviour, vital to good health and well-being, and assessment of sleep and sleep disorders should be a core component of all public health research.
- Sleep is an active state, defined behaviourally by changes in posture and arousal threshold and defined electrophysiologically by changes in the frequency and synchronization of EEG recordings.
- Sleep consists of REM and NREM sleep which cycle approximately every ~45 minutes, causing changes in breathing rate, heart rate, blood pressure, body and brain temperature over each ~90-minute cycle.
- NREM sleep has three stages (N1, N2, and N3) which represent increasingly 'deep' sleep states. Stage N3, or SWS is highly correlated with prior time awake and is a measure of sleep deprivation.

Summary box *(continued)*

- Sleep timing and structure are controlled by two oscillatory processes, an intrinsic 24-hour rhythm determined by the circadian ('about a day') pacemaker in the hypothalamus (Process C), and a homeostatic process, which monitors the duration of time spent awake and the duration of time spent asleep (Process S).

- The relationship between Process C and Process S determines diurnal preference (morningness-eveningness) and the time course of daytime alertness, mood, and performance and underpins changes in sleep that occur in adolescence and ageing.

- There are direct effects of sleep and circadian rhythms on a number of biomarkers of interest to epidemiologists that should be taken into account when developing protocols and interpreting findings.

- Single time-point assessment of biomarkers that have a rhythmic component may be misleading if not interpreted with respect to circadian phase or time of day. Knowledge of prior sleep may also be important for other biomarkers.

References

Aeschbach, D., Cajochen, C., Landolt, H.-P. & Borbély, A.A. (1996). Homeostatic sleep regulation in habitual short sleepers and long sleepers. *Am J Physiol*, **270**, R41–R53.

Aeschbach, D., Postolache, T.T., Sher, L., Matthews, J.R., Jackson, M.A. & Wehr, T.A. (2001). Evidence from the waking electroencephalogram that short sleepers live under higher homeostatic sleep pressure than long sleepers. *Neuroscience*, **102**, 493–502.

Åkerstedt, T., Ingre, M., Kecklund, G., Folkard, S. & Axelsson, J. (2008). Accounting for partial sleep deprivation and cumulative sleepiness in the Three-Process Model of alertness regulation. *Chronobiol Int*, **25**, 309–319.

Archer, S.N., Robilliard, D.L., Skene, D.J., et al. (2003). A length polymorphism in the circadian clock gene Per3 is linked to delayed sleep phase syndrome and extreme diurnal preference. *Sleep*, **26**, 413–415.

Arendt, J. & Deacon, S. (1996). Adapting to phase shifts I. An experimental model for jet lag and shift work. *Physiol Behav*, **59**, 665–673.

Baehr, E.K., Revelle, W. & Eastman, C.I. (2000). Individual differences in the phase and amplitude of the human circadian temperature rhythm: with an emphasis on morningness-eveningness. *J Sleep Res*, **9**, 117–127.

Barbosa, A.A., Pedrazzoli, M., Koike, B.D. & Tufik, S. (2010). Do Caucasian and Asian clocks tick differently? *Braz J Med Biol Res*, **43**, 96–99.

Barger, L.K., Cade, B.E., Ayas, N.T., et al. (2005). Extended work shifts and the risk of motor vehicle crashes among interns. *N Engl J Med*, **352**, 125–134.

Belenky, G., Wesensten, N.J., Thorne, D.R., et al. (2003). Patterns of performance degradation and restoration during sleep restriction and subsequent recovery: a sleep dose-response study. *J Sleep Res*, **12**, 1–12.

Benedetti, F., Dallaspezia, S., Colombo, C., Pirovano, A., Marino, E. & Smeraldi, E. (2008). A length polymorphism in the circadian clock gene Per3 influences age at onset of bipolar disorder. *Neurosci Lett*, **445**, 184–187.

Berson, D.M., Dunn, F.A. & Takao, M. (2002). Phototransduction by retinal ganglion cells that set the circadian clock. *Science*, **295**, 1070–1073.

Blask, D.E., Dauchy, R.T., Sauer, L.A., Krause, J.A. & Brainard, G.C. (2002). Light during darkness, melatonin suppression and cancer progression. *Neuroendocrinol Lett*, **23**, 52–56.

Boivin, D.B., Czeisler, C.A., Dijk, D.J., et al. (1997). Complex interaction of the sleep-wake cycle and circadian phase modulates mood in healthy subjects. *Arch Gen Psychiatry*, **54**, 145–152.

Borbély, A.A. (1982). A two process model of sleep regulation. *Human Neurobiol*, **1**, 195–204.

Bouatia-Naji, N., Bonnefond, A., Cavalcanti-Proenca, C., et al. (2009). A variant near MTNR1B is associated with increased fasting plasma glucose levels and type 2 diabetes risk. *Nat Genet*, **41**(1), 89–94.

Brainard, G.C. & Hanifin, J.P. (2005). Photons, clocks, and consciousness. *J Biol Rhythms*, **20**, 314–325.

Brainard, G.C., Hanifin, J.P., Greeson, J.M., et al. (2001). Action spectrum for melatonin regulation in humans: evidence for a novel circadian photoreceptor. *J Neurosci*, **21**(16), 6405–6412.

Cajochen, C. (2007). Alerting effects of light. *Sleep Med Rev*, **11**(6), 453–464.

Cajochen, C., Khalsa, S.B.S., Wyatt, J.K., Czeisler, C.A. & Dijk, D.J. (1999). EEG and ocular correlates of circadian melatonin phase and human performance decrements during sleep loss. *Am J Physiol*, **277**, R640–R649.

Cajochen, C., Zeitzer, J.M., Czeisler, C.A. & Dijk, D.J. (2000). Dose-response relationship for light intensity and ocular and electroencephalographic correlates of human alertness. *Behav Brain Res*, **115**, 75–83.

Cajochen, C., Wyatt, J.K., Czeisler, C.A. & Dijk, D.J. (2002). Separation of circadian and wake duration-dependent modulation of EEG activation during wakefulness. *Neuroscience*, **114**, 1047–1060.

Carpen, J.D., Archer, S.N., Skene, D.J., Smits, M. & von Schantz, M. (2005). A single-nucleotide polymorphism in the 5′-untranslated region of the hPER2 gene is associated with diurnal preference. *J Sleep Res*, **14**, 293–297.

Carpen, J.D., von Schantz, M., Smits, M., Skene, D.J. & Archer, S.N. (2006). A silent polymorphism in the PER1 gene associates with extreme diurnal preference in humans. *J Hum Genet*, **51**, 1122–1125.

Carskadon, M.A., Acebo, C. & Jenni, O.G. (2004). Regulation of adolescent sleep: implications for behavior. *Ann N Y Acad Sci*, **1021**, 276–291.

Cavallero, C. & Versace, F. (2003). Stage at awakening, sleep inertia and performance. *Sleep Res Online*, **5**, 89–97.

Chu, L.W., Zhu, Y., Yu, K., et al. (2008). Variants in circadian genes and prostate cancer risk: a population-based study in China. *Prostate Cancer Prostatic Dis*, **11**, 342–348.

Cohen, D.A., Wang, W., Wyatt, J.K., et al. (2010). Uncovering residual effects of chronic sleep loss on human performance. *Science Translat Med*, **2**, 14ra3.

Czeisler, C.A. & Klerman, E.B. (1999). Circadian and sleep-dependent regulation of hormone release in humans. *Recent Prog Horm Res*, **54**, 97–132.

Czeisler, C.A. & Gooley, J.J. (2007). Sleep and circadian rhythms in humans. *Cold Spring Harb Symp Quant Biol*, **72**, 579–597.

Czeisler, C.A., Weitzman, E.D., Moore-Ede, M.C., Zimmerman, J.C. & Knauer, R.S. (1980). Human sleep: its duration and organization depend on its circadian phase. *Science*, **210**, 1264–1267.

Czeisler, C.A., Kronauer, R.E., Allan, J.S., et al. (1989). Bright light induction of strong (type 0) resetting of the human circadian pacemaker. *Science*, **244**, 1328–1333.

Czeisler, C.A., Shanahan, T.L., Klerman, E.B., et al. (1995). Suppression of melatonin secretion in some blind patients by exposure to bright light. *N Engl J Med*, **332**, 6–11.

Czeisler, C.A., Duffy, J.F., Shanahan, T.L., et al. (1999). Stability, precision, and near-24-hour period of the human circadian pacemaker. *Science*, **284**, 2177–2181.

Czeisler, C.A., Buxton, O.M. & Khalsa, S.B.S. (2005). The human circadian timing system and sleep-wake regulation. In: Kryger, M.H., Roth, T. & Dement, W.C. (eds.), *Principles and Practices of Sleep Medicine*. Fourth edition. Philadelphia, PA: W.B. Saunders, pp. 375–394.

Daan, S., Beersma, D.G.M. & Borbély, A.A. (1984). Timing of human sleep: recovery process gated by a circadian pacemaker. *Am J Physiol*, **246**, R161–R183.

Dacey, D.M., Liao, H.W., Peterson, B.B., et al. (2005). Melanopsin-expressing ganglion cells in primate retina signal colour and irradiance and project to the LGN. *Nature*, **433**, 749–754.

Davis, S., Mirick, D.K. & Stevens, R.G. (2001). Night shift work, light at night, and risk of breast cancer. *J Natl Cancer Inst*, **93**, 1557–1562.

Dijk, D.J. (2009). Regulation and functional correlates of slow wave sleep. *J Clin Sleep Med*, 5(2 Suppl), S6–S15.

Dijk, D.J. & Czeisler, C.A. (1994). Paradoxical timing of the circadian rhythm of sleep propensity serves to consolidate sleep and wakefulness in humans. *Neurosci Lett*, **166**, 63–68.

Dijk, D.J. & Czeisler, C.A. (1995). Contribution of the circadian pacemaker and the sleep homeostat to sleep propensity, sleep structure, electroencephalographic slow waves, and sleep spindle activity in humans. *J Neurosci*, **15**, 3526–3538.

Dijk, D.J. & Cajochen, C. (1997). Melatonin and the circadian regulation of sleep initiation, consolidation, structure, and the sleep EEG. *J Biol Rhythms*, **12**, 627–635.

Dijk, D.J. & Lockley, S.W. (2002). Integration of human sleep-wake regulation and circadian rhythmicity. *J Appl Physiol*, **92**, 852–862.

Dijk, D.J., Duffy, J.F. & Czeisler, C.A. (2000). Contribution of circadian physiology and sleep homeostasis to age-related changes in human sleep. *Chronobiol Int*, **17**(3), 285–311.

Duffy, J.F. & Czeisler, C.A. (2002). Age-related change in the relationship between circadian period, circadian phase, and diurnal preference in humans. *Neurosci Lett*, **318**, 117–120.

Duffy, J.F. & Dijk, D.J. (2002). Getting through to circadian oscillators: why use constant routines? *J Biol Rhythms*, **17**, 4–13.

Duffy, J.F., Dijk, D.J., Klerman, E.B. & Czeisler, C.A. (1998). Later endogenous circadian temperature nadir relative to an earlier wake time in older people. *Am J Physiol*, **275**, R1478–R1487.

Duffy, J.F., Dijk, D.J., Hall, E.F. & Czeisler, C.A. (1999). Relationship of endogenous circadian melatonin and temperature rhythms to self-reported preference for morning or evening activity in young and older people. *J Investig Med*, **47**, 141–150.

Duffy, J.F., Rimmer, D.W. & Czeisler, C.A. (2001). Association of intrinsic circadian period with morningness-eveningness, usual wake time, and circadian phase. *Behav Neurosci*, **115**, 895–899.

Duffy, J.F., Zeitzer, J.M., Rimmer, D.W., Klerman, E.B., Dijk, D.J. & Czeisler, C.A. (2002). Peak of circadian melatonin rhythm occurs later within the sleep of older subjects. *Am J Physiol*, **282**, E297–E303.

Dumont, M., Benhaberou-Brun, D. & Paquet, J. (2001). Profile of 24-h light exposure and circadian phase of melatonin secretion in night workers. *J Biol Rhythms*, **16**, 502–511.

Ebisawa, T., Uchiyama, M., Kajimura, N., et al. (2001). Association of structural polymorphisms in the human period3 gene with delayed sleep phase syndrome. *EMBO J*, **2**, 342–346.

Elliott, D.L. & Kuehl, K.S. (2007). Effects of sleep deprivation on fire fighters and EMS responders. International Association of Fire Chiefs (IAFC) and the United States Fire Administration (USFA).

Ellis, J., von Schantz, M., Jones, K.H. & Archer, S.N. (2009). Association between specific diurnal preference questionnaire items and PER3 VNTR genotype. *Chronobiol Int*, **26**, 464–473.

Everson, C.A., Bergmann, B.M. & Rechtschaffen, A. (1989). Sleep deprivation in the rat: III. Total sleep deprivation. *Sleep*, **12**, 13–21.

Feychting, M., Österland, B. & Ahlbom, A. (1998). Reduced cancer incidence among the blind. *Epidemiology*, 9, 490–494.

Figueiro, M.G., Brainard, G.C., Lockley, S.W., Revell, V.L. & White, R. (2008). *Light and Human Health: An Overview of the Impact of Optical Radiation on Visual, Ciarcadian, Neuroendocrine, and Neurobehavioral Responses*. New York, NY: Illuminating Engineering Society of North America.

Filipski, E., Innominato, P.F., Wu, M., et al. (2005). Effects of light and food schedules on liver and tumor molecular clocks in mice. *J Natl Cancer Inst*, **97**, 507–517.

Flynn-Evans, E.E., Stevens, R.G., Tabandeh, H., Schernhammer, E.S. & Lockley, S.W. (2009a). Effect of light perception on menarche in blind women. *Ophthalmic Epidemiol*, **16**, 243–248.

Flynn-Evans, E.E., Stevens, R.G., Tabandeh, H., Schernhammer, E.S. & Lockley, S.W. (2009b). Total visual blindness is protective against breast cancer. *Cancer Causes Control*, **20**, 1753–1756.

Folkard, S. & Åkerstedt, T. (1987). Towards a model for the prediction of alertness and/or fatigue on different sleep/wake schedules. In: Oginski, A., Pokorski, J. & Rutenfranz, J. (eds.), *Contemporary Advances in Shiftwork Research*. Krakow: Medical Academy, pp. 231–240.

Folkard, S. & Lombardi, D.A. (2006). Modeling the impact of the components of long work hours on injuries and "accidents". *Am J Ind Med*, **49**(11), 953–963.

Gooley, J.J., Lu, J., Fischer, D. & Saper, C.B. (2003). A broad role for melanopsin in nonvisual photoreception. *J Neurosci*, **23**, 7093–7106.

Groeger, J.A., Zijlstra, F.R.H. & Dijk, D.J. (2004). Sleep quantity, sleep difficulties and their perceived consequences in a representative sample of some two thousand British adults. *J Sleep Res*, **13**, 359–371.

Groeger, J.A., Viola, A.U., Lo, J.C.Y., von Schantz, M., Archer, S.N. & Dijk, D.J. (2008). Early morning executive functioning during sleep deprivation is compromised by a PERIOD3 polymorphism. *Sleep*, **31**, 1159–1167.

Gronfier, C., Wright Jr., K.P., Kronauer, R.E., Jewett, M.E. & Czeisler, C.A. (2004). Efficacy of a single sequence of intermittent bright light pulses for delaying circadian phase in humans. *Am J Physiol*, **287**, E174–E181.

Gronfier, C., Wright Jr., K.P., Kronauer, R.E. & Czeisler, C.A. (2007). Entrainment of the human circadian pacemaker to longer-than-24h days. *Proc Natl Acad Sci U S A*, **104**, 9081–9086.

Hahn, R.A. (1991). Profound bilateral blindness and the incidence of breast cancer. *Epidemiology*, **2**, 208–210.

Hankins, M.W. & Lucas, R.J. (2002). The primary visual pathway in humans is regulated according to long-term light exposure through the action of a nonclassical photopigment. *Curr Biol*, **12**, 191–198.

Hattar, S., Liao, H.-W., Takao, M., Berson, D.M. & Yau, K.-W. (2002). Melanopsin-containing retinal ganglion cells: architecture, projections, and intrinsic photosensitivity. *Science*, **295**, 1065–1070.

Hébert, M., Martin, S.K., Lee, C. & Eastman, C.I. (2002). The effects of prior light history on the suppression of melatonin by light in humans. *J Pineal Res*, **33**, 198–203.

Higuchi, S., Motohashi, Y., Ishibashi, K. & Maeda, T. (2007). Less exposure to daily ambient light in winter increases sensitivity of melatonin to light suppression. *Chronobiol Int*, **24**, 31–43.

Hilton, M.F., Umali, M.U., Czeisler, C.A., Wyatt, J.K. & Shea, S.A. (2000). Endogenous circadian control of the human autonomic nervous system. *Comput Cardiol*, **27**, 197–200.

Honma, K. & Honma, S. (1988). A human phase response curve for bright light pulses. *Jpn J Psychiatry Neurol*, **42**, 167–168.

Horne, J.A. & Östberg, O. (1976). A self-assessment questionnaire to determine morningness-eveningness in human circadian rhythms. *Int J Chronobiol*, **4**, 97–110.

Horne, J.A., Brass, C.G. & Pettitt, A.N. (1980). Circadian performance differences between morning and evening 'types'. *Ergonomics*, **23**, 29–36.

Iber, C., Ancoli-Israel, S., Chesson, A. & Quan, S.F. (2007). *The AASM Manual for the Scoring of Sleep and Associated Events: Rules, Terminology and Technical Specifications*. Westchester, IL: American Academy of Sleep Medicine.

Iwase, T., Kajimura, N., Uchiyama, M., et al. (2002). Mutation screening of the human Clock gene in circadian rhythm sleep disorders. *Psychiatry Res*, **109**, 121–128.

Jewett, M.E., Wyatt, J.K., Ritz-De Cecco, A., Khalsa, S.B., Dijk, D.J. & Czeisler, C.A. (1999). Time course of sleep inertia dissipation in human performance and alertness. *J Sleep Res*, **8**, 1–8.

Johansson, C., Willeit, M., Smedh, C., et al. (2003). Circadian clock-related polymorphisms in seasonal affective disorder and their relevance to diurnal preference. *Neuropsychopharmacology*, **28**, 734–739.

Johnson, M.P., Duffy, J.F., Dijk, D.J., Ronda, J.M., Dyal, C.M. & Czeisler, C.A. (1992). Short-term memory, alertness and performance: a reappraisal of their relationship to body temperature. *J Sleep Res*, **1**, 24–29.

Jones, K.H., Ellis, J., von Schantz, M., Skene, D.J., Dijk, D.J. & Archer, S.N. (2007). Age-related change in the association between a polymorphism in the PER3 gene and preferred timing of sleep and waking activities. *J Sleep Res*, **16**, 12–16.

Katzenberg, D., Young, T., Finn, L., et al. (1998). A clock polymorphism associated with human diurnal preference. *Sleep*, **21**, 569–576.

Kerkhof, G.A. (1998). The 24-hour variation of mood differs between morning-and evening-type individuals. *Percept Motor Skills*, **86**, 264–266.

Kerkhof, G.A. & Van Dongen, H.P.A. (1996). Morning-type and evening-type individuals differ in the phase position of their endogenous circadian oscillator. *Neurosci Lett*, **218**, 153–156.

Khalsa, S.B.S., Jewett, M.E., Cajochen, C. & Czeisler, C.A. (2003). A phase response curve to single bright light pulses in human subjects. *J Physiol (Lond)*, **549**, 945–952.

Klein, T., Martens, H., Dijk, D.J., Kronauer, R.E., Seely, E.W. & Czeisler, C.A. (1993). Chronic non-24-hour circadian rhythm sleep disorder in a blind man with a regular 24–hour sleep-wake schedule. *Sleep*, **16**, 333–343.

Kleitman, N. (1963). Sleep and wakefulness. Chicago, IL: University of Chicago Press.

Klerman, E.B. & Dijk, D.J. (2008). Age-related reduction in the maximal capacity for sleep—implications for insomnia. *Curr Biol*, **18**, 1118–1123.

Kloog, I., Haim, A., Stevens, R.G., Barchana, M. & Portnov, B.A. (2008). Light at night co-distributes with incident breast but not lung cancer in the female population of Israel. *Chronobiol Int*, **25**, 65–81.

Kneisley, L.W., Moskowitz, M.A. & Lynch, H.J. (1978). Cervical spinal cord lesions disrupt the rhythm in human melatonin excretion. *J Neural Transm Suppl*, **13**, 311–323.

Knutson, K.L., Ryden, A.M., Mander, B.A. & Van Cauter, E. (2006). Role of sleep duration and quality in the risk and severity of type 2 diabetes mellitus. *Arch Intern Med*, **166**, 1768–1774.

Knutson, K.L., Spiegel, K., Penev, P. & Van Cauter, E. (2007). The metabolic consequences of sleep deprivation. *Sleep Med Rev*, **11**, 163–178.

Kryger, M.H., Roth, T., Dement, W.C. (2005). *Principles and Practice of Sleep Medicine*, The Netherlands: Elsevier.

Lavie, P. (1986). Ultrashort sleep-waking schedule III. "Gates" and "forbidden zones" for sleep. *Electroencephal Clin Neurophysiol*, **63**, 414–425.

Lavie, P. (1997). Melatonin: role in gating nocturnal rise in sleep propensity. *J Biol Rhythms*, **12**, 657–665.

Lockley, S.W. (2007). Human circadian rhythms: influence of light on circadian rhythmicity in humans. In: Squire, L. (ed.), *New Encyclopedia of Neuroscience*. Oxford: Elsevier.

Lockley, S.W. & Gooley, J.J. (2006). Circadian photoreception: spotlight on the brain. *Curr Biol*, **16**, R795–R797.

Lockley, S.W., Skene, D.J., Tabandeh, H., Bird, A.C., Defrance, R. & Arendt, J. (1997). Relationship between napping and melatonin in the blind. *J Biol Rhythms*, **12**, 16–25.

Lockley, S.W., Skene, D.J., Butler, L.J. & Arendt, J. (1999). Sleep and activity rhythms are related to circadian phase in the blind. *Sleep*, **22**, 616–623.

Lockley, S.W., Cronin, J.W., Evans, E.E., et al. (2004). Effect of reducing interns' weekly work hours on sleep and attentional failures. *N Engl J Med*, **351**, 1829–1837.

Lockley, S.W., Arendt, J. & Skene, D.J. (2007). Visual impairment and circadian rhythm disorders. *Dialogues Clin Neurosci*, **9**, 301–314.

Lockley, S.W., Dijk, D.J., Kosti, O., Skene, D.J. & Arendt, J. (2008). Alertness, mood and performance rhythm disturbances associated with circadian sleep disorders in the blind. *J Sleep Res*, **17**, 207–216.

Lyssenko, V., Nagorny, C.L., Erdos, M.R., et al. (2009). Common variant in MTNR1B associated with increased risk of type 2 diabetes and impaired early insulin secretion. *Nat Genet*, **41**(1), 82–88.

Macchi, M.M. & Bruce, J.N. (2004). Human pineal physiology and functional significance of melatonin. *Front Neuroendocrinol*, **25**, 177–195.

Megdal, S.P., Kroenke, C.H., Laden, F., Pukkala, E. & Schernhammer, E.S. (2005). Night work and breast cancer risk: a systematic review and meta-analysis. *Eur J Cancer*, **41**, 2023–2032.

Mills, J.N. (1964). Circadian rhythms during and after three months in solitude underground. *J Physiol (Lond)*, **174**, 217–231.

Mills, J.N., Minors, D.S. & Waterhouse, J.M. (1978). Adaptation to abrupt time shifts of the oscillator[s] controlling human circadian rhythms. *J Physiol (Lond)*, **285**, 455–470.

Mongrain, V., Lavoie, S., Selmaoui, B., Paquet, J. & Dumont, M. (2004). Phase relationships between sleep-wake cycle and underlying circadian rhythms in morningness-eveningness. *J Biol Rhythms*, **19**, 248–257.

Mongrain, V., Carrier, J. & Dumont, M. (2005). Chronotype and sex effects on sleep architecture and quantitative sleep EEG in healthy young adults. *Sleep*, **28**, 819–827.

Mongrain, V., Carrier, J. & Dumont, M. (2006). Circadian and homeostatic sleep regulation in morningness-eveningness. *J Sleep Res*, **15**, 162–166.

Mongrain, V., Noujaim, J., Blais, H. & Dumont, M. (2008). Daytime vigilance in chronotypes: diurnal variations and effects of behavioral sleep fragmentation. *Behavioural Brain Res*, **190**, 105–111.

Morgan, L., Arendt, J., Owens, D., et al. (1998). Effects of the endogenous clock and sleep time on melatonin, insulin, glucose and lipid metabolism. *J Endocrinol*, **157**, 443–451.

Munch, M., Kobialka, S., Steiner, R., Oelhafen, P., Wirz-Justice, A. & Cajochen, C. (2006). Wavelength-dependent effects of evening light exposure on sleep architecture and sleep EEG power density in men. *Am J Physiol*, **290**(5), R1421–R1428.

Nakagawa, H., Sack, R.L. & Lewy, A.J. (1992). Sleep propensity free-runs with the temperature, melatonin and cortisol rhythms in a totally blind person. *Sleep*, **15**, 330–336.

Pedrazzoli, M., Louzada, F.M., Pereira, D.S., et al. (2007). Clock polymorphisms and circadian rhythms phenotypes in a sample of the Brazilian population. *Chronobiol Int*, **24**, 1–8.

Peirson, S. & Foster, R.G. (2006). Melanopsin: another way of signaling light. *Neuron*, **49**, 331–339.

Pereira, D.S., Tufik, S., Louzada, F.M., et al. (2005). Association of the length polymorphism in the human Per3 gene with the delayed sleep-phase syndrome: does latitude have an influence upon it? *Sleep*, **28**, 29–32.

Phipps-Nelson, J., Redman, J.R., Dijk, D.J. & Rajaratnam, S.M. (2003). Daytime exposure to bright light, as compared to dim light, decreases sleepiness and improves psychomotor vigilance performance. *Sleep*, **26**, 695–700.

Prokopenko, I., Langenberg, C., Florez, J.C., et al. (2009). Variants in MTNR1B influence fasting glucose levels. *Nat Genet*, **41**(1), 77–81.

Provencio, I., Rodriguez, I.R., Jiang, G., Hayes, W.P., Moreira, E.F. & Rollag, M.D. (2000). A novel human opsin in the inner retina. *J Neurosci*, **20**, 600–605.

Pukkala, E., Ojamo, M., Sirkka-Liisa, R., Stevens, R.G. & Verkasalo, P. (2006). Does incidence of breast cancer and prostate cancer decrease with increasing degree of visual impairment. *Cancer Causes Control*, **17**, 573–576.

Rafnsson, V., Tulinius, H., Jonasson, J.G. & Hrafnkelsson, J. (2001). Risk of breast cancer in female flight attendants: a population-based study (Iceland). *Cancer Causes Control*, **12**, 95–101.

Rajaratnam, S.M., Middleton, B., Stone, B.M., Arendt, J. & Dijk, D.J. (2004). Melatonin advances the circadian timing of EEG sleep and directly facilitates sleep without altering its duration in extended sleep opportunities in humans. *J Physiol (Lond)*, **561**, 339–351.

Rechtschaffen, A. & Kales, A. (1968). *A Manual of Standardized Terminology, Techniques and Scoring System for Sleep Stages of Human Subjects*. Washington, DC: U.S. Government Printing Office.

Rechtschaffen, A., Bergmann, B.M., Everson, C.A., Kushida, C.A. & Gilliland, M.A. (1989). Sleep deprivation in the rat: X. Integration and discussion of the findings. *Sleep*, **12**, 68–87.

Reiter, R.J., Tan, D.X., Korkmaz, A., et al. (2007). Light at night, chronodisruption, melatonin suppression, and cancer risk: a review. *Crit Rev Oncog*, **13**, 303–328.

Rimmer, D.W., Boivin, D.B., Shanahan, T.L., Kronauer, R.E., Duffy, J.F. & Czeisler, C.A. (2000). Dynamic resetting of the human circadian pacemaker by intermittent bright light. *Am J Physiol*, **279**, R1574–R1579.

Robilliard, D.L., Archer, S.N., Arendt, J., et al. (2002). The 3111 clock gene polymorphism is not associated with sleep and circadian rhythmicity in phenotypically characterized human subjects. *J Sleep Res*, **11**, 305–312.

Roenneberg, T., Wirz-Justice, A. & Merrow, M. (2003). Life between clocks: daily temporal patterns of human chronotypes. *J Biol Rhythms*, **18**, 80–90.

Roenneberg, T., Kumar, C. J. & Merrow, M. (2007). The human circadian clock entrains to sun time. *Curr Biol*, **17**, R44–R45.

Rothschild, J.M., Keohane, C.A., Rogers, S., et al. (2009). Risks of complications by attending physicians after performing nighttime procedures. *JAMA*, **302**, 1565–1572.

Rüger, M., Gordijn, M.C., Beersma, D.G., de Vries, B. & Daan, S. (2006). Time-of-day-dependent effects of bright light exposure on human psychophysiology: comparison of daytime and nighttime exposure. *Am J Physiol*, **290**, R1413–R1420.

Sahar, S. & Sassone-Corsi, P. (2009). Metabolism and cancer: the circadian clock connection. *Nat Rev Cancer*, **9**, 886–896.

Satoh, K., Mishima, K., Inoue, Y., Ebisawa, T. & Shimizu, T. (2003). Two pedigrees of familial advanced sleep phase syndrome in Japan. *Sleep*, **26**, 416–417.

Scheer, F.A., Zeitzer, J.M., Ayas, N.T., Brown, R., Czeisler, C.A. & Shea, S.A. (2006). Reduced sleep efficiency in cervical spinal cord injury; association with abolished night time melatonin secretion. *Spinal Cord*, **44**, 78–81.

Scheer, F.A., Shea, T.J., Hilton, M.F. & Shea, S.A. (2008). An endogenous circadian rhythm in sleep inertia results in greatest cognitive impairment upon awakening during the biological night. *J Biol Rhythms*, **23**, 353–361.

Scheer, F.A., Hilton, M.F., Mantzoros, C.S. & Shea, S.A. (2009). Adverse metabolic and cardiovascular consequences of circadian misalignment. *Proc Natl Acad Sci U S A*, **106**, 4453–4458.

Schernhammer, E.S. & Hankinson, S.E. (2005). Urinary melatonin levels and breast cancer risk. *J Natl Cancer Inst*, **97**, 1084–1087.

Schernhammer, E.S., Laden, F., Speizer, F.E., et al. (2001). Rotating night shifts and risk of breast cancer in women participating in the nurses' health study. *J Natl Cancer Inst*, **93**, 1563–1568.

Shea, S.A., Hilton, M.F., Orlova, C., Ayers, R.T. & Mantzoros, C.S. (2005). Independent circadian and sleep/wake regulation of adipokines and glucose in humans. *J Clin Endocrinol Metab*, **90**, 2537–2544.

Siegel, J.M. (2005). Clues to the functions of mammalian sleep. *Nature*, **437**, 1264–1271.

Smith, K.A., Schoen, M.W. & Czeisler, C.A. (2004). Adaptation of human pineal melatonin suppression by recent photic history. *J Clin Endocrinol Metab*, **89**, 3610–3614.

Spengler, C.M., Czeisler, C.A. & Shea, S.A. (2000). An endogenous circadian rhythm of respiratory control in humans. *J Physiol (Lond)*, **526**, 683–694.

Spiegel, K., Leproult, R. & Van Cauter, E. (1999). Impact of sleep debt on metabolic and endocrine function. *Lancet*, **354**, 1435–1439.

Spiegel, K., Leproult, R., Tasali, E., Penev, P. & Van Cauter, E. (2004). Sleep curtailment results in decreased leptin levels, elevated ghrelin levels and increased hunger and appetite. *Ann Intern Med*, 141, 846–850.

Stevens, R.G. (2005). Circadian disruption and breast cancer: from melatonin to clock genes. *Epidemiology*, 16, 254–258.

Stevens, R.G., Blask, D.E., Brainard, G.C., et al. (2007). Meeting report: the role of environmental lighting and circadian disruption in cancer and other diseases. *Environ Health Perspect*, **115**, 1357–1362.

Straif, K., Baan, R., Grosse, Y., et al. (2007). Carcinogenicity of shift-work, painting, and fire-fighting. *Lancet Oncol*, **8**, 1065–1066.

Thapan, K., Arendt, J. & Skene, D.J. (2001). An action spectrum for melatonin suppression: evidence for a novel non-rod, non-cone photoreceptor system in humans. *J Physiol (Lond)*, 535, 261–267.

Van Dongen, H.P.A., Maislin, G., Mullington, J.M. & Dinges, D.F. (2003). The cumulative cost of additional wakefulness: dose-response effects on neurobehavioral functions and sleep physiology from chronic sleep restriction and total sleep deprivation. *Sleep*, **26**, 117–126.

Verkasalo, P.K., Lillberg, K., Stevens, R.G., et al. (2005). Sleep duration and breast cancer: a prospective cohort study. *Cancer Res*, **65**, 9595–9600.

Viola, A.U., Archer, S.N., James, L.M., et al. (2007). PER3 polymorphism predicts sleep structure and waking performance. *Curr Biol*, **17**, 1–6.

Von Schantz, M. (2008). Phenotypic effects of genetic variability in human clock genes on circadian and sleep parameters. *J Genet*, **87**, 513–519.

Wehr, T.A., Moul, D.E., Barbato, G., et al. (1993). Conservation of photoperiod-responsive mechanisms in humans. *Am J Physiol*, **265**, R846–R857.

Wertz, A.T., Ronda, J.M., Czeisler, C.A. & Wright Jr., K.P. (2006). Effects of sleep inertia on cognition. *JAMA*, **295**, 163–164.

Wever, R.A. (1979). *The Circadian System of Man: Results of Experiments Under Temporal Isolation.* New York, NY: Springer-Verlag.

Wright Jr., K.P., Gronfier, C., Duffy, J.F. & Czeisler, C.A. (2005). Intrinsic period and light intensity determine the phase relationship between melatonin and sleep in humans. *J Biol Rhythms*, **20**, 168–177.

Wyatt, J.K., Ritz-De Cecco, A., Czeisler, C.A. & Dijk, D.J. (1999). Circadian temperature and melatonin rhythms, sleep, and neurobehavioral function in humans living on a 20-h day. *Am J Physiol*, **277**, R1152–R1163.

Wyatt, J.K., Cajochen, C., Ritz-De Cecco, A., Czeisler, C.A. & Dijk, D.J. (2004). Low-dose repeated caffeine administration for circadian-phase-dependent performance degradation during extended wakefulness. *Sleep*, **27**, 374–381.

Wyatt, J.K., Dijk, D.J., Ritz-De Cecco, A., Ronda, J.M. & Czeisler, C.A. (2006). Sleep facilitating effect of exogenous melatonin in healthy young men and women is circadian-phase dependent. *Sleep*, **29**, 609–618.

Zaidi, F.H., Hull, J.T., Peirson, S.N., et al. (2007). Short-wavelength light sensitivity of circadian, pupillary, and visual awareness in humans lacking an outer retina. *Curr Biol*, **17**, 2122–2128.

Zeitzer, J.M., Ayas, N.T., Shea, S.A., Brown, R. & Czeisler, C.A. (2000a). Absence of detectable melatonin and preservation of cortisol and thyrotropin rhythms in tetraplegia. *J Clin Endocrinol Metab*, **85**, 2189–2196.

Zeitzer, J.M., Dijk, D.J., Kronauer, R.E., Brown, E.N. & Czeisler, C.A. (2000b). Sensitivity of the human circadian pacemaker to nocturnal light: melatonin phase resetting and suppression. *J Physiol (Lond)*, **526**, 695–702.

Zhu, Y., Brown, H.N., Zhang, Y., Stevens, R.G. & Zheng, T. (2005). Period 3 structural variation: a circadian biomarker associated with breast cancer in young women. *Cancer Epidemiol Biomarkers Prev*, **14**, 268–270.

Zhu, Y., Stevens, R.G., Leaderer, D., et al. (2008). Non-synonymous polymorphisms in the circadian gene NPAS2 and breast cancer risk. *Breast Cancer Res Treat*, **107**, 421–425.

Chapter 3

Sleep duration: risk factor or risk marker for ill-health?

N.S. Marshall and S. Stranges

Introduction

Epidemiologists and non-epidemiologists in many parts of the world are now investigating whether variability in human sleep duration is a determinant of various diseases. Self-reported sleep duration appears to be a *risk marker* for various diseases and conditions. But is it really the sleep that causes disease (*a risk factor*) or is the real causative agent or agents just peripherally associated with sleep duration (*a confounder*)? This issue is not merely academic, as alleviation of the supposed problem hinges vitally on whether we are observing a risk factor or a risk marker/confounder. Treatment to improve a risk marker will be an expensive waste of time because it is not the real cause of the disease, merely a correlate.

Observational epidemiology owes much to life insurance companies. In many cases, we use identical tools to ask very similar questions about death and disease. But we do it for very different reasons. Sometimes, as biological researchers interested in sleep, we can forget the difference between something that causes death and something that merely announces its impending presence.

The insurance industry is interested in the quantification of risk. As accurately as possible they want to determine the likelihood of death or ill-health in a given person. Essentially, they are betting against the policy holder on the likelihood of death or ill-health in a specific person. Any piece of information about that person that improves the accuracy of their mortality/morbidity models is thus of use. It does not matter whether that piece of information is an accurate representation of an underlying piece of biological pathophysiology that we would recognize as having a real cause-and-effect relationship with death. For insurance purposes it only needs to be a marker-of-risk not a causal factor in that risk.

In a simplified example, the insurance industry does not care *how* blood pressure actually kills people, they are only interested in the marked *association* with death. Even if hypertension had no causal relationship to death, the insurance industry would still care about it if it still had predictive value.

On the other hand, we as biological scientists need to be very careful not to confuse ourselves about what is a risk factor and what is a risk marker/confounder. Luckily we have a number of tools that we can use to differentiate the two. Firstly, we have an established set of loose criteria that can be applied to environmental exposures, such as sleep duration, in order to infer causality. Secondly, and more importantly in the case of sleep duration, we have the ability to employ scientifically rigorous experimentation—the only method we have for demonstrating causality conclusively.

We need to do this because the label 'risk factor' hides a great deal of complexity. Sleep is both a biological and psychosocial behaviour that we spend a relatively large proportion of our lives undertaking. Despite this, it is a relatively poorly understood process compared with more discrete health-related behaviours such as sex, eating, smoking, or drinking. We are not sure how sleep interacts with other factors to cause adverse outcomes (effect modification or interaction) and we are not sure whether other factors may need to be present or absent in order that sleep duration can have an effect on health (multi-causality chains).

If established as a modifiable risk factor, sleep gives us two potential levers we can control to improve health. We can remove or reduce abnormal sleep in order to prevent disease developing (primary prevention) or we can improve sleep in those who already have the disease in order to treat that disease or stop it recurring (treatment or secondary prevention of, for instance, stroke or myocardial infarction [MI]).

In this chapter, we will critically revise available literature on the association between sleep duration and health outcomes. Furthermore, we will address pending issues surrounding the nature of this association. The present problem is that the evidence for sleep duration being a risk factor for ill-health is largely based on subjective reports from cross-sectional observational studies. It is not currently strong enough to act upon because causality has not been demonstrated.

Sleep duration, ill-health, and obesity: a brief overview

Sleep duration and ill-health

The current avalanche of papers devoted to examining sleep duration as an exposure variable probably traces its origins to a paper published by Daniel Kripke and two small experiments published by Eve Van Cauter's group. Kripke et al. (2002) analyzed the Cancer Prevention Study II of the American Cancer Society with a sample of 1.1 million people, and found that short and long sleep were both independently associated with higher risk of death after control for an extensive range of potential confounders (see also Chapter 4). A systematic review and meta-analysis of studies linking death with sleep duration has also recently been published showing this U-shaped association (Gallicchio and Kalesan, 2009; Grandner and Patel, 2009). One of us recently reviewed a sample of such studies showing U-shaped relationships between self-reported sleep duration and various morbidity or mortality outcomes (Trenell et al., 2007). Together these studies suggested that there might exist an optimal duration of sleep by which people might be able to lower their risk of mortality, diabetes, obesity, hypertension, and perhaps even MI. The continually observed association between short sleep and harm was not expected, but the association with long sleep still lacks obvious biological plausibility to some commentators (Knutson and Turek, 2006; Patel et al., 2006a; Grandner and Drummond, 2007). Some have hypothesized that the association is causal: that long sleep causes harm (Youngstedt and Kripke, 2004). Experimental reduction of long sleep duration in older people that did not produce beneficial effects on glucose tolerance or insulin sensitivity does not refute this hypothesis but does fail to confirm it (Zielinski et al., 2008). It is also possible that long sleep duration may represent an epiphenomenon of other co-morbid conditions, particularly in the elderly (Stranges et al., 2008b).

Short sleep, on the other hand, presents a number of potential biological pathways between exposure and poor outcomes. Two outcomes, supported by short-term experimental studies from Van Cauter's group, are obesity and diabetes.

The first study (Spiegel et al., 1999) observed the effect of sleep restriction for 6 days (4 hours sleep opportunity/night) followed by 7 days recovery sleep (12 hours sleep opportunity/night) in 11 healthy young men. After sleep restriction the area under the curve of the integrated glucose and insulin curves was 50% greater than sleep extension. They also observed a similar pattern after only 2 days of 4 hours-per-night sleep in 12 healthy young men (Spiegel et al., 2004). These participants deteriorated from normal glucose control when fully rested, to levels comparable to older individuals with impaired glucose tolerance when sleep restricted. If this effect persists over the longer term it offers a causal pathway to diabetes.

The second (Spiegel et al., 2004) of these studies also provides evidence that sleep restriction might be obesigenic. Concentrations of both leptin and ghrelin, two hunger regulating hormones, were significantly perturbed by sleep restriction. The ratio of these two hormones was also subsequently increased by about 70%. The hormone change was closely associated with subjective hunger reports and participants also reported greater desire for calorie-dense foods, such as potatoes or cakes. A confirmatory association between these hunger hormones and sleep duration measured by polysomnography the night before has also been reported by Taheri et al. (2004) in the Wisconsin Sleep Cohort Study. However, it is not clear whether this effect will persist in other sub-populations, or over the longer term. For instance, Patel et al. (2006b) did not find an association between short sleep and higher caloric intake in the Nurses Health Study. Replication of these findings by other research groups and in different populations, such as older people, children, women, or those with common co-morbidities are required (Trenell et al., 2007).

Various other interesting observations have added weight to the hypothesis that short sleep might be harmful. As an example, Janszky and Ljung (2008) noted that MI hospitalizations in Sweden are 5% higher in the week after the Spring-shift in daylight savings reduces the time available for sleep by 1 hour. Conversely, the Autumn shift to an hour longer in the day is associated with a slight decrease in the MI incidence in the following week, particularly the following Monday.

Sleep duration and obesity

The bulk of the scientific evidence has addressed the potential links with obesity. This might be because of the general availability of data in many extant studies that regularly make measurements of both sleep duration and obesity as standard confounding variables. Because of the combination of availability and interest (perhaps newsworthiness) there are now a large number of epidemiological sleep-obesity papers and the fascination with, and importance of, the topic of sleep duration attracts a great deal of editorial (e.g. Bliwise and Young, 2007; Bliwise, 2008; Horne, 2008a, b; Knutson and Turek, 2006; Laffan and Punjabi, 2008; Grandner and Patel, 2009; Hale, 2005) and press interest (see also Chapter 5).

A number of investigators, including our research groups, have attempted to collate this output into a series of independent and nearly simultaneously published systematic and semi-systematic reviews (Chen et al., 2008; Horne, 2008a; Cappuccio et al., 2008; Patel and Hu, 2008). These reviews have taken a number of different approaches. Chen et al. (2008) chose to concentrate on paediatric studies perhaps because this is where the evidence is the most consistent. Cappuccio et al.'s (2008) (including the author S. Stranges) systematic review and meta-analysis chose to look at cross-sectional associations in short sleep only because of the heterogeneity in long sleep. Another systematic review also focussed on short sleep duration, but the authors (Patel and Hu, 2008) did not feel that the heterogeneity in the data allowed them to present their attempted meta-analysis. Horne (2008a, b), in a traditional qualitative review, chose to highlight that even at its most extreme levels, sleep restriction only has a weak association with weight gain. He concluded that this probably does not offer a large margin with which to treat obesity in the general community. One of our research groups (Marshall et al., 2008) wrote a critical epidemiological review that noted many of these same problems but chose instead to focus on how these sources of uncertainty might be remedied.

This heterogeneity in approaches to reviewing the field probably arises because of the heterogeneity in the dose-response curve between sleep and risk. Because some studies find long sleep is harmful and others find that long sleep is helpful, selecting a reference category can be very difficult. Because of this problem, systematic reviewers face a difficult decision as the totality of the data cannot really be quantitatively combined in a meta-analysis. Concentrating on the short sleep end of the spectrum means that quantitative summaries can be calculated with a meta-analysis, but it also means disregarding long sleep data. Given that long sleep data are collected using the same measurement technique as the short sleep data, neither approach is ideal.

The reviews we co-authored, for instance, have used both approaches. The first (Cappuccio et al., 2008) was a systematic review and meta-analysis that provided a quantitative estimate of the potential size of the association between sleep duration and obesity in cross-sectional studies in adults ($n = 18$ studies) and children ($n = 12$ studies) separately. This meta-analysis showed a consistent pattern of increased odds of being short sleeper if you are obese, both in childhood and in adulthood. This meta-analysis showed a consistent pattern of increased odds of being a short sleeper if you are obese, both in childhood and in adulthood. Specifically, in children the pooled odds ratio (OR) for obesity in short sleep duration (<10 hours per night was short sleep in children) was 1.89 (1.46–2.43; P < 0.0001). In adults, the pooled OR for obesity in short sleep duration (<5 hours per night) was 1.55 (1.43–1.68; P < 0.0001). Furthermore, a pooled regression analysis in adults also suggested that one hour less of sleep per day was associated with a 0.35 kg/m^2 increase in body mass index (BMI). For a person approximately 178 cm tall it would be equivalent to approximately 1.4 kg in weight.

Although the meta-analysis (Cappuccio et al., 2008) found no evidence of publication bias through use of the standard statistical tests, there remains the possibility that a large number of negative studies have not been published. Because there are currently no studies specifically designed to test associations between sleep duration and ill-health that are yet old enough to report conclusive longitudinal findings, we must rely on studies where sleep was incidentally measured. Publication bias (Kavvoura et al., 2007), where positive studies are preferentially written up and pass peer review for publication, may be a particular problem in this field. As far as we are aware, no negative studies of cross-sectional associations between sleep duration and obesity have yet been published.

However, a number of studies that have linked sleep duration to other outcomes have been published, with confounder tables listing obesity as not being associated with sleep duration in cross-sectional analyses (Marshall et al., 2008). This suggests that there may be a number of very important cohort studies where sleep duration does not predict obesity that cannot be included in a systematic review because they have not been published or the authors cannot get them published past a peer-review barrier that preferentially accepts positive studies.

There are also a number of examples of studies that have found baseline cross-sectional associations that have become non-significant in longitudinal analyses. For example, in cross-sectional analyses from the Whitehall II Study there were significant, inverse associations between duration of sleep and both BMI and waist circumference. However, in prospective analyses a short duration of sleep was not associated with significant changes in BMI ($\beta = -0.06$; 95% confidence interval [CI]: −0.26, 0.14) or waist circumference ($\beta = 0.44$; 95% CI: −0.23, 1.12), nor with the incidence of obesity (OR: 1.05; 95% CI: 0.60, 1.82). These findings suggest that there is no temporal relation between short duration of sleep and future changes in measures of body weight and central adiposity (Stranges et al., 2008a).

Likewise, Gangwisch et al. (2005) reported inconsistent findings from cross-sectional and longitudinal analyses of the large US sample from the NHANES-I (National Health and Nutrition Examination Survey). Similar to the Whitehall II Study, the authors found significant cross-sectional associations between short sleep duration and body weight and obesity, whereas sleep duration at baseline was not associated with significant future changes in BMI over a mean follow-up of 8–10 years ($\beta = -0.053$; $P = 0.27$). In agreement with this, there were no significant associations between sleep duration at baseline and weight gain (or incident type 2 diabetes) in a population-based study of 1,462 Swedish women followed for 32 years (Björkelund et al., 2005). It should be noted that in this study the authors did find significant, inverse associations between sleep duration and BMI and waist-to-hip ratio in cross-sectional analyses at baseline, which is consistent with the Whitehall findings. In summary, these three studies are consistent in showing inverse cross-sectional relationships between short sleep and obesity but no prospective associations.

Conversely, Hasler et al. (2004) found that short sleep duration was associated with subsequent obesity in subjects younger than 35 years, but the association diminished in older participants. However, this study was based on a small sample ($n = 496$) with over-representation of cases with psychiatric disorders and, thus, with a limited generalizability. In addition, in this study, the potential for reverse causality could not be excluded because the authors also found an association between earlier obesity and future short sleep duration. Moreover, findings from the large Nurses Health Study ($n = 68,183$) (Patel et al., 2006b) showed that a habitual sleep time of less than 7 hours predicted a modest increase in weight over a mean follow-up of 16 years. In addition, the relative risks for incident obesity were 1.15 (95% CI: 1.04, 1.26) and 1.06 (95% CI: 1.01, 1.11) for women sleeping 5 and 6 hours, respectively, compared with those sleeping 7 hours. However, this analysis was based on self-reported measures of body weight, did not include measures of body fat distribution, and was limited to a large cohort of middle-aged women from the nursing profession, thus with a limited generalizability.

In the second review by one of us, these and other issues left us with the opinion that a systematic review or a meta-analysis would not be necessarily the best approach (Marshall et al., 2008). Thus, our review was not a traditional systematic review, but may have resulted in wider inclusion because of additional flexibility in literature gathering. We chose 34 observational studies to review and categorized studies into adult or paediatric, cross-sectional or longitudinal, and objective versus subjective sleep duration measurement. We attempted to highlight some of the less often noted problems with the extant literature and the large amount of replication without substantive improvements in methodology.

The problems we found resulted in our choosing to focus on suggestions for improving the evidence base rather than making strong conclusions about whether sleep duration causes obesity or not. Some biases we identified in the literature could have been causing false positive associations. Other biases may have been masking associations that were actually stronger than was evident. As such, we were unable to determine whether sleep duration was a risk factor or a risk marker for obesity. We concluded that, given the constraints with epidemiological observational studies thus far, experimental studies would offer the most fruitful way forward in the determination of causality. This is especially warranted in childhood obesity where the epidemiological evidence is notably consistent. Many epidemiological questions do not have experimentation as a potential solution to issues of inferring causality (Rothman and Greenland, 2005). But the present debate does have viable experimental solutions and we felt that these offered a clear pathway to reduce uncertainty about causality.

In summary, there are now a substantial number of publications implicating sleep duration as a risk marker for ill-health and in particular obesity. Short sleep duration and sometimes long sleep duration are often associated with obesity or other poor outcomes. But it is still not clear whether sleep duration is a causal risk factor which we can manipulate in order to improve health. Is the association due to confounding, perhaps?

Uncontrolled confounders: could the association be explained by another factor we have not controlled for?

Sleeping seems to be a deeply social as well as biological behaviour and poor sleep seems to be particularly common in disadvantaged people and in people with chronic diseases (Hale, 2005; Adams, 2006; Moore et al., 2002; Krueger and Friedman, 2009). Recently researchers, including one of us (Stranges et al., 2008b), have tried to investigate potential confounders of the relationships between sleep duration and ill-health in order to provide an inventory of other health-related behaviours that might help us decide whether sleep duration is a risk factor or a risk marker (see also Chapter 4). An easily grasped example of this potential problem is provided by ethnic differences in the United States. African American people report different sleep durations than Caucasian Americans (Lauderdale et al., 2006; Hale and Do, 2007; Krueger and Friedman, 2009), tend to be poorer, live in the inner-city (which is a health risk in America), and have worse health and lower life expectancy (<<www.cdc.gov>>). So is sleep duration causing the poor health (Van Cauter and Spiegel, 1999) or is it simply an incidental part of being disadvantaged and in reality other associated factors are causing the ill-health? In short, is sleep duration one of the reasons poor people have worse health?

Currently, long sleep duration is sometimes found to be associated with harm but without a clear biological rationale for why this might occur. Because of this, most researchers currently seem to think of it as a risk marker. Patel et al. (2006a) attempted to explain why this might occur by investigating what other health-related behaviours are associated with long sleep in the Nurses Health Study. In 60,000 nurses reporting more than 7 hours of sleep per night, long sleep was associated with a range of diseases and risk factors including multiple sclerosis, systemic lupus erythematosus, poverty, low societal status, sedentary lifestyle, benzodiazepine use, and use of antidepressants. The authors concluded that depression and low socioeconomic status were the most likely candidates for confounders or intermediate steps between sleep and morbidity/mortality. Although this provides a list of potential correlates, it is still unclear as to whether these are confounders or part of a coherent causal chain of events.

One of us has extended these findings by investigating the correlates of both long and short sleep duration. In an attempt to guard against cohort-specific associations or the possibility of specific cultural and social context, we analyzed data from two cohorts, one in the United States and one in the United Kingdom (Stranges et al., 2008b). In 6,500 members of the Whitehall II Study and 3,000 members of the Western New York Health Study we found that, compared to typical sleep length, short sleep (<6 hours) was associated with being unmarried, having higher BMI, and worse health-related quality of life (QOL) (SF-36 scores on both the physical and mental component summary scales) in both cohorts. Long sleep (>8 hours) was associated with age (among men only), low physical activity, and lower health-related QOL (physical SF-36 scores). The association with age-ing suggests that a larger burden of undiagnosed chronic co-morbid conditions (e.g. cancer, neu-rodegenerative disease, osteomuscular problems), which are common in the elderly, may contribute to the association between long sleep and mortality. It is therefore possible that long duration of sleep might be a consequence of, rather than a causative risk factor for, unrecognized chronic co-morbidities, which in turn could explain the higher risk of morbidity and mortality observed in many studies (Gallicchio and Kalesan, 2009; Patel et al., 2004; Ferrie et al., 2007). Therefore, long sleep duration could represent a useful diagnostic tool (i.e. a risk *marker*) for detecting other sub-clinical or undiagnosed mental or physical co-morbidity (Knutson and Turek, 2006).

There is clearly a range of important confounders between sleep duration and ill-health that needs to be taken into account when deciding if sleep duration causes ill-health. However, care needs to be taken when assessing the role of potential confounders. For instance, when we con-sider the long-term effects of sleep apnoea on morbidity and mortality we should control for the effects of hypertension because it is an important determinant of cardiovascular disease and mor-tality. However, sleep apnoea is a recognized cause of hypertension (Peppard et al., 2000; Giles et al., 2006) and thus controlling for blood pressure will probably understate the true role of sleep apnoea in ill-health. Although sleep apnoea contributes to hypertension, it is not the sole cause of the problem. So not controlling for high blood pressure may overstate the importance of sleep apnoea for morbidity/mortality. Thus, relevant epidemiological investigations tend to present statistical models that both control and do not control for hypertension side-by-side

(Peppard et al., 2000; Giles et al., 2006). The true strength of the association is probably somewhere in the middle.

The same situation may exist between sleep restriction and diabetes. Poor glucose control may be caused by sleep restriction, but sleep alone is not the only causal risk factor at play. Thus, if sleep restriction causes diabetes through other mechanisms than directly through glycaemic control (it could also be through the hypothesized promotion of obesity), then controlling for glycaemic indices may give the impression that sleep is less important than it really is.

The possibility of residual confounding (left over confounding that we have not controlled for because we have not measured that variable or we have not measured it very well) is a stock critique of all observational studies. In some cases, this critique is well-founded when later experimental evidence overturns earlier conclusions based on observational data. Whether this is the case for the various effects hypothesized to be attributable to sleep is not currently clear. When considering the strength of observational data we should always keep this possibility in mind.

Subjective versus objective: are we measuring sleep when we only ask?

Subjective health reports may be unreliable. Patients might provide inaccurate information to their doctors, to researchers, or to their families about their health-related behaviours. Sometimes this is outright deception, sometimes self-deception, and sometimes people simply do not remember the information needed in an accurate fashion. Sleep behaviour is no different (see also Chapter 4). Indeed there is a diagnostic category for people who think they have insomnia but on objective testing of their sleep have completely normal sleep durations: sleep state misperception (now known as paradoxical insomnia) (AASM, 2005).

In epidemiology, random measurement error is caused when a test or marker of an exposure is inaccurate when compared to a gold standard measurement of that exposure and these errors are not predictable given other things we might know about the person (i.e. they are random). Imagining this in the case of cancer, a randomly inaccurate test might place some people who really have cancer in the non-cancer group and *vice versa*. The effect on the statistical model would be to underestimate the true size of the effect of that particular cancer on mortality. One can still detect the significance of the effect with a larger sample size but it will always appear to be of a smaller magnitude than it actually is.

A greater problem is when data are systematically biased. This is where the amount of the error is not random but instead correlates with other important characteristics. In our cancer example this might be because the test is more likely to miss cancer in people who are younger. This would cause a larger proportion of younger people to be assigned to the no cancer group when they actually did have cancer. This could give us the false impression that this cancer is harmless because the death of these young people would even out the death rate attributable to the cancer group. This effect could not be removed simply by controlling for age.

We appear to have a similar problem with systematic bias in the estimation of sleep duration by self-report compared to objective sleep duration measurements. Lauderdale et al. (2006, 2008) have collected objective sleep duration data using actigraphy for 3 days in 669 participants in the CARDIA study. They found that objectively measured sleep duration is shorter in African Americans than in Caucasians and that women sleep more than men. However, when they compared the amount of sleep they measured in people versus the amount of sleep people self-reported they found systematic bias. People tended to say they slept more than was measured by actigraphy, but the amount of this over-report was associated with some very important health-related characteristics. The amount of error also differed between people who slept long or short.

Someone who slept 5 hours/night was wrong by around 1.2 hours, whereas someone really sleeping 7 hours overestimated by only 0.4 hours. The amount of error also varied by race and sex; African American men had the least sleep but also overestimated by the largest amount. Caucasian women had the longest sleep duration and also over-reported by the least. Other correlates of this systematic bias included age, self-reported health, education, and income. The authors concluded that '*heath itself influences reports of habitual sleep*'. We cannot disregard the likelihood that disease conditions may influence reports of habitual sleep habits (Lauderdale et al., 2008) and impair sleep quality (Sahlin et al., 2009) and not *vice versa*. Thus, it may not be wise to interpret subjective reports of sleep duration as if they were accurate measures of biological sleep duration.

An additional issue in prospective epidemiological studies is the single time assessment of sleep habits, commonly at the baseline examination, as with many other environmental exposures. It is likely that that a single measure of exposure may not fully capture the sustained effects of sleep duration over time. Changes in sleep duration over time may represent a better measure of exposure, as shown by their prospective association with cause-specific mortality in the Whitehall II Study (Ferrie et al., 2007). Therefore, further prospective studies with objective assessment of long-term exposure (e.g. repeated actigraphy) and better control for confounders are needed before causality can be determined for the associations of sleep duration with morbidity and mortality outcomes.

Sir Austin Bradford Hill's criteria for causality

In 1965, Austin Bradford Hill proposed nine criteria (Hill, 1965) whereby an environmental exposure might be considered to be a causative agent in disease. Hill himself stated that these were only guidelines and not strict and specific rules, and they have been subject to substantive critique since (Rothman and Greenland, 2005), partially because of their overuse. Given these provisos, they may still provide a useful set of criteria for the current debate because the data cited in support of sleep duration causing ill-health fail to pass most of the criteria. It is important to remember however that these are aetiological criteria, not treatment criteria. Even assuming there is a causal relationship, it cannot be assumed that sleep duration alone can be successfully manipulated to improve health or avoid disease developing, especially in the case of chronic diseases which have a multi-factorial nature. Undoing the putative damage, or avoiding development of disease through healthy sleep length, is a treatment/prevention question that requires randomized controlled trials or careful public health intervention studies.

Hill's criteria

i. *Strength*: Strong associations are more likely to be causal, and weak associations are more likely to be explained by some uncontrolled factor. In the sleep duration-obesity debate, the only positive longiudinal association comes from the Nurses Health Study where only a 1.14 kg difference in weight gain was seen between the best (7 hours) and worst (5 hours or fewer) sleep duration categories over 16 years in 68,000 women (Patel et al., 2006b). There does not appear to be a strong association between sleep duration and obesity—although there are some relatively strong associations reported in paediatric studies. Regardless, a weak association is not compelling evidence against the existence of a true casual effect. Uncontrolled confounding variables can also help to obscure the observation to true causal effects as much as they can be responsible for falsely inflating associations.

ii. *Consistency*: '*Has it been repeatedly observed by different persons, in different places, circumstances, and times*'? The association is consistent in children: long sleep is often reported to be associated with obesity and this has been observed in a number of different countries and in children of different ages and ethnicities. However, because of the problems with biological gradient (i.e. dose-response curves), it is not consistently observed in adults (see point v. below). The observations that find long sleep either harmful, harmless, or helpful in adults do not provide a picture that is consistent.

iii. *Specificity*: This criterion is less applicable in this argument because sleep duration and body mass are universal characteristics and multi-factorial in nature. An example where the specificity criterion is met is the link between asbestos and mesothelioma where asbestos is usually implicated.

iv. *Temporality*: Is the exposure measured before the outcome? The evidence is mostly from cross-sectional studies. Cohort studies where sleep is measured at baseline and used to predict the onset of ill-health later (or weight gain) avoids this important criticism (see also Chapters 4 and 5). However, findings from cohort studies are quite mixed (Marshall et al., 2008). For instance, some cohorts report cross-sectional associations that are not apparent longitudinally (Stranges et al., 2008a; Björkelund et al., 2005; Gangwisch et al., 2005). We await prospective findings from cohorts with objectively measured sleep duration. Some of these may soon be able to report their findings (Patel et al., 2008; van den Berg et al., 2008; Lauderdale et al., 2006; Nixon et al., 2008).

v. *Biological gradient*: Is there a clear dose-response relationship? In children: Yes. In adults: No. In adults, the observed dose-response curve seems to differ from study to study among findings of no association, negative linear association, and U-shaped association. In children, the association does exhibit a clear and consistent biological gradient whereby more sleep is usually associated with less obesity (see Fig. 3.1).

vi. *Biological plausibility*: Is this a biological plausible hypothesis? The current data about the effects of sleep restriction on hunger hormones and the logical increase in time available to

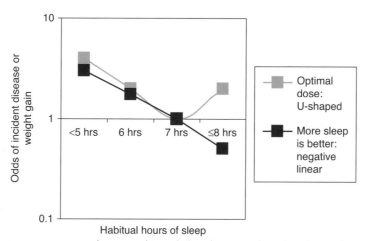

Fig. 3.1 The two most commonly reported associations between sleep duration and obesity/disease/mortality. The first is the U-shaped association (grey line) where sleep durations that are longer or shorter than about 7–7.5 h/night were associated with greater obesity. This leads to the optimal dose theory of habitual sleep duration. The other pattern is a negative linear pattern where the longest sleep durations are associated with the least likelihood and the lowest sleep durations are associated with the greatest likelihood of obesity/disease/mortality (black line). This suggests the more sleep is better theory of habitual sleep duration

Source: Reproduced from Marshall, N.S., Glozier, N. & Grunstein, R.R. (2008). Is sleep duration related to obesity? A critical review of the epidemiological evidence. *Sleep Med Rev*, **12**, 289–298, with permission from Elsevier.

eat make it biologically plausible that sleep restriction might cause obesity. However, other than reduced energy expenditure during extended sleep hours, at the present time there is not a solid, supporting argument for the biological plausibility of long sleep causing obesity.

vii. *Coherence*: '*…the cause-and-effect interpretation of our data should not seriously conflict with the generally known facts of the natural history and biology of the disease.*' The hypothesis is coherent because of the observed rise in both obesity and sleep restriction in the general community (CDC, 2005) (ecological correlation) and because of the effects of sleep restriction on hunger regulating hormones.

viii. *Experimental evidence*: Hill was not explicit about what precisely he meant by this criterion (Rothman and Greenland, 2005), since experimentation can take many forms. Direct compelling experimental evidence between the exposure and the ultimate condition is not often available for epidemiological problems. But in this situation there are no compelling reasons why experimental evidence could not be gathered. One could argue that the changes in leptin and ghrelin after sleep restriction (Spiegel et al., 2004) meet this criterion when discussing obesity because they present a biologically plausible pathway, for instance. Alternatively, because there is no experimental study to show that sleep duration modification causes weight change one could also argue that the evidence does not meet Hill's experimental criterion. Some examples of experiments that might meet this criterion are underway (e.g. www.clinicaltrials.gov NCT00261898) or recently published (Zielinski et al., 2008). Other hypothesized outcomes of sleep restriction such as hypertension could also be subject to direct experimental confirmation.

ix. *Analogy*: Given what we know about another accepted exposure, can we accept that we have enough evidence now? The clear candidate here is the effects of diet and exercise on weight. Experimental evidence for these two factors clearly indicate causality even where cohorts may fail to detect the link. We do not have the same level of evidence for sleep duration. However, analogy is probably the weakest of the criteria as it calls for imagining parallel situations which might be pertinent to whatever is being discussed. As has previously been stated: '*At best, analogy provides a source of more elaborate hypotheses about the associations under study; absence of such analogies only reflects lack of imagination or experience, not falsity of the hypothesis*' (Rothman and Greenland, 2005).

Summary

Hill's criteria provide a potentially useful lens for examination of the hypotheses that sleep duration causes obesity or ill-health. Although some of the criteria are met in certain circumstances, most of them are currently not. Checklist criteria may not be useful for definitive conclusions about causality but they could be useful here for thinking about how to improve the evidence base. This is required because at present it is still not clear whether sleep duration is a risk factor or merely a risk marker for ill-health. Other than addressing some of the concerns we have raised earlier (see sections 'Uncontrolled confounders: could the association be explained by another factor we have not controlled for?' and 'Subjective versus objective: are we measuring sleep when we only ask?'), the obvious way to improve the evidence base is experimentation.

Experiments: how to demonstrate causality

In-laboratory experiments: demonstrating causality

There is currently a paucity of any type of in-laboratory experiments that might demonstrate that shifting sleep durations might cause changes in short-term markers of long-term ill-health.

For instance, there is no study to demonstrate that sleep restriction of normal sleepers over a week or two causes weight gain (presumably through excess consumption mediated by the hormone-related changes we have discussed) (Spiegel et al., 2004). Nor is there a study showing weight loss in obese people who have their abnormal sleep duration modified. Such tightly controlled, in-laboratory experiments might provide a rationale for clinical trials in the real world by demonstrating that sleep duration modification can cause weight change. Similar experiments could also usefully address the possibility that sleep duration may cause changes in blood pressure (Cappuccio et al., 2007). Clearly we cannot undertake a study that directly shows increases in MI or diabetes, for instance, but one can easily imagine early markers of these diseases being shown to worsen.

Clinical trials: demonstrating reversibility

We are only aware of one published trial where a real-world intervention to change sleep duration has been attempted in order to study a marker of ill-health. Zielinski et al. (2008) recently tested whether healthy longer sleeping people (mean age 60) might improve their fasting glucose levels by reducing their sleep from over 9 to around 7 hours/day. Although sleep duration, as measured by actigraphy, was significantly shortened, this did not seem to have any effect on fasting glucose levels.

Another trial based at the National Institute of Health (NIH) is also trying to reduce sleep duration in long sleepers. Listed as being in the recruitment phase, it aims to reduce body mass in obese long-sleeping patients (<<www.clinicaltrials.gov NCT00261898>>).

Such a positive trial would provide good evidence affirming the hypothesis. Unfortunately, a negative clinical trial would not falsify the hypothesis that sleep duration causes obesity. A trial might fail to show a positive effect for many reasons. The intervention might not have sufficiently changed sleep duration. The investigators might have chosen to lengthen sleep by either too much or too little because they had chosen the wrong pattern (U-shaped or linear). Alternatively, sleep duration might affect weight in a way that is not reversible—once the damage has been done it cannot be undone. Such trials may tell us that sleep duration is a modifiable risk factor for morbidity (not merely a risk marker) but they cannot tell us definitively that sleep duration is not a causal risk factor in the development of morbidity. An obvious candidate for one of these trials would be reducing obesity by reducing sleep in obese long sleepers or increasing sleep in obese short sleepers.

An important feature of clinical trials of this type would be to show the feasibility of changing real-world sleep behaviours. Equally important will be in cataloguing the adverse event profile of the programmes that are used to change sleep. Potential adverse events may include increased insomnia or anxiety and depression in people who become overly focussed on 'getting the right amount of sleep'. Adverse event profiles will be extremely important in assessing the potential for public health interventions aimed at non-clinical populations.

Public health interventions: demonstrating prevention

If the clinical trials show that sleep duration can be effectively changed and that this caused improved health (or markers) without undue side effects, then we may be in a position to change the behaviour of whole populations in order to prevent disease development. Care needs to be taken when spreading public health messages as the sleep community has done this before without proper evidence and this is a likely cause of a substantial number of cot death cases (Gilbert et al., 2005).

Before we design these interventions we do need to be sure of causation and that the benefits outweigh the risks and costs. How we design these interventions is likely to be extremely complex, multi-factorial, and tailored to the needs of each target population.

Conclusion

Self-reports of sleep duration are regularly associated with ill-health. However, most of these studies are cross-sectional and thus fail to rule out reverse causality. Many are unable to control for the wide variety of confounders that are known to influence health and are also associated with abnormal sleep durations. Most studies find that short sleep is associated with higher risk but there are divergent findings about long sleep, which have been reported to be both helpful and harmful. There are a number of longitudinal studies with objective measurements of sleep duration that are ongoing and there may be others we are unaware of (Patel et al., 2008; van den Berg et al., 2008; Lauderdale et al., 2006; Nixon et al., 2008). These may help alleviate the confusion between the biological effects of sleep and the psychosocial factors that are associated with self-reported sleep. As stated in a 2007 editorial (Bliwise and Young, 2007):

> In essence, "how many hours of sleep do you get at night" and the rejoinder of "7 to 8" might be the ersatz equivalent of uttering "how ya doin" and hearing the mundane banality of a "good" or "OK" response. Anything falling outside that category puts the questioner on notice for something, but we are just not sure on notice for what.

Sleep medicine can be prone to appearing atheoretical. This is not necessarily because we do not employ underlying hypotheses but that these are rarely explicitly stated. This lack of explicit theory results in a lack of clearly defined testable hypotheses that numerous research groups can investigate with a reference standard in mind. Our underlying theory tends to be that more sleep is better but many sleep duration studies find that intermediate sleep is associated with the lowest risk. It is unclear why some studies find linear associations and why some studies find U-shape associations. That these two patterns can exist is incompatible with a biologically plausible theory. This is very rarely discussed in print. This problem in the observational data may not be rectifiable by yet more observational investigations. In order to demonstrate that sleep duration is a modifiable risk factor, we require innovative experiments both in the laboratory and in the real world. We will also need to know whether this applies to everybody or only to specific sub-populations. If sleep duration is a widely modifiable risk factor, then we may be able to design public health interventions that may have real effects on important determinants of population health, such as the obesity epidemic.

Summary box

+ Increasing evidence from observational epidemiological studies identifies sleep duration as a risk marker for obesity, poor health, or even death. These findings attract widespread public and professional attention because of our professional and personal biases (i.e. sleep is good for you) and because of the apparent ease and pleasurable implementation of a remedy (i.e. sleep more). In support of these observations, laboratory-based physiological studies also provide biological plausibility to claims of a causal link.

+ There is still considerable uncertainty from an epidemiological standpoint as to whether sleep duration is simply an associated risk marker or a causal risk factor in any disease process. Problematically, although all published studies find short sleep to be associated with worse health, some studies find long sleep to be beneficially associated while others find it to be a marker of harm. Studies to date have largely been cross-sectional and therefore do not disentangle the potential for obesity and other health conditions to have caused the sleep problems. Most studies also rely on self-report of sleep duration which appears to be incorrectly reported

Summary box *(continued)*

in most people, but more worryingly becomes systematically more underreported the lower an individual's socioeconomic status. Only few studies have linked objectively measured sleep duration to a disease outcome or obesity. Furthermore, there are no experimental studies or clinical trials in either the laboratory or in a community setting that have demonstrated that any health-related measure can be changed via sleep duration modification. We simply cannot be certain that the variation in sleep duration seen in the population is causing ill-health or that we can remedy this situation through changing sleep durations. If causation can be demonstrated we would also need reasonable certainty that any proposed public health intervention has a positive cost-benefit ratio and that it could be targeted at the appropriate segments of the population. The potential for harm of such schemes should not be dismissed out of hand as sudden infant death syndrome and sleeping position advice has already taught us.

References

American Academy of Sleep Medicine (AASM)(2005). *International Classification of Sleep Disorders*. Second edition. Westchester, IL: AASM.

Adams, J. (2006). Socioeconomic position and sleep quantity in UK adults. *J Epidemiol Community Health*, **60**, 267–269.

Björkelund, C., Bondyr-Carlsson, D., Lapidus, L., et al. (2005). Sleep disturbances in midlife unrelated to 32-year diabetes incidence: the prospective population study of women in Gothenburg. *Diabetes Care*, **28**, 2739–2744.

Bliwise, D.L. (2008). Invited commentary: cross-cultural influences on sleep—broadening the environmental landscape. *Am J Epidemiol*, **168**, 1365–1366.

Bliwise, D. & Young, T. (2007). The parable of parabola: what the U-shaped curve can and cannot tell us about sleep. *Sleep*, **30**, 1614–1615.

Cappuccio, F.P., Stranges, S., Kandala, N.-B., et al. (2007). Gender-specific associations of short sleep duration with prevalent and incident hypertension: the Whitehall II study. *Hypertension*, **50**, 693–700.

Cappuccio, F.P., Taggart, F., Kandala, N.-B., et al. (2008). Meta-analysis of short sleep duration and obesity in children and adults. *Sleep*, **31**, 619–626.

Centres for Disease Control (CDC) (2005). Percentage of adults who reported an average of less than or equal to 6 hours of sleep per 24-hour period by sex and age group—United States 1985 and (2004). *MMWR Morb Mortal Wkly Rep*, **54**, 933.

Chen, X., Beydoun, M. & Wang, Y. (2008). Is sleep duration associated with childhood obesity? A systematic review and meta-analysis. *Obesity*, **16**, 265–274.

Ferrie, J., Shipley, M. & Cappuccio, F.P., et al. (2007). A prospective study of change in sleep duration: associations with mortality in the Whitehall II cohort. *Sleep*, **30**, 1659–1666.

Gallicchio, L. & Kalesan, B. (2009). Sleep duration and mortality: a systematic review and meta-analysis. *J Sleep Res*, **18**, 148–158.

Gangwisch, J.E., Malaspina, D., Boden-Albala, B. & Heymsfield, S.B. (2005). Inadequate sleep as a risk factor for obesity: analyses of the NHANES I. *Sleep*, **28**, 1289–1296.

Gilbert, R., Salanti, G., Harden, M. & See, S. (2005). Infant sleeping position and the sudden infant death syndrome: systematic review of observational studies and historical review of recommendations from 1940 to 2002. *Int J Epidemiol*, **34**, 874–887.

Giles, T., Lasserson, T., Smith, B., White, J., Wright, J. & Cates, C. (2006). Continuous positive airways pressure for obstructive sleep apnoea in adults. *Cochrane Database Syst Rev*, Issue 3., Art. No. CD001106; DOI: 10.1002/14651858.CD001106.pub3.

Grandner, M.A. & Drummond, S.P.A. (2007). Who are the long sleepers? Towards an understanding of the mortality relationship. *Sleep Med Rev*, **11**, 341–360.

Grandner, M.A. & Patel, N.P. (2009). From sleep duration to mortality: implications of meta-analysis and future directions. *J Sleep Res*, **18**, 145–147.

Hale, L. (2005). Who has time to sleep? *Am J Public Health*, **27**, 205–211.

Hale, L. & Do, D.P. (2007). Racial differences in self-reports of sleep duration in a population-based study. *Sleep*, **30**, 1096–1103.

Hasler, G., Buysse, D.J., Klaghofer, R., et al. (2004). The association between short sleep duration and obesity in young adults. *Sleep*, **24**, 661–666.

Hill, A.B. (1965). The environment and disease: association or causation? *Proc R Soc Med*, **58**, 295–300.

Horne, J.A. (2008a). Short sleep is a questionable risk factor for obesity and related disorders: statistical versus clinical significance. *Biol Psychol*, **77**, 266–276.

Horne, J.A. (2008b). Too weighty a link between short sleep and obesity? *Sleep*, **31**, 595–596.

Janszky, I. & Ljung, R. (2008). Shifts to and from daylight saving time and incidence of myocardial infarction. *N Engl J Med*, **359**, 1966–1968.

Kavvoura, F.K., Liberopoulos, G. & Ioannidis, J.P.A. (2007). Selection in reported epidemiological risks: an empirical assessment. *PLoS Med*, **4**, e79.

Knutson, K. & Turek, F.W. (2006). The U-shaped association between sleep and heath: the 2 peaks do not mean the same thing. *Sleep*, **29**, 878–879.

Kripke, D., Garfinkel, L., Wingard, D., Klauber, M. & Marler, M. (2002). Mortality associated with sleep duration and insomnia. *Arch Gen Psychiatry*, **59**, 131–136.

Krueger, P.M. & Friedman, E.M. (2009). Sleep duration in the United States: a cross-sectional population-based study. *Am J Epidemiol*, **169**, 1052–1063.

Laffan, A.M. & Punjabi, N.M. (2008). Sleep: a nourisher in life's feast? *Sleep Med Rev*, **12**, 253–255.

Lauderdale, D.S., Knutson, K.L., Yan, L.L., et al. (2006). Objectively measured sleep characteristics among early-middle-aged adults. *Am J Epidemiol*, **164**, 5–16.

Lauderdale, D.S., Knutson, K.L., Yan, L.L., Liu, K. & Rathouz, P.J. (2008). Self-reported and measured sleep duration: how similar are they? *Epidemiology*, **19**, 838–845.

Marshall, N.S., Glozier, N. & Grunstein, R.R. (2008). Is sleep duration related to obesity? A critical review of the epidemiological evidence. *Sleep Med Rev*, **12**, 289–298.

Moore, P.J., Adler, N.E., Williams, D.R. & Jackson, J.S. (2002). Socioeconomic status and health: the role of sleep. *Psychosom Med*, **64**, 337–344.

Nixon, G., Thompson, J., Han, et al. (2008). Short sleep duration in middle-childhood: risk factors and consequences. *Sleep*, **31**, 71–78.

Patel, S., Ayas, N., Malhotra, M., et al. (2004). A prospective study of sleep duration and mortality risk in woman. *Sleep*, **27**, 440–444.

Patel, S.R. & Hu, F. (2008). Short sleep duration and weight gain: a systematic review. *Obesity*, **16**, 643–653.

Patel, S., Malhotra, A.D.J.G., White, D.P. & Hu, F. (2006a). Correlates of long sleep duration. *Sleep*, **29**, 883–889.

Patel, S.R., Malhotra, A., White, D.P., Gottlieb, D.J. & Hu, F.B. (2006b). Association between reduced sleep and weight gain in women. *Am J Epidemiol*, **164**, 947–954.

Patel, S.R., Blackwell, T., Redline, S., et al. (2008). The association between sleep duration and obesity in older adults. *Int J Obes*, **32**, 1825–1834.

Peppard, P., Young, T., Palta, M. & Skatrud, J. (2000). Prospective study of the association between sleep-disordered breathing and hypertension. *N Engl J Med*, **342**, 1378–1384.

Rothman, K.J. & Greenland, S. (2005). Causation and causal inference in epidemiology. *Am J Public Health*, **95**, S144–S150.

Sahlin, C., Franklin, K.A., Stenlund, H. & Lindberg, E. (2009). Sleep in women: normal values for sleep stages and position and the effect of age obesity sleep apnea smoking alcohol and hypertension. *Sleep Med*, **10**(9), 1025–1030.

Spiegel, K., Leproult, R. & Van Cauter, E. (1999). Impact of sleep debt on metabolic and endocrine function. *Lancet*, **354**, 1435–1439.

Spiegel, K., Tasali, E., Penev, P. & Van Cauter, E. (2004). Brief communication: sleep curtailment in healthy young men is associated with decreased leptin levels elevated ghrelin levels and increased hunger and appetite. *Ann Intern Med*, **141**, 846–850.

Stranges, S., Cappuccio, F.P., Kandala, N.-B., et al. (2008a). Cross-sectional versus prospective associations of sleep duration with changes in relative weight and body fat distribution: the Whitehall II Study. *Am J Epidemiol*, **167**, 321–329.

Stranges, S., Dorn, J.M., Shipley, M.J., et al. (2008b). Correlates of short and long sleep duration: a cross-cultural comparison between the United Kingdom and the United States: the Whitehall II Study and the Western New York Health Study. *Am J Epidemiol*, **168**, 1353–1364.

Taheri, S., Lin, L., Austin, D., Young, T. & Mignot, E. (2004). Short sleep duration is associated with reduced leptin elevated ghrelin and increased body mass index. *PLoS Med*, **1**, e62.

Trenell, M.I., Marshall, N.S. & Rogers, N.L. (2007). Sleep and metabolic control: waking to a problem? *Clin Exp Pharmacol Physiol*, **34**, 1–9.

Van Cauter, E. & Spiegel, K. (1999). Sleep as a mediator of the relationship between socioeconomic status and health: a hypothesis. In: Adler, N., Marmot, M., McEwen, B. & Stewart, J. (eds.), *Socioeconomic Status and Health in Industrial Nations: Social Psychological and Biological Pathways*. New York, NY: New York Academy of Sciences.

van den Berg, J.F., Knvistingh Neven, A., Tulen, J.H.M., et al. (2008). Actigraphic sleep duration and fragmentation are related to obesity in the elderly: the Rotterdam Study. *Int J Obes*, **32**, 1083–1090.

Youngstedt, S. & Kripke, D. (2004). Long sleep and mortality: rationale for sleep restriction. *Sleep Med Rev*, **8**, 159–174.

Zielinski, M.R., Kline, C.E., Kripke, D.F., Bogan, R.K. & Youngstedt, S.D. (2008). No effect of 8-week time in bed restriction on glucose tolerance in older long sleepers. *J Sleep Res*, **17**, 412–419.

Chapter 4

Sleep and death

J.E. Ferrie, M. Kivimäki, and M. Shipley

Introduction

Sleep that knits up the ravel'd sleeve of care,
The death of each day's life, sore labour's bath,
Balm of hurt minds, great nature's second course,
Chief nourisher in life's feast.

W. Shakespeare, *Macbeth*, Act 2 Scene 2

Although poets and philosophers have painted varying images of sleep, its kinship with death is a recurring theme. In his 'Theogony' written in 800 BC the Greek poet Hesiod describes Thánatos (Death) and Hypnos (Sleep) as twin brothers, the sons of Nyx (Night) and Erebos (Darkness). According to legend Hypnos's palace is a dark cave where the sun never shines and which has poppies and other hypnogogic plants at the entrance. Through this cave flows Lethe, the river of forgetfulness and Hypnos is attended by Morpheus who prevents noises from waking him. In the Odyssey, Homer (c. 700 BC) uses sleep to represent the idea of death, making the struggle to remain conscious and the struggle to remain alive the same. This representation appears again in the *Aeneid* in which the Roman poet Virgil (70–19 BC) has sleep (Somnus) as a kinsman to death (Finger, 1994). Indeed, the prone position, separation from consciousness, diminished movement and response to stimuli characterize sleep, coma, and death. What separates sleep from coma and death, however, is reversibility; the sleeper can wake or be woken.

This chapter examines epidemiological evidence on associations between sleep and death in adults. It includes sections on sleep duration, sleep disorders, and the implications of associations between sleep and death for health policy and health promotion. Although many of the sleep disorders affect children as well as adults, most sleep-related deaths are due to vehicle crashes, accidents at work, or long-term chronic diseases, so deaths in children, fortunately, are rare. A few disorders, such as sudden infant death syndrome (SIDS), found only in children are not included in this chapter.

To a certain extent, the separation of sleep duration from the sleep disorders is arbitrary as most disorders will affect duration and some disorders may coexist or be difficult to distinguish from one another. Classification of the sleep disorders for the purpose of this chapter is based on the International Classification of Sleep Disorders, Version 2 (ICSD-2) (2005). Although most disorders result in inadequate sleep in terms of duration or quality, for many specific disorders there is no evidence yet of any direct association with premature mortality. These disorders have only been included where prevalence or suspected prevalence is high.

Eight categories of sleep disorders are included in ICSD-2, of which 7 are considered in the following sections: insomnia, parasomnia, hypersomnia, sleep-related breathing disorder, sleep-related movement disorder, circadian rhythm sleep disorder, and other sleep disorders (isolated symptoms not included).

Sleep duration

Evidence accumulated over nearly 40 years indicates a strong association between usual duration of nighttime sleep and risk of premature death. In general, sleep duration is associated with mortality in a U-shaped fashion, with the lowest risk most often found in the group who report durations of around 7 hours (Youngstedt and Kripke, 2004). However, strong evidence that sleep duration is associated with premature death tends to be reserved for sleep durations of ≤5 hours and ≥9 hours; short or long sleep. Associations with mortality and other serious outcomes, such as cardiovascular disease (CVD), have led to the classification of short and long sleep as sleep disorders under the catch-all heading 'Isolated symptoms, apparently normal variants and unresolved issues' in ICSD-2 (2005; Zee and Turek, 2006).

A monophasic pattern of sleep is one of the main features of human behaviour. However, outside the main sleep period, short periods of sleep (naps), can occur spontaneously in response to sleepiness or be taken actively to maintain performance and alertness. Brief naps have been shown to counteract the negative effects of sleep deficit in sleep-deprived healthy people (Takahashi and Kaida, 2006). Although the terms tend to be used interchangeably, siestas tend to be longer in duration and are taken deliberately on a regular basis, often during the afternoon in hot countries (Dhand and Sohal, 2006).

Usual sleep duration and all-cause mortality

Apart from accidental deaths, any association between sleep and death emerges over a relatively long period of time. Sleep duration has been shown to be associated with serious chronic diseases, such as CVD and diabetes, and risk factors for these diseases, such as hypertension and obesity (Zee and Turek, 2006) (see also Chapter 5). To organize the literature and determine whether associations evolve over time, associations between sleep duration and all-cause mortality are examined in the following sub-sections by length of follow-up.

Mortality follow-up to 5 years

Five of the older studies have mortality follow-up of <5 years (Branch and Jette, 1984; Hammond, 1964; Pollak, et al., 1990; Ruigomez et al., 1995; Tsubono et al., 1993). In 1959–1960, questions on sleep were asked of participants in the American Cancer Society's Cancer Prevention Study I (CPSI) (Hammond, 1964). Participants were a convenience sample of ≈1 million women and men aged ≥30, mainly friends and relatives of American Cancer Society volunteers. One-year mortality rates for men aged ≥45 showed that in every age group crude death rates for men who reported 7 hours sleep were lower than for those whose sleep was shorter or longer (Hammond, 1964). Three further studies in middle-aged and older Unites States (US), Japanese, and Spanish samples with 3.5, 4, and 4.6 years follow-up similarly found higher mortality rates in short and long sleepers. However, in every case these risks were attenuated and became statistically non-significant after adjusting for covariates including health indicators (Pollak et al., 1990; Ruigomez et al., 1995; Tsubono et al., 1993) (see also Chapter 5). In another elderly sample from the US, 5-year mortality rates were higher for short and long sleepers, but even the crude odds ratios (ORs) provided no firm evidence of associations with mortality; OR (95% confidence interval [CI]) 1.34 (0.85–1.83) and 1.60 (0.94–2.29), respectively (Branch and Jette, 1984).

These findings show that while short and long sleepers appear to have higher mortality rates over the short term, this excess risk may be partly or wholly attributed to other health-related behaviours or health indicators. Consequently, evidence of a firm independent association between sleep duration and mortality over the short term is lacking.

Mortality follow-up 5–10 years

Associations between sleep duration and mortality over a follow-up period from 5 up to 10 years have been reported by studies from the UK, US, and Japan (Amagai et al., 2004; Gangwisch et al., 2008; Huppert and Whittington, 1995; Kripke et al., 1979, 2002; Rumble and Morgan, 1992; Suzuki et al., 2009; Tamakoshi and Ohno, 2004). Further analyses of deaths from CPSI over a 6-year follow-up period provided strong evidence of a U-shaped association with 7.0–7.9 hours sleep associated with the lowest risk in every age group. These analyses included both sexes and all ages groups (35–85+), and excluded participants with a history of diabetes, heart disease, stroke, or hypertension (Kripke et al., 1979). CPSII, comprising a similar convenience sample of 1.1 million adults, revisited the association between sleep duration and mortality over 6 years, but included more extensive control for confounding. After adjustment for socio-demographic factors, health-related behaviours, health status, disease history, and medications, mortality hazard ratios (HRs for 4, 5, 6, 8, 9, and ≥10 hours sleep were all significantly above the reference group (7 hours) and ranged from 1.11 and 1.17 (4 hours) to 1.41 and 1.34 (≥10 hours) in women and men, respectively (Kripke et al., 2002). These findings contrast with a smaller UK study in which neither very short (<4 hours) nor very long (≥10 hours) sleep were associated with mortality in people aged 65+. However, sleep for the reference group, 4.0–9.9 hours, covered a broad range, including durations normally classified as short and long sleep (Rumble and Morgan, 1992).

Several large-scale studies have examined associations between sleep duration and mortality in the general Japanese population (Amagai et al., 2004; Suzuki et al., 2009; Tamakoshi and Ohno, 2004). A 6-year mortality follow-up of 12,601 participants aged 65–85 found no association between short sleep and mortality in either sex (Suzuki et al., 2009). These findings for short sleep were replicated for women in a study of 11,325 people aged 19–93 followed for 8 years (Amagai et al., 2004) and in the largest Japanese study of sleep duration and mortality, the Japan Collaborative Cohort study (JACC) of over 100,000 adults aged 40–79 followed for 9.9 years (Tamakoshi and Ohno, 2004). In the latter two studies, analyses were adjusted for a wide range of potential covariates and mediators. One study showed an association between long sleep and death only in women (Amagai et al., 2004), but another found that, while very long sleep (≥10 hours) was associated with a twofold increased risk of death in both sexes, in men 8 and 9 hours were also associated with an increased relative risk (RR): 1.36 and 1.52, respectively (Suzuki et al., 2009). In JACC, all sleep durations above the 7 hour reference category (8, 9, and ≥10 hours) were associated with an increased risk of mortality in both sexes, findings which remained unchanged after exclusion of deaths in the first 2 years (Tamakoshi and Ohno, 2004).

A study over 6.9 years in 8,101 US women aged ≥69 years observed no associations between all-cause mortality and shorter (<6 hours) or longer (>8 hours) sleep compared to the reference category (6–8 hours). However, long sleep (9–9.9 hours) and very long sleep (≥10 hours) were associated with an increased risk of death; HR (95% CI) 1.28 (1.08–1.52) and 1.58 (1.27–1.95), respectively (Stone et al., 2009). In a UK study that included younger participants (aged 18+ years), sleep duration was not related to mortality in women, but very long sleep (>9 hours) predicted mortality in men compared to the reference group who slept 6–9 hours (Huppert and Whittington, 1995). A recent analysis of data from the first National Health and Nutrition Examination Survey (NHANES I) explored the relationship between sleep duration and mortality over an 8- to 10-year follow–up period for nearly 10,000 participants divided into two age categories: 32–59 and 60–86. In younger participants, long sleep was only associated with increased mortality in the crude analyses. However, among older participants short sleep and sleep durations above the reference category (7 hours) were associated with mortality in analyses adjusted for socio-demographic factors, health-related behaviours, health status, insomnia, and use of sleeping tablets (Gangwisch et al., 2008).

Taken together, these studies indicate that associations between long sleep and premature death are stronger and more ubiquitous than those for short sleep. Contrary to the widely held belief that 8 hours sleep is optimal, those who regularly sleep 8 hours are at a somewhat higher risk of death than those who sleep 7 hours (Kripke, 2004).

Mortality follow-up 10–15 years

Studies across several continents have examined associations between sleep duration and mortality over a follow-up period from 10 up to 15 years (Burazeri et al., 2003a; Goto et al., 2003; Ikehara et al., 2009; Kojima et al., 2000; Lan et al., 2007; Mallon et al., 2002; Patel et al., 2004). A 10-year study of 3,079 Taiwan Chinese aged ≥64 found no association between short sleep (<7 hours) and mortality relative to the reference group (7–7.9 hours). However, sleep durations longer than the reference category were associated with an increased risk of mortality in analyses adjusted for socio-demographic factors, health-related behaviours, and disease history; findings virtually unaltered by removal of deaths in the first 2 years of follow-up (Lan et al., 2007). No associations between sleep duration and mortality over 9–11 years were observed for women in a small study of Israelis aged ≥50. However, there was a higher risk of mortality in men sleeping more than 8 hours compared with the reference group (6–8 hours), in analyses adjusted for socio-demographic factors, health-related behaviours, health status, and siestas (Burazeri et al., 2003a).

Among Japanese people over age 65 years <6 and >7 hours sleep were associated with increased mortality over 10 years in analyses adjusted for age and health-related behaviours. After adjustment for health status, functional status, and coronary heart disease (CHD), only the relationship with <6 hours sleep remained (Goto et al., 2003). In another study of the Japanese general population aged 20–67 with 12 years follow-up, no association between sleep duration and mortality was observed in women. In men there was an age-adjusted association between short (<7 hours, relative to 7–8.9 hours) sleep and mortality which was not attenuated when additionally adjusted for health-related behaviours, disease history, and use of sleeping tablets (Kojima et al., 2000). Another study with 12 years mortality follow-up for Swedes aged 45–65 similarly showed no associations between sleep duration and death in women. However, in men long sleep (>8 hours, relative to 7 hours) was associated with an increased risk of mortality, but contrary to the Japanese findings there was no association with short sleep (<6 hours) (Mallon et al., 2002).

One of the largest studies to have examined longer-term associations between sleep duration and mortality, the Nurses Health Study, only has data for women. The 14-year follow-up for 82,969 US nurses aged 30–55 showed that short sleep (relative to 7 hours) was associated with an increased risk of mortality in analyses adjusted for age, health-related behaviours, depression, snoring, and history of cancer and CVD. The association weakened on additional adjustment for hypertension and diabetes, but 8 hours sleep and long sleep remained associated with an increased risk of mortality in analyses adjusted for shift-work in addition to all the other covariates; RR (95% CI) 1.11 (1.03–1.19) and 1.40 (1.25–1.55), respectively (Patel et al., 2004). A recent analysis that extended mortality follow-up from the JACC study to 14.3 years showed that very short sleep (≤4 hours) and all sleep durations above the 7 hours reference category (8, 9, and ≥10 hours) were associated with an increased risk of mortality in both sexes in the multivariate analyses; findings that remained little changed after the exclusion of deaths in the first 5 years (Fig. 4.1) (Ikehara et al., 2009).

As in studies with shorter follow-up, studies that have examined associations between sleep duration and mortality over periods of 10–15 years indicate that longer sleep is more strongly associated

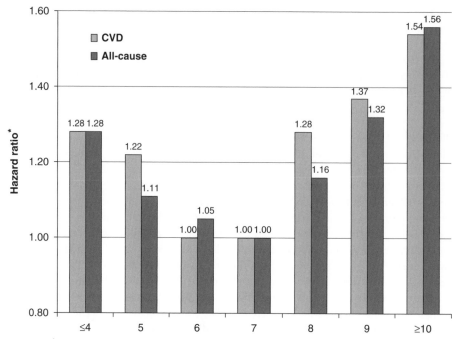

*Adjusted for age, education, employment status, exercise, smoking, alcohol, fresh fish consumption, depressive symptoms, mental stress, BMI, hypertension, and diabetes.

Fig. 4.1 Hazard ratio (95% CI) for CVD and all-cause mortality in women by sleep duration. *Source*: Data from Ikehara, S., Iso, H., Date, C., et al. (2009). Association of sleep duration with mortality from cardiovascular disease and other causes for Japanese men and women: the JACC study. *Sleep*, **32**, 295–301.

with premature death than shorter sleep. Although it has been proposed that longer sleep may simply reflect terminal illness, the observation from JACC that findings remain robust after exclusion of the first 5 years of follow-up argue against this as a sole explanation (Patel, 2009).

Mortality follow-up over 15 years

At least five large-scale studies have published data on sleep duration and mortality over a follow-up period of over 15 years (Ferrie et al., 2007; Gale and Martyn, 1998; Heslop et al., 2002; Hublin et al., 2007; Kaplan et al., 1987). A 17-year follow-up study from the US of 4,174 participants aged ≥38, which compared those who sleep 7–8 hours with those who do not (shorter and longer sleepers combined) observed an increased risk of mortality exclusively in the 50–59 age group (Kaplan et al., 1987). Associations with mortality were examined over 17 years from a baseline measure of sleep and over 12 years from a follow-up measure of sleep in a large occupational cohort, the Whitehall II Study of UK civil servants. Despite a U-shaped association across the sleep categories with the lowest risk at 7 hours, there was little evidence that either short or long sleep was associated with an increased risk of mortality over 17 years in analyses adjusted for socio-demographic factors, health-related behaviours, health indicators, CVD risk factors, and prevalent CHD. However, both short and long sleep at follow-up were associated with mortality over 12 years in the multivariate-adjusted analyses; HR (95% CI) 1.78 (1.17–2.71) and 1.95 (1.15–3.31), respectively (Ferrie et al., 2007).

A large Finnish study, the Finnish Twin study, also examined associations between sleep duration on two occasions 6 years apart and mortality among 21,268 twins. Sleep duration was categorized as short (<7 hours), average (7–8 hours), and long (>8 hours). Compared to average sleep and after adjustment for socio-demographic factors, health-related behaviours, and life satisfaction, both short and long sleep were associated with an increased risk of mortality over the 22-year follow-up period; HR (95% CI) 1.21 (1.05–1.40) and 1.17 (1.03–1.34), respectively (Hublin et al., 2007).

In a small UK study of women and men aged ≥65, long hours in bed (10, 11, and ≥12 hours, relative to 9 hours) were associated with an increased risk of mortality over 23 years in analyses adjusted for socio-demographic factors, geriatrician-diagnosed illness, blood pressure, and body mass index (BMI) (Gale and Martyn, 1998). Although these findings chime with reports of increased mortality in long sleepers, time in bed is not the same as time asleep. The study with the longest follow-up of sleep duration and mortality was carried out among working-age Scots. Sleep duration was measured on two occasions between 4 and 7 years apart and associations with mortality examined over 25 years. In women, short sleep (<7 hours) was associated with an increased risk of all-cause mortality, relative to 7–8 hours, in analyses adjusted for socio-demographic factors, health-related behaviours, and disease risk factors. However, in men short sleep was associated with mortality only in age-adjusted analyses and there was no evidence of any association with long sleep (>8 hours) (Heslop et al., 2002).

Thus, most of the studies with the longest follow-up appear to provide evidence in favour of associations between short sleep and an increased risk of mortality. However, recent reviews and a meta-analysis concur with the view that long sleep is the stronger predictor of all-cause mortality, having a higher risk and more prevalent associations across studies than short sleep (Gallicchio and Kalesan, 2009; Grandner and Drummond, 2007; Youngstedt and Kripke, 2004).

Usual sleep duration and cause-specific mortality

Some of the larger studies that have examined associations between sleep duration and all-cause mortality have had sufficient data to examine cause-specific mortality, at least for a few major cause-specific categories. Approximately half the studies use data from western industrialized populations, while the other half are from populations of Chinese or Japanese origin (see also Chapter 5).

In common with all-cause mortality, mortality rates in CPSI were higher in all sleep duration groups relative the 7.0–7.9 hours group for CHD, stroke, cancer, and suicide with women and men at the extreme ends of the distribution (≤4 hours and ≥10 hours) at highest risk (Kripke et al., 1979). Both cancer deaths and CVD deaths in the Nurses Health Study were associated with long sleep; RR (95% CI) 1.21 (1.03–1.43) and 1.56 (1.25–1.96), respectively, while death from other causes was associated with both short and long sleep (Patel et al., 2004). Another study of US women reported no associations between short (<6 hours) or longer (>8 hours) sleep and CVD death or death from other causes, but long (9–9.9 hours) and very long (≥10 hours) sleep durations were associated with an increased risk of both CVD and 'other' (non-CVD/non-cancer) deaths (Stone et al., 2009). Apart from these three US studies, evidence of associations between sleep duration and cause-specific mortality in western samples is limited. In the UK Whitehall II Study, there was evidence for an association between short sleep and CVD death over 12 years; HR (95% CI) 2.25 (1.15–4.38) (Ferrie et al., 2007) and in Israeli men aged ≥50 there was a higher risk of non-CVD mortality in short sleepers (>8 hours, relative to 6–8 hours); HR (95% CI) 2.02 (1.01–4.03) (Burazeri et al., 2003a).

The evidence from Chinese populations comes from two studies conducted in Chinese communities outside China. One from Singapore that included 58,044 participants aged 45–74 specifically examined associations between sleep duration and CHD mortality. In participants free of CHD, stroke, and cancer at baseline, there was strong evidence that, relative to 7 hours, short and long sleep were associated with an increased risk of CHD death; RR (95% CI) 1.57 (1.32–1.88) and 1.79 (1.48–2.17), respectively. These findings remained in analyses stratified by sex and BMI and after adjustment for hypertension and diabetes and exclusion of the first 4 years of follow-up (Shankar et al., 2008). The second study of Chinese people was based in Taiwan and covered deaths from cancer, CVD, respiratory conditions, and 'other'. Short sleep (<7 hours) was not associated with mortality from any cause in either sex. However, in women, all sleep durations above 7.9 hours were associated with CVD deaths and long (9–9.9 hours) and very long sleep (>10 hours) were associated with cancer, respiratory, and other deaths. In men, the only associations were between very long sleep and an increased risk of mortality from CVD or respiratory disease (Lan et al., 2007).

At least three studies of cause-specific mortality have been undertaken in Japan. Short sleep was associated with an increased risk of stroke mortality and long sleep with CVD mortality in Japanese women. Among men, short sleep was associated with an increased risk of CVD and cancer deaths and deaths from external causes; HR (95% CI) 6.2 (1.3–29.5), 3.1 (1.3–7.5), and 3.1 (1.0–9.7), respectively (Amagai et al., 2004). A study limited to older participants (Suzuki et al., 2009) found no association between short sleep and CVD mortality in either sex. In women, 8 hours sleep, relative to 7 hours, was associated with a higher risk of CVD mortality; HR (95% CI) 2.83 (1.39–5.76). Although the HRs for 9 and ≥10 hours of sleep were also over 2, the CIs included 1.0. In men, no association between sleep duration and CVD death was observed (Suzuki et al., 2009). Analyses of data from the JACC study for people aged 40–79, found short sleep and very short sleep (≤4 hours) in women were associated with an increased risk of CHD and non-CVD/non-cancer deaths. Sleep durations of 8, 9, and ≥10 hours, relative to 7 hours, were all associated with stroke, CVD and non-CVD/non-cancer deaths. In men, very long sleep (≥10 hours) was associated with stroke, in particular ischaemic stroke, and all sleep durations above 7 hours were associated with an increased risk of CVD mortality. Sleep durations above and below 7 hours were associated with non-CVD/non-cancer deaths in men, with findings little changed after exclusion of deaths in the first 5 years (Ikehara et al., 2009).

In summary, associations between sleep duration and cause-specific mortality present a mixed picture with associations between CVD, cancer, and 'other' deaths observed both for short and long sleep. As for all-cause mortality, the strength and prevalence of associations across studies appears to provide more evidence in favour of associations with long sleep.

Change in sleep duration and mortality

Despite concern about sleep curtailment to create more time for leisure and shift-work, only three studies appear to have examined associations between change in sleep duration and mortality; two from the United Kingdom and one from Finland (Ferrie et al., 2007; Heslop et al., 2002; Hublin et al., 2007). In the Whitehall II Study, a reduction in sleep duration at follow-up among those who regularly slept 6, 7, or 8 hours at baseline was associated with an increased risk of mortality, HR 1.62, mainly due to CVD deaths. An increase in usual sleep duration from 7 hours to 8 hours at baseline was also associated with a 75% increased risk of mortality, but this was mainly due to non-cardiovascular deaths (Fig. 4.2) (Ferrie et al., 2007). Observation of change in sleep duration over a period of 4–7 years in the other UK study produced no associations of note (Heslop et al., 2002).

In the study of Finnish twins, moves from average to short, long to short, and average to long sleep durations were associated with an increased risk mortality in women, relative to those who had average durations at both time points. Men who moved from average to short or average to long sleep, or who were short or long sleepers at both time points, were also at a higher risk of mortality. When deaths were broken down into natural and external causes, associations with natural deaths mirrored those for all-cause mortality in women, and a move from short to long

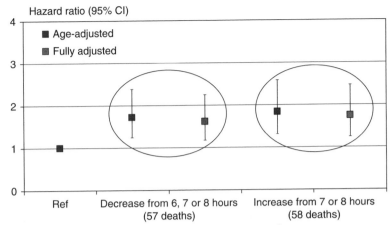

Fig. 4.2 Change in sleep duration over 5 years and all-cause mortality.
Source: Adapted with permission from Ferrie, J.E., Shipley, M.J., Cappuccio, F.P., et al. (2007). A prospective study of change in sleep duration: associations with mortality in the Whitehall II cohort. *Sleep*, **30**, 1659–1666.

sleep was associated with an excess risk of death from external causes; HR (95% CI) 6.30 (1.96–20.3). In men, excess risk of death from external causes was associated with short-short, average-short, and long-short sleep durations, while an excess risk of death from natural causes existed only in those who were short or long sleepers at both time points (Hublin et al., 2007).

Reviews and meta-analysis

Although several qualitative reviews have examined the literature on sleep duration and mortality (Grandner and Drummond, 2007; Youngstedt and Kripke, 2004), there appears to be only one systematic review that has characterized the magnitude of these associations (Gallicchio and Kalesan, 2009) (see also Chapter 5). The meta-analysis by Gallicchio and Kalesan includes data for most of the studies described above. Using random-effects meta-analysis, the authors report that the pooled RR (95% CI) for the association between sleep duration and all-cause mortality, relative to 7 hours sleep, is 1.10 (1.06–1.15) and 1.23 (1.17–1.30) for short and long sleep, respectively. In 13 of the 16 studies included in the pooled analyses for short sleep, the risk of mortality was increased and in 4 the evidence was strong. For long sleep, mortality was increased in 16 out of the 17 studies included, and in half the evidence was strong (Fig. 4.3). Findings were similar in both sexes for short and long sleep and in analyses limited to studies that either adjusted for co-morbidity or excluded participants with co-morbid conditions.

In addition to all-cause mortality, Gallicchio and Kalesan estimated associations between sleep duration and cause-specific mortality from the five studies with data. Pooled RRs (95% CI) for associations between short sleep and CVD and cancer mortality are 1.06 (0.94–1.30) and 0.99 (0.88–1.13), and for long sleep are 1.38 (1.13–1.69) and 1.21 (1.11–1.32), respectively (see also Chapter 5).

Some of the excess mortality observed in this meta-analysis among short and long sleepers is due to individual differences, such as poor health, depression, and obesity. However, as recent studies have taken account of socio-demographic factors, health-related behaviours, health status, and disease history, these factors do not entirely explain the association between sleep duration and mortality. Although this does not rule out the potential for residual confounding due to unmeasured factors or the existence at baseline of prodromal disease in apparently 'healthy'

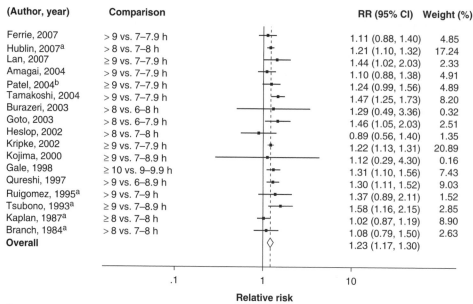

(Author, year)	Comparison		RR (95% CI)	Weight (%)
Ferrie, 2007	> 9 vs. 7–7.9 h		1.11 (0.88, 1.40)	4.85
Hublin, 2007[a]	> 8 vs. 7–8 h		1.21 (1.10, 1.32)	17.24
Lan, 2007	≥ 9 vs. 7–7.9 h		1.44 (1.02, 2.03)	2.33
Amagai, 2004	> 9 vs. 7–7.9 h		1.10 (0.88, 1.38)	4.91
Patel, 2004[b]	≥ 9 vs. 7–7.9 h		1.24 (0.99, 1.56)	4.89
Tamakoshi, 2004	> 9 vs. 7–7.9 h		1.47 (1.25, 1.73)	8.20
Burazeri, 2003	> 8 vs. 6–8 h		1.29 (0.49, 3.36)	0.32
Goto, 2003	> 8 vs. 6–7.9 h		1.46 (1.05, 2.03)	2.51
Heslop, 2002	> 8 vs. 7–8 h		0.89 (0.56, 1.40)	1.35
Kripke, 2002	≥ 9 vs. 7–7.9 h		1.22 (1.13, 1.31)	20.89
Kojima, 2000	≥ 9 vs. 7–8.9 h		1.12 (0.29, 4.30)	0.16
Gale, 1998	≥ 10 vs. 9–9.9 h		1.31 (1.10, 1.56)	7.43
Qureshi, 1997	> 9 vs. 6–8.9 h		1.30 (1.11, 1.52)	9.03
Ruigomez, 1995[a]	> 9 vs. 7–9 h		1.37 (0.89, 2.11)	1.52
Tsubono, 1993[a]	≥ 9 vs. 7–8.9 h		1.58 (1.16, 2.15)	2.85
Kaplan, 1987[a]	≥ 8 vs. 7–8 h		1.02 (0.87, 1.19)	8.90
Branch, 1984[a]	> 8 vs. 7–8 h		1.08 (0.79, 1.50)	2.63
Overall			1.23 (1.17, 1.30)	

.1   1   10

Relative risk

Fig. 4.3 Forest plot of RR (95% CI) for long sleep versus reference category in prospective studies. [a]No adjustment for or exclusions based on co-morbid conditions. [b]Women only.

Source: Reproduced with permission from Gallicchio, L. & Kalesan, B. (2009). Sleep duration and mortality: a systematic review and meta-analysis. *J Sleep Res*, **18**, 148–158.

participants, the results from these studies, together with the consistency of the evidence overall, suggests an increased risk of mortality in both short and long sleepers, with the higher risk in long sleepers (Gallicchio and Kalesan, 2009).

Limitations

A limitation common to most of the studies is reliance on a single, self-reported questionnaire-based measure of sleep duration (see also Chapter 3). Generally, it is not feasible to obtain more detailed and objective measures of sleep from large populations. However, small-scale investigations have shown high correlations between subjective estimates of sleep duration and diary, actigraph, or polysomnography data (Patel et al., 2004; Signal et al., 2005). This suggests that questionnaire-based measures do have good validity, and there are probably more data available for the simple self-reported question 'how many hours do you sleep on an average night?' than for any other measure of sleep. In addition, assessments of sleep durations in the primary healthcare setting rely on self-reported data from patients. The only study to have examined sleep duration and mortality using an objective measure of sleep, electroencephalography, collated data from small studies of people aged ≥55. Inclusion was restricted to those with no sleep problems, or mental or physical health problems. Unfortunately, the total sample was small, 184 individuals, and the data provided no conclusive evidence of associations between sleep duration and mortality over an average follow-up of 13 years (Dew et al., 2003).

Comparisons between studies are limited because categories defined as 'short' and 'long' sleep are inconsistent across studies (see also Chapter 5). As in most comparisons between studies, further heterogeneity is introduced by choice of covariate adjustment, which varies from

0 to 31 covariates, in addition to age, and variously includes other socio-demographic factors, health-related behaviour, pre-existing morbidity and/or disease history, and medication (see also Chapter 3). Both under- and over-adjustment may bias interpretation. Not adjusting for potential confounders could mean that some relationships are driven by exogenous factors and not by sleep duration, while over-adjustment may remove some of the effects of sleep if the covariate is on the causal pathway between sleep and mortality. Additionally, most of the studies lack accurate measures of sleep apnoea, making residual confounding by this prevalent and major sleep disorder a concern, despite adjustment for BMI, a correlate of sleep apnoea (Patel, 2009).

Naps and siestas

Due to cultural norms, sleep deprivation, sleep disorders, or shift-work, millions of people across the world take a nap or a siesta during the day (Dhand and Sohal, 2006). Once past childhood, napping tends to be observed with increasing prevalence in the elderly, and most studies of naps or siestas and mortality have been carried out in older populations. In a widely studied population of 70-year-old Israelis, the HR (95% CI) for 12-year mortality associated with taking a daily nap was 1.63 (1.03–2.58). These analyses, which excluded deaths in the first 2 years, were adjusted for sex, health-related behaviours, disease history, activities of daily living, nighttime sleep duration, and sleep satisfaction (Bursztyn and Stessman, 2005). Analyses of cause-specific mortality showed the all-cause findings were mainly due to CVD and 'other' deaths rather than cancer (Bursztyn et al., 1999). Stratification of these findings by sex showed that, in women, siestas of ≤1 hour or of 1–2 hours were associated with an increased risk of all-cause mortality; OR (95% CI) 4.67 (1.22–17.80) and 5.57 (1.05–29.49), respectively. In men, siestas ≤1 hour were not associated with an increased risk of mortality, but siestas of 1–2 hours were: 2.61 (1.01–6.80) (Bursztyn et al., 2002). A study of 1,859 slightly younger Israelis (≥50 years) with 10 years of follow-up provided no conclusive evidence of an association between siesta and mortality in women. In men, long siestas (>2 hours) were associated with an increased risk of both all-cause and CVD mortality; HR (95% CI) 2.01 (1.24–3.27) and 2.60 (1.30–5.21), respectively in analyses adjusted for health-related behaviours, blood markers, disease history, and nighttime sleep duration. For all-cause mortality, findings were little changed in analyses restricted to men disease-free at baseline (Burazeri et al., 2003b).

In 3,962 US women and men aged ≥65, frequent napping was associated with an increased risk of all-cause mortality over a 6-year follow-up period; OR (95% CI) 1.30 (1.08–1.58), after adjustment for health-related behaviours, diseases, and activities of daily living (Hays et al., 1996). These findings are supported by data showing that among US women disease-free at study entry daily napping was associated with an increased risk of all-cause, CVD, and 'other' deaths; HR (95% CI) 1.67 (1.26–2.20), 1.96 (1.26–3.06), and 1.82 (1.19–2.78), respectively in the multivariate-adjusted analyses (Stone et al., 2009). Contrary to these findings no association between an afternoon nap and mortality was observed in a population of elderly Chinese (Lan et al., 2007). The only cohort study that appears to have examined associations between naps and mortality across a wide age range (20–86) similarly found no association between midday naps and CHD mortality over 6.3 years. Rather, compared to men who did not nap, men who napped regularly for ≥30 minutes at least three times/week had a lower risk of mortality; HR (95% CI) 0.50 (0.31–0.82), a finding observed only among men currently in employment, but not among the retired (Naska et al., 2007). However, concerns have been raised about the lack of analyses of all-cause mortality in this study and the failure to take account of nighttime sleep duration (Bangalore et al., 2007; Patel, 2007).

In summary, despite null associations, there is some evidence to suggest that taking a daytime nap or siesta might be associated with an increased risk of all-cause mortality, CVD death in particular.

Sleep disorders

Insomnia

Insomnia is the most common of the sleep disorders. Its prevalence is higher in women and it increases with age in both sexes (Brown, 2006; Lichstein et al., 2004) (see also Chapters 8 and 9). Short-term insomnia, often the result of stressful life events or the recent onset of medical disorders, usually resolves itself once the original cause is removed. However, chronic insomnia, often psychological in origin, over time can become a separate, self-sustaining disorder (Vgontzas and Kales, 1999). Population-based studies across a number of countries have found that approximately 30% of individuals report some difficulty in sleeping over the past year and approximately 10% report chronic insomnia (Brown, 2006). Furthermore, insomnia has been shown to be on the increase, especially in the employed middle-aged population (Kronholm et al., 2008).

Insomnia and mortality

Although short sleep duration has repeatedly been associated with an increased risk of mortality, the literature on associations between insomnia and serious outcomes remains relatively sparse. This may be because findings from two extremely large early studies appeared to provide little support for an association and may have stymied subsequent research.

In CPSI, women and men who reported frequent insomnia appeared to be at slightly increased risk of mortality, RR 1.17 and 1.34, respectively, over a 6-year follow-up period. However, once stratified by use of sleeping tablets, the association in women disappeared among those who did not use sleeping tablets, although men who did not use sleeping tablets remained at a 30% increased risk (Kripke et al., 1979). At baseline 40.4% of the 636,095 women and 24.1% of the 480,841 men in CPSII reported occasional insomnia (≥ once per month), while 4.3% and 2.6%, respectively reported frequent insomnia (≥10 times per month). Mortality follow-up over 6 years provided strong evidence that women who reported insomnia 1, 2, 3, 4–9, and ≥10 times per month all had a lower risk of death; minimum-maximum HRs (95% CI) 0.81–0.87 (0.76–0.85 to 0.85–0.91). Findings for men were similar in analyses adjusted for 26 covariates, including sleep duration, insomnia frequency, and prescription sleeping tablets (Kripke et al., 2002). In addition to fully-adjusted analyses, the authors report findings from 'simplified models without full covariate control for co-morbidities'. When sleeping tablet use was removed from these simplified models the HRs for mortality associated with insomnia increased slightly; for example, for frequent insomnia removal of sleeping pill use increased the HR for women from 0.99 (0.94–1.05) to 1.05 (0.99–1.10) and for men from 1.15 (1.09–1.21) to 1.24 (1.17–1.30). These findings for men indicate that an association may exist in analyses unadjusted for co-morbidities, such as heart disease, which may be on the causal pathway and could be considered an over-adjustment (Kripke et al., 2002). An alternative explanation is that insomnia is a consequence of CVD which is driving the observed excess mortality.

A similar problem applies to a more recent examination of associations between insomnia and mortality in 13,563 women and men (45–69 years). Prevalence of insomnia defined as two of three symptoms—difficulty falling asleep or difficulty staying asleep plus non-restorative sleep—was 23%; 9.6% if all three symptoms were reported. The association between insomnia and mortality was examined over the subsequent 6.3 years. After controlling for a wide range of covariates, including hypnotics, insomnia was not associated with an increased mortality risk;

OR (95% CI) 0.9 (0.8–1.1), but again no findings from basic models are presented (Phillips and Mannino, 2005). The absence of an association between insomnia and increased mortality risk has also been observed in previous, smaller studies in the elderly (Althuis et al., 1998; Brabbins et al., 1993; Foley et al., 1995; Ganguli et al., 1996; Jensen et al., 1998; Rockwood et al., 2001; Rumble and Morgan, 1992) as well as in studies of the general population (Huppert and Whittington, 1995; Kojima et al., 2000; Mallon et al., 2000). However, a number of other studies do provide evidence in favour of an association with mortality and evidence of an association between insomnia and suicide appears to be unequivocal (Mahgoub, 2009; Taylor et al., 2003).

In the Framingham study, there was a strong association between trouble falling asleep in women (aged 45–64) and fatal/non-fatal myocardial infarction over 20 years (Eaker et al., 1992). A Swedish population-based study of 1,870 women and men, aged 45–65, examined associations between insomnia problems and all-cause, coronary artery disease (CAD), and non-CAD/non-cancer mortality over 12 years. In age-adjusted analyses, difficulty in falling asleep was associated with all-cause mortality in both sexes and CAD, and non-CAD/non-cancer deaths in men. Sleep maintenance was not associated with mortality in women but was associated with all-cause and non-CAD/non-cancer deaths in men. In analyses adjusted for a wide range of covariates and potential mediating factors, including habitual sleeping tablet use, the association between difficulty falling asleep and all-cause mortality in women was attenuated, but a strong association with non-CAD/non-cancer deaths emerged; RR (95% CI) 2.9 (1.3–6.3). In men, the association between difficulty falling asleep and CAD death, 3.1 (1.5–6.3) and between sleep maintenance and non-CAD/non-cancer deaths, 3.1 (1.3–7.6) remained, although the association of both insomnia problems with all-cause mortality was attenuated (Mallon et al., 2002). Similar findings come from another, much larger Swedish study with mortality follow-up over 12 years for 10,902 women and over 17 years for 22,444 men. In analyses adjusted for age and health-related behaviours, insomnia was associated with all-cause and non-CVD mortality in women, HRs (95% CI) 1.40 (1.07–1.84) and 2.43 (1.48–4.00), respectively, and with all-cause, CVD, and non-CVD mortality (HRs 1.76, 1.71, and 2.78) in men (Fig. 4.4) (Nilsson et al., 2001).

Over a 3.5-year follow-up period, a study of 1,855 US residents aged 65–98 found no association between insomnia and premature death in women, but a strong association in men; HR (95% CI) 3.15 (1.63–6.07). The association between insomnia frequency and mortality in men was U-shaped with a higher risk of death in those reporting frequent insomnia and those reporting no insomnia (Pollak et al., 1990), possibly a reflection of the U-shaped association observed between sleep duration and mortality. In the study of Finnish twins, there were no associations between insomnia measured as poor sleep quality and all-cause mortality in analyses adjusted for age and other covariates including sleep duration and sleeping tablet use. However, in analyses stratified by age there was a strong association in men aged 24–39. Change in sleep quality over a 6-year interval measured with items on insomnia symptoms was associated with an increased risk of mortality in age-adjusted analyses in men, but in fully-adjusted models there was no association in either sex (Hublin et al., 2007).

Mixed findings regarding the association between insomnia and mortality may be the result of a combination of factors, including the degree of covariate adjustment and measurement problems in the ascertainment of insomnia (Buysse and Ganguli, 2002; Ohayon, 2005). Due to the strong association between psychological distress and insomnia, self-reports of insomnia symptoms are likely to be subject to recall bias and reporting bias. A study of elderly people in a geriatric hospital that examined sleep onset and sleep maintenance problems reported by an observer provided strong evidence of associations with mortality over a 2-year follow-up period. HRs (95% CI) for delayed onset and poor sleep maintenance were 1.83 (1.22–2.75) and 1.59 (1.05–2.40), respectively in analyses adjusted for age, sex, and activities of daily living (Manabe et al., 2000).

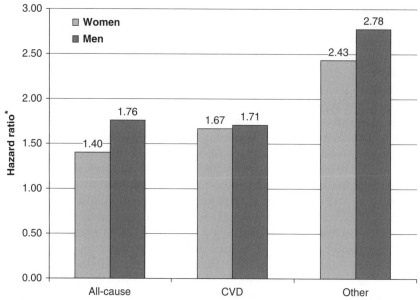

*In healthy women and men after adjustment for age, smoking, alcohol, BMI, cholesterol, and systolic blood pressure.

Fig. 4.4 Hazard ratio (95% CI) for all-cause, CVD, and other mortality in relation to insomnia. *Source*: Data from Nilsson, P.M., Nilsson, J.A., Hedblad, B. & Berglund, G. (2001). Sleep disturbance in association with elevated pulse rate for prediction of mortality—consequences of mental strain? *J Intern Med*, **250**, 521–529.

In a sample of 184 healthy, community-dwelling older people (aged 58–91), electroencephalographic data on sleep showed that delays in sleep onset of ≥30 minutes and poor sleep maintenance were associated with an increased risk of mortality; HR (95% CI) 2.14 (1.25–3.66) and 1.93 (1.14–3.25), respectively over 12.8 years (Dew et al., 2003). These findings provide strong support for an association between insomnia and premature death. The authors suggest that use of electroencephalographic data and the exclusion of individuals with health complaints or sleeping problems at baseline indicate that sleep itself may have an effect on mortality independent of health factors and co-morbidities known to affect both sleep quality and mortality rates (Dew et al., 2003).

Specific insomnia categories

Although ICSD-2 identifies 11 categories of insomnia, epidemiological studies generally do not differentiate between these. In most large-scale studies, insomnia is identified via responses to batteries of questions on sleep latency, arousals, early waking, and non-restorative sleep, such as the Jenkins scale or the Pittsburgh Sleep Quality Index (Buysse et al., 1989; Jenkins et al., 1988). However, of the 11 categories, two specific categories, in which insomnia is generated by extrinsic factors, are worthy of separate mention in relation to premature mortality: 'inadequate sleep hygiene' and 'insomnia due to drug or substance'.

Inadequate sleep hygiene is a sleep disorder arising from the performance of daily living activities, such as staying up very late, that are inconsistent with the maintenance of good quality sleep and full daytime alertness. Prevalence of this disorder in the general population is unknown, although it is believed to be a fairly common primary cause of sleep disturbance or a contributing factor.

Shorter sleep durations and the reported increased prevalence of sleeping problems in our 24/7 society have prompted concern that chronic sleep deprivation may come to prominence as a health-related behaviour with sequelae for serious adverse outcomes, including premature death, equal in importance to alcohol (Bonnet and Arand, 1995).

Hypnotic-dependent sleep disorder is characterized by insomnia or excessive sleepiness that is associated with tolerance to or withdrawal from hypnotic medications. The prevalence of hypnotic-induced sleep disorder in the general population is unknown, but the prevalence of frequent hypnotic use appears to be 2–5%. Use is higher in women (Hausken et al., 2007; Hublin et al., 2007; Kripke et al., 2002; Mallon et al., 2009; Phillips and Mannino, 2005) and use and dependency increase with age (Reynolds III et al., 1999; Rumble and Morgan, 1992). A high suicide rate has been observed among patients originally hospitalized for primary sedative-hypnotic dependence (Allgulander et al., 1984, 1987). Although the most recent pharmacotherapies for insomnia appear to be safe and effective for use up to a year (see section 'Public health and health promotion'), chronic insomnia is a long-term problem for many people and hypnotic dependency remains a serious consideration (Neubauer, 2007).

Premature death and pharmacotherapy for insomnia

Concern over the safety of pharmacotherapies for insomnia has been expressed since opium was combined with alcohol, patented in the 1800s, and sold as laudanum. Used as a potent hypnotic it was associated with many deaths (Neubauer, 2007). Studying the mortality effects of pharmacotherapy for insomnia with observational data is particularly challenging given the difficulty in disentangling this effect from the increased likelihood of taking sleeping tablets among patients with more severe sleeping problems. CPSI and CPSII both provided strong evidence that the use of sleeping pills is associated with premature mortality (Kripke et al., 1979, 2002). Although the main prescription hypnotics at the time of CPSI were barbiturates and at CPSII benzodiazepines, the second study endorsed the findings of the first. In analyses adjusted for a wide range of covariates and potential mediating factors, HRs associated with reported sleeping tablet use 1–29 times/month and ≥30 times/month were 1.10 (1.03–1.17) and 1.24 (1.12–1.38) in women and 1.15 (1.08–1.22) and 1.25 (1.14–1.38) in men (Kripke et al., 2002). Stronger associations were observed in a large Norwegian study of 7,726 women and 7,225 men aged 40–42. Self-reported daily use of anxiolytics or hypnotics as sleep medication (4.5% women, 1.9% men) was associated with an increased risk of all-cause mortality over a follow-up period of 18 years; HR (95% CI) 2.7 (1.9–4.0) and 3.1 (2.0–4.8) in women and men, respectively. Adjustment for use of painkillers, health-related behaviours, and sick-leave or disability pension attenuated these hazards to 1.7 (1.1–2.6) and 1.5 (0.9–2.7), respectively (Hausken et al., 2007). However, after controlling for a wide range of covariates and potential mediating factors, no association between sleeping tablet use and premature death was observed in another large study from the United States and a smaller, population-based study in Japan (Kojima et al., 2000; Phillips and Mannino, 2005).

Two tranquilisers, often used as sleeping tablets, diazepam and chlordiazepoxide, were not associated with an increased risk of mortality in CPSII (Kripke et al., 1998). Similarly, in a 5-year follow-up of people in the United Kingdom aged ≥65, use of medication with sedative properties or benzodiazepine hypnotics was not associated with an increase in mortality. However, there was a strong association between analgesics and over-the-counter medications for sleep and increased risk of death, after adjustment for sex, health risk, and sleep duration. One of the unique features of this study is that medication use was verified by inspection of containers and prescriptions. The authors suggest that self-medication marks out a group of people with high levels of morbidity who are possibly poorly managed medically (Rumble and Morgan, 1992). A large study in Sweden that also used an objective measure of use, register-based data on the purchase of prescriptions from pharmacies found higher mortality rates for users among women aged 45–64 and men in most age groups. Most hypnotics sold at that time were benzodiazepines. However, no adjusted analyses are presented so it is possible that associations are generated by confounding factors such as depression (Isacson et al., 1992). Benzodiazepine use has been associated in other large studies with a high risk of attempted suicide (Neutel and Patten, 1997).

Differences in findings between studies may be related to frequency of use. In the Finnish study of twins, frequent use of hypnotics and/or sedatives (3.7% women, 2.9% men) was associated with an increased risk of mortality in both sexes and across all age categories, with the highest risk in the youngest category (24–39 years). After adjustment for socio-demographic factors and health-related behaviours, HRs (95% CI) were 1.39 (1.11–1.75) in women and 1.31 (1.02–1.69) in men (Hublin et al., 2007). Similarly, in multivariate-adjusted analyses regular sleeping tablet use in Swedes aged 45–56 was associated with non-CAD/non-cancer deaths in women; RR (95% CI) 3.3 (1.1–10.1) and cancer deaths in men, 5.3 (1.8–15.4), over 12 years (Mallon et al., 2002). Observations on the effects of hypnotic use over 20 years were based on the same middle-aged population, augmented by a younger sample aged 30–44 at baseline. Although most participants used hypnotics seldom or never, 4.8% used them occasionally and 2% regularly. In analyses adjusted for a range of covariates and potential mediators, regular hypnotic use was associated with all-cause mortality in women; HR (95% CI) 2.03 (1.07–3.86). In men, it was associated with mortality from all-causes 4.54 (2.47–8.37), CAD 4.55 (1.65–12.58), cancer 3.99 (1.25–12.72), and other causes 3.64 (1.14–11.59). Hypnotic use was associated with a very high risk of suicide; HR (95% CI) 24.27 (4.36–135.20) and 21.18 (2.58–173.74) in women and men, respectively. However, these associations were based on small numbers and the findings remain uncertain. Occasional use was not associated with an increased risk of mortality (Mallon et al., 2009).

Although a number of studies have shown that hypnotic use increases the risk of motor-vehicle accidents (Gustavsen et al., 2008), few appear to have examined fatal accidents. One cross-sectional study examined data provided by coroners for 3,803 drug-related intentional and unintentional deaths in England. Median age at death was 33. The ratio of deaths in men relative to women was 4.5:1 and of intentional to unintentional deaths was 2:1. For intentional deaths the main cause was suffocation, while the main causes of unintentional deaths were falls and motor-vehicle accidents. Sedative-hypnotics were implicated in 25% of deaths in women and 17% of deaths in men and were more frequently implicated in older than younger victims, in unintentional than intentional deaths, and were most frequently implicated in motor-vehicle accidents compared with other types of fatal accident (Oyefeso et al., 2006).

Overall, existing evidence seems to support an association between sleeping tablet use and premature death. However, a limitation of most existing studies is reliance on self-reported, non-specific information on sleeping tablet use. More problematic is that information gathered once at baseline provides no indication of duration of treatment or change in type of pharmacotherapy as treatments of choice have changed over time. Compared with older insomnia treatments, the current generation of pharmacotherapies have greatly improved safety profiles and were approved for long-term use of up to a year in 2005 (Kripke, 2009; Neubauer, 2007). A further problem that occurs during data analysis relates to adjustment for covariates. People usually use medicines in response to illness, but many studies have neither data on the illnesses, mental and physical, that could result both in the use of sleep medication and a higher risk of mortality, nor on lifestyle factors or other medications. For such reasons, it is difficult to rule out the possibility that sleep medication is merely a marker of other risk factors and illnesses and acts as a confounder or causal intermediate in the association with mortality. However, epidemiological studies can never control for all possible confounders, and hence controlling for risk factors may lead to either under- or overestimation of mortality risks (Kripke et al., 1998). Randomized controlled studies would therefore provide more definite evidence but would need to be very large to achieve sufficient power to detect moderate effects.

Disorders of parasomnia and hypersomnia

Parasomnias

Parasomnias are a category of sleep disorders that involve abnormal and unnatural movements, behaviours, emotions, perceptions, and dreams that occur while falling asleep, during sleep, between sleep stages, or on arousal from sleep (see also Chapter 2).

Self-reported sleepwalking and sleep terrors have been found to have a prevalence of 2% in adults in the United Kingdom (Ohayon et al., 1999). Although the incidence of violent acts during sleep is higher in men than women, under-reporting means that actual figures are unknown. However, the high profile coverage of cases of homicidal somnambulism indicates that fatalities are very rare (Broughton et al., 1994).

Hypersomnias

The terms hypersomnia and excessive daytime sleepiness (EDS) are often used interchangeably. EDS is the predominant complaint of patients evaluated in sleep clinics and often reflects organic dysfunction. Many patients with neurodegenerative and neuromuscular diseases also suffer from sleep disturbances associated with EDS and patients with other diseases, such as stroke, experience EDS as a secondary symptom or drug-related side effect. Although the largest group of sleep disorders causing EDS are those related to sleep-disordered breathing (SDB), the most severe cases of EDS occur amongst people with narcolepsy and hypersomnia. Both are chronic neurological diseases that tend to onset at a young age (Vgontzas and Kales, 1999). Narcolepsy and hypersomnia are both rare diseases in that they affect less than 0.1% of the population. A major difference between them is that people with narcolepsy experience a sudden onset of sleepiness and find daytime sleep refreshing, while people with hypersomnia experience persistent sleepiness but do not find sleep refreshing (Brooks, 2006).

Narcolepsy and mortality

Although people with narcolepsy have an even higher risk of motor-vehicle accidents due to sleepiness than people with SDB (Powell et al., 2007), there appear to be no studies that have examined associations specifically between narcolepsy and mortality, accidental or otherwise. This lack of studies is probably due to the low prevalence of the disease.

Idiopathic hypersomnia and mortality

Although EDS is much more prevalent than narcolepsy, there appear to be few publications specifically examining whether it is an independent predictor of mortality in large population or patient samples. EDS and fatigue have been identified as the causal factors in 10–15% of fatal car crashes (Radun and Summala, 2004). A case-control study from the United States based on data from police department records for commercial vehicles similarly showed 13% of fatal crashes were due to sleepiness or fatigue. After adjusting for other human factors, seatbelt use and age, the OR (95% CI) for a fatal compared to a non-fatal crash related to sleepiness or fatigue was 21.0 (4.2–106.1) (Bunn et al., 2005).

The most recent and comprehensive study of EDS and all-cause mortality, the French Three City Study (Empana et al., 2009), builds on three previous studies from North America, all in populations aged ≥65 (Hays et al., 1996; Newman et al., 2000; Rockwood et al., 2001). The earliest of these demonstrated an association between EDS and mortality over a 4-year follow-up period that was independent of a wide range of socio-demographic factors, health-related behaviours,

and health and functioning measures. However, EDS was measured as frequency of daytime napping and was not adjusted for other sleep disorders, such as SDB (Hays et al., 1996). In the
remaining North American studies, EDS was assessed using a single-item question on sleeping
during the day (Newman et al., 2000; Rockwood et al., 2001). An association between daytime
sleepiness and mortality was observed in US women free of CVD, HR (95% CI) 1.46 (1.11–1.91),
but not in men. Analyses were adjusted for socio-demographic characteristics, health-related
behaviours, obesity, arthritis, lung function, depression, medication, and disability. Among 9,000
Canadians, daytime sleepiness was associated with an increased risk of mortality over 5 years in
both sexes in analyses adjusted for age, depression, and cognitive function. However, it was
attenuated on further adjustment for marital status, smoking, functioning, height, weight, and
cardiac symptoms (Rockwood et al., 2001).

The Three Cities multi-centre study has data on EDS for 8,269 women and men aged ≥65, with
mortality follow-up over 6 years (Empana et al., 2009). In analyses adjusted for a range of covariates and potential mediating factors, including obesity and sleeping tablets, EDS was associated
with an increased risk of all-cause mortality; HR (95% CI) 1.29 (1.07–1.55) (Fig. 4.5). These associations were strong both in snorers and non-snorers, and in insomniacs and normal sleepers.
The study also examined cause-specific mortality and found EDS to be associated with an
increased risk of CVD, 1.46 (1.02–2.09), but not cancer mortality (Empana et al., 2009). Although
this study adjusts for a large number of potential confounders and presents separate analyses for
those with insomnia and for those who snore, a marker of potential apnoea, it has a low response

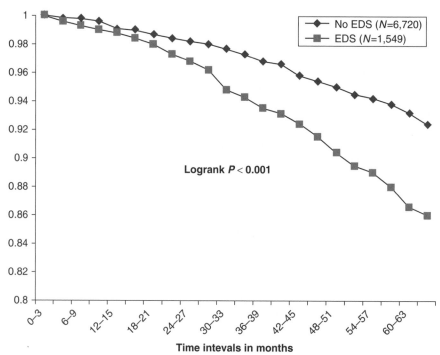

Fig. 4.5 Kaplan-Meier curve of 6-year mortality of participants with and without EDS at baseline.
Source: Reproduced from Empana, J.P., Dauvilliers, Y., Dartigues, J.F., et al. (2009). Excessive
daytime sleepiness is an independent risk indicator for cardiovascular mortality in community-dwelling
elderly: the three city study. *Stroke*, **40**, 1219–1224, with permission from Wolters Kluwer Health.

rate, 37%. Also, while obesity and loud snoring will partially account for presence of SDB, they are less powerful predictors in elderly than middle-aged populations (Empana et al., 2009). As already indicated, establishing unequivocally that EDS or hypersomnia is associated with mortality independent of other sleep disorders and other diseases remains a challenge, both in relation to death from disease and accidental death.

Sleep-related breathing disorder and sleep-related movement disorder

Sleep-disordered breathing

Sleep-disordered breathing describes a group of disorders characterized by respiratory abnormalities or lack of ventilation during sleep. Prevalence of SDB, defined as an apnoea-hypopnoea index (AHI) of $\geq$5 events per hour. There are three major types of SDB with respect to prevalence and health consequences: obstructive sleep apnoea (OSA), central sleep apnoea (CSA), and obesity hyperventilation syndrome (OHS) (see also Chapters 5 and 7) (Levy et al., 2008). The most common are the sleep apnoeas, in particular OSA, characterized by apnoeic and hypopnoeic events during sleep.

Sleep-disordered breathing and cardiovascular mortality

Due to strong associations between SDB and CVD, most mortality studies have focussed on CVD mortality (see also Chapter 5). Associations with all-cause mortality have, in general, been reported in addition to CVD mortality, or instead of CVD mortality in studies that are underpowered for this outcome. For this reason, findings for CVD mortality and all-cause mortality are presented together, while accidental death, which has its own literature, is presented separately.

Sleep-disordered breathing and mortality in sleep clinic patients

Several studies of sleep clinic patients suggest that OSA results in increased CVD and all-cause mortality (see also Chapters 5 and 7). A study of 198 patients showed all-cause and CVD mortality rates were higher in patients who had been treated conservatively (weight loss) than those who had undergone surgical treatment for OSA (tracheostomy). The crude mortality rate (95% CI) over 5 years for conservatively treated patients was 11.0 (6.0–18.5)/100 for all-cause and 6.3 (2.5–11.6)/100 for CVD mortality (Partinen et al., 1988). In another study of 385 men tracked over 8 years, survival was related to OSA severity, particularly in men aged <50 among whom death from other causes is uncommon (He et al., 1988). The observation of particularly high relative rates of mortality in sleep apnoea patients aged <50 has been confirmed in a number of subsequent patient studies in Israel (Lavie et al., 1995), Japan (Noda et al., 1998), and Spain (Marti et al., 2002).

Although a couple of small studies in patients with obstructive sleep apnoea syndrome (OSAS) have reported null findings, underlying illnesses in the control group could provide alternative explanations of the null effects (Gonzalez-Rothi and Block, 1988a, b). A larger, more recent study compared the incidence of fatal CVD events between men categorized as: simple snorers, mild-moderate OSAS, severe untreated OSAS, and treated OSAS, with healthy men from the general population matched for age and body mass. There was good evidence that risk of CVD death was higher in men with severe untreated OSAS compared to healthy controls; OR (95% CI) 2.9 (1.2–7.5), but there was no firm evidence of higher risks in other groups (Marin et al., 2005). Findings in this study contrast with the finding that habitual snorers are at greater risk of death, CVD death in particular, than those who snore occasionally or never (Seppala et al., 1991). However, retrospective reports of snoring by the closest co-habiting individual will be open to recall bias.

OSA has also been shown to increase CVD events and mortality in patients with pre-existing CAD (Mooe et al., 2001; Peker et al., 2000), and untreated OSA (Wang et al., 2007) and CSA in particular are independent risk factors for mortality in patients with heart failure (Ancoli-Israel et al., 2003; Hanly and Zuberi-Khokhar, 1996; Javaheri et al., 2007; Lanfranchi et al., 1999; Sin et al., 2000). However, not all studies support an association between CSA and mortality (Roebuck et al., 2004) and as yet a causal role has not been proven (Garcia-Touchard et al., 2008). A recent study differentiated heart failure patients into those with ischaemic heart failure and those with non-ischaemic cardiomyopathy. Among patients with non-ischaemic cardiomyopathy there was no difference in survival between those with and without moderate-severe sleep apnoea. However, in those with ischaemic heart failure there was evidence that moderate-severe apnoea increased the risk of mortality; HR (95% CI) 3.0 (1.0–8.8) after adjustment for age, sex, BMI, and other potential confounding factors (Yumino et al., 2009). Studies that have examined stroke patients show that SDB is generally associated with increased long-term mortality, although null findings have also been reported (Bassetti et al., 2006). A recent study that measured OSAS using polysomnography examined associations with a composite measure comprising incident stroke and all-cause mortality over 3 years. A strong trend was observed with increasing quartiles of AHI; HR (95% CI) for patients in the highest versus the lowest quartile 3.3 (1.74–6.26) (Yaggi et al., 2005). Another study showed OSA, but not CSA, to be associated with a higher risk of post-stroke mortality; HR (95% CI) 1.76 (1.05–2.95) (Sahlin et al., 2008).

Taken together, these clinic-based studies appear to provide evidence that people with untreated OSA are at greater risk of premature mortality and that OSA is a prognostic factor associated with an increased likelihood of further events, including death, in patients with CAD, heart failure, or stroke. However, it is possible that observed differences at follow-up merely reflect disease severity at study entry rather than any causal effects. Furthermore, findings in patients experiencing severe OSA may not be applicable to OSA of mild or moderate severity which is more prevalent, often undiagnosed, in the general population.

Sleep-disordered breathing and mortality in community samples

The association between snoring or sleep apnoea and CVD or all-cause mortality has been examined in several cohort and population-based studies (see also Chapter 5). In the first published prospective study of snoring, the age-adjusted RR (95% CI) for CVD mortality among habitual and frequent snorers relative to light snorers was 1.58 (1.05–2.38) in 3,847 men aged 40–69 over 35 months. Ischaemic heart disease mortality (rate/100,000/year) followed a dose-response relationship: 503 in habitual/frequent snorers, 354 in occasional snorers, and 143 in non-snorers; RR 3.52 ($P < 0.05$) for habitual/frequent snorers relative to non-snorers. The RR for stroke mortality was also high, 3.59, but the estimate was imprecise due to small numbers and the findings did reach conventional levels of statistical significance ($P > 0.05$) (Koskenvuo et al., 1987).

In contrast, a prospective study of 2,937 Danish men (aged 54–74) provided no evidence that snorers were at a higher risk of all-cause mortality than non-snorers (Jennum et al., 1995). A study of a random sample of 3,100 Swedish men aged 30–69 that combined data on snoring with EDS did not support these findings. In analyses restricted to men aged 30–59, those with snoring and EDS were nearly three times as likely to die over the follow-up period as men without those symptoms; age-adjusted RR (95% CI), 2.7 (1.6–4.5) for all-cause and 2.9 (1.3–6.7) for CVD mortality. Neither snoring nor EDS alone were associated with excess mortality in any age group (Lindberg et al., 1998).

Associations between self-reported snoring and CVD were examined among nearly 72,000 female US nurses over 8 years (Hu et al., 2000). Occasional and frequent snoring were associated with an increased risk of fatal CHD and stroke, but adjustment for multiple potential confounders attenuated these associations; RR (95% CI) 1.33 (0.90–1.96) and 1.35 (0.80–2.26), for occasional and regular snoring, respectively. Although the evidence is weak after adjustment, these findings are similar to the RRs observed for fatal and non-fatal events combined: 1.20 and 1.33 for occasional and regular snoring, indicating that the lack of an association with fatal CVD may be due to the low number of outcomes (Hu et al., 2000).

Study of a random sample of 233 elderly people in nursing homes also demonstrated a strong association between the AHI and all-cause mortality in women, but not in men. Participants with OSA also had a greater tendency to die in their sleep (Ancoli-Israel et al., 1989). In contrast, population-based studies of community-dwelling older people present a more mixed picture of associations between OSA and mortality. A study that followed a representative sample of 426 people aged ≥65 for mortality over a period of 9.5 years measured sleep apnoea using recordings taken at night in the home. In unadjusted analyses, participants with severe apnoea had a much shorter survival time, dying as much as 2 years earlier than others. However, in multiple regression analyses that adjusted for age, sex, BMI, and disease history there was no evidence of an association with mortality (Ancoli-Israel et al., 1996). Adjustment for CVD, assumed to be on the causal pathway, may in fact be an over-adjustment, but other small studies of older participants have not found evidence of associations between sleep apnoea and mortality (Bliwise et al., 1988; Mant et al., 1995).

Irrespective of adjustments, these findings may simply reflect an association of OSA with mortality only in younger to middle-aged adults, as data from other studies have suggested (He et al., 1988; Lindberg et al., 1998). Although the prevalence of sleep apnoea increases with age, it is possible that it is less threatening in older people or that those reaching older ages are already selected on their ability to withstand the adverse effects of the disorder.

Two recent studies add support to the importance of sleep apnoea as a predictor of premature death in younger age groups. A mortality follow-up (mean 14 years) of 1,522 participants, aged 30–60, in the Wisconsin Sleep Cohort Study provided strong evidence of an association between severe sleep apnoea and all-cause mortality in analyses adjusted for age, sex, and BMI; HR (95% CI) 3.0 (1.4–6.3). In analyses restricted to untreated participants, severe sleep apnoea was associated with both all-cause and CVD mortality: 3.8 (1.6–9.0) and 5.2 (1.4–19.2), respectively; associations that were not attenuated by further adjustment for self-reported sleepiness. Some further evidence of the association was provided by the observation of a dose-response relationship between sleep apnoea severity and survival over a 20-year follow-up (Fig. 4.6) (Young et al., 2008).

The other, much smaller, Australian study followed 380 participants, aged 40–65, over 13 years. In unadjusted analyses those with moderate-severe apnoea had an HR of 5 for all-cause mortality relative to those without apnoea. This increased to 6.2 (2.0–19.4), after adjustment for age, sex, BMI, and a range of other potential confounding factors. No association between mild apnoea and mortality was observed (Marshall et al., 2008).

The results from these mainly community-dwelling samples add further weight to evidence from patient samples that severe sleep apnoea syndrome is an important risk factor for all-cause and CVD mortality. Although some studies have observed a dose-response association between AHI and mortality, evidence that moderate sleep apnoea is an important determinant of mortality remains equivocal. The observation in a number of studies that the risk of mortality among those with sleep apnoea is reduced or eliminated by treatment, mainly continuous positive airways pressure (CPAP), further strengthens support for an association and illustrates the importance, in terms of premature death, of diagnosis and treatment (Doherty et al., 2005; Marin et al., 2005; Pack et al., 2008).

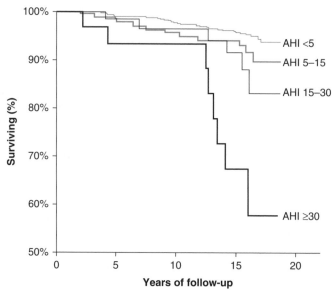

Fig. 4.6 Kaplan-Meier estimates of survival probability according to SDB severity.
Source: Reproduced from Young, T., Finn, L., Peppard, P.E., et al. (2008). Sleep disordered breathing and mortality: eighteen-year follow-up of the Wisconsin sleep cohort. *Sleep*, **31**, 1071–1078, with permission.

Sleep-disordered breathing and accidental death

Recognition of the contribution of sleep loss and sleepiness to traumatic or fatal accidents has increased over the last two decades (see also Chapters 15 and 16) (Rosa, 2006). The majority of these accidents occur in healthy young people who have had insufficient sleep (Pack et al., 1995), or in people who are driving or working at their circadian nadir. However, when a pathological cause is present this tends to be a sleep disorder, most commonly sleep apnoea syndrome (Horne and Reyner, 1999; Rodenstein, 2008). Unlike the other outcomes of sleep apnoea, in which serious outcomes are restricted to the individual sufferer, accidents at work and motor-vehicle accidents also endanger the lives of other people (Desai et al., 2003).

People with SDB have problems with concentration, attention, and cognitive function during the day, with performance inversely related to the level of sleep disruption (Rosa, 2006). Although more than 10 people per day die at work in the United States, little research has examined associations between SDB and fatal accidents at work and there are no large population-based studies of associations between SDB measured objectively and occupational accidents. Patients with OSA have high crash rates, but again studies that have determined the proportion that are fatal appear to be rare. In a study of 4,333 crashes between 1990 and 1992 in North Carolina in which the driver was judged to be asleep, 13.5% involved the severest category of injury and 1.4% were fatal (Pack et al., 1995). One report covering two separate studies in the United Kingdom found sleep-related crashes accounted for 16% and 23% of all accidents and, of these, 23% and 22%, respectively resulted in either death or serious injury to the driver. One of the studies also reported on accidents unrelated to sleep. In these accidents, the proportion resulting in death or serious injury was 15% (Horne and Reyner, 1995).

A problem with examining associations between SDB and motor-vehicle crashes in patient samples is the potential for overestimation of risk due to selection bias. Although most of the few reported population-based studies appear to confirm the findings from patient studies of a role for OSA (Masa et al., 2000; Teran-Santos et al., 1999; Young et al., 1997), a case-control study that examined the contribution of driver sleepiness to vehicle crashes involving hospitalization or death found no firm evidence of an association with self-reported sleep apnoea symptoms (Connor et al., 2002).

Sleep-related movement disorder

Five separate categories of sleep-related movement disorder are listed in ICSD-2: restless legs syndrome (RLS), periodic limb movement disorder (PLMD), sleep-related leg cramps, sleep-related bruxism, and sleep-related rhythmic movement disorder (Benz et al., 2000). There appear to be no published studies of associations between the latter three disorders and serious health outcomes, although they are likely to be associated with some level of sleep disturbance in sufferers and their bed partners.

Restless legs syndrome, periodic limb movement disorder and mortality

Restless legs syndrome is a disorder characterized by disagreeable leg sensations, usually prior to sleep onset, which cause an almost irresistible urge to move the legs. Definitive data for prevalence are not available, but symptoms of RLS have been identified in 5–10% of the general population in western countries (Allen et al., 2005). Prevalence is higher in women and increases significantly with age (Allen et al., 2005; Ohayon and Roth, 2002). Chronic insomnia, together with daytime fatigue, distress, depression, and reduced quality of life are common problems for people with RLS and sleep problems are considered to be characteristic of the disorder (Allen et al., 2005; Becker, 2006; Broman et al., 2008). Although RLS has been associated with decreased concentration and deficits in cognitive functioning, it is questionable whether it is associated with a tendency to fall asleep during the day (Allen, 2006).

PLMD, previously known as nocturnal myoclonus, is a sleep disorder characterized by periodic episodes of repetitive, involuntary movement of the arms and/or legs during sleep with symptoms, such as insomnia, related to the movement (Khassawneh, 2006). Although the exact prevalence is unknown, it has been estimated to occur in approximately 4% of adults aged 15–100 (Ohayon and Roth, 2002). Like RLS, PLMD is more common in women and the elderly, with up to 11% of elderly women experiencing symptoms (Hornyak and Trenkwalder, 2004). A person who moves his/her limbs during sleep but suffers no consequences is classified as having periodic limb movements of sleep (PLMS). Most people with PLMS do not have PLMD or any disorder that requires treatment, but a study of 133 people found that 80% of those with RLS also had PLMS (Montplaisir et al., 1997). PLMD is associated with other sleep disorders, such as OSA, and with the use of certain drugs or withdrawal from sedative-hypnotics (Khassawneh, 2006).

Despite the relatively high prevalence of RLS and PLMD, little work appears to have examined associations between these sleep disorders and mortality. A general population study in Sweden of just over 5,000 people aged 30–65 examined associations between restless legs symptoms combined with daytime sleepiness and mortality (Broman et al., 2008; Mallon et al., 2000, 2002, 2008, 2009). Restless legs symptoms with daytime sleepiness were reported by about 10% of women and men. Relative to controls, women with restless legs symptoms and daytime sleepiness had an increased risk of all-cause mortality; HR (95% CI) 1.89 (1.35–2.66), but there was no association in men, 1.23 (0.89–1.70). Daytime sleepiness alone, reported by 19.3% of the participants, was not associated with an increased risk of mortality in women but with a 50% increase in men, while the HR for restless legs symptoms alone, reported by 17.5% of women and 12.5% of men, were indicative of an association only in men: 1.31 (0.98–1.74). However, in analyses adjusted for age, living alone, obesity, disease history, short sleep duration, and snoring, only evidence for the association between restless legs symptoms with daytime sleepiness and mortality in women remained convincing: 1.85 (1.20–2.85) (Mallon et al., 2008).

There appear to be no published studies of associations between PLMS or PLMD and mortality in the general population, but they have been shown to be strong, independent predictors of mortality in patients with end-stage renal disease (Benz et al., 2000).

Circadian rhythm sleep disorders and other sleep disorders

Circadian rhythm sleep disorders

The circadian rhythm sleep disorders (CRSD) is a group of disorders characterized by a mismatch between the sleep-wake schedule required by a person's environment and his/her circadian sleep-wake pattern (see also Chapter 2). There are four main types: delayed sleep phase syndrome, advanced sleep phase syndrome, free-running sleep-wake pattern, and irregular sleep-wake pattern. By far the most common is delayed sleep phase syndrome, the disorder diagnosed in 85% of patients presenting with CRSD. Population prevalence appears to be very low, but is actually unknown. Onset is usually in childhood or adolescence and there appear to be no sex differences in prevalence (Åkerstedt, 2006; Dagan, 2002).

Other conditions classified under the CRSD category in ICSD-2 are disruptions to the normal sleep-wake pattern induced by medical conditions, drugs or alcohol, shift-work sleep disorder, and jet lag (ICSD-2, 2005). Although many shift-workers experience difficulties with sleep and remaining alert at work, a subset experience difficulty severe enough to warrant the diagnosis shift-work sleep disorder. This disorder has been shown to have a prevalence of approximately 14% among night shift-workers and 8% among those on rotating shifts (Richardson, 2006).

Jet lag results from rapid travel across multiple time zones and consists of varying degrees of difficulties in initiating or maintaining sleep, daytime sleepiness, decrements in alertness and performance, and somatic symptoms. Work in mice has demonstrated a potential role for the circadian clock in the progression of vascular disease (Anea et al., 2009) and shown repeated advances of the light-dark cycle to be associated with increased mortality in old but not in young mice (Fig. 4.7) (Davidson et al., 2006). However, premature deaths, in particular fatal accidents, among people with CRSDs are more likely to result from the insomnia and daytime sleepiness generated by the persistent or recurrent patterns of sleep disruption that are their hallmark (Åkerstedt, 2006). There appears to be little published on the possible contribution of CRSDs to mortality independent of insomnia and EDS.

Other sleep disorders

Sudden unexplained death during sleep

This condition which occurs in healthy young adults, particularly of Southeast Asian descent is characterized by unexpected death during sleep. First noted in 1977 among Hmong refugees in the United States (Parrish et al., 1987), the disease was again noted in Singapore, when a retrospective survey of records showed that 230 otherwise healthy Thai men died suddenly of unexplained causes between 1982 and 1990 (Goh et al., 1990). In the Philippines, the disease affects 43/100,000 people per year, mostly young men (Gervacio-Domingo et al., 2007).

Sleeping sickness (African trypanosomiasis)

Sleeping sickness is caused by trypanosomes transmitted by the tsetse fly. It occurs only in sub-Saharan Africa with populations aged 15–45 in remote rural areas most affected. In the early 1960s, prevalence had been reduced to very low levels. However, due to lack of regular surveillance and reduced resource allocation the disease was neglected for several decades. This led to a resurgence of the disease, a trend that began to be reversed toward the end of the 1990s. In 2006, the

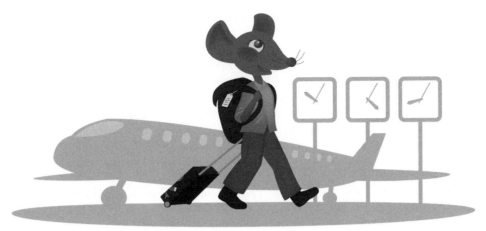

Fig. 4.7 Jet lag is not associated with mortality in young mice.
Source: Reproduced with kind permission of Hung Ho Thanh, Loaloa Studio.

WHO estimated the number of cases as 50,000–70,000. When the infection spreads to the central nervous system, it causes the symptoms typical of sleeping sickness; the sleep cycle is disturbed with bouts of fatigue punctuated with manic periods progressing to daytime slumber and nighttime insomnia. Without treatment, the disease is invariably fatal, with progressive mental deterioration leading to coma and death (WHO, 2006).

Public health and health promotion

Although sleep is a potentially modifiable health-related behaviour, it has received little attention in terms of health policy and promotion compared to other health-related behaviours, such as smoking, physical exercise, diet, and alcohol use.

Existing policy measures

Motor-vehicle crashes are the main cause of sleep-related death at present, but little legislation is addressed to the problem (see also Chapters 15–18). This is probably partly due to civil liberties issues and the impossibility of monitoring adherence were regulations to be put in place. In most countries, regulations are in force to restrict the number of hours commercial drivers can drive without an adequate rest or break. However, there appears to have been limited study of adherence to or benefits from these strategies (Committee on Sleep Medicine and Research Board on Health Sciences Policy, 2006) and no restrictions apply to non-commercial drivers.

In some countries, people with specific sleep disorders, such as narcolepsy, are required to inform driving licence authorities of their condition and licences are restricted according to compliance with treatment. However, there is huge variation between countries. For example, there is no consistency in the way that OSA is considered by the national 'Physical Fitness to Drive' legislation within the member countries of the European Union, although harmonization has been proposed (Rodenstein, 2008).

In the United States, a number of campaigns have aimed at increasing awareness of the importance of sleep for children and adolescents, but there is a need for studies adequately to evaluate the impact of these campaigns. There has been less effort directed towards adults, in particular susceptible sub-populations like shift-workers and the elderly, although the National Heart Blood and Lung Institute produced a general guide aimed at adults in 2005 called 'Your Guide to Healthy Sleep'. Private organizations, professional societies, and patient advocacy groups have also developed a number of health education programmes. One of the most innovative is the US National Sleep Foundation's 'National Sleep Awareness Week' campaign, which coincides annually with the start of daylight savings and includes activities such as sleep health fairs and a public policy and sleep leadership forum (Committee on Sleep Medicine and Research Board on Health Sciences Policy, 2006). Sleep research societies, such as the British Sleep Society, also contribute to increasing awareness mainly among researchers and clinicians, but also the general public.

The 'Back to Sleep' programmes in the United States and United Kingdom are examples of successful public awareness campaigns based on evidence of a strong association between infant sleeping position and SIDS. Since the early 1990s, parents have been advised to place babies on their backs when laying them down to sleep—the 'Back to Sleep' position. This has been shown to significantly reduce the risk of SIDS. Since the campaigns were launched in 1991, the rate of cot deaths in the United Kingdom has fallen by 70%; equivalent to 12 babies/week (<<www.parentscentre.gov.uk/familymatters/havingababy/cotdeath/>>)—and by 50% in the United States (National Institute of Child Health and Development, 2003).

Implications for future policy and health promotion

Many of the main sleep disorders have fairly specific symptoms and can be treated on diagnosis. However, many people are either unaware they have a problem or fail to seek diagnosis and treatment. In addition, the 24/7 society encourages people to skimp on sleep and neglect basic sleep hygiene. A well-coordinated, three-pronged approach to these problems needs to be implemented comprised of education and training for healthcare professionals, improved surveillance and monitoring of the general population, and a public awareness campaign.

Misperceptions about the need for sleep and under-reporting of sleep disorders partly stem from lack of professional understanding of the benefits of adequate sleep and of the symptoms of sleep disorders. In this way, patient contacts with the primary healthcare system are often missed opportunities to diagnose sleep disorders and provide advice on sleep needs and sleep hygiene. All healthcare professionals consulted by patients require greater exposure to the public health burden of sleep loss and sleep disorders. Although the data are limited, they suggest that focussed training on sleep increases the likelihood that medical students will seek sleep histories from patients (Committee on Sleep Medicine and Research Board on Health Sciences Policy, 2006). However, at present, the number of specialist diagnostic and treatment sleep centres available in most countries is far below demand. For example, in France the number of patients diagnosed with OSAS and receiving CPAP treatment is increasing by 20% per year.

Adequate public health education not only requires informing and training the public and healthcare professionals, but also adequate monitoring of the public health burden; in particular serious outcomes, including premature mortality. In many countries, national surveys, such as the Health Survey for England and NHANES in the United States, are used to monitor the population disease burden. Although such surveys from time to time have panel data relevant to sleep patterns and sleep disorders, birth cohort and other longitudinal, prospective studies require funding to incorporate sleep components so that changes in sleep patterns and disorders can be monitored over time in the same individuals. Researchers also need to be encouraged to make use of sleep datasets through increased funding for sleep research.

Summary box

◆ With the exception of fatal accidents caused by falling asleep and a small number of fatal sleep-related diseases, debate remains with regard to the 'independent' contribution of sleep to premature death.

◆ It is generally considered that the associations observed between sleep duration and many of the sleep disorders and premature death is due to effects mediated via risk factors for disease or suicide, or because inadequate sleep is a marker of existing morbidity.

◆ Fatal sleep-related diseases in adults are rare. Sleeping sickness (African trypanosomiasis) has the highest prevalence, but rates are currently falling after three decades in which prevalence increased due to inadequate surveillance and resource allocation.

◆ Fatalities directly attributable to sleep disorders, such as somnambulism, are rare.

◆ In population health terms, fatal accidents resulting from EDS or fatigue are probably the most serious sleep-related public health problem.

◆ It has been estimated that 10–15% of fatal motor-vehicle crashes are due to sleepiness or driver fatigue.

◆ By 2020, the WHO estimate there will be 2.3 million deaths per annum due to motor-vehicle crashes worldwide, of which approximately 230,000–345,000 will be due to sleepiness or fatigue.

◆ Public awareness campaigns need to be implemented alongside increased training of health-care professionals and increased monitoring and surveillance.

References

Åkerstedt, T. (2006). Sleepiness and circadian rhythm sleep disorders. *Sleep Med Clin*, **1**, 17–30.

Allen, R.P. (2006). Periodic leg movements in sleep and restless legs syndrome relation to daytime alertness and sleepiness. *Sleep Med Clin*, **1**, 157–163.

Allen, R.P., Walters, A.S., Montplaisir, J., et al. (2005). Restless legs syndrome prevalence and impact: REST general population study. *Arch Intern Med*, **165**, 1286–1292.

Allgulander, C., Borg, S. & Vikander, B. (1984). A 4-6-year follow-up of 50 patients with primary dependence on sedative and hypnotic drugs. *Am J Psychiatry*, **141**, 1580–1582.

Allgulander, C., Ljungberg, L. & Fisher, L.D. (1987). Long-term prognosis in addiction on sedative and hypnotic drugs analyzed with the Cox regression model. *Acta Psychiatr Scand*, **75**, 521–531.

Althuis, M.D., Fredman, L., Langenberg, P.W. & Magaziner, J. (1998). The relationship between insomnia and mortality among community-dwelling older women. *J Am Geriatr Soc*, **46**, 1270–1273.

Amagai, Y., Ishikawa, S., Gotoh, T., et al. (2004). Sleep duration and mortality in Japan: the Jichi Medical School Cohort Study. *J Epidemiol*, **14**, 124–128.

Ancoli-Israel, S., Klauber, M.R., Kripke, D.F., Parker, L. & Cobarrubias, M. (1989). Sleep apnea in female patients in a nursing home. Increased risk of mortality. *Chest*, **96**, 1054–1058.

Ancoli-Israel, S., Kripke, D.F., Klauber, M.R., et al. (1996). Morbidity, mortality and sleep-disordered breathing in community dwelling elderly. *Sleep*, **19**, 277–282.

Ancoli-Israel, S., DuHamel, E.R., Stepnowsky, C., Engler, R., Cohen-Zion, M. & Marler, M. (2003). The relationship between congestive heart failure, sleep apnea, and mortality in older men. *Chest*, **124**, 1400–1405.

Anea, C.B., Zhang, M., Stepp, D.W., et al. (2009). Vascular disease in mice with a dysfunctional circadian clock. *Circulation*, **119**, 1510–1517.

Bangalore, S., Sawhney, S. & Messerli, F.H. (2007). Siesta, all-cause mortality, and cardiovascular mortality: is there a "siesta" at adjudicating cardiovascular mortality? *Arch Intern Med*, **167**, 2143.

Bassetti, C.L., Milanova, M. & Gugger, M. (2006). Sleep-disordered breathing and acute ischemic stroke: diagnosis, risk factors, treatment, evolution, and long-term clinical outcome. *Stroke*, 37, 967–972.

Becker, P.M. (2006). Restless legs syndrome. In: Lee-Chiong, T. (ed.), *Sleep: A Comprehensive Handbook*. Hoboken, NJ: John Wiley & Sons, pp. 473–481.

Benz, R.L., Pressman, M.R., Hovick, E.T. & Peterson, D.D. (2000). Potential novel predictors of mortality in end-stage renal disease patients with sleep disorders. *Am J Kidney Dis*, 35, 1052–1060.

Bliwise, D.L., Bliwise, N.G., Partinen, M., Pursley, A.M. & Dement, W.C. (1988). Sleep apnea and mortality in an aged cohort. *Am J Public Health*, **78**, 544–547.

Bonnet, M.H. & Arand, D.L. (1995). We are chronically sleep deprived. *Sleep*, **18**, 908–911.

Brabbins, C.J., Dewey, M.E., Copeland, J.R.M., et al. (1993). Insomnia in the elderly—prevalence, gender differences and relationships with morbidity and mortality. *Int J Geriatr Psychiatry*, **8**, 473–480.

Branch, L.G. & Jette, A.M. (1984). Personal health practices and mortality among the elderly. *Am J Public Health*, 74, 1126–1129.

Broman, J.E., Mallon, L. & Hetta, J. (2008). Restless legs syndrome and its relationship with insomnia symptoms and daytime distress: epidemiological survey in Sweden. *Psychiatry Clin Neurosci*, **62**, 472–475.

Brooks, S.N. (2006). Idiopathic hypersomnia. In: Lee-Chiong, T. (ed.), *Sleep: A Comprehensive Handbook*. Hoboken, NJ: John Wiley & Sons, pp. 151–156.

Broughton, R., Billings, R., Cartwright, R., et al. (1994). Homicidal somnambulism: a case report. *Sleep*, 17, 253–264.

Brown, W.D. (2006). Insomnia: prevalence and daytime consequences. In: Lee-Chiong, T. (ed.), *Sleep: A Comprehensive Handbook*. Hoboken, NJ: John Wiley & Sons, pp. 93–98.

Bunn, T.L., Slavova, S., Struttmann, T.W. & Browning, S.R. (2005). Sleepiness/fatigue and distraction/inattention as factors for fatal versus nonfatal commercial motor vehicle driver injuries. *Accid Anal Prev*, 37, 862–869.

Burazeri, G., Gofin, J. & Kark, J.D. (2003a). Over 8 hours of sleep—marker of increased mortality in Mediterranean population: follow-up population study. *Croat Med J*, **44**, 193–198.

Burazeri, G., Gofin, J. & Kark, J.D. (2003b). Siesta and mortality in a Mediterranean population: a community study in Jerusalem. *Sleep*, **26**, 578–584.

Bursztyn, M. & Stessman, J. (2005). The siesta and mortality: twelve years of prospective observations in 70-year-olds. *Sleep*, **28**, 345–347.

Bursztyn, M., Ginsberg, G., Hammerman-Rozenberg, R. & Stessman, J. (1999). The siesta in the elderly: risk factor for mortality? *Arch Intern Med*, **159**, 1582–1586.

Bursztyn, M., Ginsberg, G. & Stessman, J. (2002). The siesta and mortality in the elderly: effect of rest without sleep and daytime sleep duration. *Sleep*, **25**, 187–191.

Buysse, D.J. & Ganguli, M. (2002). Can sleep be bad for you? Can insomnia be good? *Arch Gen Psychiatry*, **59**, 137–138.

Buysse, D.J., Reynolds, C.F., III, Monk, T.H., Berman, S.R. & Kupfer, D.J. (1989). The Pittsburgh Sleep Quality Index: a new instrument for psychiatric practice and research. *Psychiatry Res*, **28**, 193–213.

Committee on Sleep Medicine and Research Board on Health Sciences Policy (2006). *Sleep Disorders and Sleep Deprivation: An Unmet Public Health Problem*. Washington, DC: The National Academies Press.

Connor, J., Norton, R., Ameratunga, S., et al. (2002). Driver sleepiness and risk of serious injury to car occupants: population based case control study. *Br Med J*, 324, 1125.

Dagan, Y. (2002). Circadian rhythm sleep disorders (CRSD). *Sleep Med Rev*, **6**, 45–54.

Davidson, A.J., Sellix, M.T., Daniel, J., Yamazaki, S., Menaker, M. & Block, G.D. (2006). Chronic jet-lag increases mortality in aged mice. *Curr Biol*, **16**, R914–R916.

Desai, A.V., Ellis, E., Wheatley, J.R. & Grunstein, R.R. (2003). Fatal distraction: a case series of fatal fall-asleep road accidents and their medicolegal outcomes. *Med J Aust*, **178**, 396–399.

Dew, M.A., Hoch, C.C., Buysse, D.J., et al. (2003). Healthy older adults' sleep predicts all-cause mortality at 4 to 19 years of follow-up. *Psychosom Med*, **65**, 63–73.

Dhand, R. & Sohal, H. (2006). Good sleep, bad sleep! The role of daytime naps in healthy adults. *Curr Opin Pulm Med*, **12**, 379–382.

Doherty, L.S., Kiely, J.L., Swan, V. & McNicholas, W.T. (2005). Long-term effects of nasal continuous positive airway pressure therapy on cardiovascular outcomes in sleep apnea syndrome. *Chest*, **127**, 2076–2084.

Eaker, E.D., Pinsky, J. & Castelli, W.P. (1992). Myocardial infarction and coronary death among women: psychosocial predictors from a 20-year follow-up of women in the Framingham Study. *Am J Epidemiol*, **135**, 854–864.

Empana, J.P., Dauvilliers, Y., Dartigues, J.F., et al. (2009). Excessive daytime sleepiness is an independent risk indicator for cardiovascular mortality in community-dwelling elderly: the three city study. *Stroke*, **40**, 1219–1224.

Ferrie, J.E., Shipley, M.J., Cappuccio, F.P., et al. (2007). A prospective study of change in sleep duration: associations with mortality in the Whitehall II cohort. *Sleep*, **30**, 1659–1666.

Finger, S. (1994). *Origins of Neuroscience*. New York, NY: Oxford University Press.

Foley, D.J., Monjan, A.A., Brown, S.L., Simonsick, E.M., Wallace, R.B. & Blazer, D.G. (1995). Sleep complaints among elderly persons: an epidemiologic study of three communities. *Sleep*, **18**, 425–432.

Gale, C. & Martyn, C. (1998). Larks and owls and health, wealth, and wisdom. *Br Med J*, **317**, 1675–1677.

Gallicchio, L. & Kalesan, B. (2009). Sleep duration and mortality: a systematic review and meta-analysis. *J Sleep Res*, **18**, 148–158.

Ganguli, M., Reynolds, C.F. & Gilby, J.E. (1996). Prevalence and persistence of sleep complaints in a rural older community sample: the MoVIES project. *J Am Geriatr Soc*, **44**, 778–784.

Gangwisch, J.E., Heymsfield, S.B., Boden-Albala, B., et al. (2008). Sleep duration associated with mortality in elderly, but not middle-aged, adults in a large US sample. *Sleep*, **31**, 1087–1096.

Garcia-Touchard, A., Somers, V.K., Olson, L.J. & Caples, S.M. (2008). Central sleep apnea: implications for congestive heart failure. *Chest*, **133**, 1495–1504.

Gervacio-Domingo, G., Punzalan, F.E., Amarillo, M.L. & Dans, A. (2007). Sudden unexplained death during sleep occurred commonly in the general population in the Philippines: a sub study of the National Nutrition and Health Survey. *J Clin Epidemiol*, **60**, 567–571.

Goh, K.T., Chao, T.C. & Chew, C.H. (1990). Sudden nocturnal deaths among Thai construction workers in Singapore. *Lancet*, **335**, 1154.

Gonzalez-Rothi, R.J. & Block, A.J. (1988a). Mortality and sleep apnea. The trouble with looking backward. *Chest*, **94**, 678–679.

Gonzalez-Rothi, R.J., Foresman, G.E. & Block, A.J. (1988b). Do patients with sleep apnea die in their sleep? *Chest*, **94**, 531–538.

Goto, A., Yasumura, S., Nishise, Y. & Sakihara, S. (2003). Association of health behavior and social role with total mortality among Japanese elders in Okinawa, Japan. *Aging Clin Exp Res*, **15**, 443–450.

Grandner, M.A. & Drummond, S.P. (2007). Who are the long sleepers? Towards an understanding of the mortality relationship. *Sleep Med Rev*, **11**, 341–360.

Gustavsen, I., Bramness, J.G., Skurtveit, S., Engeland, A., Neutel, I. & Morland, J. (2008). Road traffic accident risk related to prescriptions of the hypnotics zopiclone, zolpidem, flunitrazepam and nitrazepam. *Sleep Med*, **9**, 818–822.

Hammond, E.C. (1964). Some preliminary findings on physical complaints from a prospective study of 1,064,004 men and women. *Am J Public Health*, **54**, 11–23.

Hanly, P.J. & Zuberi-Khokhar, N.S. (1996). Increased mortality associated with Cheyne-Stokes respiration in patients with congestive heart failure. *Am J Respir Crit Care Med*, **153**, 272–276.

Hausken, A.M., Skurtveit, S. & Tverdal, A. (2007). Use of anxiolytic or hypnotic drugs and total mortality in a general middle-aged population. *Pharmacoepidemiol Drug Saf*, **16**, 913–918.

Hays, J.C., Blazer, D.G. & Foley, D.J. (1996). Risk of napping: excessive daytime sleepiness and mortality in an older community population. *J Am Geriatr Soc*, **44**, 693–698.

He, J., Kryger, M.H., Zorick, F.J., Conway, W. & Roth, T. (1988). Mortality and apnea index in obstructive sleep apnea. Experience in 385 male patients. *Chest*, **94**, 9–14.

Heslop, P., Smith, G.D., Metcalfe, C., Macleod, J. & Hart, C. (2002). Sleep duration and mortality: the effect of short or long sleep duration on cardiovascular and all-cause mortality in working men and women. *Sleep Med*, **3**, 305–314.

Horne, J.A. & Reyner, L.A. (1995). Sleep related vehicle accidents. *Br Med J*, **310**, 565–567.

Horne, J. & Reyner, L. (1999). Vehicle accidents related to sleep: a review. *Occup Environ Med*, **56**, 289–294.

Hornyak, M. & Trenkwalder, C. (2004). Restless legs syndrome and periodic limb movement disorder in the elderly. *J Psychosom Res*, **56**, 543–548.

Hu, F.B., Willett, W.C., Manson, J.E., et al. (2000). Snoring and risk of cardiovascular disease in women. *J Am Coll Cardiol*, **35**, 308–313.

Hublin, C., Partinen, M., Koskenvuo, M. & Kaprio, J. (2007). Sleep and mortality: a population-based 22-year follow-up study. *Sleep*, **30**, 1245–1253.

Huppert, F.A. & Whittington, J.E. (1995). Symptoms of psychological distress predict 7-year mortality. *Psychol Med*, **25**, 1073–1086.

Ikehara, S., Iso, H., Date, C., et al. (2009). Association of sleep duration with mortality from cardiovascular disease and other causes for Japanese men and women: the JACC study. *Sleep*, **32**, 295–301.

International Classification of Sleep Disorders, Version 2 (2005). *Diagnostic and Coding Manual*. Rochester, MN: American Academy of Sleep Medicine.

Isacson, D., Carsjo, K., Bergman, U. & Blackburn, J.L. (1992). Long-term use of benzodiazepines in a Swedish community: an eight-year follow-up. *J Clin Epidemiol*, **45**, 429–436.

Javaheri, S., Shukla, R., Zeigler, H. & Wexler, L. (2007). Central sleep apnea, right ventricular dysfunction, and low diastolic blood pressure are predictors of mortality in systolic heart failure. *J Am Coll Cardiol*, **49**, 2028–2034.

Jenkins, C.D., Stanton, B.A., Niemcryk, S.J. & Rose, R.M. (1988). A scale for the estimation of sleep problems in clinical research. *J Clin Epidemiol*, **41**, 313–321.

Jennum, P., Hein, H.O., Suadicani, P. & Gyntelberg, F. (1995). Risk of ischemic heart disease in self-reported snorers. A prospective study of 2,937 men aged 54 to 74 years: the Copenhagen Male Study. *Chest*, **108**, 138–142.

Jensen, E., Dehlin, O., Hagberg, B., Samuelsson, G. & Svensson, T. (1998). Insomnia in an 80-year-old population: relationship to medical, psychological and social factors. *J Sleep Res*, **7**, 183–189.

Kaplan, G.A., Seeman, T.E., Cohen, R.D., Knudsen, L.P. & Guralnik, J. (1987). Mortality among the elderly in the Alameda County Study: behavioral and demographic risk factors. *Am J Public Health*, **77**, 307–312.

Khassawneh, B.Y. (2006). Periodic limb movement disorder. In: Lee-Chiong, T. (ed.), *Sleep: A Comprehensive Handbook*. Hoboken, NJ: John Wiley & Sons, pp. 483–486.

Kojima, M., Wakai, K., Kawamura, T., et al. (2000). Sleep patterns and total mortality: a 12-year follow-up study in Japan. *J Epidemiol*, **10**, 87–93.

Koskenvuo, M., Kaprio, J., Telakivi, T., Partinen, M., Heikkila, K. & Sarna, S. (1987). Snoring as a risk factor for ischaemic heart disease and stroke in men. *Br Med J (Clin Res Ed)*, **294**, 16–19.

Kripke, D.F. (2004). Do we sleep too much? *Sleep*, **27**, 13–14.

Kripke, D.F. (2009). Do hypnotics cause death and cancer? The burden of proof. *Sleep Med*, **10**, 275–276.

Kripke, D.F., Simons, R.N., Garfinkel, L. & Hammond, E.C. (1979). Short and long sleep and sleeping pills. Is increased mortality associated? *Arch Gen Psychiatry*, **36**, 103–116.

Kripke, D.F., Klauber, M.R., Wingard, D.L., Fell, R.L., Assmus, J.D. & Garfinkel, L. (1998). Mortality hazard associated with prescription hypnotics. *Biol Psychiatry*, **43**, 687–693.

Kripke, D.F., Garfinkel, L., Wingard, D.L., Klauber, M.R. & Marler, M.R. (2002). Mortality associated with sleep duration and insomnia. *Arch Gen Psychiatry*, **59**, 131–136.

Kronholm, E., Partonen, T., Laatikainen, T., et al. (2008). Trends in self-reported sleep duration and insomnia-related symptoms in Finland from 1972 to 2005: a comparative review and re-analysis of Finnish population samples. *J Sleep Res*, **17**, 54–62.

Lan, T.Y., Lan, T.H., Wen, C.P., Lin, Y.H. & Chuang, Y.L. (2007). Nighttime sleep, Chinese afternoon nap, and mortality in the elderly. *Sleep*, **30**, 1105–1110.

Lanfranchi, P.A., Braghiroli, A., Bosimini, E., et al. (1999). Prognostic value of nocturnal Cheyne-Stokes respiration in chronic heart failure. *Circulation*, **99**, 1435–1440.

Lavie, P., Herer, P., Peled, R., et al. (1995). Mortality in sleep apnea patients: a multivariate analysis of risk factors. *Sleep*, **18**, 149–157.

Levy, P., Pepin, J.L., Arnaud, C., et al. (2008). Intermittent hypoxia and sleep-disordered breathing: current concepts and perspectives. *Eur Respir J*, **32**, 1082–1095.

Lichstein, K.L., Durrance, H.H., Riedel, B.W., Taylor, D.J. & Bush, A.J. (2004). *Epidemiology of Sleep: Age, Gender, and Ethnicity*. Mahwah, NJ: Lawrence Erlbaum Associates.

Lindberg, E., Janson, C., Svardsudd, K., Gislason, T., Hetta, J. & Boman, G. (1998). Increased mortality among sleepy snorers: a prospective population based study. *Thorax*, **53**, 631–637.

Mahgoub, N.A. (2009). Insomnia and suicide risk. *J Neuropsychiatry Clin Neurosci*, **21**, 232–233.

Mallon, L., Broman, J.E. & Hetta, J. (2000). Relationship between insomnia, depression, and mortality: a 12-year follow-up of older adults in the community. *Int Psychogeriatr*, **12**, 295–306.

Mallon, L., Broman, J.E. & Hetta, J. (2002). Sleep complaints predict coronary artery disease mortality in males: a 12-year follow-up study of a middle-aged Swedish population. *J Intern Med*, **251**, 207–216.

Mallon, L., Broman, J.E. & Hetta, J. (2008). Restless legs symptoms with sleepiness in relation to mortality: 20-year follow-up study of a middle-aged Swedish population. *Psychiatry Clin Neurosci*, **62**, 457–463.

Mallon, L., Broman, J.E. & Hetta, J. (2009). Is usage of hypnotics associated with mortality? *Sleep Med*, **10**, 279–286.

Manabe, K., Matsui, T., Yamaya, M., et al. (2000). Sleep patterns and mortality among elderly patients in a geriatric hospital. *Gerontology*, **46**, 318–322.

Mant, A., King, M., Saunders, N.A., Pond, C.D., Goode, E. & Hewitt, H. (1995). Four-year follow-up of mortality and sleep-related respiratory disturbance in non-demented seniors. *Sleep*, **18**, 433–438.

Marin, J.M., Carrizo, S.J., Vicente, E. & Agusti, A.G. (2005). Long-term cardiovascular outcomes in men with obstructive sleep apnoea-hypopnoea with or without treatment with continuous positive airway pressure: an observational study. *Lancet*, **365**, 1046–1053.

Marshall, N.S., Wong, K.K., Liu, P.Y., Cullen, S.R., Knuiman, M.W. & Grunstein, R.R. (2008). Sleep apnea as an independent risk factor for all-cause mortality: the Busselton Health Study. *Sleep*, **31**, 1079–1085.

Marti, S., Sampol, G., Munoz, X., et al. (2002). Mortality in severe sleep apnoea/hypopnoea syndrome patients: impact of treatment. *Eur Respir J*, **20**, 1511–1518.

Masa, J.F., Rubio, M. & Findley, L.J. (2000). Habitually sleepy drivers have a high frequency of automobile crashes associated with respiratory disorders during sleep. *Am J Respir Crit Care Med*, **162**, 1407–1412.

Montplaisir, J., Boucher, S., Poirier, G., Lavigne, G., Lapierre, O. & Lesperance, P. (1997). Clinical, polysomnographic, and genetic characteristics of restless legs syndrome: a study of 133 patients diagnosed with new standard criteria. *Mov Disord*, **12**, 61–65.

Mooe, T., Franklin, K.A., Holmstrom, K., Rabben, T. & Wiklund, U. (2001). Sleep-disordered breathing and coronary artery disease: long-term prognosis. *Am J Respir Crit Care Med*, **164**, 1910–1913.

Naska, A., Oikonomou, E., Trichopoulou, A., Psaltopoulou, T. & Trichopoulos, D. (2007). Siesta in healthy adults and coronary mortality in the general population. *Arch Intern Med*, **167**, 296–301.

Neubauer, D.N. (2007). The evolution and development of insomnia pharmacotherapies. *J Clin Sleep Med*, 3(5 Suppl), S11–S15.

Neutel, C.I. & Patten, S.B. (1997). Risk of suicide attempts after benzodiazepine and/or antidepressant use. *Ann Epidemiol*, 7, 568–574.

Newman, A.B., Spiekerman, C.F., Enright, P., et al. (2000). Daytime sleepiness predicts mortality and cardiovascular disease in older adults. The Cardiovascular Health Study Research Group. *J Am Geriatr Soc*, 48, 115–123.

Nilsson, P.M., Nilsson, J.A., Hedblad, B. & Berglund, G. (2001). Sleep disturbance in association with elevated pulse rate for prediction of mortality—consequences of mental strain? *J Intern Med*, 250, 521–529.

Noda, A., Okada, T., Yasuma, F., Sobue, T., Nakashima, N. & Yokota, M. (1998). Prognosis of the middle-aged and aged patients with obstructive sleep apnea syndrome. *Psychiatry Clin Neurosci*, 52, 79–85.

Ohayon, M.M. (2005). Insomnia: a dangerous condition but not a killer? *Sleep*, 28, 1043–1044.

Ohayon, M.M. & Roth, T. (2002). Prevalence of restless legs syndrome and periodic limb movement disorder in the general population. *J Psychosom Res*, 53, 547–554.

Ohayon, M.M., Guilleminault, C. & Priest, R.G. (1999). Night terrors, sleepwalking, and confusional arousals in the general population: their frequency and relationship to other sleep and mental disorders. *J Clin Psychiatry*, 60, 268–276.

Oyefeso, A., Schifano, F., Ghodse, H., Cobain, K., Dryden, R. & Corkery, J. (2006). Fatal injuries while under the influence of psychoactive drugs: a cross-sectional exploratory study in England. *BMC Public Health*, 6, 148.

Pack, A.I., Pack, A.M., Rodgman, E., Cucchiara, A., Dinges, D.F. & Schwab, C.W. (1995). Characteristics of crashes attributed to the driver having fallen asleep. *Accid Anal Prev*, 27, 769–775.

Pack, A.I., Platt, A.B. & Pien, G.W. (2008). Does untreated obstructive sleep apnea lead to death? A commentary on Young et al., *Sleep* 2008;31:1071–1078 and Marshall et al., *Sleep* 2008;31:1079–1085. *Sleep*, 31, 1067–1068.

Parrish, R.G., Tucker, M., Ing, R., Encarnacion, C. & Eberhardt, M. (1987). Sudden unexplained death syndrome in Southeast Asian refugees: a review of CDC surveillance. *MMWR CDC Surveill Summ*, 36, 43SS–53SS.

Partinen, M., Jamieson, A. & Guilleminault, C. (1988). Long-term outcome for obstructive sleep apnea syndrome patients. Mortality. *Chest*, 94, 1200–1204.

Patel, S.R. (2007). Is siesta more beneficial than nocturnal sleep? *Arch Intern Med*, 167, 2143–2144.

Patel, S.R. (2009). Sleep—an affair of the heart. *Sleep*, 32, 289–290.

Patel, S.R., Ayas, N.T., Malhotra, M.R., et al. (2004). A prospective study of sleep duration and mortality risk in women. *Sleep*, 27, 440–444.

Peker, Y., Hedner, J., Kraiczi, H. & Loth, S. (2000). Respiratory disturbance index: an independent predictor of mortality in coronary artery disease. *Am J Respir Crit Care Med*, 162, 81–86.

Phillips, B. & Mannino, D.M. (2005). Does insomnia kill? *Sleep*, 28, 965–971.

Pollak, C.P., Perlick, D., Linsner, J.P., Wenston, J. & Hsieh, F. (1990). Sleep problems in the community elderly as predictors of death and nursing home placement. *J Community Health*, 15, 123–135.

Powell, N.B., Schechtman, K.B., Riley, R.W., Guilleminault, C., Chiang, R.P. & Weaver, E.M. (2007). Sleepy driver near-misses may predict accident risks. *Sleep*, 30, 331–342.

Radun, I. & Summala, H. (2004). Sleep-related fatal vehicle accidents: characteristics of decisions made by multidisciplinary investigation teams. *Sleep*, 27, 224–227.

Reynolds, C.F., III, Buysse, D.J. & Kupfer, D.J. (1999). Treating insomnia in older adults: taking a long-term view. *JAMA*, 281, 1034–1035.

Richardson, G.S. (2006). Shift work sleep disorder. In: Lee-Chiong, T. (ed.), *Sleep: A Comprehensive Handbook*. Hoboken, NJ: John Wiley & Sons, pp. 395–399.

Rockwood, K., Davis, H.S., Merry, H.R., MacKnight, C. & McDowell, I. (2001). Sleep disturbances and mortality: results from the Canadian Study of Health and Aging. *J Am Geriatr Soc*, **49**, 639–641.

Rodenstein, D. (2008). Driving in Europe: the need of a common policy for drivers with obstructive sleep apnoea syndrome. *J Sleep Res*, **17**, 281–284.

Roebuck, T., Solin, P., Kaye, D.M., Bergin, P., Bailey, M. & Naughton, M.T. (2004). Increased long-term mortality in heart failure due to sleep apnoea is not yet proven. *Eur Respir J*, **23**, 735–740.

Rosa, R.R. (2006). Sleep loss, sleepiness, performance, and safety. In: Lee-Chiong, T. (ed.), *Sleep: A Comprehensive Handbook*. Hoboken, NJ: Wiley-Liss, pp. 203–207.

Ruigomez, A., Alonso, J. & Anto, J.M. (1995). Relationship of health behaviours to five-year mortality in an elderly cohort. *Age Ageing*, **24**, 113–119.

Rumble, R. & Morgan, K. (1992). Hypnotics, sleep, and mortality in elderly people. *J Am Geriatr Soc*, **40**, 787–791.

Sahlin, C., Sandberg, O., Gustafson, Y., et al. (2008). Obstructive sleep apnea is a risk factor for death in patients with stroke: a 10-year follow-up. *Arch Intern Med*, **168**, 297–301.

Seppala, T., Partinen, M., Penttila, A., Aspholm, R., Tiainen, E. & Kaukianen, A. (1991). Sudden death and sleeping history among Finnish men. *J Intern Med*, **229**, 23–28.

Shankar, A., Koh, W.P., Yuan, J.M., Lee, H.P. & Yu, M.C. (2008). Sleep duration and coronary heart disease mortality among Chinese adults in Singapore: a population-based cohort study. *Am J Epidemiol*, **168**, 1367–1373.

Signal, T.L., Gale, J. & Gander, P.H. (2005). Sleep measurement in flight crew: comparing actigraphic and subjective estimates to polysomnography. *Aviat Space Environ Med*, **76**, 1058–1063.

Sin, D.D., Logan, A.G., Fitzgerald, F.S., Liu, P.P. & Bradley, T.D. (2000). Effects of continuous positive airway pressure on cardiovascular outcomes in heart failure patients with and without Cheyne-Stokes respiration. *Circulation*, **102**, 61–66.

Stone, K.L., Ewing, S.K., Ancoli-Israel, S., et al. (2009). Self-reported sleep and nap habits and risk of mortality in a large cohort of older women. *J Am Geriatr Soc*, **57**, 604–611.

Suzuki, E., Yorifuji, T., Ueshima, K., et al. (2009). Sleep duration, sleep quality and cardiovascular disease mortality among the elderly: a population based cohort study. *Prev Med*, **49**, 135–141.

Takahashi, K. & Kaida, K. (2006). Napping. In: Lee-Chiong, T. (ed.), *Sleep: A Comprehensive Handbook*. Hoboken, NJ: John Wiley & Sons, pp. 197–201.

Tamakoshi, A. & Ohno, Y. (2004). Self-reported sleep duration as a predictor of all-cause mortality: results from the JACC study, Japan. *Sleep*, **27**, 51–54.

Taylor, D.J., Lichstein, K.L. & Durrence, H.H. (2003). Insomnia as a health risk factor. *Behav Sleep Med*, **1**, 227–247.

Teran-Santos, J., Jimenez-Gomez, A. & Cordero-Guevara, J. (1999). The association between sleep apnea and the risk of traffic accidents. Cooperative Group Burgos-Santander. *N Engl J Med*, **340**, 847–851.

Tsubono, Y., Fukao, A. & Hisamichi, S. (1993). Health practices and mortality in a rural Japanese population. *Tohoku J Exp Med*, **171**, 339–348.

Vgontzas, A.N. & Kales, A. (1999). Sleep and its disorders. *Annu Rev Med*, **50**, 387–400.

Wang, H., Parker, J.D., Newton, G.E., et al. (2007). Influence of obstructive sleep apnea on mortality in patients with heart failure. *J Am Coll Cardiol*, **49**, 1625–1631.

WHO Media Centre (2006). Fact sheet N°259: African trypanosomiasis or sleeping sickness.

Yaggi, H.K., Concato, J., Kernan, W.N., Lichtman, J.H., Brass, L.M. & Mohsenin, V. (2005). Obstructive sleep apnea as a risk factor for stroke and death. *N Engl J Med*, **353**, 2034–2041.

Young, T., Blustein, J., Finn, L. & Palta, M. (1997). Sleep-disordered breathing and motor vehicle accidents in a population-based sample of employed adults. *Sleep*, **20**, 608–613.

Young, T., Finn, L., Peppard, P.E., et al. (2008). Sleep disordered breathing and mortality: eighteen-year follow-up of the Wisconsin sleep cohort. *Sleep*, **31**, 1071–1078.

Youngstedt, S.D. & Kripke, D.F. (2004). Long sleep and mortality: rationale for sleep restriction. *Sleep Med Rev*, **8**, 159–174.

Yumino, D., Wang, H., Floras, J.S., et al. (2009). Relationship between sleep apnoea and mortality in patients with ischaemic heart failure. *Heart*, **95**, 819–824.

Zee, P.C. & Turek, F.W. (2006). Sleep and health: everywhere and in both directions. *Arch Intern Med*, **166**, 1686–1688.

Chapter 5

The epidemiology of sleep and cardiovascular risk and disease

F.P. Cappuccio and M.A. Miller

Introduction

Sleep patterns of quantity and quality are affected by a variety of cultural, social, psychological, behavioural, pathophysiological, and environmental influences. Changes in the modern society include longer working hours, more shift-work, and 24/7 availability of commodities. These changes have been paralleled by secular trends of curtailed duration of sleep to fewer hours per day across westernized populations (Åkerstedt and Nilsson, 2003). This has led to increased reporting of fatigue, tiredness, and excessive daytime sleepiness (EDS) (Bliwise, 1996). Lack of sleep exerts deleterious effects on a variety of systems with detectable changes in metabolic (Knutson et al., 2007; Spiegel et al., 2009), endocrine (Spiegel et al., 1999; Taheri et al., 2004), and immune pathways (Miller and Cappuccio, 2007).

One of the most significant developments in the field of epidemiology and sleep medicine has been the growing evidence that not only are sleep-related breathing disorders, such as obstructive sleep apnoea syndrome (OSAS), contributing factors for the development of cardiovascular disease (CVD), but more importantly from a societal perspective that variations of quantity and quality of sleep may also be risk factors for, or markers of, CVD. This notion is gathering momentum and it adds to the better known relationships of CVD as a cause of sleep disorders. The present chapter summarizes the wealth of recent evidence to support the epidemiological link between quantity of sleep (short and long duration of sleep) and quality of sleep (like difficulties in falling asleep or of maintaining sleep) and both fatal and non-fatal cardiovascular outcomes, like myocardial infarction (MI) and stroke, and cardiovascular risk factors, namely hypertension, obesity, type 2 diabetes and other disturbances of glucose metabolism, and lipids. There will be reference to gender differences in the risk, to the meaning of U-shaped relationships, particularly as the associations between short and long duration of sleep with cardiovascular risk may reflect different pathways, and to potential mechanisms.

The epidemiology of sleep

Sleep problems and sleep restriction are popular topics of discussion, but until recently there have been few data available on representative population samples. A British study based on a nationally representative sample of 16–93 years old, who participated in 1997 in face-to-face interviews, provides a descriptive picture of the basic epidemiology of sleep (Groeger et al., 2004).

More than half of respondents reported sleep problems on one or more nights the previous week and 18% reported that the sleep they obtained was insufficient on the majority of nights. Sleep durations were longest in the youngest participants (16–24 years), who slept on average 1 hour longer than the 7.04 hour sample average. Sleep duration showed no appreciable change beyond middle age. Men and women reported sleeping similar amounts but women reported more sleep problems. Men reported sleeping less when there were more children in their household. Participants in regular employment reported sleeping less on workdays than on non-workdays, but those based at home and those not employed did not. Inability to switch off from work was related to sleep duration on non-workdays. Across all participants average sleep duration exhibited a non-linear association with quality of life (QOL) (i.e. contribution of sleep to energy, satisfaction and success in work, home and leisure activities). QOL was positively associated with sleep duration, for durations up to 9 hours, but negatively associated with QOL beyond this. Comparison with the US National Sleep Poll suggests that Britain sleeps as little or less. In conclusion, when we report sleeping less we also tend to associate that lack of sleep with poor performance and QOL.

Both long and short sleep durations have been associated with negative health outcomes. This is true in young, middle-aged, and older adults. Using anonymous questionnaires, Steptoe et al. (2006) collected data from 17,465 university students aged 17–30 years who were taking non–health-related courses at 27 universities in 24 countries worldwide. Sleep duration was measured by self-report, the health outcome was self-rated health, and a number of confounders were also controlled for. Sixty-three percent of respondents slept for 7–8 hours; 21% were short sleepers (6%, <6 hours; 15%, 6–7 hours); and 16% were long sleepers (10%, 8–10 hours; 6%, >10 hours) (Fig. 5.1).

The proportion of people reporting ill-health increased significantly in those who reported sleeping <6 hours per night.

Compared with the reference category (7–8 hours), the adjusted odds ratio (OR) of poor health was 1.56 (95% confidence interval [CI]: 1.22–1.99) for respondents sleeping 6–7 hours and 1.99 (95% CI: 1.31–3.03) for those sleeping <6 hours. The same significant pattern was seen when the results were analyzed separately by sex. Interestingly, the short sleepers were predominantly from

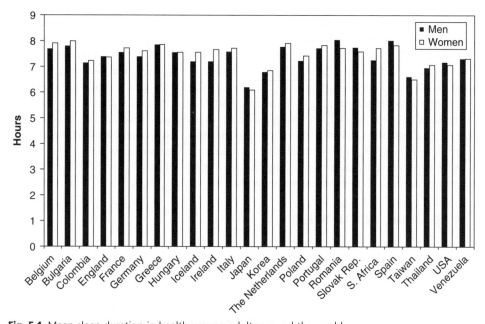

Fig. 5.1 Mean sleep duration in healthy young adults around the world.
Source: Re-drawn from Steptoe, A., Peacey, V. & Wardle, J. (2006). Sleep duration and health in young adults. *Arch Intern Med*, **166**(16), 1689–1692.

East Asian countries (i.e. Japan, Korea, Taiwan, and Thailand) (Fig. 5.2), indicating the possibility of cultural and behavioural patterns. There were no significant associations between self-rated health and long sleep duration. Short sleep may be more of a concern than long sleep in young adults.

The relationship between sleep disturbances and poor health, however, changes in later life. This is reflected in the unambiguous association with health outcomes, including all-cause mortality. Chapter 4 has described in detail the association between both short and long sleep with all-cause mortality. A recent meta-analysis (Cappuccio et al., 2010b) has quantified such relationship pooling numerous cohort studies involving more than 1.3 million participants and over 110,000 deaths. Short duration of sleep was associated with a greater risk of death (relative risk [RR]: 1.12; 95% CI: 1.06–1.18; $P < 0.01$) with no evidence of publication bias (Fig. 5.3).

Long duration of sleep was also associated with a greater risk of death (RR: 1.30; 95% CI: 1.22–1.38; $P < 0.0001$) with no evidence of publication bias (Fig. 5.4).

There was some indication that the mean effects for both short and long duration of sleep were stronger in studies carried out in East Asia, predominantly Japan (Cappuccio et al., 2010b). The explanations may be different. For short sleep, some cross-cultural comparisons have shown that the average duration of sleep is shorter in countries of East Asia, possibly as a result of societal pressures. For long sleep, the stronger association with mortality may, at least in part, be the result of longer life expectancy in countries like Japan compared to Europe and the United States. It is likely that the shape of the relationship between sleep duration and mortality is heavily influenced by deaths in elderly participants. This view is supported by a stronger effect of long duration of sleep on all-cause mortality in older cohorts (>60 years) (Cappuccio et al., 2010b).

In conclusion, both short and long duration of sleep are significant predictors of all-cause mortality.

The epidemiology of cardiovascular diseases

Cardiovascular diseases (including coronary heart disease [CHD], stroke, and heart failure) are the major cause of death and disability among people aged over 60 years, and second among those aged 15–59 years. Below is a brief summary of the epidemiology of CVD and related global health statistics.

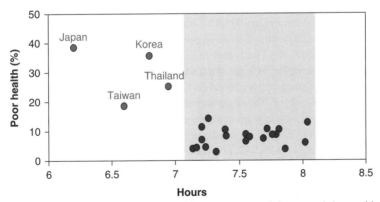

Fig. 5.2 Sleep duration and self-rated health problems in young adults around the world. *Source*: Re-drawn from Steptoe, A., Peacey, V. & Wardle, J. (2006). Sleep duration and health in young adults. *Arch Intern Med*, **166**(16), 1689–1692.

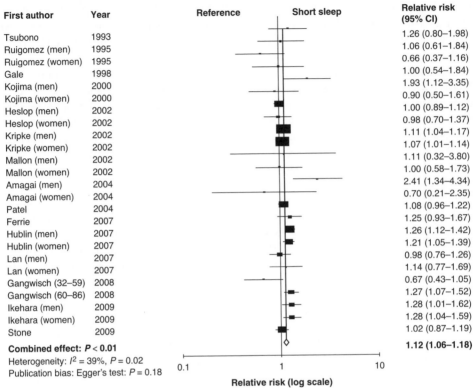

Fig. 5.3 Forest plot of the risk of all-cause mortality amongst people with short duration of sleep in a meta-analysis of prospective population-based study including 1,381,324 participants with 112,324 events.

Source: Re-drawn from Cappuccio, F.P., D'Elia, L., Strazzullo, P. & Miller, M.A. (2010b). Sleep duration and all-cause mortality: a systematic review and meta-analysis of prospective studies. *Sleep*, **33**(5), 585–592.

Burden

According to the WHO estimates in 2003, 16.7 million people around the globe die of CVD each year. This is over 29% of all deaths globally. Eighty percent of chronic disease deaths occur in low and middle income countries and half are women. CVD alone will kill five times as many people as HIV/AIDS in these countries. At least 20 million people survive heart attacks and strokes every year; many require continuing costly clinical care. CVD accounted for more than 216,000 deaths in the United Kingdom in 2004. Thirty-seven percent of deaths are from CVD, and 32% of premature deaths in men and 24% in women are from CVD. Each year CVD causes over 4.35 million deaths in Europe and over 1.9 million deaths in the EU. CVD causes nearly half of all deaths in Europe (49%) and in the EU (42%). CVD is the main cause of death in women in all countries of Europe and is the main cause of death in men in all countries except France and San Marino. CVD is the main cause of years of life lost from early death in Europe and the EU—around a third of years of life lost are due to CVD. Mortality rates for CHD and acute myocardial infarction (AMI) continue to decrease, but mortality rates for stroke have not changed significantly during

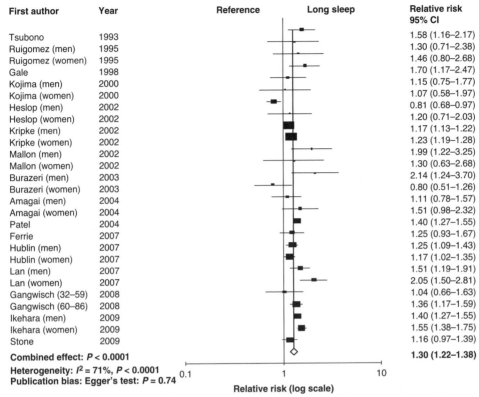

First author	Year	Reference	Long sleep	Relative risk 95% CI
Tsubono	1993			1.58 (1.16–2.17)
Ruigomez (men)	1995			1.30 (0.71–2.38)
Ruigomez (women)	1995			1.46 (0.80–2.68)
Gale	1998			1.70 (1.17–2.47)
Kojima (men)	2000			1.15 (0.75–1.77)
Kojima (women)	2000			1.07 (0.58–1.97)
Heslop (men)	2002			0.81 (0.68–0.97)
Heslop (women)	2002			1.20 (0.71–2.03)
Kripke (men)	2002			1.17 (1.13–1.22)
Kripke (women)	2002			1.23 (1.19–1.28)
Mallon (men)	2002			1.99 (1.22–3.25)
Mallon (women)	2002			1.30 (0.63–2.68)
Burazeri (men)	2003			2.14 (1.24–3.70)
Burazeri (women)	2003			0.80 (0.51–1.26)
Amagai (men)	2004			1.11 (0.78–1.57)
Amagai (women)	2004			1.51 (0.98–2.32)
Patel	2004			1.40 (1.27–1.55)
Ferrie	2007			1.25 (0.93–1.67)
Hublin (men)	2007			1.25 (1.09–1.43)
Hublin (women)	2007			1.17 (1.02–1.35)
Lan (men)	2007			1.51 (1.19–1.91)
Lan (women)	2007			2.05 (1.50–2.81)
Gangwisch (32–59)	2008			1.04 (0.66–1.63)
Gangwisch (60–86)	2008			1.36 (1.17–1.59)
Ikehara (men)	2009			1.40 (1.27–1.55)
Ikehara (women)	2009			1.55 (1.38–1.75)
Stone	2009			1.16 (0.97–1.39)
Combined effect: *P* < 0.0001				**1.30 (1.22–1.38)**

Heterogeneity: I^2 = 71%, *P* < 0.0001
Publication bias: Egger's test: *P* = 0.74

0.1   1   10
Relative risk (log scale)

Fig. 5.4 Forest plot of the risk of all-cause mortality amongst people with long duration of sleep in a meta-analysis of prospective population-based study including 1,382,999 participants with 112,566 events.
Source: Re-drawn from Cappuccio, F.P., D'Elia, L., Strazzullo, P. & Miller, M.A. (2010b). Sleep duration and all-cause mortality: a systematic review and meta-analysis of prospective studies. *Sleep*, **33**(5), 585–592.

the past 10 years. As a result of population ageing, the number of deaths due to stroke and CHD has increased. This trend is expected to continue for the next 15 years.

Risk factors

A number of traditional risk factors are considered singly as long-term causes of morbidity, disability, and mortality from CVD. The most important are: high serum cholesterol, high blood pressure, smoking, obesity, and diabetes. It is beyond the scope of this book to expand on these factors. We refer to Marmot and Elliott (2005) for a full account.

High blood cholesterol

Circulating blood cholesterol levels predict CVD (CHD, stroke, and other vascular events) and their lowering (whether with diet or with drugs) reduces the risk. A blood cholesterol level <5.0 mmol/L is recommended for both primary and secondary prevention of CHD. About 66% of men and women in the United Kingdom have blood cholesterol levels >5.0 mmol/L. High-density lipoprotein (HDL)-cholesterol level for men aged 16 and above in England is 1.4 mmol/L and for women 1.6 mmol/L. Overall, about 6% of men and 2% of women have HDL-cholesterol levels <1.0 mmol/L.

Hypertension

High blood pressure or hypertension is an important cause of stroke and other CVDs. Blood pressure reduction through both non-pharmacological means and drug therapy reduces the risk significantly. In England, 34% of men and 30% of women have hypertension (blood pressure 140/90 mmHg or higher) or are being treated for hypertension. About 78% of men and 67% of women with hypertension are not being treated. Of those being treated, just under 60% remain hypertensive. It has been estimated recently that the prevalence of hypertension will soar to 1.56 billion by the year 2025 (Kearney et al., 2005).

Smoking

There is a dose-dependent causal relationship between cigarette smoking and cardiovascular outcomes, reversible upon quitting. The number of smokers in the world is estimated at 1.3 billion. In Great Britain in 2004, 26% of men and 23% of women aged 16 and older smoked cigarettes. Mortality from CHD is 60% higher in smokers (and 80% higher in heavy smokers) than in non-smokers. In 2000, smoking caused about 14% of CVD deaths in men and 12% in women. According to the WHO, 1 year after quitting, the risk of CHD decreases by 50%. Within 15 years, the relative risk of dying from CHD for an ex-smoker approaches that of a long-time (lifetime) non-smoker. The WHO estimates that by 2020, tobacco is expected to be the single greatest cause of death and disability worldwide, accounting for about 10 million deaths per year. Smoking results in a 100% increase in the risk of stroke and CHD, and a 300% increase in the risk of death from undiagnosed CHD. Each year, smoking kills over 1.2 million people in Europe (450,000 from CVD) and about 650,000 people in the EU (185,000 from CVD).

Overweight and obesity

Using a body mass index (BMI) of 25–30 kg/m^2 as overweight, 44% of men and 35% of women in the United Kingdom are overweight. An additional 23% of men and 24% of women are obese (BMI > 30 kg/m^2). The International Obesity Task Force estimates that about 200 million of the 350 million adults living in the EU may be overweight or obese. From Greece to Germany, the proportion of overweight or obese men is higher than in the United States. Obesity is especially common in Mediterranean countries. Among the EU's 103 million children, the number of those overweight rises by 400,000 each year. The WHO estimates that if current trends continue, the number of overweight people globally will increase to 1.5 billion by 2015. Raised BMI is a major risk factor for heart disease, stroke, type 2 diabetes, and other chronic diseases. The WHO estimates that over the next 10 years, CVD—primarily CHD and stroke—will increase most notably in the regions of the Eastern Mediterranean and Africa, where CVD-related deaths are predicted to rise by over 25%.

Diabetes

The number of adults with diabetes in the world is estimated to be 170 million in 2000. It is estimated that just under 1.9 million people in the United Kingdom. have been diagnosed with diabetes (4% of men and 3% of women). An estimated additional 589,000 have undiagnosed diabetes, accounting for a total of 2.5 million adults. The rising prevalence of type 2 diabetes mellitus (T2DM) in children and adolescents was initially recognized in the United States in the 1990s. T2DM, which 15 years ago accounted for less than 3% of all cases of new-onset diabetes in children and adolescents, today accounts for up to 45% of new-onset cases among adolescents.

Over 48 million adults in Europe and 23 million adults in the EU have diabetes and the prevalence is increasing.

Metabolic syndrome

The metabolic syndrome (MetS) is a cluster of the most dangerous cardiovascular risk factors: diabetes or pre-diabetes, abdominal obesity, serum cholesterol, and high blood pressure. Although up to 80% of the almost 200 million adults worldwide with diabetes will die of CVD, people with MetS are also at increased risk, being twice as likely to die from and three times as likely to have a heart attack or stroke compared to people without the syndrome. Preliminary estimates suggest that 550,000 youngsters may be affected by MetS in the EU.

Energy balance and diet

In 2004, only 37% of men and 25% of women in the United Kingdom met the government's physical activity guidelines. In addition, in 2003 over one-third of adults were inactive. Levels of physical inactivity are high in many European countries. In 2003–2004, British adults derived between 36% and 37% of their food energy (calories) from total fat and between 14% and 15% from saturated fat. About 13% of men and 15% of women consume the recommended five or more portions of fruits and vegetables daily. Among British children ages 4–11 the average food energy derived from fat is 35.4% for boys and 35.9% for girls. The total worldwide mortality currently attributable to inadequate consumption of fruits and vegetables is estimated to be up to 2.635 million deaths per year. Increasing individual fruit and vegetable consumption to up to 600 g/day could reduce the total worldwide burden of disease by 1.8%, and reduce the burden of CHD and ischaemic stroke by 31% and 19%, respectively.[1]

Costs

Cardiovascular disease on average costs every EU citizen €230 in healthcare, but it led to 268.8 million lost working days, 2 million deaths, and 4.4 million whose daily lives were affected. Some 1.4 million people were involved in providing unpaid care to sufferers of CHD and stroke alone, which together account for 47% of costs and two-thirds of deaths (Leal et al., 2006).

Compared to 2000, the number of years of productive life lost to CVD will have increased in 2030 by only 20% in the United States and by 30% in Portugal. For Brazil the figure is 64%, 57% for China, and 95% for India. The increase in South Africa is 28%, greater than that for the United States and comparable to Portugal. Only in Russia does the number of years lost lag, largely because death rates are already at such high levels and the size of the population at risk is falling.

Coronary heart disease and heart failure

Projected global CHD deaths by sex, all ages, 2005, show that 53% are in men and 47% are in women. About 231,000 MIs occur annually in the United Kingdom (128,000 in men and 103,000 in women in 2004). It is estimated that almost 1.3 million people living in the United Kingdom have had a heart attack (870,000 men and 419,000 women). Overall, it is estimated that just over 1.5 million men and 1.1 million women who have had CHD (either heart attack or angina) are living in the United Kingdom.

---

[1] The above statistics are derived by the BHF Coronary Heart Disease Statistics (www.bhf.org.uk/profesionals/index.asp?secondlevel=519), Eurostat (europa.eu.int/en/comm./eurostat/eurostat.html), and WHO Statistical Information System (WHOSIS) (www.who.int/whosis/en).

The total prevalence of heart failure (definite and probable) in the United Kingdom is estimated at 912,000 in people aged 45 and older (506,000 men and 406,000 women). In 2002–2003, there were just under 30,000 coronary bypass procedures performed in the United Kingdom. In addition, 62,780 percutaneous coronary intervention (PCI) procedures were performed in 2004.

According to the WHO, in 2002 there were 7.22 million deaths from CHD globally. CHD alone is the most common cause of death in the United Kingdom, causing just under 105,000 deaths in 2004. One in five deaths of men and one in six deaths of women are from CHD. Other forms of heart disease cause more than 32,000 deaths. Total deaths from heart disease in the United Kingdom in 2004 were just over 137,500. The premature death rate from CHD for male manual workers is 58% higher than for non-manual workers. For female manual workers the death rate is more than twice as high as that for female non-manual workers. The WHO predicts 11.1 million deaths from CHD in 2020.

Stroke

According to the WHO estimates, 15 million people each year suffer strokes and 5 million are left permanently disabled. The WHO estimates 5.5 million deaths from stroke worldwide in 2002. Stroke accounts for a higher proportion of deaths among women than men (11% vs. 8.4%). Among women, 3 million deaths from stroke occur annually. In England, the death rates for stroke for people under 65 fell by 25% in the last 10 years. Recently, rates have declined at a slower rate, particularly in the younger age groups. Stroke killed 60,458 people in 2004 in the United Kingdom.

Socioeconomic consequences of CVD

Low socioeconomic status is associated with increased risk of CVD. CVD affects people in their peak mid-life years, disrupting the future of the families dependent on them and undermining the development of nations by depriving them of workers in their most productive years. In developed countries, lower socioeconomic groups have a greater prevalence of risk factors, higher incidence of disease, and higher disability and mortality. In developing countries, as the CVD epidemic matures, the burden will shift to the lower socioeconomic groups. CVD is estimated to cost the UK economy a total of £26 billion a year in direct and indirect costs. Overall CVD is estimated to cost the EU economy £169 billion a year. Of the total cost of CVD in the EU, around 62% is due to healthcare costs, 21% due to productivity losses, and 17% due to the informal care of people with CVD.

Sleep and coronary heart disease, stroke, and total cardiovascular disease

The relationship between duration of sleep and vascular events has been often described as a U-shaped association, although other studies have not found such a uniform effect or have found no association. It is believed that different mechanisms may underlie such associations at either end of the distribution of sleep duration. Given the variety of studies, the large differences in the types and sizes of populations examined, the duration of follow-up, and the size of the effects, it is difficult to draw immediate conclusions on the consistency of the associations at either end of the distribution of sleep duration and at its effect size. The latter is important in public health to ascertain the likely impact at population level, if amenable to modification.

A recent study systematically reviewed published prospective population-based studies, assessed whether the global evidence supports the presence of a relationship between either short or long

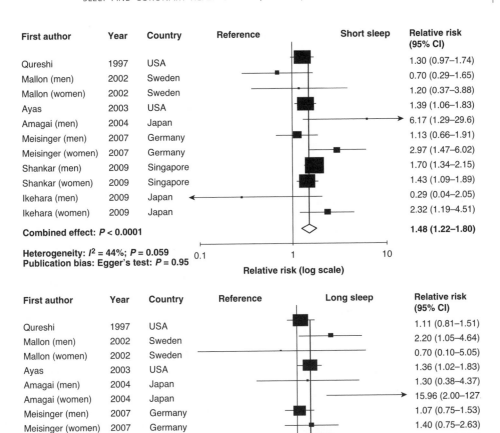

Fig. 5.5 Forest plot of the risk of developing or dying of CHD amongst short sleepers (top) and long sleepers (bottom). The meta-analysis of short sleepers includes 249,324 participants with 4,141 fatal and non-fatal CHD events. That of long sleepers includes 256,230 participants with 4,169 fatal and non-fatal CHD events.

duration of sleep and incidence of CHD, stroke, and total CVD and obtained a quantitative estimate of the risk. The study included only population-based prospective studies in adults with a follow-up period of more than 3 years. Twenty-four cohorts were included in the meta-analysis for three separate end-points, CHD, stroke, and CVD (all fatal and non-fatal). The analysis included 474,684 male and female participants (follow-up range 6.9–25 years), and 16,067 fatal and non-fatal events (4,169 for CHD, 3,478 for stroke, and 8,420 for total CVD).

Short duration of sleep was associated with greater risk of developing or dying of CHD (RR: 1.48; 95% CI: 1.22–1.80; $P < 0.0001$) with no evidence of publication bias (Fig. 5.5, top).

Long duration of sleep was also associated with greater risk of developing or dying of CHD (RR: 1.38; 95% CI: 1.15–1.66; $P = 0.0005$) with no evidence of publication bias (Fig. 5.5, bottom).

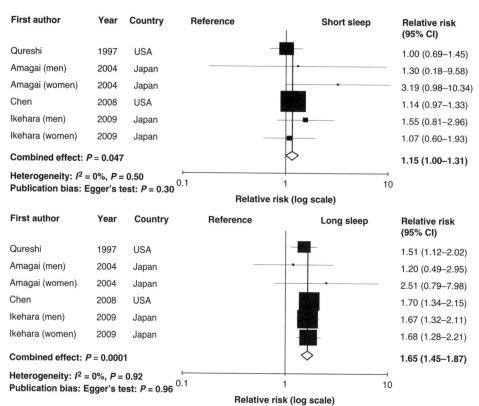

Fig. 5.6 Forest plot of the risk of developing or dying of stroke amongst short sleepers (top) and long sleepers (bottom). The meta-analysis of short sleepers includes 210,978 participants with 3,478 fatal and non-fatal stroke events. That of long sleepers includes 210,978 participants with 3,478 fatal and non-fatal stroke events.

Short duration of sleep was associated with greater risk of developing or dying of stroke (RR: 1.15; 95% CI: 1.00–1.31; $P = 0.047$) with no evidence of publication bias (Fig. 5.6, top).

Long duration of sleep was associated with greater risk of developing or dying of stroke (RR: 1.65; 95% CI: 1.45–1.87; $P < 0.0001$) with no evidence of publication bias (Fig. 5.6, bottom).

Short duration of sleep was weakly and not significantly associated with a greater risk of developing or dying of total CVD (RR: 1.03; 95% CI: 0.93–1.15; $P = 0.52$) with no evidence of publication bias ($P = 0.97$) (Fig. 5.7, top).

Long duration of sleep was associated with greater risk of developing or dying of total CVD (RR: 1.41; 95% CI: 1.19–1.68, $P < 0.0001$) with no evidence of publication bias (Fig. 5.7, bottom).

Obstructive sleep apnoea syndrome and cardiovascular disease

According to the latest Joint Expert Consensus Document of the American Heart Association and the American College of Cardiology (Somers et al., 2008), OSAS is a clinical condition characterized by repetitive interruption of ventilation during sleep caused by collapse of the pharyngeal airway (see also Chapter 7). An obstructive apnoea is a ≥10-second pause in respiration associated with ongoing ventilatory effort. Obstructive hypopnoea are decreases in—but not complete

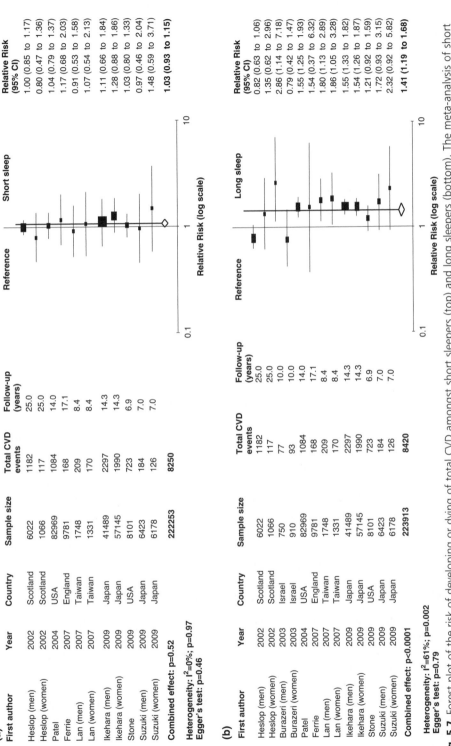

Fig. 5.7 Forest plot of the risk of developing or dying of total CVD amongst short sleepers (top) and long sleepers (bottom). The meta-analysis of short sleepers includes 222,253 participants with 8,250 fatal and non-fatal CVD events. That of long sleepers includes 223,913 participants with 8,420 fatal and non-fatal CVD events.

cessation of—ventilation, with an associate fall in oxygen saturation and/or arousal. A diagnosis of OSAS is accepted when a patient has an apnoea-hypopnoea index (AHI = number of apnoeas and hypopnoeas per hour of sleep) >5 and symptoms of EDS. Other signs and symptoms include disruptive snoring, obesity and/or enlarged neck size, and hypersomnolence (Guilleminault, 1985). It is beyond the scope of this chapter to describe the pathophysiology, clinical presentations, diagnostic criteria, and management strategies of OSAS (see also Chapter 7). This chapter will summarize the epidemiology of OSAS, its relation with CVD, and the public health aspects that arise.

It is estimated that approximately 4% of middle-aged men and 2% of middle-aged women are affected by OSAS (Duran et al., 2001; Young et al., 1993), estimated over 15 million adult Americans. The large majority have concomitant risk factors for CVD or prevalent disease.

This syndrome is associated with high rates of morbidity and mortality, mostly due to CVD (Ancoli-Israel et al., 1996; He et al., 1988; Partinen et al., 1988) and traffic accidents (Barbe et al., 1998) resulting from daytime sleepiness. Continuous positive airway pressure (CPAP) represents its most effective treatment (Ballester et al., 1999; Farre et al., 1999). Recently, two large observational prospective studies reported cardiovascular fatal and non-fatal event rates in patients with OSAS. In the first study carried out in Spain, a large cohort of men was recruited and followed up for over 10 years (Marin et al., 2005). There were 1,651 men, including 403 with untreated mild-to-moderate OSAS, 235 with untreated severe disease, and 372 with OSAS and treated with CPAP. When allowing for potential confounders, patients with untreated severe disease had a higher incidence of fatal cardiovascular events (death from MI and stroke; OR: 2.87, 95% CI: 1.17–7.51; $P = 0.025$) and non-fatal cardiovascular events (non-fatal MI, stroke, and acute coronary insufficiency requiring either coronary bypass surgery or percutaneous transluminal coronary angiography or both; OR: 3.17; 95% CI: 1.12–7.52; $P = 0.001$) than did patients with untreated mild-to-moderate OSAS (OR: 1.15; 95% CI: 0.34–2.69 and OR: 1.57; 95% CI: 0.62–3.16, respectively), patients treated with CPAP (OR: 1.05; 95% CI: 0.39–2.21 and OR: 1.42; 95% CI: 0.52–3.40, respectively), and simple snorers (OR: 1.03; 95% CI: 0.31–1.84 and OR: 1.32; 95% CI: 0.64–3.01, respectively) when compared to healthy controls. Earlier studies suggested an association between snoring and CVD (Koskenvuo et al., 1985, 1987; Palomaki, 1991); however, more recent studies indicate that snoring is not in itself a risk factor, unless it is a symptom of OSAS (Lindberg et al., 1998; Marin et al., 2005). In the second study carried out at the Yale Centre for Sleep Medicine, 1,022 patients (68% with OSAS) were enrolled and followed up for a median duration of 3.4 years (Yaggi et al., 2005). They were men and women. After adjustment for confounders, patients with OSAS had an increased risk of stroke or death (hazard ratio [HR]: 1.97; 95% CI: 1.12–3.48; $P = 0.01$). Moreover, increased severity of OSAS was associated with increased risk of developing stroke or death ($P = 0.005$).

Obstructive sleep apnoea syndrome, stroke, and heart failure

Studies evaluating the presence of OSAS in patients with stroke are inherently biased as they only study stroke survivors. Several studies have reported a high prevalence of sleep apnoea in subjects shortly after a stroke. The prevalence of OSAS in stroke patients, however, is as common as central apnoea (Somers et al., 2008). The concept of OSAS as a risk factor for primary ischaemic stroke is mainly inferred from the effect of OSAS on the risk factors for stroke, like hypertension and heart disease. The concept is further supported by prospective studies in stroke patients. In a 10-year follow-up study of patients with stroke, recurrence was more common amongst patients with OSAS (adjusted HR: 1.76; 95% CI: 1.05–2.95; $P = 0.03$). In contrast, central sleep apnoea was not associated with an increased incidence of stroke recurrence (Sahlin et al., 2008).

Since the early descriptions of John Cheyne (1818) and William Stokes (1846) on the distinctive pattern of breathing in severe cases of heart failure (Cheyne-Stokes breathing), later studied by John Hunter (Ward, 1973) who described its characteristics of gradual crescendo-decrescendo, changes in tidal volume and central apnoea, heart failure has been known to be associated with abnormal breathing patterns. Periodic breathing consists of cycles of apnoea or hypopnoea, or both, followed by hyperpnoea. The apnoeas and hypopnoeas can be obstructive or central (the predominant form). Central apnoea is characterized by repetitive cessation of ventilation during sleep, like in OSAS (Somers et al., 2008). The main difference is that there is no associated respiratory effort and, in people with central apnoea and heart failure, no EDS (Somers et al., 2008). Sleep-related breathing disorders may contribute to the progressively declining course of heart failure in some patients. Treatment of sleep-related breathing disorders may improve morbidity and mortality of patients with heart failure.

The epidemiology of sleep and cardiovascular risk

Growing epidemiological evidence indicates that reduced sleep duration and/or sleep deprivation may be associated with a number of cardiovascular risk factors and this would explain in part the association with vascular outcomes. Amongst many, hypertension, obesity, type 2 diabetes and other abnormalities of glucose metabolism, and lipids have received particular attention.

Sleep and hypertension

Sleep-disordered breathing (SDB) has been linked to elevated blood pressure and risk of hypertension in several epidemiological observational studies (Duran et al., 2001; Haas et al., 2005; Nieto et al., 2000; Peppard et al., 2000; Young et al., 1997).

For example, in a recent longitudinal analysis of the first National Health and Nutrition Examination Survey (NHANES-I), short sleep duration (<5 hours per night) was associated with a 60% higher risk of incident hypertension in middle-aged (32–59 years) American adults without apparent sleep disorders during a mean follow-up of 8–10 years (Gangwisch et al., 2006). No association was found in individuals >60 years of age. However, the outcome was based on self-reported diagnosis of incident hypertension, and no gender-specific analyses were included. Furthermore, a cross-sectional analysis from the Sleep Heart Health Study on a sample of more than 6,000 US adults showed a significant higher prevalence of hypertension among individuals with usual sleep duration above or below the median of 7–8 hours per night (Gottlieb et al., 2006). The association was stronger, that is, a 66% higher risk of hypertension, among short sleepers (<6 hours per night). Although this study attempted to account for a number of potential confounders, including psychiatric and cardiovascular co-morbidities, the cross-sectional design did not allow inference on the temporal relationship between sleep duration and hypertension.

Recent findings from the Coronary Artery Risk Development in Young Adults (CARDIA) study show that reduced sleep duration, measured by wrist actigraphy, predicts higher blood pressure levels and adverse changes in blood pressure over 5 years among 578 African Americans and Whites aged 33–45 years at baseline (Knutson et al., 2009).

We recently examined both the cross-sectional and prospective associations of sleep duration with prevalent and incident hypertension in the Whitehall II Study, a prospective cohort of 10 308 white-collar British civil servants aged 35–55 at baseline (phase 1: 1985–1988) (Cappuccio et al., 2007). Because reduced durations of sleep might be associated with more detrimental effects on cardiovascular outcomes among women (Ayas et al., 2003a, b; Meisinger et al., 2007; Patel et al., 2004, 2006), unlike previous investigations, we conducted gender-specific analyses with the inclusion of a number of potential confounding variables.

In cross-sectional analyses at phase 5 ($n = 5,766$), short duration of sleep (<5 hours per night) was associated with higher risk of hypertension compared with the group sleeping 7 hours, among women (OR: 1.72; 95% CI: 1.07–2.75), independent of confounders, with an inverse linear trend across decreasing hours of sleep ($P < 0.003$). No association was detected in men. In prospective analyses (mean follow-up: 5 years), the cumulative incidence of hypertension was 20.0% ($n = 740$) among 3,691 normotensive individuals at phase 5. In women, short duration of sleep was associated with a higher risk of hypertension in a reduced model (age and employment) (6 hours per night: OR: 1.56; 95% CI: 1.07–2.27; <5 hours per night: OR: 1.94; 95% CI: 1.08–3.50 vs. 7 hours). The associations were attenuated after accounting for cardiovascular risk factors and psychiatric co-morbidities (OR: 1.42; 95% CI: 0.94–2.16 and OR: 1.31; 95% CI: 0.65–2.63, respectively).

The study indicated for the first time that sleep deprivation may produce detrimental cardiovascular effects among women. Similar results have since been confirmed in a cross-sectional analysis of the Heinz Nixdorf Recall Study in Germany (Stang et al., 2008). They showed a significant association between reduced sleep duration (≤5 hours per night) and hypertension only among women (OR: 1.24; 95% CI: 1.04–1.46).

Altogether, these findings have raised concern that reduced sleep duration might produce detrimental cardiovascular effects particularly in women, as supported by several independent studies evaluating gender-specific effects of sleep duration on CVD-related morbidity and mortality (Ayas et al., 2003a, b; Meisinger et al., 2007; Patel et al., 2004, 2006).

In a recent analysis, we examined the cross-sectional gender-specific association of sleep duration with hypertension in the Western New York Health Study, a large, well-characterized population-based sample from the United States (Stranges et al., 2010).

In chronic diseases, menopause represents an important effect modifier of the relation between exposure to endogenous factors and disease risk. Therefore, unlike previous studies, we decided *a priori* to perform subgroup analyses by menopausal status among women to further investigate potential mechanisms for the observed gender-specific effect of reduced sleep duration on the risk of hypertension. Participants were 3,027 White men (43.5%) and women (56.5%) without prevalent CVD (median age: 56 years). In multivariate analyses, <6 hours of sleep was associated with a significant increased risk of hypertension compared to sleeping ≥6 hours per night, only among women (OR: 1.66; 95% CI: 1.09–2.53). No significant association was found among men (OR: 0.93; 95% CI: 0.62–1.41). In subgroup analyses by menopausal status, the effect was stronger among pre-menopausal women (OR: 3.25; 95% CI: 1.37–7.76) than among post-menopausal women (OR: 1.49; 95% CI: 0.92–2.41) (Stranges et al., 2010).

Several studies in humans indicate potential pathophysiological mechanisms supporting the biological plausibility of the association between sleep deprivation and hypertension. For example, acute curtailments of sleep may induce an overactivity of the sympathetic nervous system leading to higher blood pressure in both normotensive and hypertensive individuals. Other contributing mechanisms may include overactivity of the renin-angiotensin-aldosterone system, pro-inflammatory responses, endothelial dysfunction, and renal impairment. On the other hand, intervention studies to improve duration and quality of sleep have been effective in reducing both daytime and nighttime blood pressures. However, there is concern that sleep habits may represent a marker of health status and QOL rather than a causal factor for hypertension and other health outcomes.

The mechanisms underlying the gender-specific association of reduced sleep duration with hypertension and other cardiovascular outcomes are unclear. Hormonal influences and psychosocial distress may contribute to the observed associations, particularly during periods marking shifts in the reproductive stages of women, such as menopause. Moreover, methodological issues such as differential self-reporting of sleep habits between men and women may also play a role. However, the possibility that reduced sleep duration may represent a risk marker rather than a causal risk factor for diseases cannot be ruled out at the present time.

Sleep and obesity

In the last few decades, there has been a significant increase in the prevalence of obesity worldwide and the WHO has declared it a global epidemic (WHO Europe, 2006). Obesity in childhood is a cause of psychosocial problems including low self-esteem, and frequently continues into adulthood where it is a cause of major morbidity and mortality including CVD and type 2 diabetes. At the same time there has been a reduction in sleep time. National surveys in the United States have shown a decline in self-reported sleep duration over the past 50 years by 1.5–2 hours (National Sleep Foundation, 2005). This sleep curtailment has been attributed to lifestyle changes.

Several studies have reported associations between duration of sleep (short as well as long) and ill-health, including relationships with self-reported well-being (Steptoe et al., 2006), morbidity and mortality (Cappuccio et al., 2010b; Ferrie et al., 2007), and with chronic conditions including type 2 diabetes (Cappuccio et al., 2010a), respiratory disorders (Somers et al., 2008), hypertension (Cappuccio et al., 2007), and obesity (Cappuccio et al., 2008). The associations between short duration of sleep and obesity, in particular, have stimulated a debate given the potential implications for children (Currie and Cappuccio, 2007; Taheri, 2006) as well as adults (Cizza et al., 2005; Stranges et al., 2007). However, given the variety of studies and the large differences in the target populations, it is difficult to draw immediate conclusions on the consistency of the association, the direction of causality, and the likely mechanisms involved. A recent systematic review and meta-analysis of cross-sectional studies in children and adults provides the global evidence in support of the presence of a relationship between short duration of sleep and obesity, providing a quantitative estimate of the risk (Cappuccio et al., 2008). Of 696 studies identified, 45 met the inclusion criteria (19 in children and 26 in adults) and 30 (12 and 18, respectively) were pooled in the meta-analysis for a total of 36 population samples. They included 634,511 participants (30,002 children and 604,509 adults) from around the world. Age ranged from 2 to 102 years and included boys, girls, men, and women. In children, the pooled OR for short duration of sleep ($\leq$10 hours per night) and obesity was 1.89 (95% CI: 1.46–2.43; $P < 0.0001$) (Fig. 5.8).

In adults (short sleep defined as <5 hours per night), the pooled OR was 1.55 (95% CI: 1.43–1.68; $P < 0.0001$) (Fig. 5.9).

There was no evidence of publication bias. In adults, the pooled regression coefficient for short sleep duration was –0.35 (95% CI: –0.57 to –0.12) unit change in BMI per hour of sleep change.

These results are of interest for several reasons. First, the association is consistent in different populations. Although the meta-analysis detected significant heterogeneity between studies, further sensitivity analyses and the exclusion of publication bias are in favour of a similar effect across the populations. Second, they indicate an effect size consistent across ages. The 60–80% increase in the odds of being short sleeper amongst obese was seen in both children and adults, even after some attenuation following sensitivity analyses. Third, the categorical results were corroborated by the meta-analysis of regression coefficients, at least in adults.

The authors highlight some limitations. First, the quality of the data cannot go beyond the quality of the individual studies included. Second, a meta-analysis of observational studies is open to important fallacies in that it cannot directly control for confounding and therefore may be open to biased estimates. Third, the results can only be representative of the studies that have been included and are unable to provide a representative inference of all studies published.

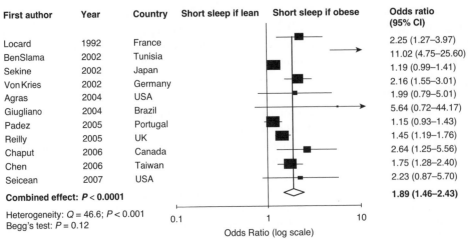

Fig. 5.8 Forest plot of the risk of obesity amongst short sleepers in population-based studies including 29,502 children (age 2–20 years) around the world.

Source: Data from Cappuccio, F.P., Taggart, F.M., Kandala, N.-B., et al. (2008). Meta-analysis of short sleep duration and obesity in children, adolescents and adults. *Sleep*, **31**(5), 619–626.

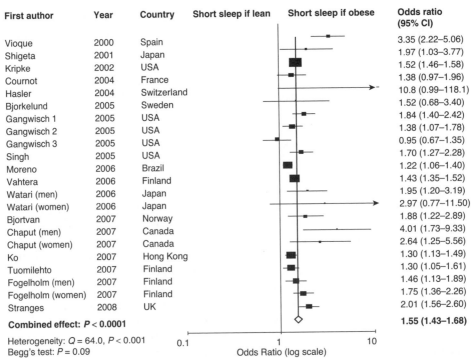

Fig. 5.9 Forest plot of the risk of obesity amongst short sleepers in population-based studies including 603,519 adults (age 15–102 years) around the world.

Source: Data from Cappuccio, F.P., Taggart, F.M., Kandala, N.-B., et al. (2008). Meta-analysis of short sleep duration and obesity in children, adolescents and adults. *Sleep*, **31**(5), 619–626.

Nevertheless, these results are important in guiding the assessment of current evidence and the definition of future research strategies.

The pooled studies are cross-sectional and cannot, therefore, determine temporal sequence, hence, causality. They also cannot examine changes in sleeping habits with time. Moreover, all studies used sleep questionnaires to determine self-reported sleep duration within their populations. The variety of methods for analyzing weight and obesity reflects our current poor understanding of what the most effective measuring scheme is. Many different methods were used to determine obesity, particularly in children, making the various studies more difficult to reconcile.

The studies varied in the degree of control for confounders such as age, gender, ethnic background, socioeconomic status, energy intake and expenditure, frequency of snacking, and other health-related behaviours and nutritional habits. A confounding factor in the relationship between sleep duration and obesity in adults is psychiatric co-morbidity, particularly depression. Chronic illness, physical disability, use of hypnotics, etc. would also be important confounders to consider.

The results of prospective studies do not provide consistency in support of the view that short sleep duration predicts the future development of obesity (Bjorkelund et al., 2005; Gangwisch et al., 2005; Lauderdale et al., 2009; Snell et al., 2007; Stranges et al., 2007) with the exception of a very large study ($n > 60,000$), carried out in women only, which shows a small effect (HR 1.15 and 1.06 for those sleeping ≤5 hours and ≤6 hours per night, respectively) (Patel et al., 2006). The relationship may be confounded by co-morbidity, such as chronic mental illness, causing a decrease in the levels of physical activity and a reduction in sleep, or by physical illnesses associated with pain—hence disrupted sleep—and severe limitation in energy expenditure through limited physical activity. More recent studies have adjusted for these potential confounders and found no prospective association (Stranges et al., 2007).

Potential mechanisms for the association between short sleep and obesity are described in detail elsewhere (see also Chapters 6 and 11). It has been suggested that short sleep may lead to obesity through the activation of hormonal responses leading to an increase in appetite and caloric intake. Short sleep is associated to reciprocal changes in leptin and ghrelin. This in turn would increase appetite and contribute to the development of obesity. The evidence in humans comes from short-lived severe sleep deprivation experiments in young volunteers that cannot be extrapolated to longer-term effects of sustained sleep curtailment in the general population. Indeed, in recent experiments in animal models, acute sleep loss and changes to the circadian clock altered metabolism, especially energy stores. However, energy stores were also altered in conditions of chronic sleep loss induced by mechanical stimuli, but not via light stimuli, suggesting that the changes in energy stores are caused by stress rather than sleep loss *per se* (Harbison and Sehgal, 2009).

Activation of inflammatory pathways by short sleep may also be implicated in the development of obesity (see also Chapter 11). Finally, it is inconceivable that short sleep may just be a marker of unfavourable health status and of lifestyle characteristics.

The potential public health implications of a causal relationship between short duration of sleep and obesity have already been widely disseminated in the media. The findings of the pooled analysis suggest that although sustained sleep curtailment and ensuing EDS are undoubtedly cause for concern, the link to obesity is of interest but still to be proven as a causal link. Many questions still need an answer to determine causality. Prospective studies in which weight, height, waist measurements, and adiposity are measured at baseline and again at subsequent data collection times together with more accurate objective measurement of sleep duration (including naps) and confounding factors or mediators, such as depression, are needed. Further prospective studies with improved assessment of long-term exposure (repeated self-reported sleep duration, repeated actigraphy, or polysomnography), more specific outcomes (including measures of adiposity) and better control for confounders are needed before causality can

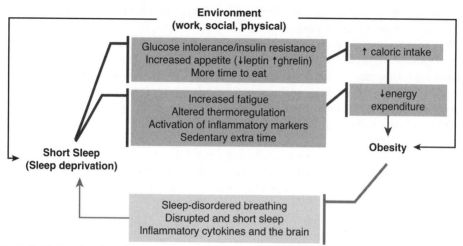

Fig. 5.10 Bi-directional model of the association between sleep deprivation and obesity.

be confirmed. Finally, the real possibility of reverse causality must not be ruled out. It is conceivable to construct a bi-directional model for the association between short sleep and obesity (Fig. 5.10).

One way would suggest that societal, socioeconomic, and physical environmental causes lead to a chronic curtailment of sleep. This in turn would activate mechanisms leading to an increase in caloric intake and a reduction in energy expenditure leading to obesity. On the other hand, it is possible that the same environmental pressures may lead to obesity that, in turn, would cause a chronic reduction of the duration of sleep via SDB and disrupted sleep and a direct effect on the brain by the activation of inflammatory cytokines.

Sleep and type 2 diabetes

Short-term, acute, laboratory, and cross-sectional observational studies have indicated that disturbed or reduced sleep is associated with glucose intolerance, insulin resistance, reduced acute insulin response to glucose, and a reduction in the disposition index (Spiegel et al., 2009), thus predisposing to type 2 diabetes (see also Chapter 6). The causality of the association and the generalizability of the results to longer-term effects of sustained sleep disturbances have been studied in prospective population studies to establish a temporal sequence between exposure and outcome. Given the variety of studies, the large differences in the types and sizes of populations examined, the duration of follow-up, and the size of the effects, it is difficult to draw immediate conclusions on the consistency of the associations and the size of effect.

A recent systematic review and meta-analysis of prospective population-based studies provides the global evidence in support of the presence of a relationship between sleep disturbances (in quantity and quality) and the development of type 2 diabetes, providing a quantitative estimate of the risk (Cappuccio et al., 2010a). Ten studies (13 independent cohort samples) were included (107,756 male and female participants, follow-up range 4.2–32 years, 3,586 incident cases of type 2 diabetes) (Ayas et al., 2003a; Beihl et al., 2009; Bjorkelund et al., 2005; Gangwisch et al., 2007; Hayashino et al., 2007; Kawakami et al., 2004; Mallon et al., 2005; Meisinger et al., 2005; Nilsson et al., 2004; Yaggi et al., 2006). The study shows an unambiguous and consistent pattern of increased risk of developing type 2 diabetes on either end of the distribution of sleep duration, and for qualitative disturbances of sleep patterns. Pooled analyses indicate that the risk varies between 28% in people who report habitual sleep of less than 5–6 hours per night and 84% in those with difficulties in maintaining their sleep. For short duration of sleep (≤5–6 hours per night), the RR was 1.28 (95% CI: 1.03–1.60; P = 0.024) (Fig. 5.11, top); for long duration of sleep (>8–9 hours per night), the RR was 1.48 (95% CI: 1.13–1.96; P = 0.005) (Fig. 5.11, bottom); for difficulty in initiating sleep, the RR was 1.57 (95% CI: 1.25–1.97; P < 0.0001) (Fig. 5.12, top); and for difficulty in maintaining sleep, the RR was 1.84 (95% CI: 1.39–2.43; P < 0.0001) (Fig. 5.12, bottom).

The study also suggests that, by and large, the effect increases with the duration of follow-up. These results confirm the suggestion originating from cross-sectional studies adding to the inference of causality due to the prospective nature of the evidence in the meta-analysis. The presence of little or no heterogeneity between studies, the absence of publication bias, and the high statistical power conferred by over 100,000 participants included with more than 3,000 incident cases of type 2 diabetes provides further strength to the results. The effects were, by and large, comparable in men and women, did not depend on the type of assessment of exposure and outcome nor on the variation in the definitions of short or long sleep. A large number of potential confounders, particularly age and BMI were considered in the primary analyses. The effect tended to increase with the duration of follow-up.

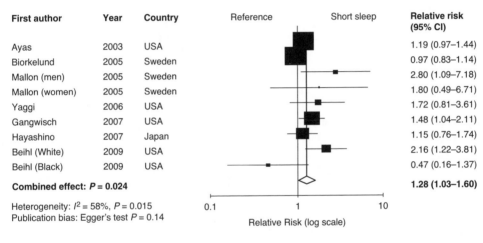

Fig. 5.11 Forest plot of the risk of developing type 2 diabetes amongst short sleepers (top) and long sleepers (bottom). The meta-analysis in short sleepers includes 90,623 participants with 3,079 incident cases of diabetes. That in long sleepers includes 88,611 participants with 2,903 incident cases of diabetes.

Source: Data from Cappuccio, F.P., D'Elia, L., Strazzullo, P., & Miller, M.A. (2010). Quantity and quality of sleep and incidence of type 2 diabetes. *Diabetes Care*, **33**, 414–420.

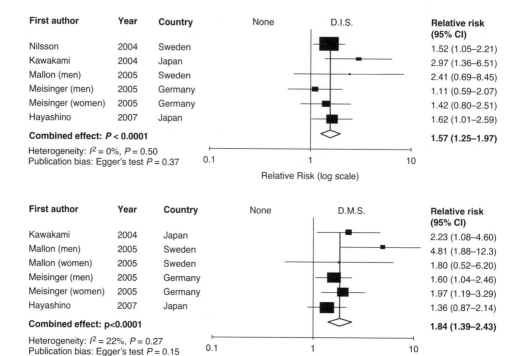

Fig. 5.12 Forest plot of the risk of developing type 2 diabetes amongst those with difficulties in initiating sleep (D.I.S.) (top) and those with difficulties in maintaining sleep (D.M.S.) (bottom). The meta-analysis in D.I.S. includes 24,192 participants with 787 incident cases of diabetes. That in D.M.S. includes 18,213 participants with 544 incident cases of diabetes.
Source: Data from Cappuccio, F.P., D'Elia, L., Strazzullo, P., & Miller, M.A. (2010). Quantity and quality of sleep and incidence of type 2 diabetes. *Diabetes Care*, **33**, 414–420.

These results are of interest for several reasons. First, the association is consistent in different populations. Although the meta-analysis detected some heterogeneity between studies (in particular in the short sleep category), further sensitivity analyses and the absence of publication bias are in favour of similar effects across populations. Second, they indicate an effect size of potential public health relevance, consistent across genders and depending on the duration of follow-up. There are limitations. First, the quality of the data cannot go beyond the quality of the individual studies included (Downs and Black, 1998). Second, a meta-analysis of observational data is open to fallacies in that it cannot directly control for confounding. We made an attempt to allow for multiple confounding by including adjusted estimates from multivariate models from each contributing study. However, residual confounding and bias remain a possibility. Third, the results can only be representative of the studies that have been included and are unable to provide a representative inference of all studies published, but not included. Nevertheless, there was no evidence of publication bias. These results are therefore important in guiding the assessment of current evidence and the definition of future research strategies and public health policy decisions.

All studies used self-reported sleep disturbances (either as quantity or as quality of sleep). These methods have limitations in that they often may not allow (unless explicitly built as additional questions) to differentiate time asleep from time in bed or to estimate number and duration of naps when assessing duration of sleep. On the other hand, formal sleep studies using objective measures of sleep are not practical and often not feasible in large prospective population studies. Sleep diaries, actigraphy, and polysomnography from some large population and small-scale investigations have shown high correlations between subjective estimates of sleep duration and more direct assessments (Lockley et al., 1999; Patel et al., 2004; Signal et al., 2005). Furthermore, assessments of sleep durations in the primary healthcare setting rely on self-reported data from patients.

Quantity and quality of sleep were assessed at one point of time in all studies. It is possible that a single measure of exposure may not fully capture the sustained effects of sleep disruption over time when relating them to long-term morbidity. The studies included in the analysis did not always exclude subjects with OSAS. These would represent approximately 4% of middle-aged men and 2% of middle-aged women (Duran et al., 2001; Young et al., 1993). This disorder is associated with obesity, disrupted and short sleep, EDS, and high rates of morbidity and mortality, predominantly due to CVD (Marin et al., 2005). Although it is possible that they may have contributed to the observed increased risk of type 2 diabetes in the categories of sleep disturbance, the adjustment for obesity or BMI in almost every study would have, at least in part, corrected for this.

Gender differences in outcomes and risk related to duration of sleep have been reported (Cappuccio et al., 2007; Meisinger et al., 2007; Stang et al., 2008; Stranges et al., 2010; Suarez, 2008). The meta-analysis was repeated after stratification by gender wherever possible. No differences were detected in the association with short duration of sleep or difficulty in maintaining sleep and the development of type 2 diabetes. Ideally, long follow-up durations would be appropriate to assess the influence of sleep on health over the life course (Gangwisch et al., 2008). Studies with short follow-up (<3 years) were excluded *a priori* to avoid measurements of sleep quantity and quality being too close to the diagnosis of type 2 diabetes. A meta-regression analysis indicated that the effect size tended to be directly related to the duration of follow-up, suggesting the possibility of a time-dependent cumulative effect.

Potential mechanisms relating sleep problems to adverse health outcomes include reciprocal changes in circulating levels of leptin and ghrelin (Spiegel et al., 2004; Taheri et al., 2004), that in turn would increase appetite, caloric intake, reduce energy expenditure (Knutson et al., 2007; Spiegel et al., 2009), and facilitate the development of obesity (Spiegel et al., 2010; Taheri et al., 2004) and impaired glycaemic control (Spiegel et al., 2005) with increased cardiovascular risk. Increased cortisol secretion and altered growth hormone metabolism have also been implicated (Copinschi, 2005). Low grade inflammation is activated during short sleep, with possible implications not only for CVD (Miller et al., 2009; Miller and Cappuccio, 2007), but also for other chronic conditions including cancer. The association of difficulty of initiating or maintaining sleep could be related to the same mechanisms, as expression of reduced total sleep duration. Finally, elevated levels of dopamine and symptoms of gastroesophageal reflux have recently been described as important contributors to difficulties in maintaining sleep and insomnia (Mody et al., 2009; Seugnet et al., 2009). Conversely, there is less clear indication of possible mechanisms mediating the effect of long duration of sleep as a cause of type 2 diabetes. Depressive symptoms, low socioeconomic status, unemployment, low level of physical activity, undiagnosed health conditions, poor general health have all been shown to be associated with long duration of sleep and to confound the association with morbidity as well as mortality (Krueger and Friedman, 2009; Stranges et al., 2008).

Sleep, both quantity and quality, should be regarded as a behavioural risk factor for the development of type 2 diabetes, heavily determined by the environment and possibly amenable to modification through both education and counselling as well as through favourable modifications of physical and working environments to allow sufficient sleep and avoid habitual and sustained sleep deprivation and disruption.

Sleep and lipids

Alterations of lipid metabolism and ensuing dyslipidaemia are strong modifiable risk factors for cardiovascular morbidity and mortality. Dyslipidaemia is characterized by high circulating levels of total, low-density lipoprotein (LDL)-cholesterol and plasma triglycerides, and low circulating levels of HDL-cholesterol. Besides genetic determinants, these factors are strongly influenced by lifestyle and dietary factors and are therefore amenable to modification. Given the relationship between sleep patterns and cardiovascular outcomes, the research interest has been directed to studying the possible relationships between sleep and lipids. One of the first population reports was within the cross-sectional occupational study of the relationships between life-style factors and lipids in 1,580 middle-aged Japanese male office workers (Nakanishi et al., 1999). They found no association between sleep duration and serum lipid and lipoprotein levels. The study was limited to working men and therefore there was limited generalizability to the population at large. Another population-based study in 935 American middle-aged women with type 2 diabetes and no presence of vascular disease at baseline, in contrast, showed that HDL-cholesterol levels were reduced in both short (<5 hours per night) and long (>9 hours per night) sleepers in normotensive, but not in hypertensive, women (Williams et al., 2007). More frequent snoring was also directly associated with triglycerides and inversely with HDL-cholesterol, when adjusted for confounders including body mass. This sample is representative of American women but has the limitation that the results could not be extrapolated to men and to women with no underlying conditions like type 2 diabetes. A more recent population study in 1,666 men and 2,329 women, aged 20 and older, from Japan, addresses the previous limitations (Kaneita et al., 2008). The study shows that, in women, both short and long durations of sleep are associated with high serum triglycerides and low serum HDL-cholesterol. On the other hand, amongst men, these associations were not detected. This study, as many others using different outcomes (Cappuccio et al., 2007; Meisinger et al., 2007; Miller et al., 2009), does point to a consistent gender difference in the cluster of cardiovascular risk as function of sleep duration. To corroborate these findings is the evidence of an association between both short and long duration of sleep with measure of the MetS (Hall et al., 2008). The MetS is a composite set of cardio-metabolic risk factors that include central adiposity, high blood pressure, dyslipidaemia, and altered glucose metabolism. There is no international consensus on the definition and on whether the strong predictive value for CVD risk improves the predictive value of the sum of each individual risk factor (Strazzullo et al., 2008), as they are physiologically interrelated within an individual. Nevertheless, it provides additional evidence to consider. The authors studied the cross-sectional relationship between sleep duration and features of the MetS in 1,214 middle-aged American men and women. The odds for presenting with the MetS increased by more than 45% in both short (<6 hours) and long (>8 hours) sleepers. The single strongest correlates with duration of sleep were abdominal adiposity, elevated fasting glucose, and high triglycerides. It is noteworthy that, when adjustment was made for use of anti-hypertensive medications (possibly a proxy for severity of hypertension as well as an indication of iatrogenic metabolic effects), the relationship remained for short sleep only. Dyslipidaemia predicts cardiovascular risk by facilitating atherosclerosis and, therefore, large vessel disease. Two well-known sub-clinical markers of generalized atherosclerosis and strong predictors of outcome are the intima-media thickness (IMT) measured with ultrasound at the level of the carotid artery and the degree of calcification of the coronary arteries (CAC) measured by computed tomography. In a general population random sample of 2,437 men and women from Germany, a J-shaped association was detected between self-reported duration of sleep and IMT (Wolff et al., 2008). In this study, age- and sex-adjusted IMT was lowest among subjects with an average duration of sleep of 7- to 8-hours per day but increased with shorter and longer duration of sleep. As part of the CARDIA cohort, the Chicago site analyzed their data on 495 participants (men and women, Blacks and Whites) who had undergone both direct measures of sleep duration with wrist actigraphy and indirect measures with self-reporting, and CAC measurements at baseline and after 5 years of follow-up (King et al., 2008). The primary end-point was the incidence of new coronary calcifications. The cumulative incidence was 12.3%. There was a highly significant inverse relationship between duration of sleep by actigraphy and incidence of CAC. Alternative sleep metrics were not significantly associated with CAC. From an epidemiological standpoint, the latter study has a number of strengths. It uses a direct measure of exposure, it establishes a temporal sequence between exposure and outcome, it employs a reliable sub-clinical marker of atherosclerosis, and it allows for important confounders. However, there are still no well-described plausible mechanisms. The results may be mediated through socioeconomic factors common to poor sleep and cardiovascular risk not well-accounted for by multivariate analyses. They may also reflect mediating mechanisms such as inflammatory mechanisms (see also Chapter 11), metabolic factors (see also Chapter 6), and other vascular risk factors, including high blood pressure.

Conclusion

Sleep disturbances of quality and quantity are highly prevalent in modern society; they vary across the life course of an individual and are more prevalent in groups according to gender, socioeconomic status, employment status, and geographical location. In the context of a high prevalence and incidence of CVD and the growing epidemics of risk factors such as hypertension, obesity, and diabetes, it has become apparent in the last decade that there is a strong epidemiological link between these common sleep-related exposures and CVD. As the potential population and public health implications may be significant, it is imperative that the causality of the associations described be determined and the reversibility of the effects tested.

Summary box

- Cardiovascular disease (including ischaemic heart disease and stroke) is the commonest cause of morbidity, mortality, and disability in the world.
- CVD accounts for high healthcare costs and loss of productive life.
- The 'epidemics' of obesity, type 2 diabetes, and hypertension, major risk factors for CVD, are paralleled by a *silent epidemic* of reduced sleep duration, detectable both in adults and in children.
- Short sleep duration is associated with increased risk of obesity both in adults and in children. Evidence from prospective studies, however, does not always confirm a temporal sequence.
- Plausible mechanisms could be the effect of short sleep on appetite through the ghrelin-leptin system.
- Quantity and quality of sleep are significant predictors of type 2 diabetes.
- Other metabolic and inflammatory pathways could be involved.
- The mechanisms mediating the effects of long sleep on diabetes are likely to be different.
- Sleep duration also predicts hypertension, CHD, stroke, and CVD.
- A decrease in sleep duration affects all-cause mortality via increases in cardiovascular deaths.
- An increase in sleep duration affects overall mortality via an increase in non-cardiovascular deaths.
- More research is needed to understand the mechanisms by which sleep disturbances are linked to chronic conditions of affluent societies.

References

Åkerstedt, T. & Nilsson, P.M. (2003). Sleep as restitution: an introduction. *J Intern Med*, **254**(1), 6–12.

Ancoli-Israel, S., Kripke, D.F., Klauber, M.R., et al. (1996). Morbidity, mortality and sleep-disordered breathing in community dwelling elderly. *Sleep*, **19**(4), 277–282.

Ayas, N.T., White, D.P., Al-Delaimy, W.K., et al. (2003a). A prospective study of self-reported sleep duration and incident diabetes in women. *Diabetes Care*, **26**(2), 380–384.

Ayas, N.T., White, D.P., Manson, J.E., et al. (2003b). A prospective study of sleep duration and coronary heart disease in women. *Arch Intern Med*, **163**, 205–209.

Ballester, E., Badia, J.R., Hernandez, L., et al. (1999). Evidence of the effectiveness of continuous positive airway pressure in the treatment of sleep apnea/hypopnea syndrome. *Am J Respir Crit Care Med*, **159**(2), 495–501.

Barbe, F., Pericas, J., Munoz, A., Findley, L., Anto, J.M. & Agusti, A.G. (1998). Automobile accidents in patients with sleep apnea syndrome. An epidemiological and mechanistic study. *Am J Respir Crit Care Med*, **158**(1), 18–22.

Beihl, D.A., Liese, A.D. & Haffner, S.M. (2009). Sleep duration as a risk factor for incident type 2 diabetes in a multiethnic cohort. *Ann Epidemiol*, **19**(5), 351–357.

Bjorkelund, C., Bondyr-Carlsson, D., Lapidus, L., et al. (2005). Sleep disturbances in midlife unrelated to 32-year diabetes incidence: the prospective population study of women in Gothenburg. *Diabetes Care*, **28**(11), 2739–2744.

Bliwise, D.L. (1996). Historical change in the report of daytime fatigue. *Sleep*, **19**(6), 462–464.

Cappuccio, F.P., Stranges, S., Kandala, N.-B., et al. (2007). Gender-specific associations of short sleep duration with prevalent and incident hypertension. The Whitehall II Study. *Hypertension*, **50**(4), 694–701.

Cappuccio, F.P., Taggart, F.M., Kandala, N.-B., et al. (2008). Meta-analysis of short sleep duration and obesity in children, adolescents and adults. *Sleep*, **31**(5), 619–626.

Cappuccio, F.P., D'Elia, L., Strazzullo, P. & Miller, M.A. (2010a). Quantity and quality of sleep and incidence of type 2 diabetes: a systematic review and meta-analysis. *Diabetes Care*, **33**, 414–420.

Cappuccio, F.P., D'Elia, L., Strazzullo, P. & Miller, M.A. (2010b). Sleep duration and all-cause mortality: a systematic review and meta-analysis of prospective studies. *Sleep*, **33**(5), 585–592.

Cheyne, J. (1818). A case of apoplexy, in which the fleshy part of the heart was converted into fat. *Dub Hosp Rep Commun*, **2**, 216–223.

Cizza, G., Skarulis, M. & Mignot, E. (2005). A link between short sleep and obesity: building the evidence for causation. *Sleep*, **28**(10), 1217–1220.

Copinschi, G. (2005). Metabolic and endocrine effects of sleep deprivation. *Essent Psychopharmacol*, **6**(6), 341–347.

Currie, A. & Cappuccio, F.P. (2007). Sleep in children and adolescents: a worrying scenario: can we understand the sleep deprivation-obesity epidemic? *Nutr Metab Cardiovasc Dis*, **17**(3), 230–232.

Downs, S.H. & Black, N. (1998). The feasibility of creating a checklist for the assessment of the methodological quality both of randomised and non-randomised studies of health care interventions. *J Epidemiol Community Health*, **52**(6), 377–384.

Duran, J., Esnaola, S., Rubio, R. & Iztueta, A. (2001). Obstructive sleep apnea-hypopnea and related clinical features in a population-based sample of subjects aged 30 to 70 yr. *Am J Respir Crit Care Med*, **163**(3 Pt 1), 685–689.

Farre, R., Hernandez, L., Montserrat, J.M., Rotger, M., Ballester, E. & Navajas, D. (1999). Sham continuous positive airway pressure for placebo-controlled studies in sleep apnoea. *Lancet*, **353**(9159), 1154.

Ferrie, J.E., Shipley, M.J., Cappuccio, F.P., et al. (2007). A prospective study of change in sleep duration: associations with mortality in the Whitehall II cohort. *Sleep*, **30**(12), 1659–1666.

Gangwisch, J.E., Malaspina, D., Boden-Albala, B. & Heymsfield, S.B. (2005). Inadequate sleep as a risk factor for obesity: analyses of the NHANES I. *Sleep*, **28**(10), 1289–1296.

Gangwisch, J.E., Heymsfield, S.B., Boden-Albala, B., et al. (2006). Short sleep duration as a risk factor for hypertension: analyses of the first National Health and Nutrition Examination Survey. *Hypertension*, **47**(5), 833–839.

Gangwisch, J.E., Heymsfield, S.B., Boden-Albala, et al. (2007). Sleep duration as a risk factor for diabetes incidence in a large U.S. sample. *Sleep*, **30**(12), 1667–1673.

Gangwisch, J.E., Heymsfield, S.B., Boden-Albala, B., et al. (2008). Sleep duration associated with mortality in elderly, but not middle-aged, adults in a large US sample. *Sleep*, **31**(8), 1087–1096.

Gottlieb, D.J., Redline, S., Nieto, F.J., et al. (2006). Association of usual sleep duration with hypertension: the Sleep Heart Health Study. *Sleep*, **29**(8), 1009–1014.

Groeger, J.A., Zijlstra, F.R. & Dijk, D.J. (2004). Sleep quantity, sleep difficulties and their perceived consequences in a representative sample of some 2000 British adults. *J Sleep Res*, **13**(4), 359–371.

Guilleminault, C. (1985). Obstructive sleep apnea. The clinical syndrome and historical perspective. *Med Clin North Am*, **69**(6), 1187–1203.

Haas, D.C., Foster, G.L., Nieto, F.J., et al. (2005). Age-dependent associations between sleep-disordered breathing and hypertension: importance of discriminating between systolic/diastolic hypertension and isolated systolic hypertension in the Sleep Heart Health Study. *Circulation*, **111**(5), 614–621.

Hall, M.H., Muldoon, M.F., Jennings, J.R., Buysse, D.J., Flory, J.D. & Manuck, S.B. (2008). Self-reported sleep duration is associated with the metabolic syndrome in midlife adults. *Sleep*, **31**(5), 635–643.

Harbison, S.T. & Sehgal, A. (2009). Energy stores are not altered by long-term partial sleep deprivation in Drosophila melanogaster. *PLoS One*, **4**(7), e6211.

Hayashino, Y., Fukuhara, S., Suzukamo, Y., Okamura, T., Tanaka, T. & Ueshima, H. (2007). Relation between sleep quality and quantity, quality of life, and risk of developing diabetes in healthy workers in Japan: the High-risk and Population Strategy for Occupational Health Promotion (HIPOP-OHP) Study. *BMC Public Health*, **7**, 129.

He, J., Kryger, M.H., Zorick, F.J., Conway, W. & Roth, T. (1988). Mortality and apnea index in obstructive sleep apnea. Experience in 385 male patients. *Chest*, **94**(1), 9–14.

Kaneita, Y., Uchiyama, M., Yoshiike, N. & Ohida, T. (2008). Associations of usual sleep duration with serum lipid and lipoprotein levels. *Sleep*, **31**(5), 645–652.

Kawakami, N., Takatsuka, N. & Shimizu, H. (2004). Sleep disturbance and onset of type 2 diabetes. *Diabetes Care*, **27**(1), 282–283.

Kearney, P.M., Whelton, M., Reynolds, K., Muntner, P., Whelton, P.K. & He, J. (2005). Global burden of hypertension: analysis of worldwide data. *Lancet*, **365**(9455), 217–223.

King, C.R., Knutson, K.L., Rathouz, P.J., Sidney, S., Liu, K. & Lauderdale, D.S. (2008). Short sleep duration and incident coronary artery calcification. *JAMA*, **300**(24), 2859–2866.

Knutson, K.L., Spiegel, K., Penev, P. & Van Cauter, E. (2007). The metabolic consequences of sleep deprivation. *Sleep Med Rev*, **11**(3), 163–178.

Knutson, K.L., Van Cauter, C.E., Rathouz, P.J., et al. (2009). Association between sleep and blood pressure in midlife: the CARDIA sleep study. *Arch Intern Med*, **169**(11), 1055–1061.

Koskenvuo, M., Kaprio, J., Partinen, M., Langinvainio, H., Sarna, S. & Heikkila, K. (1985). Snoring as a risk factor for hypertension and angina pectoris. *Lancet*, **1**(8434), 893–896.

Koskenvuo, M., Kaprio, J., Telakivi, T., Partinen, M., Heikkila, K. & Sarna, S. (1987). Snoring as a risk factor for ischaemic heart disease and stroke in men. *Br Med J (Clin Res Ed)*, **294**(6563), 16–19.

Krueger, P.M. & Friedman, E.M. (2009). Sleep duration in the United States: a cross-sectional population-based study. *Am J Epidemiol*, **169**(9), 1052–1063.

Lauderdale, D.S., Knutson, K.L., Rathouz, P.J., Yan, L.L., Hulley, S.B. & Liu, K. (2009). Cross-sectional and longitudinal associations between objectively measured sleep duration and body mass index: the CARDIA Sleep Study. *Am J Epidemiol*, **170**(7), 805–813.

Leal, J., Luengo-Fernandez, R., Gray, A., Petersen, S. & Rayner, M. (2006). Economic burden of cardiovascular diseases in the enlarged European Union. *Eur Heart J*, **27**(13), 1610–1619.

Lindberg, E., Janson, C., Svardsudd, K., Gislason, T., Hetta, J. & Boman, G. (1998). Increased mortality among sleepy snorers: a prospective population based study. *Thorax*, **53**(8), 631–637.

Lockley, S.W., Skene, D.J. & Arendt, J. (1999). Comparison between subjective and actigraphic measurement of sleep and sleep rhythms. *J Sleep Res*, **8**(3), 175–183.

Mallon, L., Broman, J.E. & Hetta, J. (2005). High incidence of diabetes in men with sleep complaints or short sleep duration: a 12-year follow-up study of a middle-aged population. *Diabetes Care*, **28**(11), 2762–2767.

Marin, J.M., Carrizo, S.J., Vicente, E. & Agusti, A.G. (2005). Long-term cardiovascular outcomes in men with obstructive sleep apnoea-hypopnoea with or without treatment with continuous positive airway pressure: an observational study. *Lancet*, **365**(9464), 1046–1053.

Marmot, M.G. & Elliott, P. (2005). *Coronary Heart Disease Epidemiology*. Second edition. Oxford: Oxford University Press.

Meisinger, C., Heier, M. & Loewel, H. (2005). Sleep disturbance as a predictor of type 2 diabetes mellitus in men and women from the general population. *Diabetologia*, **48**(2), 235–241.

Meisinger, C., Heier, M., Lowel, H., Schneider, A. & Doring, A. (2007). Sleep duration and sleep complaints and risk of myocardial infarction in middle-aged men and women from the general population: the MONICA/KORA Augsburg Cohort Study. *Sleep*, **30**(9), 1121–1127.

Miller, M.A. & Cappuccio, F.P. (2007). Inflammation, sleep, obesity and cardiovascular disease. *Curr Vasc Pharmacol*, **5**, 93–102.

Miller, M.A., Kandala, N.-B., Kivimaki, M., et al. (2009). Gender differences in the cross-sectional relationships between sleep duration and markers of inflammation: Whitehall II study. *Sleep*, **32**(7), 857–864.

Mody, R., Bolge, S.C., Kannan, H. & Fass, R. (2009). Effects of gastroesophageal reflux disease on sleep and outcomes. *Clin Gastroenterol Hepatol*, **7**(9), 953–959.

Nakanishi, N., Nakamura, K., Ichikawa, S., Suzuki, K. & Tatara, K. (1999). Relationship between lifestyle and serum lipid and lipoprotein levels in middle-aged Japanese men. *Eur J Epidemiol*, **15**(4), 341–348.

National Sleep Foundation (2005). *Sleep in America Poll*. Washington, DC: National Sleep Foundation.

Nieto, F.J., Young, T.B., Lind, B.K., et al. (2000). Association of sleep-disordered breathing, sleep apnea, and hypertension in a large community-based study. Sleep Heart Health Study. *JAMA*, **283**(14), 1829–1836.

Nilsson, P.M., Roost, M., Engstrom, G., Hedblad, B. & Berglund, G. (2004). Incidence of diabetes in middle-aged men is related to sleep disturbances. *Diabetes Care*, **27**(10), 2464–2469.

Palomaki, H. (1991). Snoring and the risk of ischemic brain infarction. *Stroke*, **22**(8), 1021–1025.

Partinen, M., Jamieson, A. & Guilleminault, C. (1988). Long-term outcome for obstructive sleep apnea syndrome patients. Mortality. *Chest*, **94**(6), 1200–1204.

Patel, S.R., Ayas, N.T., Malhotra, M.R., et al. (2004). A prospective study of sleep duration and mortality risk in women. *Sleep*, **27**(3), 440–444.

Patel, S.R., Malhotra, A., White, D.P., Gottlieb, D.J. & Hu, F.B. (2006). Association between reduced sleep and weight gain in women. *Am J Epidemiol*, **164**(10), 947–954.

Peppard, P.E., Young, T., Palta, M. & Skatrud, J. (2000). Prospective study of the association between sleep-disordered breathing and hypertension. *N Engl J Med*, **342**(19), 1378–1384.

Sahlin, C., Sandberg, O., Gustafson, Y., et al. (2008). Obstructive sleep apnea is a risk factor for death in patients with stroke: a 10-year follow-up. *Arch Intern Med*, **168**(3), 297–301.

Seugnet, L., Suzuki, Y., Thimgan, M., et al. (2009). Identifying sleep regulatory genes using a Drosophila model of insomnia. *J Neurosci*, **29**(22), 7148–7157.

Signal, T.L., Gale, J. & Gander, P.H. (2005). Sleep measurement in flight crew: comparing actigraphic and subjective estimates to polysomnography. *Aviat Space Environ Med*, **76**(11), 1058–1063.

Snell, E.K., Adam, E.K. & Duncan, G.J. (2007). Sleep and the body mass index and overweight status of children and adolescents. *Child Dev*, **78**(1), 309–323.

Somers, V.K., White, D.P., Amin, R., et al. (2008). Sleep apnea and cardiovascular disease: an American Heart Association/American College of Cardiology Foundation Scientific Statement from the American Heart Association Council for High Blood Pressure Research Professional Education Committee, Council on Clinical Cardiology, Stroke Council, and Council on Cardiovascular Nursing. *J Am Coll Cardiol*, **52**(8), 686–717.

Spiegel, K., Leproult, R. & Van Cauter, E. (1999). Impact of sleep debt on metabolic and endocrine function. *Lancet*, **354**(9188), 1435–1439.

Spiegel, K., Tasali, E., Penev, P. & Van Cauter, E. (2004). Sleep curtailment in healthy young men is associated with decreased leptin levels, elevated ghrelin levels, and increased hunger and appetite. *Ann Intern Med*, **141**(11), 846–850.

Spiegel, K., Knutson, K., Leproult, R. & Van Cauter, E. (2005). Sleep loss: a novel risk factor for insulin resistance and type 2 diabetes. *J Appl Physiol*, **99**(5), 2008–2019.

Spiegel, K., Tasali, E., Leproult, R. & Van Cauter, C.E. (2009). Effects of poor and short sleep on glucose metabolism and obesity risk. *Nat Rev Endocrinol*, **5**(5), 253–261.

Stang, A., Moebus, S., Mohlenkamp, S. & Erbel, R. (2008). Gender-specific associations of short sleep duration with prevalent hypertension. *Hypertension*, **51**(3), e15–e16.

Steptoe, A., Peacey, V. & Wardle, J. (2006). Sleep duration and health in young adults. *Arch Intern Med*, **166**(16), 1689–1692.

Stokes, W. (1846). Observations on some cases of permanently slow pulse. *Dub Q J Med Sci*, **2**, 73–85.

Stranges, S., Cappuccio, F.P., Kandala, N.-B., et al. (2007). Cross-sectional versus prospective associations of sleep duration with changes in relative weight and body fat distribution: the Whitehall II study. *Am J Epidemiol*, **167**(3), 321–329.

Stranges, S., Dorn, J.M., Shipley, M.J., et al. (2008). Correlates of short and long sleep duration: a cross-cultural comparison between the United Kingdom and the United States: the Whitehall II Study and the Western New York Health Study. *Am J Epidemiol*, **168**(12), 1353–1364.

Stranges, S., Dorn, J.M., Cappuccio, F.P., et al. (2010). A population-based study of reduced sleep duration and hypertension: the strongest association may be in premenopausal women. *J Hypertens*, **28**, 896–902.

Strazzullo, P., Barbato, A., Siani, A., et al. (2008). Diagnostic criteria for metabolic syndrome: a comparative analysis in an unselected sample of adult male population. *Metabolism*, **57**(3), 355–361.

Suarez, E.L. (2008). Gender-specific associations between disturbed sleep and biomarkers of inflammation, coagulation and insulin resistance. *Brain Behav Immun*, **22**, 29–35.

Taheri, S. (2006). The link between short sleep duration and obesity: we should recommend more sleep to prevent obesity. *Arch Dis Child*, **91**(11), 881–884.

Taheri, S., Lin, L., Austin, D., Young, T. & Mignot, E. (2004). Short sleep duration is associated with reduced leptin, elevated ghrelin, and increased body mass index. *PLoS Med*, **1**(3), e62.

Ward, M. (1973). Periodic respiration. A short historical note. *Ann R Coll Surg Engl*, **52**(5), 330–334.

WHO Europe (2006). *WHO European Ministerial Conference on Counteracting Obesity. Diet and Physical Activity for Health* EUR/06/5062700/9.

Williams, C.J., Hu, F.B., Patel, S.R. & Mantzoros, C.S. (2007). Sleep duration and snoring in relation to biomarkers of cardiovascular disease risk among women with type 2 diabetes. *Diabetes Care*, **30**(5), 1233–1240.

Wolff, B., Volzke, H., Schwahn, C., Robinson, D., Kessler, C. & John, U. (2008). Relation of self-reported sleep duration with carotid intima-media thickness in a general population sample. *Atherosclerosis*, **196**(2), 727–732.

Yaggi, H.K., Concato, J., Kernan, W.N., Lichtman, J.H., Brass, L.M. & Mohsenin, V. (2005). Obstructive sleep apnea as a risk factor for stroke and death. *N Engl J Med*, **353**(19), 2034–2041.

Yaggi, H.K., Araujo, A.B. & McKinlay, J.B. (2006). Sleep duration as a risk factor for the development of type 2 diabetes. *Diabetes Care*, **29**(3), 657–661.

Young, T., Palta, M., Dempsey, J., Skatrud, J., Weber, S. & Badr, S. (1993). The occurrence of sleep-disordered breathing among middle-aged adults. *N Engl J Med*, **328**(17), 1230–1235.

Young, T., Peppard, P., Palta, M., et al. (1997). Population-based study of sleep-disordered breathing as a risk factor for hypertension. *Arch Intern Med*, **157**(15), 1746–1752.

Chapter 6

Sleep and metabolic disease

J. Broussard and K.L. Knutson

Introduction

Metabolic diseases include diabetes and obesity, both of which are associated with reduced quality of life (QOL), decreased life expectancy, and increased economic burden on both the individual and on society (Solomon and Manson, 1997; Wolf and Colditz, 1998; Ettaro et al., 2004; Franco et al., 2007). Rates of obesity in the United States have doubled since 1980 (Flegal et al., 1998, 2002) and the age-adjusted percentage of persons with diagnosed diabetes has also nearly doubled in the United States between 1980 and 2006 (Ioannou et al., 2007; Centers for Disease Control, 2006; Gregg et al., 2004) (see Fig. 6.1). The epidemics of obesity and diabetes are not limited to the United States, however. Rates of both conditions are increasing rapidly worldwide (Wild et al., 2004). Obesity and diabetes, and their consequences, are truly a global problem.

Due to the potentially devastating consequences of these metabolic diseases, it is imperative that modifiable causes of both diabetes and obesity be identified as potential areas of intervention. Because this increase in prevalence was so rapid, occurring over a mere 20- to 30-year period, changes in the genetic composition of the population cannot be blamed. Therefore, environmental and/or behavioural factors must be responsible for the increased rates of obesity and diabetes in the United States and worldwide. Although changes in diet and exercise have played an important role, another possible explanation for the epidemic is reduced sleep duration and quality. There is some evidence that average sleep duration in the United States has declined over the same time period as the increase in obesity and diabetes (Gallup Organization, 1995, 1979; Breslau et al., 1997; Kripke et al., 1979; National Sleep Foundation, 2001). For example, a report from the National Health Interview Survey indicated the percentage of adults reporting sleeping 6 hours or less increased by approximately 5–6% between 1985 and 2004 (National Center for Health Statistics, 2005). Sleep loss may be the result of either a voluntary restriction of time spent in bed or as a result of a sleep disorder, particularly obstructive sleep apnoea (OSA), the prevalence of which has increased in association with the increase in obesity. This chapter will explore the evidence for an association between metabolic diseases and sleep duration and quality.

Three potential pathways leading from insufficient or disturbed sleep to diabetes and obesity are presented in Fig. 6.2. First, short or disturbed sleep may impair glucose metabolism thereby increasing the risk of developing insulin resistance and diabetes independently of changes in weight. Second, short or disturbed sleep may lead to an increase in appetite, which would increase the risk of weight gain if food intake increased without a compensatory increase in energy expenditure. If the weight gain is substantial, it could lead to the development of obesity, which is a major risk factor for the development of insulin resistance and type 2 diabetes. Finally, the third pathway would involve a reduction in energy expenditure after sleep loss, which could also increase the risk of weight gain. This third pathway, however, remains understudied and is only proposed here as a possibility.

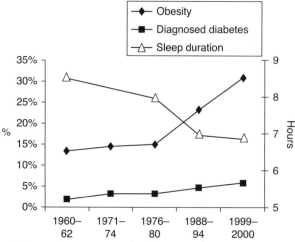

Fig. 6.1 Prevalence of obesity (BMI > 30 kg/m²), prevalence of diabetes and average self-reported sleep duration in the US between 1960 and 2000 (Gallup Organization, 1979,1995; Kripke et al., 1979; Breslau et al., 1997; Flegal et al., 1998; National Sleep Foundation, 2001; Flegal et al., 2002; Gregg et al., 2004).

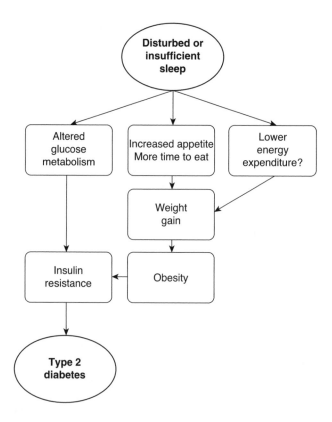

Fig. 6.2 Potential pathways linking disturbed or insufficient sleep to the development of obesity and diabetes.

Sleep and glucose metabolism—an overview

In healthy individuals, glucose levels in the blood are tightly regulated through a balance between glucose production (either from the liver or from nutrient-derived glucose in the gut) and glucose utilization by tissues. Insulin plays a key role in this process by inhibiting glucose production in the liver and by stimulating glucose uptake by insulin-sensitive tissues (i.e. muscle, liver, and fat cells). Glucose tolerance refers to the ability of the body's tissues to absorb exogenous glucose from the blood and return blood glucose levels to baseline values. Glucose tolerance is assessed in response to either oral glucose administration, intravenous glucose administration, or meals containing carbohydrates. Insulin sensitivity (SI) and insulin resistance refer to the ability of insulin to exert its effects in target cells and is the best predictor of future development of diabetes. The cellular response elicited by insulin depends on the cell type involved. For example, following a meal, there is an increase in blood glucose, which leads to insulin secretion by pancreatic beta (β)-cells. Insulin binding to its receptor in muscle cells leads to glucose uptake by the muscle to be used as immediate energy or stored as glycogen for use by the muscle cell during times of fasting. When muscle cells become insulin resistant, the same amount of secreted insulin does not induce glucose uptake into the cell, and therefore glucose remains in the blood at elevated concentrations.

In the liver, insulin signalling suppresses gluconeogenesis, which is the production of *de novo* glucose from precursor molecules and is unnecessary in the face of glucose ingestion. Insulin resistance in this tissue results in a lack of inhibition of gluconeogenesis, leading to further elevations of blood glucose. Reduced muscle glucose uptake and increased liver glucose production both contribute to elevated blood glucose levels and decreased insulin action. High blood glucose can have a number of deleterious health consequences, including blood vessel damage, kidney disease, glaucoma, and nerve damage if not controlled. An inadequate reduction of blood glucose then leads to additional insulin secretion by the pancreas, a phenomenon known as β-cell compensation. In this situation, only a higher amount of insulin will result in the desired amount of glucose clearance. Muscle, kidney, and liver account for ~75–85% of glucose disposal. Brain glucose uptake has been reported to use up to ~15–20% of ingested glucose, resulting in at least 90% of glucose disposal accounted for by liver, muscle, brain, and kidney (Meyer et al., 2002) thus even small changes in these tissues' sensitivity to insulin signalling could robustly affect global energy metabolism.

Another important insulin sensitive tissue is the adipose tissue, in which the main function of insulin is to inhibit the mobilization and release of triglycerides into the blood stream (lipolysis). Adipose tissue can account for 2–10% of glucose uptake (Marin et al., 1992), which is partially metabolized to triglyceride precursors for storage and subsequent release into circulation when necessary. The critical role of adipose tissue is as a lipid storage depot. Insulin resistance in these cells impairs the ability of insulin to inhibit lipolysis, which leads to elevated blood fatty acid levels. Fatty acids in the blood can result in the inappropriate accumulation in other tissues, such as muscle and liver. The presence of fatty acids in these areas further impairs insulin action through various mechanisms. In the fed state, insulin acts on adipocytes (fat cells) to inhibit lipolysis and adipocytes respond to glucose uptake by secreting leptin, an adipocyte-derived satiety hormone which signals to the hypothalamus to inhibit feeding in the presence of adequate energy intake. The characterization of leptin as an adipocyte-derived factor was the pivotal discovery that established adipose tissue as not just a lipid storage depot, but an entire endocrine organ responsible for secreting a variety of adipokines, which are important regulators of energy balance and metabolism. Adipokines can affect feeding through proximal signalling to nearby tissues as well as more distal signalling in the hypothalamus of the brain. This will be further discussed in a later section regarding appetite regulation and the effects of sleep on these functions.

Glucose metabolism in relation to normal sleep

During normal sleep, glucose tolerance is highest in the morning and lowest in the middle of the night (Van Cauter et al., 1997). This fluctuation appears to be related to reduced SI combined with reduced insulin secretion, resulting in elevated glucose levels in the middle of the sleep period. Optimal glucose tolerance is observed in the morning and decreases throughout the day and into the sleep period.

Exogenous glucose injection will inhibit glucose production by the liver. Therefore, changes in plasma glucose levels during constant glucose infusion reflect changes in glucose effectiveness, which is the ability of glucose to mediate its own disposal independently of insulin. In these studies, higher plasma levels of glucose would indicate reduced glucose effectiveness. In one such study, during 8 hours of nocturnal sleep, plasma glucose levels rose at the beginning of the sleep period, peaked around midsleep, and then declined back to pre-sleep levels (Scheen et al., 1996), indicating reduced glucose effectiveness during sleep. The insulin secretory rate (ISR) followed a very similar pattern to the plasma glucose levels, except that these changes occurred approximately 9 minutes after the changes in glucose levels (Scheen et al., 1996). When subjects were allowed to sleep in the daytime after a night of total sleep deprivation, plasma glucose levels increased abruptly (Scheen et al., 1996). The glucose increase during sleep was positively correlated with stages 2–4 of non-rapid eye movement (NREM) sleep, while glucose levels declined during periods of prolonged wakefulness (Scheen et al., 1996). Rapid eye movement (REM) sleep did not appear to impact glucose levels since they remained stable during REM. Thus, the pattern of glucose levels observed during sleep reflects the pattern of sleep stages during the night: greater NREM sleep in the early part of the night and greater wake and less NREM sleep during the later part of the night. Results from positron emission tomography (PET) demonstrated that whole-brain glucose metabolism declined significantly from wake to NREM sleep (Nofzinger et al., 2002). Since the brain glucose utilization is not mediated by insulin, this decline in brain glucose utilization would result in reduced glucose effectiveness. The increase in glucose levels during sleep may also partly reflect decreased glucose utilization by peripheral tissues. Glucose regulation is thus markedly affected by the sleep-wake cycle.

Glucose metabolism in response to experimental manipulations of sleep

The effects of acute total sleep deprivation over one night have been examined using constant glucose infusion. The typical pattern of plasma glucose levels during sleep (described above) was not observed during total sleep deprivation. During total sleep deprivation, plasma glucose levels do not exhibit the large increase that is observed during sleep (Scheen et al., 1996). Also, plasma glucose levels were higher in the morning after sleep deprivation than after a night of sleep despite similar insulin levels, suggesting that total sleep deprivation may impair insulin action. The pattern of glucose secretion during nocturnal sleep deprivation may be partly due to the absence of slow wave sleep (SWS) and growth hormone (GH) secretion at the beginning of the night. The effects of total sleep deprivation on metabolism or endocrine profiles are not the same as the effects of partial sleep deprivation (Knutson et al., 2007).

Total sleep deprivation can only be maintained for a brief period of time and does not reflect typical real-world behaviour. Chronic partial sleep restriction, on the other hand, is practiced by many people throughout the United States and the world. Recent estimates from the National

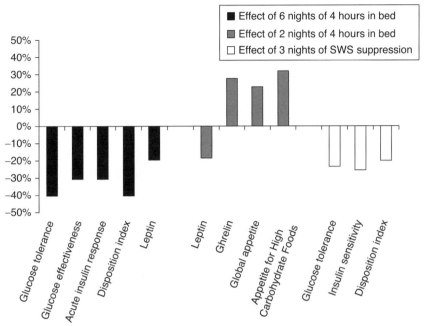

Fig. 6.3 Summary of results from 3 laboratory studies that manipulated sleep (Spiegel et al., 1999; Spiegel et al., 2004; Tasali et al., 2008).

Sleep Foundation indicate that 16% of adults who work at least 30 hours per week report sleeping less than 6 hours per night on weekdays (National Sleep Foundation, 2008). The first detailed laboratory study of the effects of partial sleep deprivation on glucose metabolism subjected healthy young men to 6 nights of 4 hours in bed followed by 7 nights of 12 hours in bed (Spiegel et al., 1999). On the last 2 days of each condition, the subjects ate identical carbohydrate-rich meals and were at continuous bed rest. Subjects had an intravenous glucose tolerance test (ivGTT) in the morning after the fifth night of each condition followed by 24 hours of blood sampling at 10- to 30-minutes interval (Spiegel et al., 1999). Glucose tolerance was 40% lower, glucose effectiveness was 30% lower, and the acute insulin response to glucose (AIR_G) was also 30% lower (Fig. 6.3). SI was lower after sleep restriction but it was not statistically significant. Comparison of the glucose tolerance values observed in this study to values obtained in different subject populations using the same ivGTT protocol indicated that the glucose tolerance values observed after 5 days of sleep restriction were similar to those observed in older adults with impaired glucose tolerance (Garcia et al., 1997), while the values observed after sleep recovery were, as expected, in the range typical of healthy young subjects (Prigeon et al., 1995). The disposition index (DI) is a marker of diabetes risk and is the product of $AIR_G \times SI$, which will remain constant in healthy individuals because β-cell function is able to compensate for insulin resistance with increased insulin release (Bergman et al., 2002). Type 2 diabetes occurs when the pancreatic β-cells are not able to compensate for insulin resistance, resulting in hyperglycaemia. Thus, lower DI values represent a higher risk of type 2 diabetes. DI values of 2,000 and above are typical of subjects with normal glucose tolerance, while DI values under 1,000 have been reported in populations at high risk for type 2 diabetes (Xiang et al., 2006). After sleep restriction, the DI was 40% lower than after sleep extension and 3 of the 11 subjects had DI values under 1,000. These results suggest that a few days of bedtimes restricted to 4 hours in bed could increase the risk of developing impaired glucose tolerance or diabetes.

One limitation to this study was that there may have been an order effect since sleep extension always followed sleep restriction (Youngstedt and Kripke, 2004). A second study compared the effect of 4 hours in bed per night for 2 nights to the effect of 10 hours in bed per night for 2 nights using a randomized cross-over design in healthy lean young subjects. After the second night of both conditions participants underwent constant glucose infusion and blood samples were collected every 20 minutes from 8:00 to 21:00 hours. These results were similar to the findings of the previous sleep restriction study. Between 9:00 and 11:00 hours, glucose levels were higher and insulin levels were lower after 2 days of 4-hour bedtimes than after 2 days of 10-hour bedtimes (Spiegel et al., 2005).

Recently, the effects of an experimental reduction in SWS on glucose metabolism in nine healthy, lean subjects aged 20–31 years were examined. Investigators in this study used noise to inhibit the transition to the SWS stages (stages 3 and 4), resulting an overall reduction in sleep *quality*, rather than quantity. Glucose metabolism after three nights of SWS suppression was compared to glucose metabolism after two nights of undisturbed sleep. Both conditions allowed for 7.5 hours in bed and total sleep time did not differ significantly between the two conditions. Suppression of SWS was associated with 23% reduction in glucose tolerance, 25% reduction in SI, and 20% reduction in the DI (Fig. 6.3) (Tasali et al., 2005). The results of this study suggest that sleep quality, in addition to sleep duration, may play an important role in glucose metabolism.

A second study of healthy, non-obese men aged 20–35 years examined the effects of sleep restricted to 5 hours per night for 7 days compared to 13 days of 10 hours in bed (Buxton et al., 2008). This study used a euglycaemic hyperinsulinaemic clamp technique, which involves measuring the amount of glucose infusion required to maintain constant blood glucose levels in the face of increased insulin administration. A higher rate of glucose infusion indicates greater SI. In this study, SI was reduced by approximately 11% after sleep restriction. This experimental study that involved less severe sleep loss further supports the hypothesis that sleep restriction, at least for one week or less, can impair glucose regulation.

Another recent study attempted to examine the effects of restricting bedtimes of elderly long sleepers on glucose metabolism (Zielinski et al., 2008). They enrolled 40 adults, 50–70 years old who reported that they slept an average of 9.5 hours or more per day. Actigraphic recordings in these individuals indicated that they averaged in fact only 7.5–7.9 hours per night. Subjects were randomly assigned to one of two groups: (1) the experimental group where bedtime was restricted by 90 minutes and (2) the control group who maintained a fixed bedtime schedule. At the end of the intervention, participants in the bedtime restriction averaged 6.55 hours of sleep per night and participants in the control group averaged 6.82 hours per night, a difference of approximately 16 minutes. Fasting glucose increased by 1% in the experimental group and decreased by 4% in the control group, which resulted in a statistically significant post-treatment effect. Pre-treatment SI, which was derived from fasting glucose and fasting insulin levels, was significantly higher in the restriction group, which suggests that randomization did not successfully lead to similar groups at baseline. Nonetheless, the results of these studies suggest that sleep restricted to 6.5 hours per night in older adults does not impair glucose metabolism. Another important finding from this study is that self-reported long sleepers may not, in fact, be long sleepers, but rather be suffering from poor sleep efficiency. Additional research is required to understand the increased morbidity and mortality risk associated with self-reported long sleep (see also Chapter 4).

Sleep and appetite regulation—an overview

As discussed above, adipokines secreted from fat cells can affect feeding in a variety of ways, including proximal signalling to nearby tissues, as well as more distal signalling in the hypothalamus of the brain. The arcuate nucleus of the hypothalamus is considered the feeding area of the brain and exerts potent effects on appetite, energy expenditure, and glucose homeostasis. Neurons in this nucleus are regulated by input from a variety of locations in the periphery, including adiposity signals (leptin), gut-derived signals (ghrelin and peptide YY [PYY]), and nutrient-derived signals (free fatty acids) (Schwartz and Porte, 2005). As with most biological systems, the arcuate nucleus contains opposing sets of neuronal circuitry: appetite simulating and appetite-inhibiting neurons (Gale et al., 2004). Ghrelin and PYY, both produced in the gut, have opposing effects on energy balance via an impact on neuronal activity in the arcuate nucleus. Ghrelin, secreted by gastric cells, stimulates appetite, whereas PYY, secreted by intestinal cells, inhibits feeding. Both leptin, produced in adipose tissue, and insulin, secreted by the pancreas in response to a meal, inhibit orexigenic neurons and activate anorexigenic neurons, leading to a decrease in feeding behaviour (Schwartz and Porte, 2005; Porte et al., 2005). Many of these hormones have been implicated as targets of sleep deprivation, specifically leptin.

Leptin is primarily a starvation signal from peripheral tissues to the hypothalamic region of the brain to indicate inadequate energy reserves (Flier, 2004). A decrease in leptin leads to a subsequent increase in feeding. The regulation of leptin is complex and is not entirely understood, however, it is known that leptin secretion is stimulated directly in response to glucose uptake. Leptin secretion requires both insulin signalling, as well as the stimulated uptake of glucose into the adipocyte. When glucose uptake and/or metabolism are impaired, leptin secretion is reduced and appetite is increased (Mueller et al., 1998). Conversely, exogenous leptin treatment inhibits feeding in animals and leptin-deficient humans (Farooqi, 2002).

Appetite regulation in response to experimental manipulations of sleep

Several laboratory studies have examined the effects of sleep restriction on one or more hormones involved in appetite regulation. The laboratory study discussed above that involved 6 nights of 4-hour bedtimes followed by 6 nights of 12-hour bedtimes reported that mean leptin levels were 19% lower during sleep restriction (Fig. 6.3) (Spiegel et al., 2004a). These changes in leptin levels occurred despite identical caloric intake and physical activity and no change in weight (Spiegel et al., 2004a). The maximal leptin level during sleep restriction was on average 1.7 ng/mL lower, which is somewhat larger than the decrease in leptin reported in young adults after 3 days of dietary intake restricted to 70% of energy requirements (Spiegel et al., 2005; Chin-Chance et al., 2000). Another group recruited eight healthy men aged 18–25 years to compare the effects of 7 days with 4-hour bedtimes to a 3-day recovery period with one night of *ad libitum* sleep followed by 2 nights with 7.5 hours in bed. They found that leptin levels were approximately 33% lower after sleep restriction ($P <.001$) (Guilleminault et al., 2003).

The impact of 2 days of 4-hour bedtimes versus 2 days of 10-hour bedtimes on leptin, ghrelin, and subjective appetite was examined in the laboratory study discussed above that used a randomized cross-over design (Fig. 6.3). Again, this study involved constant glucose infusion after the 2 nights of sleep restriction or extension and 20-minute blood sampling (Spiegel et al., 2004b). Mean leptin levels were 18% lower and mean ghrelin levels were 28% higher in the sleep restriction condition relative to sleep extension (Spiegel et al., 2004b). Appetite was measured using visual analogue scales and was 23% higher during sleep restriction. Furthermore, the increase in appetite for high calorie, carbohydrate-rich foods (including sweets, salty snacks, and starchy foods) was greater than for other food types (Spiegel et al., 2004b). Finally, the change in the ratio of ghrelin-to-leptin between the two conditions was strongly correlated to the change in hunger ratings ($r = 0.87$; $P = 0.01$), suggesting that the changes observed in these appetite hormones was partially responsible for the increase in subjective appetite. These observed changes would suggest that these subjects would have increased their food intake if they had been allowed *ad libitum* food, and a more recent study has confirmed this. Ten young lean subjects underwent two nights of base-line sleep with 8.5 hours in bed and four nights of 4.5 hours in bed in a randomized order (Tasali et al., 2009). At the end of each condition, subjects had access to a buffet lunch, buffet dinner, and unrestricted snacks. Caloric intake after sleep restriction was increased by approximately 460 kcal ($P = 0.04$), and was particularly increased for carbohydrate-rich foods (Tasali et al., 2009).

A separate laboratory study enrolled 11 sedentary men and women aged 34–49 years who were overweight (body mass index [BMI] between 24 and 29 kg/m^2) to examine the effects of more mild sleep restriction (Nedeltcheva et al., 2009). These subjects completed two 14-day periods consisting of either 5.5 hours or 8.5 hours in bed in a randomized order. Average daily caloric consumption from meals across the 14 days did not differ significantly between the two conditions, however, caloric intake from snacks was significantly increased in the sleep restriction condition (Nedeltcheva et al., 2009). Average 24-hour leptin and total ghrelin levels as well as energy expenditure did not differ significantly between the two conditions. Subjects in both conditions gained an average of 2 kg of weight, reflecting the obesogenic environment of the laboratory that included sedentary activity combined with unlimited palatable food. The absence of an effect of sleep restriction on leptin and ghrelin may reflect differences in the effects of this more mild sleep restriction on overweight individuals. Alternatively, the effects of the obesogenic environment and subsequent weight gain may have been so large that they masked any potential effects of mild sleep restriction.

Potential mechanisms

The deleterious effects of sleep perturbations on health outcomes are unlikely to be attributed to an alteration of a single metabolic variable. Rather these effects are more likely due to a constellation of changes that in their gestalt result in an increased risk of diabetes and obesity if the behaviour should become chronic. It has been postulated that the increase in blood glucose levels in studies of subjects undergoing total sleep deprivation is a result of decreased brain glucose utilization, as seen in studies using PET (Thomas et al., 2000). The reductions observed in insulin-independent glucose disposal in studies of restricted sleep are consistent with this hypothesis since, as mentioned above, brain glucose uptake is a non–insulin-mediated phenomenon.

Another mechanism by which sleep restriction increases the risk of obesity and subsequently diabetes is the observed increase in hunger and appetite in the laboratory studies. It has been suggested that this subjective increase in hunger may be a result of decreased inhibition of hypothalamic activity following sleep restriction. A loss of inhibition on orexigenic neurons in the hypothalamus would result in increased hunger and decreased ability to control that hunger (Gautier et al., 2001; Thomas et al., 2000).

Additionally, 6 days of sleep restriction were associated with an extended duration of elevated nighttime GH concentrations (Spiegel et al., 2000) and with an increase in evening cortisol levels (Spiegel et al., 1999), both of which could exacerbate already deleterious alterations in glucose regulation. For example, elevated evening cortisol concentrations are likely to result in reduced SI on the following morning, leading to an additional increase in blood glucose following sleep restriction (Van Cauter et al., 1997). Increased levels of GH can lead to an induction of a transient insulin resistance in muscle cells, resulting in decreased glucose uptake, elevated blood glucose levels, and subsequent increases in insulin resistance in other tissues. Finally, acute total sleep loss or even a 2-hour reduction of sleep per night for 1 week is associated with increased levels of proinflammatory cytokines and low grade inflammation, a condition known to predispose to insulin resistance and diabetes (Vgontzas et al., 1999, 2004) (see also Chapter 11).

Lastly, increased sympathetic nervous activity is a likely contributor to the increased risk of diabetes and obesity following chronic partial sleep restriction. Increased sympathetic nervous activity at the level of the pancreas could result in a reduction of insulin secretion from pancreatic β-cells. In both laboratory studies of sleep restriction described above, cardiac sympatho-vagal balance, derived from estimations of heart rate variability, was elevated (likely reflecting an increased influence of sympathetic tone) when sleep was restricted (Spiegel et al., 1999, 2004a). However, sympatho-vagal balance at the level of the pancreas has not yet been assessed in any study, but the findings mentioned above would suggest an alteration at this site as well.

Observational studies of sleep and metabolic disease

Laboratory studies of sleep restriction provide essential insight into potential mechanisms because they are typically conducted in well-controlled environments and involve detailed physiological measurements. One limitation, however, is that laboratory studies can only be short term, lasting a few weeks at most. This leads to the question of whether the associations observed in the laboratory persist in the real world when sleep restriction becomes chronic. Observational studies, especially large population-based epidemiological studies, can provide some insight into the associations between sleep and health outside of the laboratory.

Several large observational studies have reported associations between sleep duration or quality and the presence of diabetes (see also Chapter 5). The Sleep Heart Health Study is a large multi-centre cohort study that has performed an overnight in-home polysomnography (PSG) in approximately 6,000 adults 40 years of age and older to determine the cardiovascular and other consequences of sleep-disordered breathing (SDB) (Quan et al., 1997). Results from this study indicated that the odds of having diabetes was significantly higher in those reporting sleeping 5 hours or less (odds ratio [OR]: 2.51; 95% confidence interval [CI]: 1.57–4.02), 6 hours (OR: 1.66; 95% CI: 1.15–2.39), and 9 or more hours (OR: 1.79; 95% CI: 1.08–2.96) compared to 7–8 hours per night (Gottlieb et al., 2005). The OR of having impaired glucose tolerance was significantly higher in those sleeping 6 hours (OR: 1.58; 95% CI: 1.15–2.18) or 9 or more hours (OR: 1.88; 95% CI: 1.21–2.91) compared to 7–8 hours (Gottlieb et al., 2005). Another study of over 1,200 American adults aged 34–54 years also found a U-shaped association between self-reported sleep duration and diabetes (Hall et al., 2008). Adults who reported sleeping less than 6 hours (OR: 1.74; 95% CI: 1.18–2.55) or more than 8 hours (OR: 1.70; 95% CI: 1.04–2.80) per night were more likely to have diabetes than those reporting 7–8 hours per night. Results from the Quebec Family Study in Canada also found a U-shaped association between self-reported sleep duration and the prevalence of type 2 diabetes or impaired glucose tolerance in both men and women (Chaput et al., 2007a). A smaller study in the United States among 210 adults aged 30–54 years used the Pittsburgh Sleep Quality Index (PSQI), which is a validated questionnaire that assesses sleep quality, and found that worse sleep quality was significantly associated with higher serum insulin and glucose levels after adjustment for age and sex (Jennings et al., 2007). The PSQI was completed in another US study of healthy men and women, and the results indicated that frequent problems falling asleep was associated with higher insulin levels in women but not in men (Suarez, 2008).

Similar studies have been conducted in Asia and Europe as well. A study in Korea of over 4,000 adults did not find a significant association between self-reported sleep duration and hyperglycaemia (fasting blood glucose ≥ 5.6 mmol/L) in adults less than 60 years old, however, there was a trend ($P = 0.07$) for higher glucose with increasing sleep duration in those aged 60 years and older (Choi et al., 2008). A Japanese study that used homeostasis model assessment-estimated insulin resistance (HOMA-IR) reported that the OR of having elevated insulin resistance (HOMA-IR > 2.0) was higher among those reporting sleeping less than 6 hours per night compared to those sleeping

6 or more hours per night (OR: 2.17; 95% CI: 1.10–4.26). After adjustment for self-reported sleep quality, only long sleep duration (≥8 hours) predicted high fasting plasma glucose (>125 mg/dL) in over 1,000 adults aged 20 years or older from rural Japan, however, the prevalence of high haemoglobin A1c (HbA1c) (≥6.5%) was significantly higher in those sleeping less than 6 hours (OR: 4.96; 95% CI: 1.03–23.96), 8 to <9 hours (OR: 2.92; 95% CI: 1.03–8.27), and ≥9 hours (OR: 4.96; 95% CI: 1.70–14.50) compared to 7 to <8 hours per night (Nakajima et al., 2008). Two studies, one from India and one from Sweden, found greater difficulty initiating sleep, maintaining sleep, and excessive daytime sleepiness among patients with diabetes compared to healthy controls (Sridhar and Madhu, 1994; Gislason and Almqvist, 1987), however, a study in Finland found no difference in self-reported sleep time or sleep complaints between patients with type 2 diabetes and controls (Hyyppa and Kronholm, 1989). Sex differences in the association between sleep duration and prevalent diabetes were observed in a Finnish study (Tuomilehto et al., 2008). Prevalence of type 2 diabetes was significantly higher in women who were short (≤6 hours) and long (≥8 hours) sleepers compared to women who slept 7 hours per night after adjustment for many covariates including BMI and probability of sleep apnoea among others, however, there was no association in men (Tuomilehto et al., 2008). One limitation to these studies is that they used self-reported sleep duration and quality, but one study used wrist activity monitoring to estimate habitual sleep duration and quality (Trento et al., 2008). They observed greater sleep fragmentation and movement time in those with type 2 diabetes as compared to healthy controls (Trento et al., 2008). A study in children also examined the association between sleep and markers of glucose metabolism. These investigators reviewed clinical charts of 40 obese children aged 3.5–18.5 years without diabetes who had one night of PSG in the sleep clinic and found that only age, total sleep time, and percent of REM sleep were significant predictors of insulin resistance as estimated by the HOMA-IR method, but apnoea-hypopnoea index (AHI), SWS, BMI, and measures of oxygen desaturation were not significant (Flint et al., 2007). The results of these studies suggest a cross-sectional association between diabetes and short sleep duration or poor sleep quality, however, the causal direction cannot be determined. Poor or insufficient sleep may increase the risk of developing diabetes, as the laboratory studies suggest, or having diabetes may impair one's sleep.

Several prospective epidemiological studies conducted in the United States have examined the association between sleep duration or disturbance and incident diabetes. The Nurses Health Study, which recruited married female nurses aged 30–55 years in 1976, found an increased risk of diabetes over 10 years among those reporting sleeping less than 6 hours or 9 or more hours per night relative to 7–8 hours, after controlling for many covariates such as shift-work, hypertension, exercise, and depression (Ayas et al., 2003). Adjusting for BMI resulted in a significant risk of incident diabetes for the long sleepers only (Ayas et al., 2003), suggesting that BMI may be on the causal pathway between short sleep and the development of diabetes. When predicting only those cases of diabetes that had symptoms, which included itching, coma, frequent urination, hunger, weight loss, and thirst, sleeping ≤5 hours (OR: 1.37; 95% CI: 1.07–1.77) and sleeping 9 or more hours (OR: 1.36; 95% CI: 1.04–1.73) were associated with a significant increase in incident symptomatic diabetes compared to sleeping 7–8 hours even after adjustment for covariates including BMI (Ayas et al., 2003). Analysis of data from the National Health and Nutrition Examination Survey also demonstrated that diabetes incidence was significantly higher in those reporting sleeping ≤5 hours (OR: 1.47; 95% CI: 1.03–2.09) and those reporting sleeping 9 or more hours (OR: 1.52; 95% CI: 1.06–2.17) compared to those reporting sleeping 7 hours per night after adjusting for covariates including physical activity, depression, alcohol, ethnicity, education, marital status, age, overweight/obesity, and hypertension (Gangwisch et al., 2007). The Massachusetts Male Aging Study recruited men aged 40–70 years in 1987–1989 and examined them again in 1995–1997 and 2002–2004 (Yaggi et al., 2006). Among men without diabetes at baseline, the odds of developing diabetes were higher among those who reported sleeping 5 hours or less (OR: 1.95; 95% CI: 0.85–4.01), 6 hours (OR: 1.95; 95% CI: 1.06–3.58), and >8 hours (OR: 3.12; 95% CI: 1.53–6.37) per night compared to 7 hours per night after adjustment for covariates such as age, hypertension, smoking, self-rated health, waist circumference, and education (Yaggi et al., 2006). All of these studies suggest a U-shaped association between self-reported sleep duration and incident diabetes in the United States.

Prospective studies of sleep and diabetes are not limited to the United States. A prospective study of adult men in Japan reported that men with either a high frequency of difficulty initiating sleep or difficulty maintaining sleep had two to three times the odds of developing type 2 diabetes over an 8-year period compared to those with a low frequency of these sleep disturbances (Kawakami et al., 2004). Another prospective study in Japan followed 6,500 men and women aged 19–69 years for an average of 4.2 years and found that difficulty initiating sleep, but not sleep duration, was significantly associated with incident diabetes (Hayashino et al., 2007). Over 6,500 Swedish men were followed for 7–22 years and an increased odds of incident diabetes was observed among those who reported difficulty falling asleep or use of sleeping pills (OR: 1.52; 95% CI: 1.05–2.20) after controlling for numerous covariates including age, BMI at baseline, physical activity, smoking, and family history of diabetes (Nilsson et al., 2004). A second prospective study conducted in Sweden followed men and women for 12 years, and found that men who reported difficulty maintaining sleep (OR: 4.8, 95% CI: 1.9–12.5) or who reported sleep duration of 5 hours or less (OR: 2.8, 95% CI: 1.1–7.3) had a significantly greater odds of developing diabetes (Mallon et al., 2005). Sleep duration or disturbances did not significantly predict incident diabetes in women in this sample. A third prospective study from Sweden followed over 1,000 women for 32 years and observed no association between self-reported sleep problems, sleep medication use or sleep duration at baseline, and the incidence of diabetes (Bjorkelund et al., 2005). A prospective study in Germany followed 8,269 men and women aged 25–74 years for an average of 7.5 years and found a significant increased odds of incident type 2 diabetes for those who reported difficulty maintaining sleep at baseline in both men (OR: 1.60; 95% CI: 1.05–2.45) and women (OR: 1.98; 95% CI: 1.20–3.29), even after adjustment for numerous covariates (Meisinger et al., 2005). These studies suggest that self-reported sleep problems and short sleep may increase the risk of developing diabetes, particularly in men.

Since short sleep may lead to the development of diabetes, some investigators questioned whether sleep is associated with glycaemic control among individuals who already have diabetes. In a study of 50 patients with type 2 diabetes from Brazil, a higher percentage of those with poor sleep quality (PSQI score >5) had elevated HbA1c (>7%) (Cunha et al., 2008). Haemoglobin A1c (HbA1c) is a measure of glycaemic control and higher values indicate worse glycaemic control. A study in the United States of 38 patients with type 2 diabetes (18 of whom had restless legs syndrome) observed a significant unadjusted correlation between the Epworth Sleepiness Score and HbA1c ($r = 0.36$), but HbA1c was not associated with PSQI score (Cuellar and Ratcliffe, 2008). Another US study found that 71% of the participants were classified as having poor quality sleep (PSQI score >5) (Knutson et al., 2006). In patients without diabetic complications, HbA1c was associated with perceived sleep debt (self-reported preferred sleep duration minus self-reported actual sleep duration) but in patients with at least one complication, HbA1c level was associated with PSQI score (Knutson et al., 2006). In the study that used wrist activity monitoring to measure sleep in patients with type 2 diabetes, higher HbA1c levels were associated with lower sleep efficiency ($r = -0.29$, $P = 0.057$) (Trento et al., 2008).

Several observational studies have examined the association between sleep duration and obesity or BMI. Table 6.1 summarizes results from studies conducted in adults and Table 6.2 summarizes

Table 6.1 Summary of published articles examining the association between sleep and BMI or obesity in adults*

Reference	Sleep measure	Sample	Association with higher BMI or overweight/obesity			Country
			Short sleep	Long sleep	No significant association	
Cross-sectional studies						
Vioque et al. (2000)	Self-report	n = 1,772 men and women Aged >15 years	✓			Spain
Shigeta et al. (2001)	Self-report	n = 453 men and women Age not reported	✓			Japan
Kripke et al. (2002)	Self-report	n = 636,095 men and women Aged 30–02 years	✓ (men and women)	✓ (women)		US
Taheri et al. (2004)	Sleep diary	n = 1,040 men and women Aged 30–60 years	✓	✓		US
Patel et al. (2004)	Self-report	n = 82,969 women Aged 40–65 years	✓	✓		US
Cournot et al. (2004)	Self-report	n = 3,236 men and women; Aged 32–62 years	✓ (women)		✓ (men)	France
Vorona et al. (2005)	Self-report	n = 924 men and women Aged 18–91 years	✓			US
Singh et al. (2005)	Self-report	n = 3,158 men and women Aged 18–65 years	✓			US
Kohatsu et al. (2006)	Self-report	n = 990 employed men and women Mean age 48.3 ± 13.0 years	✓			Rural US
Gortmaker et al. (1990)	Self-report	n = 712 men and women Age not reported			✓	US
Heslop et al. (2002)	Self-report	n = 5,819 men <65 years; n = 978 women <60 years	✓			UK
Tamakoshi and Ohno (2004)	Self-report	n = 110,792 men and women Aged 40–79 years			✓	Japan
Amagai et al. (2004)	Self-report	n = 11,325 men and women Aged 19–93 years			✓	Japan

Table 6.1 (continued) Summary of published articles examining the association between sleep and BMI or obesity in adults*

Reference	Sleep measure	Sample	Association with higher BMI or overweight/obesity			Country
			Short sleep	Long sleep	No significant association	
Ohayon (2004)	Self-report	n = 8,091 men and women Aged 55–101 years			✓	Europe
Bjorkelund et al. (2005)	Self-report	n = 1,447 women Aged 38–60 years				Sweden
Ohayon and Vecchierini (2005)	Self-report	n = 1,026 men and women Aged ≥60 years	✓			France
Gottlieb et al. (2006)	Self-report	n = 5,910 men and women Aged 40–100 years	✓	✓		US
Lauderdale et al. (2006)	Actigraphy	n = 612 men and women Aged 35–50 years	✓			US
Moreno et al. (2006)	Self-report	n = 4,878 men (truck drivers)Mean age 40 ± 10 SD years	✓			Brazil
Chaput et al. (2007a)	Self-report	n = 740 men and women Aged 21–64 years	✓			Canada
Ko et al. (2007)	Self-report	n = 4,793 men and women Aged 17–83 years	✓			China
Rontoyanni et al. (2007)	Self-report	n = 30 women Aged 30–60 years	✓			Greece
Bjorvatn et al. (2007)	Self-report	n = 8,860 men and women Aged 40–45 years	✓			Norway
Asplund and Aberg (2001)	Self-report	n = 3,712 women Aged 40–64 years				Sweden
Jennings et al. (2007)	Self-report (PSQI)	n = 210 men and women Aged 30–54 years				US
Stamatakis and Brownson (2008)	Self-report	n = 1,258 men and women Aged 20–92 years	✓	✓		Rural US
Patel et al. (2008)	Actigraphy	n = 3,135 men ≥65 years n = 3,219 women ≥65 years	✓(obesity and body fat %)	✓(body fat %)		US

Table 6.1 (continued) Summary of published articles examining the association between sleep and BMI or obesity in adults*

Reference	Sleep measure	Sample	Association with higher BMI or overweight/obesity			Country
			Short sleep	Long sleep	No significant association	
Choi et al. (2008)	Self-report	n = 4,222 men and women Aged >20 years	✓(<60 years)	✓(<60 years)	✓(>60 years)	Korea
Buscemi et al. (2007)	Self-report	n = 199 men and women (internal medicine patients) Aged 18–89 years	✓(women)	✓(women)	✓(men)	US
Chaput et al. (2007b)	Self-report	n = 90 women Aged 60–75 years			✓	Quebec
Hall et al. (2008)	Self-report	n = 1,295 men and women Aged 30–54 years	✓			US
Fogelholm et al. (2007)	Self-report	n = 7,641 men and women Aged ≥30 years	✓(men)		✓(women)	Finland
Park et al. (2009)	Self-report	n = 8,717 men and women Aged ≥20 years	✓			Korea
Gangwisch et al. (2005)	Self-report	n = 9,588 men and women Aged 32–86 years	✓(32–49 years)		✓(≥50 years)	US
Lopez-Garcia et al. (2008)	Self-report	n = 4,008 men and women Aged ≥60 years	✓	✓		Spain
Stranges et al. (2008)	Self-report	n = 10,308 men and women Aged 44–65 years	✓			UK
Prospective studies						
Gangwisch et al. (2005)	Self-report	n = 9,588 men and women Aged 32–86 years			✓	US
Lopez-Garcia et al. (2008)	Self-report	n = 3,235 men and women Aged ≥60 years	✓	✓		Spain
Stranges et al. (2008)	Self-report	n = 10,308 men and women Aged 44–65 years			✓	UK
Patel et al. (2006)	Self-report	n = 68,183 women Aged 39–65 years	✓			US

Table 6.1 (continued) Summary of published articles examining the association between sleep and BMI or obesity in adults*

Reference	Sleep measure	Sample	Association with higher BMI or overweight/obesity			Country
			Short sleep	Long sleep	No significant association	
Chaput et al. (2008)	Self-report	n = 276 men and women Aged 21–64 years	✓			Canada
Gunderson et al. (2008)	Self-report	n = 940 women Mean age 33.0 (SD 4.7) years	✓			US
Hasler et al. (2004)	Self-report	n = 496 men and women Aged 19 years at baseline	✓			Switzerland
Littman et al. (2006)	Self-report	n = 173 women Aged 50–75 years			✓	US
Lauderdale et al. (2006)	Actigraphy	n = 612 men and women Aged 35–50 years			✓	US
Total			**34**	**10**	**13**	

*A check indicates a significant association between higher BMI or prevalence of overweight/obesity and either short sleep, long sleep, or no significant association. Groups in parentheses indicate that the associations were significant only for that group or outcome measure.

Table 6.2 Summary of published articles examining the association between sleep and BMI or obesity in children*

Reference	Sleep measure	Sample	Association with higher BMI or overweight/obesity			Country
			Short sleep	Long sleep	No significant association	
Cross-sectional studies						
Locard et al. (1992)	Parental report	n = 327 obese boys and girls, n = 704 non-obese boys and girls Aged 5 years	✓			France
Gupta et al. (2002)	Actigraphy	n = 383 boys and girls Aged 11–16 years	✓			US
von Kries et al. (2002)	Parental report	n = 6,862 boys and girls Aged 5–6 years	✓			Germany
Sekine et al. (2002)	Parental report	n = 8,274 boys and girls Aged 6–7 years	✓			Japan

Table 6.2 (continued) Summary of published articles examining the association between sleep and BMI or obesity in children*

Reference	Sleep measure	Sample	Association with higher BMI or overweight/obesity			Country
			Shortsleep	Long sleep	No significant association	
Chaput et al. (2006)	Parental report	n = 422 boys and girls Aged 5–10 years	✓			Canada
Knutson (2005)	Self-report	n = 4,555 boys and girls Aged 11–21 years	✓(boys)		✓(girls)	US
Ben Slama et al. (2002)	Parental report	n = 3,148 boys Aged 6–10 years	✓			Tunisia
Benefice et al. (2004)	Actigraphy	n = 40 girls Aged 13–14 years	✓			Senegal
Giugliano and Carneiro (2004)	Parental report	n = 452 boys and girls Aged 6–10 years	✓(overweight children only)			Brazil
Padez et al. (2009)	Parental report	n = 4,511 boys and girls Aged 7–9 years	✓			Portugal
Chen et al. (2006)	Self-report	n = 656 boys and girls Aged 13–18 years	✓			Taiwan
Nixon et al. (2008)	Waist Actigraphy	n = 519 boys and girls Aged 7 years	✓			New Zealand
Yu et al. (2007)	Self-report	n = 500 boys and girls (twins) Aged 10–20 years	✓(girls)	✓(boys)		China
Kohyama et al. (2002)	Parental report	n = 1,105 boys and girls Aged 3–3.8 years			✓	Japan
Kuriyan et al. (2007)	Parental/ self-report	n = 598 boys and girls Aged 6–16 years	✓			India
Eisenmann et al. (2006)	Self-report	n = 6,324 boys and girls Aged 7–15 years	✓(boys)		✓(girls)	Australia
Liu et al. (2008)	3 nights PSG	n = 335 boys and girls Aged 7–17 years	✓			US
Seicean et al. (2007)	Self-report	n = 529 boys and girls Aged 14–18 years	✓			US
Dieu et al. (2007)	Parental report	n = 670 boys and girls Aged 4–5 years	✓			Vietnam
Hitze et al. (2008)	Parental/self-report	n = 414 boys and girls Aged 6–20 years	✓			Germany
Beebe et al. (2006)	Actigraphy	n = 60 overweight boys and girls n = 22 healthy controls boys and girls Aged 10–17 years	✓			US

Table 6.2 (continued) Summary of published articles examining the association between sleep and BMI or obesity in children*

Reference	Sleep measure	Sample	Association with higher BMI or overweight/obesity			Country
			Short sleep	Long sleep	No significant association	
Wells et al. (2008)	Self-report	n = 4,452 boys and girls Aged 11–12 years	✓(BMI)		✓(obesity)	Brazil
Lumeng et al. (2007)	Maternal report	n = 785 boys and girls Aged 11–12 years (6th grade)	✓			US
Prospective studies						
Lumeng et al. (2007)	Maternal report	n = 785 boys and girls Aged 9–10 years (3rd grade) and 11–12 years (6th grade)	✓			US
Agras et al. (2004)	Parental report	n = 150 boys and girls Sleep measured at 3–5 years Weight measured at 9.5 years	✓			US
Reilly et al. (2005)	Parental report	n = 7,758 boys and girls Sleep measured at 38 months Obesity measured at 7 years	✓			UK
Taveras et al. (2008)	Parental report	n = 915 boys and girls Sleep measured at 6 months, 1 year and 2 years; BMI z-score measured at 3 years	✓			US
Touchette et al. (2008)	Parental report	n = 1,138 boys and girls Sleep duration reported yearly from 2.5–6 years and BMI measured at 2.5 and 6 years	✓			Quebec
Sugimori et al. (2004)	Self-report	n = 8,170 boys and girls Sleep and BMI measured at ages 3 and 6 years	✓(boys)		✓(girls)	Japan
Snell et al. (2007)	Time diaries	n = 2,281 boys and girls Aged 3–12 years at baseline	✓(3–8 year olds)			US
Total			29	1	5	

*A check indicates a significant association between higher BMI or prevalence of overweight/obesity and either short sleep, long sleep, or no significant association. Groups in parentheses indicate that the associations were significant only for that group or outcome measure.

results from studies in children. Many studies have reported a significant cross-sectional association between short sleep duration and increased prevalence of obesity or higher BMI in both adults and children. Some of these studies also observed higher BMI and obesity associated with longer sleep durations as well, and this U-shaped association between sleep and morbidity has yet to be fully explained. Other studies examined self-reported measures of sleep quality and their association with BMI or obesity. A Swedish study found differences between ages in the association between obesity and sleep problems (Asplund and Aberg, 2001). In 40- to 49-year olds, obesity ($\geq$30 kg/m^2) was associated with worse sleep quality, while in 60- to 64-year olds, underweight (<20 kg/m^2) was associated with worse sleep quality. A US study that administered the PSQI found that worse sleep quality was associated with higher waist circumference, BMI, and body fat percentage (Jennings et al., 2007). Of note, many studies have reported differences in these associations by gender, by age group, or by outcome measures. In particular, the effect of sleep on BMI appears stronger at younger ages, and fewer studies in children have reported a U-shaped association (Table 6.2). Although we need to consider that the study methodology, sample demographics, and the analytical methods vary between these studies, most have found a cross-sectional association between sleep and BMI. There have also been a few prospective studies of sleep and weight gain (see Tables 6.1 and 6.2), however, these results are more mixed and the effects of sleep have been generally small or non-significant.

Two recent meta-analyses have examined data from studies on the cross-sectional association between sleep and BMI or obesity. Cappuccio et al. (2008) analyzed data from 17 studies including 22 different population samples in adults. Short sleep duration (<5 hours) significantly predicted obesity in 17 of the 22 population samples, and the pooled OR was 1.55 (95% CI: 1.43–1.68). Sleep duration as a continuous variable was significantly associated with BMI in all seven studies for which these data were available, and the pooled regression coefficient was -0.35 kg/m^2 change in BMI for every hour more sleep. Cappuccio et al. (2008) also identified 13 different population samples in children Short sleep duration (<10 hours) in children significantly predicted obesity (BMI > 95th percentile) in 7 of the 11 studies and the pooled OR was 1.89 (95% CI: 1.46–2.43). A second meta-analysis also examined sleep and obesity in children (Chen et al., 2008). They identified 17 observational studies in children and the pooled OR predicting obesity from short sleep duration was 1.58 (95% CI: 1.26–1.98). Thus, both meta-analyses found a significant overall association between short sleep duration and increased likelihood of being obese (see also Chapter 5).

A few observational studies have also examined the association between habitual sleep and levels of leptin and/or ghrelin. The Wisconsin Sleep Cohort Study was a population-based study that enrolled Wisconsin State employees aged 30–60 years (Taheri et al., 2004). Investigators collected sleep diaries to assess habitual sleep, conducted one night of PSG in the laboratory, and in the morning following the PSG, a single blood sample was obtained. The results indicated that total sleep time from PSG was negatively associated with ghrelin levels (β coefficient = -0.69, P = 0.008), while average habitual sleep duration was positively associated with leptin levels independently of BMI (β coefficient = 0.11; P = 0.01) (Taheri et al., 2004). Data from the Quebec Family Study of 740 men and women aged 21–64 years found that leptin levels in 5–6 hours were approximately 15–17% lower than expected based on fat mass in both men and women (Chaput et al., 2007b). Two studies in women, however, did not observe similar associations. The Nurses Health Study, which asked participants to mail back a blood sample, did not observe a significant association between self-reported sleep duration and leptin levels (Williams et al., 2007). A randomized trial of moderate-intensity exercise among obese, sedentary post-menopausal women aged 50–74 found no cross-sectional associations between self-reported sleep duration and leptin or total ghrelin levels at baseline nor any significant associations between change in sleep duration and changes in leptin or ghrelin (Littman et al., 2006). The lack of significant associations may reflect differences in the effects of sleep on appetite regulation in women, particularly obese older women, or may be due to methodological issues such as self-reported sleep duration or sample collection.

Although there are some consistent findings among the numerous observational studies described above, we must consider the methodological limitations of these studies. First, the vast majority of these studies relied on a self-reported measure of sleep duration, which may not be very accurate. Recent analysis comparing actigraphically recorded sleep to self-reported sleep in a sample of over 600 middle-aged adults indicated only moderate agreement between these measures ($r = 0.47$) (Lauderdale et al., 2008). In addition, there may be important confounders that are not taken into account in these analyses, including race, socioeconomic status, physical activity, alcohol and caffeine consumption, and psychological disorders (Lauderdale et al., 2008; Magee et al., 2008). Future studies need to incorporate objective measures of sleep and include detailed measures of potential confounding variables.

The result of these studies, which originated from different countries and cultures, generally agreed that short or poor sleep may increase the risk of developing type 2 diabetes, which is consistent with the findings from the laboratory studies. However, some studies did find differences by sex such that associations were not always observed in women. Furthermore, many studies found that self-reported long sleep (>8 or 9 hours) was associated with diabetes or obesity, and the mechanisms underlying this association need to be determined. Additional prospective and intervention studies that use objective measures of sleep are required to determine if sleep loss is on the causal pathway to the development of diabetes and obesity.

Obstructive sleep apnoea and metabolic disease

Reduced sleep duration and quality can also be a consequence of a sleep disorder, and one such disorder that has been associated with metabolic disturbances is OSA. OSA is characterized by SDB and involves an obstruction in the upper airway that leads to repeated episodes of increased breathing effort and a reduction (hypopnoea) or complete cessation (apnoea) of air flow (Thorpy, 2009). These episodes are often associated with reduced blood oxygen saturation and sleep fragmentation, and, in some, excessive daytime sleepiness. A diagnosis of OSA requires a minimum of five apnoeas or hypopnoeas per hour of sleep (the AHI). OSA is most common in people aged 40–65 years, and is also more common in men, although post-menopausal women appear to have similar risk of OSA as men of similar ages. A major risk factor for OSA is obesity and the current obesity epidemic has likely led to an increase in the prevalence of OSA. Estimates of the prevalence of SDB (defined as AHI > 5 events per hour) among 30- to 60-year olds in the United States in the early 1990s was 9% for women and 24% for men and the prevalence of OSA (defined as AHI > 5 events per hour plus daytime sleepiness) was 2% for women and 4% for men (Young et al., 1993). Approximately 26% of obese men and women (BMI > 30 kg/m^2) have AHI >15 events per hour and 60% have an AHI >5 events per hour (Gami et al., 2003).

Numerous studies have reported a close association between the presence of OSA and the presence of type 2 diabetes. For example, the Wisconsin Sleep Cohort Study found that almost 15% of participants who had an AHI of 15 events per hour or more had diagnosed diabetes compared to only 3% of those with an AHI <5 events per hour (Reichmuth et al., 2005). Another report found that 48% of patients with type 2 diabetes had an AHI of 10 events per hour or higher and 29% had an AHI of 20 events per hour or higher (Einhorn et al., 2007). In fact, the International Diabetes Federation Taskforce on Epidemiology and Prevention recently recommended that patients with either diabetes or SDB be examined for the other condition (Shaw et al., 2008).

The potential mechanisms linking OSA to metabolic disturbances include reduced sleep duration and quality. The impact of short or disturbed sleep on glucose metabolism and appetite regulation discussed previously could also contribute to impaired metabolism in patients with OSA. A few studies have examined glucose metabolism in relation to the presence and severity of SDB. The Sleep Heart Health Study reported that compared to those without SDB (AHI < 5 events per hour), adults with moderate-to-severe SDB (AHI ≥ 15 events per hour) were more likely to have glucose intolerance based on both a fasting blood sample and the 2-hour post-glucose ingestion sample from an oral glucose tolerance test (Punjabi et al., 2004). Furthermore, both a greater degree and a longer duration of oxyhaemoglobin desaturation were associated with glucose intolerance (Punjabi et al., 2004), suggesting that hypoxia may play a role in the disturbances in glucose metabolism. The Wisconsin Sleep Cohort Study also observed a significant cross-sectional association where increasing severity of SDB was associated with a greater prevalence of diabetes, but they did not observe a significant association between the presence of SDB and the development of diabetes over a 4-year period (Reichmuth et al., 2005). These results do not support a causal connection between SDB and impaired glucose metabolism, however, it is possible that a follow-up period of 4 years is not long enough to detect an association. Another study among approximately 2,500 adults without diagnosed diabetes found a significant cross-sectional association between increased SDB and the prevalence of impaired fasting glucose, impaired glucose tolerance, and occult diabetes even after adjustment for age, sex, race, BMI, and waist circumference (Seicean et al., 2008). In a study of 118 non-diabetic adults, SI, DI, and glucose effectiveness all decreased with increasing SDB, particularly in the moderate-to-severe SDB groups (Punjabi and Beamer, 2009). The reduction in SI compared to those without SDB ranged from 26.7% in those with mild SDB (AHI of 5–15 events per hour) to 43.7% in those with severe SDB (AHI of 30 or greater events per hour) independent of age, sex, race, and percent body fat (Punjabi and Beamer, 2009). The decreases in the DI and SI were associated with the average degree of oxyhaemoglobin desaturation (Punjabi and Beamer, 2009). Typically, a hypopnoea is defined as a reduction in airflow that is accompanied by an oxyhaemoglobin desaturation of at least 4%, however, investigators from the Sleep Heart Health Study examined whether a more mild oxyhaemoglobin desaturation was associated with metabolic measures. They reported that greater SDB associated with oxyhaemoglobin desaturation as low as 2% was associated with increased fasting glucose levels (Stamatakis and Brownson, 2008). Of particular concern is that these associations are not found only in adults. Two studies among children found that severity of OSA was associated with greater insulin resistance (Flint et al., 2007) and higher fasting insulin levels (de la Eva et al., 2002). Together these studies suggest an association between SDB or OSA and the prevalence of impaired glucose metabolism or diabetes, however, a causal link remains to be established.

Continuous positive airway pressure (CPAP) is a commonly used treatment for OSA. While sleeping, patients wear a mask that delivers continuous air flow at a pressure sufficient to keep the airways open. Several studies have examined the effects of CPAP treatment on glucose metabolism and appetite regulation in patients with OSA. In patients who have both type 2 diabetes and OSA, most studies observed an improvement in glucose regulation after CPAP (Dawson et al., 2008; Hassaballa et al., 2005; Babu et al., 2005; Schahin et al., 2008; Harsch et al., 2004a; Brooks et al., 1994), but one did not (West et al., 2007). In OSA patients without diabetes, the results are more mixed. Several studies have seen improvements in insulin sensitivity after CPAP use in patients with SDB (Harsch et al., 2004b; Lindberg et al., 2006; Dorkova et al., 2008). Other studies, did not observe an effect of CPAP on measures of glucose regulation (Vgontzas et al., 2008; Smurra et al., 2001; Coughlin et al., 2007; Trenell et al., 2007; Saarelainen et al., 1997). Patients with OSA typically have both higher ghrelin and higher leptin levels compared to BMI-matched controls without OSA (Takahashi et al., 2008; Phillips et al., 2000; Harsch et al., 2003; Ip et al., 2000). The higher levels of leptin are not consistent with the laboratory models of sleep loss, and may in fact reflect greater leptin resistance among OSA patients. Most studies that examined the effect of CPAP use on either leptin or ghrelin levels have observed a decline in these hormones (Saarelainen et al., 1997; Trenell et al., 2007; Takahashi et al., 2008; Harsch et al., 2003; Ip et al., 2000; Sanner et al., 2004; Chin et al., 1999), but some studies saw no change in leptin levels after CPAP use (Harsch et al., 2004b; Drummond et al., 2008; Rubinsztajn et al., 2006). Finally, OSA is also often associated with recent weight gain (Phillips et al., 1999) and greater visceral adiposity (Vgontzas et al., 2008) compared to BMI-matched controls, however studies that examined the effects of CPAP use on weight loss are also inconclusive. One study observed that those who used CPAP for at least 4 hours per night for 6 months were more likely to lose more than 4.5 kg of weight compared to those who did not meet this minimum use criterion for CPAP compliance (Loube et al., 1997). Two other studies reported a significant reduction in visceral adiposity after CPAP use (Trenell et al., 2007; Chin et al., 1999), but other studies saw no effect of CPAP on weight loss or visceral adiposity (Redenius et al., 2008; Vgontzas et al., 2008; Kajaste et al., 2004). One problem with these studies is the length of time that CPAP is used each night can be quite low. In fact, many of these studies defined compliance as use of CPAP for at least 4 hours, which probably does not allow the patients to achieve a sufficient amount of good quality sleep. In fact, one of the laboratory studies discussed above saw significant deleterious effects on glucose metabolism and appetite regulation when bedtimes were restricted to only 4 hours. Future research is still required to determine if a minimum number of hours of CPAP use can ameliorate metabolic disturbances among patients with OSA.

Summary

The accumulated evidence from both laboratory and observational studies suggest that insufficient or impaired sleep may play a role in the development of metabolic diseases such as diabetes and obesity. We have discussed the pathways through which sleep could lead to the development of obesity and diabetes. In particular, these pathways involve impairments in both glucose metabolism and appetite regulation, however, sleep's potential impact on energy expenditure warrants further examination.

Despite the large number of studies published to date in support of a link between sleep and metabolic disease, we must keep in mind some of the limitations of these studies. The primary limitation of the laboratory studies is the necessarily short duration of the sleep restriction, which can last a few weeks at most. These studies leave one wondering whether the effects of sleep restriction observed in the laboratory will persist if sleep restriction becomes chronic, or whether one's physiology can adapt to the sleep restriction. The evidence from the observational and large epidemiological studies suggest that one does not adapt to sleep durations less than 6 hours per night. There are, however, limitations to the epidemiological evidence as well. The majority of these studies relied on self-reported sleep duration, which may not be an accurate measure of actual sleep duration. Furthermore, most of the observational studies were cross-sectional so causality cannot be determined. In order to verify the importance of sleep's role in metabolism, future studies need to be designed to address these limitations. Prospective epidemiological studies need to include objective measures of habitual sleep duration and quality and consider important confounders. Finally, intervention studies that test the impact of sleep extension on metabolic health are critical for determining the causal link between sleep and metabolism.

Given the enormous impact obesity and diabetes have on QOL, life expectancy, and economic burden, it is very important to understand what factors influence the development of one or both of these conditions. Evidence reviewed here suggest that sleep duration or quality may play a role, thus future research into the causes and consequences of metabolic disease should include an examination of the impact of impaired or insufficient sleep. If sleep extension is an effective intervention, it would be an inexpensive behavioural modification that may be amenable to many at-risk people.

Summary box

♦ Sleep plays an important role in the release of many hormones, including glucose and cortisol. Sleep disturbances can therefore disrupt endocrine function.

♦ Laboratory studies have observed that sleep restriction is associated with impairments in glucose metabolism and appetite regulation. Sleep restriction is associated with decreased glucose tolerance, lower leptin levels (an appetite suppressant), higher ghrelin levels (an appetite stimulant), and increased subjective appetite.

♦ Epidemiological studies have found significant associations between shorter self-reported sleep durations and increased diabetes prevalence and higher body mass indices or increased obesity prevalence. Most of these studies have been cross-sectional, however a few longitudinal studies have reported increased weight gain among short sleepers.

♦ Potential mechanisms underlying these associations include increased sympathetic nervous activity, alterations in GH and cortisol profiles, and decreased inhibition of hypothalamic activity.

♦ OSA is a sleep disorder that is associated with obesity and appears to increase the risk of impaired glucose metabolism and diabetes. It is not yet known whether this increased risk is due to sleep loss, sleep fragmentation, and/or hypoxia, all of which characterize OSA.

♦ Future research needs to be conducted to fully understand sleep's role in obesity and diabetes risk. In particular, future studies should be prospective, include objective, detailed measures of habitual sleep, and an examination of energy expenditure. Intervention studies that involve extending or improving sleep are especially important.

References

Agras, W.S., Hammer, L.D., McNicholas, F. & Kraemer, H.C. (2004). Risk factors for childhood overweight: a prospective study from birth to 9.5 years. *J Pediatr*, **145**, 20–25.

Amagai, Y., Ishikawa, S., Gotoh, T., et al. (2004). Sleep duration and mortality in Japan: the Jichi Medical School Cohort Study. *J Epidemiol*, **14**, 124–128.

Asplund, R. & Aberg, H. (2001). Sleep complaints in women of ages 40-64 years in relation to sleep in their parents. *Sleep Med*, **2**, 233–237.

Ayas, N.T., White, D.P., Al-Delaimy, W.K., et al. (2003). A prospective study of self-reported sleep duration and incident diabetes in women. *Diabetes Care*, **26**, 380–384.

Babu, A.R., Herdegen, J., Fogelfeld, L., Shott, S. & Mazzone, T. (2005). Type 2 diabetes, glycemic control, and continuous positive airway pressure in obstructive sleep apnea. *Arch Intern Med*, **165**, 447–452.

Beebe, D.W., Lewin, D., Zeller, M., et al. (2006). Sleep in overweight adolescents: shorter sleep, poorer sleep quality, sleepiness, and sleep-disordered breathing. *J Pediatr Psychol,* **32**(1), 69–79.

Ben Slama, F., Achour, A., Belhadj, O., Hsairi, M., Oueslati, M. & Achour, N. (2002). Obesity and life style in a population of male school children aged 6 to 10 years in Ariana (Tunisia). *Tunis Med*, **80**, 542–7.

Benefice, E., Garnier, D. & Ndiaye, G. (2004). Nutritional status, growth and sleep habits among Senegalese adolescent girls. *Eur J Clin Nutr*, **58**, 292–301.

Bergman, R.N., Ader, M., Huecking, K. & Van Citters, G. (2002). Accurate assessment of beta-cell function: the hyperbolic correction. *Diabetes*, **51**(Suppl 1), S212–S220.

Bjorkelund, C., Bondyr-Carlsson, D., Lapidus, L., et al. (2005). Sleep disturbances in midlife unrelated to 32-year diabetes incidence: the prospective population study of women in Gothenburg. *Diabetes Care*, **28**, 2739–2744.

Bjorvatn, B., Sagen, I.M., Oyane, N., et al. (2007). The association between sleep duration, body mass index and metabolic measures in the Hordaland Health Study. *J Sleep Res*, **16**, 66–76.

Breslau, N., Roth, T., Rosenthal, L. & Andreski, P. (1997). Daytime sleepiness: an epidemiological study of young adults. *Am J Public Health*, **87**, 1649–1653.

Brooks, B., Cistulli, P.A., Borkman, M., et al. (1994). Obstructive sleep apnea in obese noninsulin-dependent diabetic patients: effects of continuous positive airway pressure treatment on insulin responsiveness. *J Clin Endocrinol Metab*, **79**, 1681–1685.

Buscemi, D., Kumar, A., Nugent, R. & Nugent, K. (2007). Short sleep times predict obesity in internal medicine clinic patients. *J Clin Sleep Med*, **3**, 681–688.

Buxton, O., Pavlova, M., Reid, E., Simonson, D. & Adler, G. (2008). Sleep restriction for one week reduces insulin sensitivity measured using the euglycemic hyperinsulinemic clamp technique [abstract]. *Sleep*, **31**, A107.

Cappuccio, F.P., Taggart, F.M., Kandala, N.B., et al. (2008). Meta-analysis of short sleep duration and obesity in children and adults. *Sleep*, **31**, 619–626.

Centers for Disease Control (2006). Diabetes: Prevalence and Trends. Available at: http://www.cdc.gov/diabetes/statistics/prev/national/figage.htm (accessed March 19, 2009).

Chaput, J.P., Brunet, M. & Tremblay, A. (2006). Relationship between short sleeping hours and childhood overweight/obesity: results from the 'Quebec en Forme' Project. *Int J Obes (Lond)*, **30**, 1080–1085.

Chaput, J.P., Despres, J.P., Bouchard, C. & Tremblay, A. (2007a). Association of sleep duration with type 2 diabetes and impaired glucose tolerance. *Diabetologia*, **50**, 2298–2304.

Chaput, J.P., Despres, J.P., Bouchard, C. & Tremblay, A. (2007b). Short sleep duration is associated with reduced leptin levels and increased adiposity: results from the Quebec family study. *Obesity (Silver Spring)*, **15**, 253–261.

Chaput, J.P., Lord, C., Aubertin-Leheudre, M., Dionne, I.J., Khalil, A. & Tremblay, A. (2007c). Is overweight/obesity associated with short sleep duration in older women? *Aging Clin Exp Res*, **19**, 290–294.

Chaput, J.P., Despres, J.P., Bouchard, C. & Tremblay, A. (2008). The association between sleep duration and weight gain in adults: a 6-year prospective study from the Quebec Family Study. *Sleep*, **31**, 517–523.

Chen, M.Y., Wang, E.K. & Jeng, Y.J. (2006). Adequate sleep among adolescents is positively associated with health status and health-related behaviors. *BMC Public Health*, **6**, 59.

Chen, X., Beydoun, M.A. & Wang, Y. (2008). Is sleep duration associated with childhood obesity? A systematic review and meta-analysis. *Obesity (Silver Spring)*, **16**, 265–274.

Chin-Chance, C., Polonsky, K.S. & Schoeller, D. (2000). Twenty-four hour leptin levels respond to cumulative short-term energy imbalance and predict subsequent intake. *J Clin Endocrinol Metab*, **85**, 2685–2691.

Chin, K., Shimizu, K., Nakamura, T., et al. (1999). Changes in intra-abdominal visceral fat and serum leptin levels in patients with obstructive sleep apnea syndrome following nasal continuous positive airway pressure therapy. *Circulation*, **100**, 706–712.

Choi, K.M., Lee, J.S., Park, H.S., Baik, S.H., Choi, D.S. & Kim, S.M. (2008). Relationship between sleep duration and the metabolic syndrome: Korean National Health and Nutrition Survey 2001. *Int J Obes (Lond)*, **32**, 1091–1097.

Coughlin, S.R., Mawdsley, L., Mugarza, J.A., Wilding, J.P. & Calverley, P.M. (2007). Cardiovascular and metabolic effects of CPAP in obese males with OSA. *Eur Respir J*, **29**, 720–727.

Cournot, M., Ruidavets, J.B., Marquie, J.C., Esquirol, Y., Baracat, B. & Ferrieres, J. (2004). Environmental factors associated with body mass index in a population of Southern France. *Eur J Cardiovasc Prev Rehabil*, **11**, 291–297.

Cuellar, N.G. & Ratcliffe, S.J. (2008). A comparison of glycemic control, sleep, fatigue, and depression in type 2 diabetes with and without restless legs syndrome. *J Clin Sleep Med*, **4**, 50–56.

Cunha, M.C., Zanetti, M.L. & Hass, V.J. (2008). Sleep quality in type 2 diabetics. *Rev Lat Am Enfermagem*, **16**, 850–855.

Dawson, A., Abel, S.L., Loving, R.T., et al. (2008). CPAP therapy of obstructive sleep apnea in type 2 diabetics improves glycemic control during sleep. *J Clin Sleep Med*, 4, 538–542.

de la Eva, R.C., Baur, L.A., Donaghue, K.C. & Waters, K.A. (2002). Metabolic correlates with obstructive sleep apnea in obese subjects. *J Pediatr*, 140, 654–659.

Dieu, H.T., Dibley, M.J., Sibbritt, D. & Hanh, T.T. (2007). Prevalence of overweight and obesity in preschool children and associated socio-demographic factors in Ho Chi Minh City, Vietnam. *Int J Pediatr Obes*, 2, 40–50.

Dorkova, Z., Petrasova, D., Molcanyiova, A., Popovnakova, M. & Tkacova, R. (2008). Effects of continuous positive airway pressure on cardiovascular risk profile in patients with severe obstructive sleep apnea and metabolic syndrome. *Chest*, 134, 686–692.

Drummond, M., Winck, J.C., Guimaraes, J.T., Santos, A.C., Almeida, J. & Marques, J.A. (2008). Autoadjusting-CPAP effect on serum leptin concentrations in obstructive sleep apnoea patients. *BMC Pulm Med*, 8, 21.

Einhorn, D., Stewart, D.A., Erman, M.K., Gordon, N., Philis-Tsimikas, A. & Casal, E. (2007). Prevalence of sleep apnea in a population of adults with type 2 diabetes mellitus. *Endocr Pract*, 13, 355–362.

Eisenmann, J.C., Ekkekakis, P. & Holmes, M. (2006). Sleep duration and overweight among Australian children and adolescents. *Acta Paediatr*, 95, 956–963.

Ettaro, L., Songer, T.J., Zhang, P. & Engelgau, M.M. (2004). Cost-of-illness studies in diabetes mellitus. *Pharmacoeconomics*, 22, 149–164.

Farooqi, I.S. (2002). Leptin and the onset of puberty: insights from rodent and human genetics. *Semin Reprod Med*, 20(2), 139–144.

Flegal, K., Carroll, M., Kuczmarski, F. & Johnson, C. (1998). Overweight and obesity in the United States: prevalence and trends, 1960-1994. *Int J Obes Relat Metab Disord*, 22, 39–47.

Flegal, K., Carroll, M., Ogden, C. & Johnson, C. (2002). Prevalence and trends in obesity among US adults, 1999-2000. *JAMA*, 288, 1723–1727.

Flier, J.S. (2004). Obesity wars: molecular progress confronts an expanding epidemic. *Cell*, 116(2), 337–350.

Flint, J., Kothare, S.V., Zihlif, M., et al. (2007). Association between inadequate sleep and insulin resistance in obese children. *J Pediatr*, 150, 364–369.

Fogelholm, M., Kronholm, E., Kukkonen-Harjula, K., Partonen, T., Partinen, M. & Harma, M. (2007). Sleep-related disturbances and physical inactivity are independently associated with obesity in adults. *Int J Obes (Lond)*, 31, 1713–1721.

Franco, O.H., Steyerberg, E.W., Hu, F.B., Mackenbach, J. & Nusselder, W. (2007). Associations of diabetes mellitus with total life expectancy and life expectancy with and without cardiovascular disease. *Arch Intern Med*, 167, 1145–1151.

Gale, S.M., Castracane, V.D. & Mantzoros, C.S. (2004). Energy homeostasis, obesity and eating disorders: recent advances in endocrinology. *J Nutr*, 134, 295–298.

Gallup Organization (1979). *The Gallup Study of Sleeping Habits*. Princeton, NJ: Gallup Organization.

Gallup Organization (1995). *Sleep in America*. Princeton, NJ: Gallup Organization.

Gami, A.S., Caples, S.M. & Somers, V.K. (2003). Obesity and obstructive sleep apnea. *Endocrinol Metab Clin North Am*, 32, 869–894.

Gangwisch, J.E., Malaspina, D., Boden-Albala, B. & Heymsfield, S.B. (2005). Inadequate sleep as a risk factor for obesity: analyses of the NHANES I. *Sleep*, 28, 1289–1296.

Gangwisch, J.E., Heymsfield, S.B., Boden-Albala, B., et al. (2007). Sleep duration as a risk factor for diabetes incidence in a large US sample. *Sleep*, 30, 1667–1673.

Garcia, G., Freeman, R., Supiano, M., Smith, M., Galecki, A. & Halter, J. (1997). Glucose metabolism in older adults: a study including subjects more than 80 years of age. *J Am Geriatr Soc*, 45, 813–817.

Gautier, J.F., Del Parigi, A., Chen, K., et al. (2001). Effect of satiation on brain activity in obese and lean women. *Obes Res*, 9, 676–684.

Gislason, T. & Almqvist, M. (1987). Somatic diseases and sleep complaints. An epidemiological study of 3,201 Swedish men. *Acta Med Scand*, 221, 475–481.

Giugliano, R. & Carneiro, E.C. (2004). Factors associated with obesity in school children. *J Pediatr (Rio J)*, **80**, 17–22.

Gortmaker, S.L., Dietz, W.H., Jr. & Cheung, L.W. (1990). Inactivity, diet, and the fattening of America. *J Am Diet Assoc*, **90**, 1247–1252, 1255.

Gottlieb, D.J., Punjabi, N.M., Newman, A.B., et al. (2005). Association of sleep time with diabetes mellitus and impaired glucose tolerance. *Arch Intern Med*, **165**, 863–867.

Gottlieb, D.J., Redline, S., Nieto, F.J., et al. (2006). Association of usual sleep duration with hypertension: the Sleep Heart Health Study. *Sleep*, **29**, 1009–1014.

Gregg, E.W., Cadwell, B.L., Cheng, Y.J., et al. (2004). Trends in the prevalence and ratio of diagnosed to undiagnosed diabetes according to obesity levels in the U.S. *Diabetes Care*, **27**, 2806–2812.

Guilleminault, C., Powell, N.B., Martinez, S., et al. (2003). Preliminary observations on the effects of sleep time in a sleep restriction paradigm. [see comment]. *Sleep Med*, **4**, 177–184.

Gunderson, E.P., Rifas-Shiman, S.L., Oken, E., et al. (2008). Association of fewer hours of sleep at 6 months postpartum with substantial weight retention at 1 year postpartum. *Am J Epidemiol*, **167**, 178–187.

Gupta, N.K., Mueller, W.H., Chan, W. & Meininger, J.C. (2002). Is obesity associated with poor sleep quality in adolescents? *Am J Hum Biol*, **14**, 762–768.

Hall, M.H., Muldoon, M.F., Jennings, J.R., Buysse, D.J., Flory, J.D. & Manuck, S.B. (2008). Self-reported sleep duration is associated with the metabolic syndrome in midlife adults. *Sleep*, **31**, 635–643.

Harsch, I.A., Konturek, P.C., Koebnick, C., et al. (2003). Leptin and ghrelin levels in patients with obstructive sleep apnoea: effect of CPAP treatment. *Eur Respir J*, **22**, 251–257.

Harsch, I., Schahin, S., Bruckner, K., et al. (2004a). The effect of continuous positive airway pressure treatment on insulin sensitivity in patients with obstructive sleep apnoea syndrome and type 2 diabetes. *Respiration*, **71**, 252–259.

Harsch, I.A., Schahin, S.P., Radespiel-Troger, M., et al. (2004b). Continuous positive airway pressure treatment rapidly improves insulin sensitivity in patients with obstructive sleep apnea syndrome. [see comment]. *Am J Respir Crit Care Med*, **169**, 156–162.

Hasler, G., Buysse, D., Klaghofer, R., et al. (2004). The association between short sleep duration and obesity in young adults: a 13-year prospective study. *Sleep*, **27**, 661–666.

Hassaballa, H.A., Tulaimat, A., Herdegen, J.J. & Mokhlesi, B. (2005). The effect of continuous positive airway pressure on glucose control in diabetic patients with severe obstructive sleep apnea. *Sleep Breath*, **9**, 176–180.

Hayashino, Y., Fukuhara, S., Suzukamo, Y., Okamura, T., Tanaka, T. & Ueshima, H. (2007). Relation between sleep quality and quantity, quality of life, and risk of developing diabetes in healthy workers in Japan: the High-risk and Population Strategy for Occupational Health Promotion (HIPOP-OHP) Study. *BMC Public Health*, **7**, 129.

Heslop, P., Smith, G., Metcalfe, C., Macleod, J. & Hart, C. (2002). Sleep duration and mortality: the effect of short or long sleep duration on cardiovascular and all-cause mortality in working men and women. *Sleep Med*, **3**, 305–314.

Hitze, B., Bosy-Westphal, A., Bielfeldt, F., et al. (2008). Determinants and impact of sleep duration in children and adolescents: data of the Kiel Obesity Prevention Study. *Eur J Clin Nutr*.

Hitze, B., Bosy-Westphal, A. et al. (2009). Determinants and impact of sleep duration in children and adolescents: data of the Kiel Obesity Prevention Study. *Eur J Clin Nutr*, **63**(6), 739–746.

Hyyppa, M.T. & Kronholm, E. (1989). Quality of sleep and chronic illnesses. *J Clin Epidemiol*, **42**, 633–638.

Ioannou, G.N., Bryson, C.L. & Boyko, E.J. (2007). Prevalence and trends of insulin resistance, impaired fasting glucose, and diabetes. *J Diabetes Complications*, **21**, 363–370.

Ip, M.S., Lam, K.S., Ho, C., Tsang, K.W. & Lam, W. (2000). Serum leptin and vascular risk factors in obstructive sleep apnea.[see comment]. *Chest*, **118**, 580–586.

Jennings, J.R., Muldoon, M.F., Hall, M., Buysse, D.J. & Manuck, S.B. (2007). Self-reported sleep quality is associated with the metabolic syndrome. *Sleep*, **30**, 219–223.

Kajaste, S., Brander, P.E., Telakivi, T., Partinen, M. & Mustajoki, P. (2004). A cognitive-behavioral weight reduction program in the treatment of obstructive sleep apnea syndrome with or without initial nasal CPAP: a randomized study. *Sleep Med*, 5, 125–131.

Kawakami, N., Takatsuka, N. & Shimizu, H. (2004). Sleep disturbance and onset of type 2 diabetes. *Diabetes Care*, 27, 282–283.

Knutson, K.L. (2005). Sex differences in the association between sleep and body mass index in adolescents. *J Pediatr*, 147, 830–834.

Knutson, K.L., Ryden, A.M., Mander, B.A. & Van Cauter, E. (2006). Role of sleep duration and quality in the risk and severity of type 2 diabetes mellitus. *Arch Intern Med*, 166, 1768–1774.

Knutson, K.L., Spiegel, K., Penev, P. & Van Cauter, E. (2007). The metabolic consequences of sleep deprivation. *Sleep Med Rev*, 11, 163–178.

Ko, G.T., Chan, J.C., Chan, A.W., et al. (2007). Association between sleeping hours, working hours and obesity in Hong Kong Chinese: the 'better health for better Hong Kong' health promotion campaign. *Int J Obes (Lond)*, 31, 254–260.

Kohatsu, N.D., Tsai, R., Young, T., et al. (2006). Sleep duration and body mass index in a rural population. *Arch Intern Med*, 166, 1701–1705.

Kohyama, J., Shiiki, T., Ohinata-Sugimoto, J. & Hasegawa, T. (2002). Potentially harmful sleep habits of 3-year-old children in Japan. *J Dev Behav Pediatr*, 23, 67–70.

Kripke, D., Simons, R., Garfinkel, L. & Hammond, E. (1979). Short and long sleep and sleeping pills. Is increased mortality associated? *Arch Gen Psychiatry*, 36, 103–116.

Kripke, D.F., Garfinkel, L., Wingard, D.L., Klauber, M.R. & Marler, M.R. (2002). Mortality associated with sleep duration and insomnia. *Arch Gen Psychiatry*, 59, 131–136.

Kuriyan, R., Bhat, S., Thomas, T., Vaz, M. & Kurpad, A.V. (2007). Television viewing and sleep are associated with overweight among urban and semi-urban South Indian children. *Nutr J*, 6, 25.

Lauderdale, D., Knutson, K., Rathouz, P., Yan, L., Hulley, S. & Liu, K. (2009). Cross-sectional and longitudinal associations between objectively measured sleep duration and body mass index: the CARDIA Sleep Study. *Am J Epidemiol*, 170(7): 805–813.

Lauderdale, D.S., Knutson, K.L., Yan, L.L., Liu, K. & Rathouz, P.J. (2008). Self-reported and measured sleep duration: how similar are they? *Epidemiology*, 19, 838–845.

Lindberg, E., Berne, C., Elmasry, A., Hedner, J. & Janson, C. (2006). CPAP treatment of a population-based sample—what are the benefits and the treatment compliance? *Sleep Med*, 7, 553–560.

Littman, A.J., Vitiello, M.V., Foster-Schubert, K., et al. (2006). Sleep, ghrelin, leptin and changes in body weight during a 1-year moderate-intensity physical activity intervention. *Int J Obes (Lond)*, 31, 466–475.

Liu, X., Forbes, E.E., Ryan, N.D., Rofey, D., Hannon, T.S. & Dahl, R.E. (2008). Rapid eye movement sleep in relation to overweight in children and adolescents. *Arch Gen Psychiatry*, 65, 924–932.

Locard, E., Mamelle, N., Billette, A., Miginiac, M., Munoz, F. & Rey, S. (1992). Risk factors of obesity in a five year old population. Parental versus environmental factors. *Int J Obes Relat Metab Disord*, 16, 721–729.

Lopez-Garcia, E., Faubel, R., Leon-Munoz, L., Zuluaga, M.C., Banegas, J.R. & Rodriguez-Artalejo, F. (2008). Sleep duration, general and abdominal obesity, and weight change among the older adult population of Spain. *Am J Clin Nutr*, 87, 310–316.

Loube, D., Loube, A. & Erman, M. (1997). Continuous positive airway pressure treatment results in weight loss in obese and overweight patients with obstructive sleep apnea. *J Am Diet Assoc*, 97, 896–897.

Lumeng, J.C., Somashekar, D., Appugliese, D., Kaciroti, N., Corwyn, R.F. & Bradley, R.H. (2007). Shorter sleep duration is associated with increased risk for being overweight at ages 9 to 12 years. *Pediatrics*, 120, 1020–1029.

Magee, C.A., Iverson, D.C., Huang, X.F. & Caputi, P. (2008). A link between chronic sleep restriction and obesity: methodological considerations. *Public Health*, 122, 1373–1381.

Mallon, L., Broman, J.E. & Hetta, J. (2005). High incidence of diabetes in men with sleep complaints or short sleep duration: a 12-year follow-up study of a middle-aged population. *Diabetes Care*, 28, 2762–2767.

Marin, P., Hogh-Kristiansen, I. et al. (1992). Uptake of glucose carbon in muscle glycogen and adipose tissue triglycerides in vivo in humans. *Am J Physiol*, **263**(3 Pt 1), E473–480.

Meisinger, C., Heier, M. & Loewel, H. (2005). Sleep disturbance as a predictor of type 2 diabetes mellitus in men and women from the general population. *Diabetologia*, **48**, 235–241.

Meyer, C., Dostou, J.M. et al. (2002). Role of human liver, kidney, and skeletal muscle in postprandial glucose homeostasis. *Am J Physiol Endocrinol Metab*, **282**(2), E419–427.

Moreno, C.R., Louzada, F.M., Teixeira, L.R., Borges, F. & Lorenzi-Filho, G. (2006). Short sleep is associated with obesity among truck drivers. *Chronobiol Int*, **23**, 1295–1303.

Mueller, W. M., Gregoire, F.M. et al. (1998). Evidence that glucose metabolism regulates leptin secretion from cultured rat adipocytes. *Endocrinology*, **139**(2), 551–558.

Nakajima, H., Kaneita, Y., Yokoyama, E., et al. (2008). Association between sleep duration and hemoglobin A1c level. *Sleep Med*, **9**, 745–752.

National Center for Health Statistics (2005). QuickStats: Percentage of adults who reported an average of ≤ 6 hours of sleep per 24-hour period, by sex and age group—United States, 1985 and 2004. *MMWR Morb Mortal Wkly Rep*, **54**, 933.

National Sleep Foundation (2001). *Sleep in America Poll*. Washington, DC: National Sleep Foundation.

National Sleep Foundation (2008). *Sleep in America* Poll. Washington, DC: National Sleep Foundation.

Nedeltcheva, A.V., Kilkus, J.M., Imperial, J., Kasza, K., Schoeller, D.A. & Penev, P.D. (2009). Sleep curtailment is accompanied by increased intake of calories from snacks. *Am J Clin Nutr*, **89**, 126–133.

Nilsson, P.M., Roost, M., Engstrom, G., Hedblad, B. & Berglund, G. (2004). Incidence of diabetes in middle-aged men is related to sleep disturbances. *Diabetes Care*, **27**, 2464–2469.

Nixon, G.M., Thompson, J.M., Han, D.Y., et al. (2008). Short sleep duration in middle childhood: risk factors and consequences. *Sleep*, **31**, 71–78.

Nofzinger, E.A., Buysse, D.J., Miewald, J.M., et al. (2002). Human regional cerebral glucose metabolism during non-rapid eye movement sleep in relation to waking. *Brain*, **125**, 1105–1115.

Ohayon, M.M. (2004). Interactions between sleep normative data and sociocultural characteristics in the elderly. *J Psychosom Res*, **56**, 479–486.

Ohayon, M.M. & Vecchierini, M.F. (2005). Normative sleep data, cognitive function and daily living activities in older adults in the community. *Sleep*, **28**, 981–989.

Padez, C., Mourao, I., Moreira, P. & Rosado, V. (2009). Long sleep duration and childhood overweight/obesity and body fat. *Am J Hum Biol*, **21**(3), 371–376.

Park, S.E., Kim, H.M., Kim, D.H., Kim, J., Cha, B.S. & Kim, D.J. (2009). The association between sleep duration and general and abdominal obesity in Koreans: data from the Korean National Health and Nutrition Examination Survey, 2001 and 2005. *Obesity (Silver Spring)*, **17**, 767–771.

Patel, S.R., Ayas, N.T., Malhotra, M.R., et al. (2004). A prospective study of sleep duration and mortality risk in women. *Sleep*, **27**, 440–444.

Patel, S.R., Malhotra, A., White, D.P., Gottlieb, D.J. & Hu, F.B. (2006). Association between reduced sleep and weight gain in women. Am J Epidemiol, **164**, 947–954.

Patel, S.R., Blackwell, T., Redline, S., et al. (2008). The association between sleep duration and obesity in older adults. *Int J Obes (Lond)*, **32**, 1825–1834.

Phillips, B.G., Hisel, T.M., Kato, M., et al. (1999). Recent weight gain in patients with newly diagnosed obstructive sleep apnea. *Am J Hypertens*, **17**, 1297–1300.

Phillips, B.G., Kato, M., Narkiewicz, K., Choe, I. & Somers, V.K. (2000). Increases in leptin levels, sympathetic drive, and weight gain in obstructive sleep apnea. *Am J Physiol Heart Circ Physiol*, **279**, H234–H237.

Porte, D., Jr., Baskin, D.G. & Schwartz, M.W. (2005). Insulin signaling in the central nervous system: a critical role in metabolic homeostasis and disease from C. elegans to humans. *Diabetes*, **54**, 1264–1276.

Prigeon, R.L., Kahn, S.E. & Porte, D., Jr. (1995). Changes in insulin sensitivity, glucose effectiveness, and B-Cell function in regularly exercising subjects. *Metabolism*, **44**, 1259–1263.

Punjabi, N.M. & Beamer, B.A. (2009). Alterations in glucose disposal in sleep-disordered breathing. *Am J Respir Crit Care Med*, **179**, 235–240.

Punjabi, N.M., Shahar, E., Redline, S., Gottlieb, D.J., Givelber, R. & Resnick, H.E. (2004). Sleep-disordered breathing, glucose intolerance, and insulin resistance: the Sleep Heart Health Study. *Am J Epidemiol*, **160**, 521–530.

Quan, S.F., Howard, B.V., Iber, C., et al. (1997). The Sleep Heart Health Study: design, rationale, and methods. *Sleep*, **20**, 1077–1085.

Redenius, R., Murphy, C., O'neill, E., Al-Hamwi, M. & Zallek, S.N. (2008). Does CPAP lead to change in BMI? *J Clin Sleep Med*, **4**, 205–209.

Reichmuth, K.J., Austin, D., Skatrud, J.B. & Young, T. (2005). Association of sleep apnea and type II diabetes: a population-based study. *Am J Respir Crit Care Med*, **172**, 1590–1595.

Reilly, J., Armstrong, J., Dorosty, A., et al. (2005). Early life risk factors for obesity in childhood: cohort study. *Br Med J*, **330**, 1357.

Rontoyanni, V.G., Baic, S. & Cooper, A.R. (2007). Association between nocturnal sleep duration, body fatness, and dietary intake in Greek women. *Nutrition*, **23**, 773–777.

Rubinsztajn, R., Kumor, M., Byskiniewicz, K. & Chazan, R. (2006). The influence of 3 weeks therapy with continuous positive airway pressure on serum leptin and homocysteine concentration in patients with obstructive sleep apnea syndrome. *Pneumonol Alergol Pol*, **74**, 63–67.

Saarelainen, S., Lahtela, J. & Kallonen, E. (1997). Effect of nasal CPAP treatment on insulin sensitivity and plasma leptin. *J Sleep Res*, **6**, 146–147.

Sanner, B.M., Kollhosser, P., Buechner, N., Zidek, W. & Tepel, M. (2004). Influence of treatment on leptin levels in patients with obstructive sleep apnoea. *Eur Respir J*, **23**, 601–604.

Schahin, S.P., Nechanitzky, T., Dittel, C., et al. (2008). Long-term improvement of insulin sensitivity during CPAP therapy in the obstructive sleep apnoea syndrome. *Med Sci Monit*, **14**, CR117– CR121.

Scheen, A.J., Byrne, M.M., Plat, L. & Van Cauter, E. (1996). Relationships between sleep quality and glucose regulation in normal humans. *Am J Physiol*, **271**, E261–E270.

Schwartz, M.W. & Porte, D., Jr. (2005). Diabetes, obesity, and the brain. *Science*, **307**, 375–379.

Seicean, A., Redline, S., Seicean, S., et al. (2007). Association between short sleeping hours and overweight in adolescents: results from a US Suburban High School survey. *Sleep Breath*, **11**, 285–293.

Seicean, S., Kirchner, H.L., Gottlieb, D.J., et al. (2008). Sleep-disordered breathing and impaired glucose metabolism in normal-weight and overweight/obese individuals: the Sleep Heart Health Study. *Diabetes Care*, **31**, 1001–1006.

Sekine, M., Yamagami, T., Hamanishi, S., et al. (2002). Parental obesity, lifestyle factors and obesity in preschool children: results of the Toyama Birth Cohort Study. *J Epidemiol*, **12**, 33–39.

Shaw, J.E., Punjabi, N.M., Wilding, J.P., Alberti, K.G. & Zimmet, P.Z. (2008). Sleep-disordered breathing and type 2 diabetes: a report from the International Diabetes Federation Taskforce on Epidemiology and Prevention. *Diabetes Res Clin Pract*, **81**, 2–12.

Shigeta, H., Shigeta, M., Nakazawa, A., Nakamura, N. & Yoshikawa, T. (2001). Lifestyle, obesity, and insulin resistance. *Diabetes Care*, **24**, 608.

Singh, M., Drake, C.L., Roehrs, T., Hudgel, D.W. & Roth, T. (2005). The association between obesity and short sleep duration: a population-based study. *J Clin Sleep Med*, **1**, 357–363.

Smurra, M., Philip, P., Taillard, J., Guilleminault, C., Bioulac, B. & Gin, H. (2001). CPAP treatment does not affect glucose-insulin metabolism in sleep apneic patients. *Sleep Med*, **2**, 207–213.

Snell, E.K., Adam, E.K. & Duncan, G.J. (2007). Sleep and the body mass index and overweight status of children and adolescents. *Child Dev*, **78**, 309–323.

Solomon, C.G. & Manson, J.E. (1997). Obesity and mortality: a review of the epidemiologic data. *Am J Clin Nutr*, **66**, 1044S–1050S.

Spiegel, K., Leproult, R. & Van Cauter, E. (1999). Impact of sleep debt on metabolic and endocrine function. *Lancet*, **354**, 1435–1439.

Spiegel, K., Leproult, R., Colecchia, E.F., et al. (2000). Adaptation of the 24-h growth hormone profile to a state of sleep debt. *Am J Physiol Regul Integr Comp Physiol*, **279**, R874–R883.

Spiegel, K., Leproult, R., L'Hermite-Baleriaux, M., Copinschi, G., Penev, P. & Van Cauter, E. (2004a). Leptin levels are dependent on sleep duration: Relationships with sympathovagal balance, carbohydrate regulation, cortisol, and thyrotropin. *J Clin Endocrinol Metab*, **89**, 5762–5771.

Spiegel, K., Tasali, E., Penev, P. & Van Cauter, E. (2004b). Sleep curtailment in healthy young men is associated with decreased leptin levels, elevated ghrelin levels and increased hunger and appetite. *Ann Intern Med*, **141**, 846–850.

Spiegel, K., Knutson, K., Leproult, R., Tasali, E. & Van Cauter, E. (2005). Sleep loss: a novel risk factor for insulin resistance and type 2 diabetes. *J Appl Physiol*, **99**, 2008–2019.

Sridhar, G.R. & Madhu, K. (1994). Prevalence of sleep disturbances in diabetes mellitus. *Diabetes Res Clin Pract*, **23**, 183–186.

Stamatakis, K.A. & Brownson, R.C. (2008). Sleep duration and obesity-related risk factors in the rural Midwest. *Prev Med*, **46**, 439–444.

Stranges, S., Cappuccio, F.P., Kandala, N.B., et al. (2008). Cross-sectional versus prospective associations of sleep duration with changes in relative weight and body fat distribution: the Whitehall II Study. *Am J Epidemiol*, **167**, 321–329.

Suarez, E.C. (2008). Self-reported symptoms of sleep disturbance and inflammation, coagulation, insulin resistance and psychosocial distress: evidence for gender disparity. *Brain Behav Immun*, **22**, 960–968.

Sugimori, H., Yoshida, K., Izuno, T., et al. (2004). Analysis of factors that influence body mass index from ages 3 to 6 years: a study based on the Toyama cohort study. *Pediatr Int*, **46**, 302–310.

Taheri, S., Lin, L., Austin, D., Young, T. & Mignot, E. (2004). Short sleep duration is associated with reduced leptin, elevated ghrelin, and increased body mass index (BMI). *Sleep*, **27**, A146–A147.

Takahashi, K., Chin, K., Akamizu, T., et al. (2008). Acylated ghrelin level in patients with OSA before and after nasal CPAP treatment. *Respirology*, **13**, 810–816.

Tamakoshi, A. & Ohno, Y. (2004). Self-reported sleep duration as a predictor of all-cause mortality: results from the JACC Study, Japan. *Sleep*, **27**, 51–54.

Tasali, E., Ehrmann, D.A. & Van Cauter, E. (2005). Experimental suppression of slow wave sleep without change in total sleep time is associated with decreased insulin sensitivity and glucose tolerance. *Sleep*, A149.

Tasali, E., Leproult, R., Ehrmann, D.A. & Cauter, E.V. (2008). Slow-wave sleep and the risk of type 2 diabetes in humans. *Proc Natl Acad Sci USA*, **105**(3), 1044–1049.

Tasali, E., Broussard, J., Day, A., Kilkus, J. & Van Cauter, E. (2009). Sleep curtailment in healthy young adults is associated with increased ad lib food intake [abstract]. *Sleep*, **32**(Abstract Supplement): A131.

Taveras, E.M., Rifas-Shiman, S.L., Oken, E., Gunderson, E.P. & Gillman, M.W. (2008). Short sleep duration in infancy and risk of childhood overweight. *Arch Pediatr Adolesc Med*, **162**, 305–311.

Thomas, M., Sing, H., Belenky, G., et al. (2000). Neural basis of alertness and cognitive performance impairments during sleepiness. I. Effects of 24 h of sleep deprivation on waking human regional brain activity. *J Sleep Res*, **9**, 335–352.

Thorpy, M.J. (2009). Classification of sleep disorders. In: Kryger, M.H., Roth, T. & Dement, W.C. (eds.), *Principles and Practice of Sleep Medicine*. Fourth edition. Philadelphia, PA: Elsevier.

Touchette, E., Petit, D., Tremblay, R.E., et al. (2008). Associations between sleep duration patterns and overweight/obesity at age 6. *Sleep*, **31**, 1507–1514.

Trends in the prevalence and incidence of self-reported diabetes mellitus—United States, 1980-1994 (1997). *MMWR Morb Mortal Wkly Rep*, **46**, 1014–1018.

Trenell, M.I., Ward, J.A., Yee, B.J., et al. (2007). Influence of constant positive airway pressure therapy on lipid storage, muscle metabolism and insulin action in obese patients with severe obstructive sleep apnoea syndrome. *Diabetes Obes Metab*, **9**, 679–687.

Trento, M., Broglio, F., Riganti, F., et al. (2008). Sleep abnormalities in type 2 diabetes may be associated with glycemic control. *Acta Diabetol*, **45**, 225–229.

Tuomilehto, H., Peltonen, M., Partinen, M., et al. (2008). Sleep duration is associated with an increased risk for the prevalence of type 2 diabetes in middle-aged women—The FIN-D2D survey. *Sleep Med*, **9**, 221–227.

Van Cauter, E., Polonsky, K.S. & Scheen, A.J. (1997). Roles of circadian rhythmicity and sleep in human glucose regulation. *Endocr Rev*, **18**, 716–738.

Vgontzas, A.N., Papanicolaou, D.A., Bixler, E.O., et al. (1999). Circadian interleukin-6 secretion and quantity and depth of sleep. *J Clin Endocrinol Metab*, **84**, 2603–2607.

Vgontzas, A.N., Zoumakis, E., Bixler, E.O., et al. (2004). Adverse effects of modest sleep restriction on sleepiness, performance, and inflammatory cytokines. *J Clin Endocrinol Metab*, **89**, 2119–2126.

Vgontzas, A.N., Zoumakis, E., Bixler, E.O., et al. (2008). Selective effects of CPAP on sleep apnoea-associated manifestations. *Eur J Clin Invest*, **38**, 585–595.

Vioque, J., Torres, A. & Quiles, J. (2000). Time spent watching television, sleep duration and obesity in adults living in Valencia, Spain. *Int J Obes Relat Metab Disord*, **24**, 1683–1688.

von Kries, R., Toschke, A.M., Wurmser, H., Sauerwald, T. & Koletzko, B. (2002). Reduced risk for overweight and obesity in 5- and 6-y-old children by duration of sleep—a cross-sectional study. *Int J Obes Relat Metab Disord*, **26**, 710–716.

Vorona, R., Winn, M., Babineau, T., Eng, B., Feldman, H. & Ware, J. (2005). Overweight and obese patients in a primary care population report less sleep than patients with a normal body mass index. *Arch Intern Med*, **165**, 25–30.

Wells, J.C., Hallal, P.C., Reichert, F.F., Menezes, A.M., Araujo, C.L. & Victora, C.G. (2008). Sleep patterns and television viewing in relation to obesity and blood pressure: evidence from an adolescent Brazilian birth cohort. *Int J Obes (Lond)*, **32**, 1042–1049.

West, S.D., Nicoll, D.J., Wallace, T.M., Matthews, D.R. & Stradling, J.R. (2007). Effect of CPAP on insulin resistance and HbA1c in men with obstructive sleep apnoea and type 2 diabetes. *Thorax*, **62**, 969–974.

Wild, S., Roglic, G., Green, A., Sicree, R. & King, H. (2004). Global prevalence of diabetes: estimates for the year 2000 and projections for 2030. *Diabetes Care*, **27**, 1047–1053.

Williams, C.J., Hu, F.B., Patel, S.R. & Mantzoros, C.S. (2007). Sleep duration and snoring in relation to biomarkers of cardiovascular disease risk among women with type 2 diabetes. *Diabetes Care*, **30**, 1233–1240.

Wolf, A.M. & Colditz, G.A. (1998). Current estimates of the economic cost of obesity in the United States. *Obes Res*, **6**, 97–106.

Xiang, A.H., Peters, R.K., Kjos, S.L., et al. (2006). Effect of pioglitazone on pancreatic beta-cell function and diabetes risk in Hispanic women with prior gestational diabetes. *Diabetes*, **55**, 517–522.

Yaggi, H.K., Araujo, A.B. & Mckinlay, J.B. (2006). Sleep duration as a risk factor for the development of type 2 diabetes. *Diabetes Care*, **29**, 657–661.

Young, T., Palta, M., Dempsey, J., Skatrud, J., Weber, S. & Badr, S. (1993). The occurrence of sleep-disordered breathing among middle-aged adults. *N Engl J Med*, **328**, 1230–1235.

Youngstedt, S.D. & Kripke, D.F. (2004). Long sleep and mortality: rationale for sleep restriction. *Sleep Med Rev*, **8**, 159–174.

Yu, Y., Lu, B.S., Wang, B., et al. (2007). Short sleep duration and adiposity in Chinese adolescents. *Sleep*, **30**, 1688–1697.

Zielinski, M.R., Kline, C.E., Kripke, D.F., Bogan, R.K. & Youngstedt, S.D. (2008). No effect of 8-week time in bed restriction on glucose tolerance in older long sleepers. *J Sleep Res*, **17**, 412–419.

Chapter 7

Sleep and respiratory diseases

A. Xie, R. Kakkar, M.C. Teodorescu, L. Herpel,
V. Krishnan, and M. Teodorescu

Sleep respiratory physiology

Introduction

It has long been known that sleep generally depresses respiration, circulation, and other vital activities such as metabolic rate. Furthermore, the currently recognized sleep-disordered breathing (SDB) reveals more complex effects of sleep on ventilation than merely depression of the respiratory function. In this section, we will briefly review the physiological principles of ventilation during sleep that may cast insight as to how the sleeping state itself can permit—or even provoke—apnoeas in an otherwise healthy respiratory system, which is precise and mechanically efficient in wakefulness.

In general, sleep may disturb breathing via the following mechanisms: (1) physiological and functional changes in the central nervous system, such as the loss of the wakefulness stimulus on breathing and the state-related fluctuations of excitatory and inhibitory influences on respiration; (2) decline of skeletal muscle tone; (3) attenuation of ventilatory response to chemical and mechanical loads (Gora et al., 1998); and (4) reduction in functional residual capacity (FRC) and mismatch of ventilation/blood (V/Q) ratio related to recumbent position (Stanchina et al., 2003). Besides, circadian rhythm and sleep-related alteration of cerebral vascular reactivity to CO_2 may contribute to changes in breathing throughout the night. The following discussion will examine the implications of these fundamental factors on breathing stability and respiratory pattern during sleep.

Loss of wakefulness drive to breathing control

The withdrawal of the wakefulness stimulus has the most important impact on ventilatory control and probably plays a critical role in the pathogenesis of SDB (Bulow, 1963). Like all oscillators, the respiratory rhythm generator requires tonic inputs to keep oscillations between inspiration and expiration, which is mainly provided by chemical drive and wakefulness stimulus. The wakefulness stimulus, a non-specific drive, might arise from suprapontine regions or the reticular activating system (Aston-Jones, 2005). During wakefulness, the tonic input from the wakefulness stimulus to the respiratory centre is sufficient to compensate for reductions in chemical stimuli and sufficient to overcome other inhibitory factors, so that apnoea rarely occurs in awake humans even in the presence of substantial hypocapnia. In contrast, a sleep-related loss of the wakefulness stimulus will leave ventilation under metabolic control. Hence, chemical drive becomes critical during sleep, and a small reduction in $PaCO_2$, readily leads to apnoea or periodic breathing (Skatrud and Dempsey, 1983). In addition, the loss of wakefulness stimulus, coupled with the reduced respiratory muscular tone during sleep may exacerbate alveolar hypoventilation in some diseases, making marginal ventilation during wakefulness inadequate during sleep.

Neurophysiological changes with sleep state and arousal on respiration

Sleep is not a homogeneous state. Dynamic changes of sleep state with alterations in the degree of alertness are also potential factors in destabilizing breathing. For example, during non-rapid eye movement (NREM) sleep, light sleep stage, especially stage N1, is characterized by unstable autonomic regulation, which may lead to ventilatory instability at sleep onset. With the deepening of sleep, autonomic regulation becomes more stable, and the behavioural system becomes more quiescent during slow wave NREM sleep. Therefore, sleep apnoeas are more often seen in light sleep stages (Xie et al., 2009).

Rapid eye movement (REM) sleep is characterized by tonic motor inhibition, and bursts of phasic events. In the tonic phase, breathing is still under chemical-metabolic control as it is in NREM sleep. However, in the phasic phase, the breathing pattern is mainly affected by behavioural system through the REM sleep processes, becoming irregular. The irregularity stems from ponto-geniculo-occipital (PGO)-driven excitatory and inhibitory influences on ventilation (Bulow, 1963). REM-related withdrawal of excitatory noradrenergic and serotonergic inputs to upper airway (UAW) motoneurons on top of the REM-related muscular hypotonia may suppress pharyngeal muscle activity, predisposing to obstructive sleep apnoea (OSA) (Fenik et al., 2005).

Moreover, sleep is fragmented by arousals and state-transitions. All of these events may also affect breathing stability (Ferre et al., 2006). Arousal is a brief awakening (3–15 seconds) from sleep induced by various external or internal influences, including chemical as well as mechanical stimuli arising from respiratory effort. This protective mechanism is often triggered by apnoeas and hypopnoeas, helping to terminate them. On the other hand, the transition from sleep to arousal provides excitatory drives to the respiratory system, enhancing chemoresponsiveness and causing a surge of ventilation and transient hypocapnoea. These changes, in turn, tend to destabilize breathing. Hence, arousal often plays dual roles in SDB as it terminates the existing apnoea, but also triggers new ones.

It appears paradoxical that sleep predisposes patients to SDB via removal of the wakefulness stimulus, while arousal facilitates SDB although it restores the wakefulness stimulus. The explanation for this paradox lies in the transient nature of arousals and the short-lived nature of this state-related excitatory respiratory drive (Horner et al., 2001). When transient arousal yields to sleep, the quick abolition of excitatory input makes the respiratory control system very sensitive to the transient hypocapnoe that results from prior arousal-provoked hyperpnoea. This effect is exaggerated when arousal occurs at the end of apnoeas or hypopnoeas. The strong chemical stimuli built up during apnoea, plus the sudden release of upper airway resistance (R_{UAW}), enhances the arousal-provoked hyperpnoea, driving $PaCO_2$ even lower. Therefore, a frequent transition between sleep and arousal/wakefulness would exaggerate the instability of the breathing controller.

Reduction in respiratory muscle function

There is usually a progressive fall in the activity of the skeletal muscles with respiratory or non-respiratory function, from wakefulness to NREM to REM sleep, and a marked motor inhibition prevails during REM sleep. The motorneurons are only slightly hyperpolarized during NREM sleep, but this change becomes more substantial during REM sleep. In addition, postsynaptic inhibition occurs during REM sleep, which is also responsible for the REM-related hypotonia/atonia of the somatic musculature (Krieger, 2005). Since most respiratory cells are more active in REM sleep than NREM (Orem et al., 2005), the REM-related hypoventilation must result from the muscle hypotonia.

More importantly, the influence of sleep on the chest wall muscles and UAW muscles does not appear to be uniform or parallel. The UAW dilator muscle activity demonstrates a progressive depression during the night. As a result, R_{UAW} undergoes a relatively small increase in the early sleep period but continues to rise with the deepening of sleep (Worsnop et al., 1998). In contrast, both the principal inspiratory muscles such as the diaphragm and scalene are relatively spared from the direct inhibitory influence of NREM sleep (Henke et al., 1992; Xie et al., 1995). For instance, diaphragm electromyography (EMG) activity is only reduced at the onset of sleep with the transition from alpha to theta (Worsnop et al., 1998), and then gradually recovers to the same or an even slightly higher level than the resting awake values during stable NREM (Tabachnik et al., 1981). The recruitment of the chest wall muscle activity as sleep progresses may at least partly result from the enhanced chemosensory stimulation of CO_2 retention in the face of increased R_{UAW}.

During REM sleep, diaphragmatic EMG activity is still able to be relatively spared from REM-related inhibition (Kline et al., 1986), but it often undergoes intermittent and brief inhibition and fractionation coincident with PGO waves or eye movements (Orem, 1980), causing a reduction of airflow. Meanwhile, phasic motor discharges also occur with PGO bursts, causing tidal volume (VT) fluctuations.

Reduced protective reflexes and compensatory mechanisms

The ability of the respiratory control system to compensate for chemical and/or mechanical loads declines during sleep because response thresholds for many modalities of stimulation (such as stimulation of bronchopulmonary stretch receptors, airway irritant receptors, etc.) increase in both NREM and REM sleep (Henke et al., 1992). Among them, the reduction of protective reflexes involving pharyngeal muscle dilators has more clinical significance because it may cause pharyngeal collapse. The REM-related muscular hypotonia/atonia further diminishes ventilatory load compensation. In addition, the low sympathetic neural tone in sleep may desensitize the carotid bodies, reducing the chemosensitivity to CO_2 and hypoxia. Unfortunately, the sleep state also imposes a variety of loads on the respiratory system, for instance, the increased airflow resistance and increased $PaCO_2$. The reduced compensation ability for these spontaneously occurring chemical/mechanical loads permits UAW occlusion and CO_2 retention.

Alterations in lung function

As one assumes the supine position to sleep, the lung volumes, especially FRC, decrease slightly in healthy humans but much more in obese individuals and asthma patients (Ballard et al., 1990a), probably because of cephalad displacement of the diaphragm resulting from the pressure of abdominal content. During sleep, respiratory muscle hypotonia, central pooling of blood, and reduced lung compliance will further decrease the end-expiratory lung volume (Hudgel and Devadatta, 1984). This postural and sleep-related reductions in FRC would decrease pharyngeal airway caliber and predispose the UAW to collapse (Stanchina et al., 2003). In addition, distribution of air and blood within the lungs changes, worsening the V/Q mismatch, particularly in obese subjects, probably due to atelectasis and less uniform distribution of air and blood in the lung bases. The reduced gas exchange and gas storage likely disturb breathing by increasing the plant gain (i.e. $PaCO_2$ response to alveolar ventilation) and contribute to the rapid fall in SaO_2 during apnoeas in obese patients.

Summary

The interaction and combination of the above changes during sleep introduce the following alterations in ventilatory parameters: (1) UAW impedance and total airway resistance could increase more than twofold compared to the resting wakefulness (Wiegand et al., 1990), whereas no alteration of the elastic properties of the respiratory apparatus occurs. If these normal changes in UAW mechanics are exaggerated by any other factors, then airflow limitation, snoring, or OSA may occur; (2) a 10–15% of reduction in minute ventilation (V_E), mainly through a decrease in tidal volume (V_T) as a result of respiratory muscles hypotonia, often causes an increase in $PaCO_2$ and slight oxygen desaturation, regardless of the reduction in metabolic rate with sleep state (Krieger, 2005); (3) under the background of a relatively low ventilation, there are several sighs (large V_T) sporadically occurring during sleep. These sighs help to open collapsed alveoli but they often trigger periodic breathing through the post-hyperventilation hypocapnia (Xie et al., 1994); (4) ventilatory response to CO_2 is attenuated during NREM and tonic REM sleep, which allows $PaCO_2$ to raise to a small extent during sleep. Moreover, ventilatory response to CO_2 is subject to modulation by circadian rhythm (Raschke and Moller, 1989). One interesting area in need for more studies is how the circadian rhythm and sleep state interact to affect breathing.

In conclusion, sleep, mainly through withdrawal of the wakefulness stimulus and alteration of reflex responses, muscular tone, lung volumes, metabolic rate, and ventilatory chemosensitivity, has a significant impact on breathing, predisposing sleepers to SDB.

Sleep-related breathing disorders

Obstructive sleep apnoea

Introduction

Obstructive sleep apnoea is a common condition affecting an estimated 15 million Americans. The effect of OSA on the health of public is increasingly being recognized. It is estimated that OSA afflicts about 24% of adult males and about 9% of adult females (Young et al., 1993). Studies from different countries have consistently shown a prevalence rate of OSA and excessive daytime sleepiness (EDS) at about 5–7% in adult males and 3–4 % in adult females. Since these publications, the incidence and prevalence of obesity, a major risk factor for OSA, has increased. Between 1980 and 2004, the prevalence of obesity increased from 15% to 33% among adults and the prevalence of overweight in children increased from more than 6% to 19% in the United States (Ogden et al., 2006). Second, the Wisconsin Sleep Cohort Study has included a predominantly Caucasian population employed with three state agencies. In general, employed people are healthier than the unemployed ones. Further, nasal pressure monitoring, which is more sensitive in detecting hypopnoeas than thermocouples used in many of the initial studies, has become widely available. Due to these factors it is reasonable to assume that both prevalence and detection rate of OSA have increased over the last two decades.

Risk factors

The prevalence of OSA increases with increasing body mass index (BMI), neck circumference, age, in certain disease states, with family history of OSA, craniofacial abnormalities, and in certain races. It is estimated that about 80–90% of all OSA and about 70% of severe OSA remains undiagnosed. OSA is most commonly seen in adults between the ages of 30 and 60 years. Middle-aged obese men are at greatest risk of developing OSA. Many other sleep apnoeics lack these characteristic features, and remain undiagnosed for this reason.

Body weight

Obesity is one of the most important risk factors for development of OSA. Studies in different countries and ethnicities have consistently shown a graded increase in the risk of OSA with increase in body weight (Bixler et al., 1998, 2001; Ogden et al., 2006; Young et al., 1993). In the Wisconsin Sleep Cohort Study, an increase in BMI by one standard deviation was associated with a fourfold increase in disease prevalence. A 10% increase in weight over a period of 4 years resulted in 32% worsening in apnoea-hypopnoea index (AHI), whereas a 10% weight loss was associated with 26% decrease in AHI. The risk of having moderate-to-severe sleep apnoea also increased 6-fold with this degree of weight change. In the Sleep Heart Health Study (SHHS), a 10-kg weight gain in men was associated with 5.2-fold the odds of an increase in the AHI by more than 15 events per hour. For women, the same amount of weight gain was associated with 2.5-fold the odds of a similar increase in their AHI. The effect of weight and age on AHI is non-linear over time with obese older men at the highest risk of increase in the severity of OSA (Redline et al., 2003). Obesity is less common among Asians, and the reported values of BMI of Asians with OSA are lower than in their Caucasian counterparts. Population-based studies have consistently demonstrated that obesity is still the major risk factor for OSA in Asians. Weight loss is associated with a decrease in the severity of OSA although in a recent meta-analysis, significant residual OSA persisted after bariatric surgery (Greenburg et al., 2009). The pooled data from 10 studies showed that an overall decrease in BMI from 55 to 38 kg/m^2 resulted in a decrease in the AHI by 38.2 events per hour. Despite a 71% decrease in AHI, more than 62% patients had residual OSA at least moderate in severity. Only 25% of individuals achieved an AHI < 5 events per hour and less than half (44%) achieved an AHI < 10 events per hour. Although it has been proposed that central distribution of obesity probably increases the risk of OSA more than the peripheral fat deposition, the close correlation between BMI, neck circumference, and waist-hip ratio make such a distinction difficult. Nevertheless, studies indicate best correlations of OSA with neck size than with BMI.

Gender

Differences in the relative proportion of male to female in clinic-based population (5–8:1) and epidemiological studies (2–3:1) have been attributed to several possible explanations (Punjabi, 2008). A possible role of different symptom profile has been suspected. Some investigators have found women to complain more often of fatigue, lack of energy, and depression (Young et al., 1996). Snoring and excessive sleepiness are similar in men and women in most studies. Female bed partners of male patients are more likely to report their symptoms than male bed partners of female patients, which may lead to preferential clinical recognition of male patients (Breugelmans et al., 2004).

Polysomnographic differences between genders have been addressed in several studies. It appears that: (a) OSA is less severe in women, being milder during NREM sleep; (b) women have a greater clustering of respiratory events during REM sleep than men do; (c) REM OSA is disproportionately more common in women than in men; and (d) supine OSA is disproportionately more common in men than in women ($P < 0.001$) (O'Connor et al., 2000). Women also have lower sleep efficiency, shorter duration of respiratory events, and lower desaturation index. The sex hormones are thought to play a role in differential predisposition to OSA in men and women. Women with AHI > 10 events per hour have been reported to have significantly lower levels of 17-OH progesterone, progesterone, and estradiol than women with AHI of < 10 events per hour (Netzer et al., 2003). Hormone replacement therapy in post-menopausal women seems to afford some protective effect against OSA. In contrast, excess endogenous or exogenous testosterone increases the predisposition to OSA in women.

Age

Obstructive sleep apnoea becomes most prevalent in midlife with most of the age-related increase in OSA occurring before the age of 65. In one study, 70% of the men and 56% of the women had OSA (AHI > 10 events per hour) (Ancoli-Israel et al., 1991). Influence of gender on REM AHI seems to wane with increasing age. REM SDB decreases with age in women and there is a disproportionate age-dependent rise in NREM in women compared to men. Younger women may be protected from OSA during NREM sleep, even in the face of obesity. Other studies have additionally found a higher prevalence of OSA in older individuals although the estimates have ranged widely. OSA in the elderly may also have a distinct clinical presentation. Excessive sleepiness, hypertension, cognitive decline, and obesity have a weaker correlation with OSA in elderly patients than in the middle-aged patients (Ancoli-Israel et al., 1991; Durán, 2001). Despite an increase in the prevalence of OSA in the elderly, self-reported snoring and excess daytime sleepiness are less common in this population, either due to the death of bed partner or due to emergence of central sleep apnoea (CSA). OSA in the elderly also appears to have less impact on the quality of life (QOL) as compared to their middle-aged counterparts. Despite these differences in symptoms, treatment of OSA with continuous positive airway pressure (CPAP) in the elderly is associated with beneficial effects on cognitive performance, alertness, memory, executive function, decreased sleep disruption due to nocturia, and positive effects on the cardiovascular system.

Ethnicity

Although studies show comparable prevalence rates of OSA in different countries and populations, important differences exist. Despite a lower prevalence of obesity in Asia, the prevalence of OSA is similar to that in the West. The disease severity in Asians is greater than Caucasians for a given age, sex, and BMI. The increased predisposition in Asians may partly be explained by craniofacial anatomy, however other factors, possibly genetic, may play a role. Middle-aged African Americans have a similar prevalence of OSA as Caucasians. BMI appears to be more strongly associated with OSA in Caucasians than in African Americans or Polynesians. There is paucity of data about OSA in other ethnicities.

Genetics

Familial aggregation of OSA is well-known (Redline et al., 1995). First-degree relatives of OSA patients have a higher risk of developing the disease than individuals without a first-degree relative with OSA. The risk increases with the number of individuals involved in the family. Quantitative apnoea-related phenotypes have also demonstrated a substantial heritability of OSA. One study of elderly twins found the heritability of both the respiratory disturbance index (RDI) and the oxygen desaturation index (ODI) to be nearly 40%. Since 78% of variation in weight can be explained by intrafamilial factors, the question arises whether familial aggregation of OSA can be explained based upon obesity or is it influenced by independent genetic factors. Familial aggregation of OSA persists even after controlling for BMI, indicating that genetic and familial factors affecting obesity do not entirely explain such aggregation. In an excellent review of shared genetics of OSA and obesity, Patel (2005) highlighted the possible interaction between genes affecting both, obesity and OSA. Accordingly, some susceptibility genes may act directly on one phenotype and may have indirect effects on the other due to bi-directional relationships between obesity and OSA. Some loci may have pleiotropic effects, affecting susceptibility to obesity and OSA via independent mechanisms (Fig. 7.1).

Another potential mechanism is a form of gene-by-environment effect where the adverse effects of obesity or OSA can be thought of as environmental stressors. It is thought that obesity may have more effect on genetically susceptible individuals in development of OSA. Increased fat deposition in the neck may have more effect on individuals with impaired pharyngeal dilator activity.

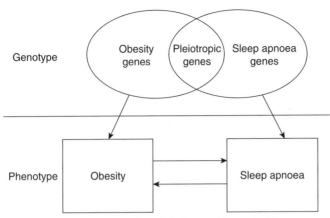

Fig. 7.1 Both obesity and sleep apnoea are heavily influenced by underlying genotype. Some susceptibility genes act directly on one phenotype and through the causal relationships between obesity and sleep apnoea have indirect effects on the other. Other loci have pleiotropic effects, impacting susceptibility to both obesity and sleep apnoea via independent mechanisms.
Source: Reproduced with kind permission from Patel, S.R. (2005). Shared genetic risk factors for obstructive sleep apnea and obesity. *J Appl Physiol*, **99**, 1600–1606.

On the other hand, sleep fragmentation may have more effect in genetically susceptible individuals by affecting leptin and ghrelin systems (Fig. 7.2). Study of non-obese OSA patients has also revealed strong genetic risk. The first linkage scans of OSA have been reported from the Cleveland Family Study. These studies have reported heritability of OSA in both Caucasians and African Americans to be ~33%, and heritability of obesity to be more than 50%. Significant heritability of OSA persisted after controlling for BMI, indicating that about half of genetic variation of OSA is obesity related and about half is independent of OSA. Other factors known to be important in the pathogenesis of OSA, like cephalometric variables, lateral pharyngeal wall fat distribution, and ventilatory control have also been demonstrated to have significant heritability (Schwab et al., 2006).

Craniofacial abnormalities

Craniofacial abnormalities associated with tonsillar hypertrophy, enlarged tongue or soft palate, inferiorly positioned hyoid bone, maxillary and mandibular retroposition, and decreased posterior airway space increase the risk of OSA (Cistulli, 1996). Mandibular body length appears to be the strongest predictor of OSA amongst various craniofacial features. Different craniofacial measures may have different effect on susceptibility of OSA across races. For example, AHI is more strongly correlated with brachycephaly in Whites, with tongue size and soft palate length in African Americans and with retrognathia in Asians. Some recent studies have shown the ability of photographic analysis in predicting OSA based on analysis of certain craniofacial features (Lee et al., 2009). Measures of face width, eye width, cervicomental angle, and mandibular length were used to classify subjects with and without OSA. In performing craniofacial phenotyping, mandibular length, mandibular nasion angle, mandibular triangular area, and anterior neck space area were smaller, while mandibular width-length angle and face width-midface depth angle were larger in the OSA group as compared with controls. More than 90% of patients in these studies were Caucasians. Clearly, more studies are needed to replicate these findings and to apply this technique to other ethnicities.

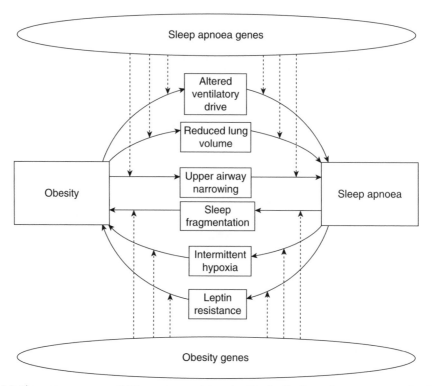

Fig. 7.2 Sleep apnoea susceptibility genes may interact with obesity through numerous mechanisms to influence sleep apnoea predisposition. Genetic polymorphisms may modulate the degree to which obesity alters ventilatory drive, reduces lung volume, or narrows the UAW. Other polymorphisms may affect the degree to which these stresses result in the development of sleep apnoea. Similarly, obesity susceptibility genes may interact with sleep apnoea in its potential effect on obesity. *Source*: Reproduced with kind permission from Patel, S.R. (2005). Shared genetic risk factors for obstructive sleep apnea and obesity. *J Appl Physiol*, **99**, 1600–1606.

Exogenous factors

Obstructive sleep apnoea is more common in smokers. Current smoking, in contrast to past smoking, is associated with increased risk of developing OSA, presumably due to increased inflammation and swelling of the UAW. Alcohol ingestion prior to bedtime can induce OSA in otherwise asymptomatic patients and can worsen the severity and oxygen desaturation in established OSA. Recreational drug use was associated with increased risk of developing OSA in truck drivers. Patients on long-term opiates are also known to have a high prevalence of OSA (39%) and combined OSA and CSA (8%). Whether some opiates are more likely to increase the risk of OSA over the others remains to be studied.

Co-morbid conditions

Medical conditions such as polycystic ovary disease (PCOD), hypothyroidism, type 2 diabetes mellitus (T2DM), pregnancy, and acromegaly are associated with high prevalence of OSA. Strong correlation between T2DM and OSA led the International Diabetes Federation Task Force on Epidemiology and Prevention to publish a consensus statement on sleep apnoea and T2DM. The report recommends screening patients with T2DM for OSA, and, conversely, screening OSA patients for hyperlipidaemia, hypertension, and T2DM.

Effect of obstructive sleep apnoea on health

Obstructive sleep apnoea has a systemic impact on health, with effects discussed throughout this chapter, including a manyfold increase in all-cause and cardiovascular mortality (Marshall et al., 2008; Young et al., 2008). Prevalence of OSA in patients with cardiovascular disease is about two to three times higher than in the reference population. Several putative mechanisms have been put forth to explain development of cardiovascular complications: sympathetic activation, cardiovascular variability, vasoactive substances, inflammation, oxidative stress, endothelial dysfunction, insulin resistance, thrombosis, elevated C-reactive protein levels, increased coagulability, and increased intrathoracic pressure changes (Somers et al., 2008).

Hypertension

The Seventh Report of Joint National Committee on prevention, detection, evaluation, and treatment of hypertension lists OSA as an important cause of secondary hypertension. About 50–60% of patients with OSA have hypertension and about 30% of patients with hypertension have OSA. In patients with refractory hypertension, the prevalence of OSA is estimated to be more than 80%. Nocturnal blood pressure dipping is absent in OSA patients and is associated with increased cardiovascular mortality (Ben-Dov et al., 2007). In the Wisconsin Sleep Cohort Study and the SHHS, a close-response relationship between AHI and risk of development of hypertension was observed. In a separate study, an increase in AHI by 1 event per hour, or a decrease in oxygen saturation nadir by 10%, increased the odds ratio (OR) of developing hypertension by 1% (Lavie et al., 2000).

Use of CPAP was associated with at least modest, but clinically significant, reductions in blood pressure; higher pretreatment blood pressure may show a more robust response to CPAP treatment. Some reports have also implicated OSA in pathogenesis of pregnancy-induced hypertension and benefit of CPAP treatment in women in their third trimester of pregnancy (Yinon et al., 2006).

Coronary artery disease

The prevalence of OSA in patients with coronary artery disease (CAD) is estimated to be two times that in the reference population. In a longitudinal study, the risk of developing fatal (OR: 2.87; 95% confidence interval [CI]: 1.17–7.51) and non-fatal (OR: 3.17; 95% CI: 1.12–7.51) cardiovascular events over a 10-year period was significantly higher in patients with untreated severe OSA as compared with healthy participants (Marin et al., 2005). In another 7-year study of 308 snorers in Sweden, CAD was observed in 16.2% with OSA compared with 5.4% snorers without OSA ($P = 0.003$) (Peker et al., 2006). Efficient treatment of OSA was associated with significant reduction in the incidence of CAD (3.2%) as compared with incidence of CAD in inefficiently treated patients (24.6%) ($P = 0.022$). Patients with OSA also have an increased incidence of subclinical CAD. In a study of 200 non-CAD patients who underwent electron-beam computed tomography within 3 years of polysomnography, the median coronary artery calcification score (Agatston units) was 9 in OSA patients and 0 in non-OSA patients (Sorajja et al., 2008). Compared with controls, patients with OSA exhibit two to six times the odds of having an acute coronary event between midnight and 6:00 a.m. (Kuniyoshi et al., 2008; Somers et al., 2008). Amongst the patients with OSA and CAD, patients with nocturnal ischaemia are older, have worse sleep efficiency, more severe CAD, deeper oxygen desaturation, and higher nocturnal systolic BP. The increased risk of CAD with OSA is evident in women as well as in men. The ongoing Randomized Intervention with CPAP in CAD and OSA (RICCADSA) trial is designed to address if CPAP treatment reduces the combined rate of new revascularization, myocardial infarction, stroke, and cardiovascular mortality over a 3-year period in CAD patients with OSA (Peker et al., 2009).

Arrhythmias

Approximately half of patients with OSA exhibit cardiac arrhythmias during sleep (Somers et al., 2008). The most common arrhythmias during sleep include non-sustained ventricular tachycardia, sinus arrest, second-degree atrioventricular conduction block, and frequent premature ventricular contractions. Obstructive apnoeic episodes elicit the diving reflex in which there is potent cardiac vagal discharge occurring simultaneously with peripheral sympathetic discharge, resulting in bradyarrhythmias or frank sinoatrial or atrioventricular blocks. In the SHHS, nocturnal cardiac arrhythmias were two- to fourfold more common in patients with severe OSA and occurred independent of other risk factors. These episodes take place more commonly during REM sleep and are associated with oxygen desaturation. The European Multicentre Polysomnographic study showed a high prevalence of OSA in patients with pacemaker implantation (59%). No significant correlation was found between AHI and Epworth Sleepiness Score (ESS), age, and BMI. In the Outcomes of Sleep Disorders in Older Men (MrOS) study, increasing severity of SDB was associated with a progressive increase in odds of atrial fibrillation (AF) (OR: 2.15; 95% CI: 1.19–3.89) and complex ventricular ectopy (OR: 1.43; 95% CI: 1.12–1.82). In other studies, AF has been shown to be a strong predictor of OSA.

A high prevalence of OSA (50%) in patients admitted to hospital with AF has been reported as compared to a prevalence of 30% in patients admitted to a general cardiology floor.

One study reported that the treatment of OSA was associated with a 50% decrease in recurrence rate of AF following cardioversion. Treatment of OSA has been shown to decrease the frequency of ventricular arrhythmias as well. In one 1-month long randomized controlled trial, treatment of OSA with CPAP resulted in a 58% reduction in the frequency of ventricular premature complexes during sleep.

Heart failure

Prevalence of OSA in patients with heart failure ranges from 11% to 37% (Somers et al., 2008). Heart failure patients with obesity and snoring are at an increased risk of having OSA. Patients with diastolic dysfunction are more likely to have OSA than patients with systolic dysfunction. EDS is not common in these patients and its absence should not be used to rule out OSA in patients with heart failure (Arzt et al., 2006). In men, the likelihood of OSA is related to BMI, whereas in women it is more closely linked to age. Although left ventricular hypertrophy has been noted to occur in patients with OSA, it is not clear if OSA by itself can cause heart failure.

The effect of treatment of OSA on heart failure outcomes has not been rigorously studied. Left ventricular ejection fraction (LVEF) improved by 5–11% in some studies following CPAP treatment for 1–3 months. Automatically adjusting CPAP (AutoPAP) has not been proven to impact the ejection fraction or 6-minute walk distance. The effect of treatment of OSA with mandibular advancement devices or UAW surgery on LVEF is unknown.

Stroke

Obstructive sleep apnoea is thought to be an independent risk factor for cerebrovascular disease (CVD) (Somers et al., 2008). In the SHHS, the OR of prevalent stroke was 1.58 among those subjects with OSA with an AHI >11 events per hour. It is proposed that the hypertension and OSA have additive effects on markers of carotid atherosclerosis. The studies on the prevalence of OSA in patients with stroke have yielded conflicting results. Excessive sleepiness has also been reported to be a predictor of stroke (OR: 3.07; 95% CI: 1.65–6.08) (Davies et al., 2003). In a study of the patients with angina pectoris referred for coronary angiography, the patients with OSA were not more likely to die or experience a myocardial infarction than were individuals without OSA, but were approximately three times more likely to experience a new stroke. There was a dose-response effect, with patients having mild OSA being 2.4 times and those with severe OSA being 3.6 times more likely to experience stroke. OSA patients who experience a stroke may have greater impairment in their rehabilitation potential and increased risk of secondary stroke and mortality. It has been shown that stroke patients with OSA spend longer time in hospital and rehabilitation centres than those without OSA. However, the treatment of patients with OSA was not associated with decreased risk of death due to stroke.

Motor vehicle and occupational accidents

Obstructive sleep apnoea is associated with increased risk of motor vehicle accidents (MVA) (Howard et al., 2004). The risk has been replicated in research studies from different countries and appears to be independent of traffic densities, topographical variation, and cultural differences. Most studies have not found much correlation between risk of accidents and excessive sleepiness. Other contributing factors like reduced alertness, impaired concentration, impaired judgment, fatigue, and slowed reflexes in sleep apnoeics may contribute to heightened risk of MVA. In studies from Sweden, patients with diagnosed OSA or with history of snoring and excessive sleepiness are two to three times more likely to have had an occupational accident within last 10 years. In another European study, there was a disproportionately increased risk of personal injury like head-on collisions or accidents involving pedestrians and cyclists in patients with OSA ($P = 0.06$) (Mulgrew et al., 2008). This study also found that the risk of MVA was high even with mild OSA, whereas the earlier studies had indicated that risk was probably high for moderate or severe sleep apnoea only. Treatment of OSA with CPAP or uvulopalatopharyngoplasty (UPPP) has been shown to improve performance on simulated driving tests and to reduce the risk of accidents. Treatment of OSA with alertness promoting agents, like modafinil, has not been shown to reduce the risk of accidents.

Summary

Obstructive sleep apnoea is an under-recognized disease with profound effects on cardiovascular and neurocognitive function. Many of these effects are preventable and reversible with proper treatment of OSA. However, high suspicion and proper recognition of OSA remains a key to success with the outcomes. Although obesity and male sex are strong risk factors, there are many patients who lack the conventional characteristics of OSA phenotype. A high index of suspicion in patients with cardiovascular disease, diabetes, hypothyroidism, and certain ethnicities could help identify those patients early and may impact the outcomes.

Sleep-related hypoventilation

Introduction

The obesity hypoventilation syndrome (OHS) is known under various names, including obesity-associated hypoventilation, alveolar hypoventilation in the obese, and the Pickwickian syndrome. OHS describes a patient with a BMI ≥30 kg/m^2 who has chronic alveolar hypoventilation leading to daytime hypercapnia, in the absence of intrinsic pulmonary or neuromuscular disease. These patients usually have concomitant hypoxaemia with an arterial partial pressure of oxygen (PaO_2) less than 70 mmHg. Although OHS can exist autonomously, it is frequently associated with OSA. Sleep-induced hypoventilation is characterized by elevated levels of $PaCO_2$ while asleep, defined as a level >45 mmHg or an increase in $PaCO_2$ during sleep by 10 mmHg above wakefulness (Mokhlesi et al., 2008). In addition, the International Classification of Sleep Disorders-2 defines sleep-related hypoxaemia as 'an SpO_2 (oxyhaemoglobin saturation) during sleep of <90% for more than 5 minutes with a nadir of at least 85%' or '>30% of total sleep time with an SpO_2 < 90%'.

Epidemiology

Obesity

Obesity is the main risk factor for OHS. Currently, obesity represents the most common metabolic disease in the world. For practical reasons, it is defined as a BMI of >30 kg/m2. The WHO estimates that more than 1 billion people are overweight and 300 million are obese. In the last decades, the prevalence of obesity showed a progressive and non-stop rising tendency. Epidemiological studies demonstrate that in the United States, between 1986 and 2000, the prevalence of adult obesity doubled, from 10% to 20% of the adult population. Also, during the same time, the prevalence of severe obesity (BMI > 40 kg/m2) quadrupled from 0.5% to 2% of the adult population and that of BMI of at least 50 kg/m2 increased by fivefold. African Americans and Hispanics have higher and increasing prevalence rates of obesity: 31% and 23%, respectively. Morbid obesity appears to be an important contributor to OHS: the prevalence of OSA has been demonstrated to be in the range of 70% and OHS in the range of upper 20%, as opposed to 60% for OSA and 10% for OHS in non-morbidly obese (Resta et al., 2003).

Obstructive sleep apnoea

Obesity hypoventilation syndrome frequently coexists with OSA. The prevalence of OHS among patients with OSA is estimated between 10% and 20%, higher in the subgroup of patients with extreme obesity (Mokhlesi et al., 2008). Approximately 90% of patients with OHS have coexistent OSA. The remaining 10% of patients have an AHI less than 5 events per hour with sleep-related hypoventilation outside obstructive apnoeas and hypopnoeas (Mokhlesi et al., 2008).

Daytime hypercapnia

The prevalence of daytime hypercapnia is related to the severity of obesity and obesity-related impairment in lung function, and is especially high (>20%) in patients with massive obesity (Laaban and Chailleux, 2005). In addition, OSA can be associated with daytime alveolar hypoventilation thought to result from an alteration of the ventilatory drive secondary to repeated episodes of nighttime hypoxaemia and hypercapnia, and sleep fragmentation. The role of OSA is supported by finding daytime hypoxaemia in 7.2% (27 of 377 patients) with OSA without obesity (BMI < 30 kg/m^2), outside of chronic obstructive pulmonary disease (COPD) and restrictive pulmonary abnormalities (Laaban and Chailleux, 2005). Furthermore, daytime hypercapnia was reported in 4.3% and daytime hypoxia in 6.5% of patients with OSA syndrome (OSAS) and normal pulmonary function tests (PFTs) (Orem et al., 2005).

In a study of 91 non-smoking obese women, 10 subjects had diurnal hypercapnia (defined as $PaCO_2$ > 43 mmHg) (Resta et al., 2003). Sleep hypoventilation was present in 70% of the hypercapnic subjects. In another population of 285 patients suspected of SDB, of whom 24 had OHS, hypercapnia ($PaCO_2$ > 45 mmHg) was associated with OSA (RDI > 10/hour) in 27% of the morbidly obese, but only in 11% of the non-morbidly obese patients (Resta et al., 2000). In a study of 1,141 patients with chronic respiratory insufficiency due to OSAS needing CPAP therapy, the prevalence of daytime hypercapnia ($PaCO_2$ > 45 mmHg) was 11% (Laaban and Chailleux, 2005). The prevalence of daytime hypercapnia was 7.2% in the non-obese (BMI < 30 kg/m^2), 9.8% in moderate obesity (BMI 30–40 kg/m^2), and 23.6% in morbidly obese (BMI > 40 kg/m^2). The prevalence of daytime hypercapnia associated with daytime hypoxaemia (PaO_2 < 70 mmHg) was 5.6%.

Patients with hypercapnia and OSA have worse ventilatory restrictive defects (forced vital capacity as % of predicted value [FVC%], total lung capacity as % of predicted [TLC%]), higher RDI, longer total sleep time with oxyhaemoglobin saturation <90% (), and a lower percentage of REM sleep than normocapnic subjects with OSA or those without OSA (Resta et al., 2000).

$PaCO_2$ level is positively associated with age, BMI, neck circumference, waist circumference, AHI, and negatively correlated with forced expiratory volume in 1 second as percentage of predicted value (FEV_1%), FVC%, and PaO_2 (Resta et al., 2003). Other contributors include mean apnoea duration and decreased functional reserve capacity (FRC) (Orem et al., 2005). Awake hypercapnia also appears to correlate with the maximum voluntary ventilation (MVV) (Sahebjami and Gartside, 1996). In a sample of 63 obese male subjects, the prevalence of OHS was much less (5.2% vs. 25%) in patients with normal as opposed to those with low MVV.

Prevalence of OHS in special populations

Bariatric surgery and hospitalized patients are two special populations that are at increased risk for OHS. In a retrospective analysis of 3,451 bariatric surgery patients (282 Medicare and 3,169 non-Medicare patients), the overall OHS prevalence was 3.3%, 9.9% in the Medicare group and 2.7% in the non-Medicare group (Yuan et al., 2009). The overall OSA prevalence was 30%. Male patients had an OHS prevalence of 9.7% and an OSA prevalence of 57.2%. Medicare patients were on average 8 years older and had a higher BMI. In another sample of 77 patients referred for bariatric surgery (mean BMI 43 ± 4 kg/m^2), OSAHS with an AHI >10 events per hour was detected in 31 patients (40%), including 17 patients (22%) with AHI above 15 events per hour (Catheline et al., 2008). Hypoxaemia <80 mmHg was observed in 27% and hypercapnia >45 mmHg in 8% of the patients. In a study evaluating 4,332 consecutive patients admitted to the hospital, 6% were severely obese (BMI > 35 kg/m^2); 31% of these (1% of all screened admissions) had hypercapnia unexplained by other disorders (Nowbar et al., 2004). Almost half of patients with a BMI >50 kg/m^2 had hypoventilation.

Pathophysiology

In a given patient with OHS, the development of chronic hypercapnia may be dependent on the relative balance between the severity of apnoea and hypopnoea, and the amount of non-apnoeic sustained hypoventilation (Berger et al., 2001). Two mechanisms have been proposed as underlying the sustained nocturnal hypoventilation: (1) obstructive hypoventilation and (2) central hypoventilation. These relationships may be illustrated by associations found between diurnal PaCO2 with the severity of AHI as well as with . The obstructive hypoventilation is present in the context of increased RUAW and subsequent flow limitation, with O2 desaturation corrected with treatment of the UAW obstruction. The central hypoventilation is associated with O2 desaturation that persists after the correction of flow limitation (Berger et al., 2001) which has been reported to be present in at least 50% of cases (Kessler et al., 2001). Non-obstructive hypoventilation in OHS may be attributed to a decrease in ventilatory drive (probably a blunted response to hypercapnia) and/or worsening ventilation/perfusion mismatch with greater effective shunt (Kessler et al., 2001). The alteration of the ventilatory drive was proposed to be secondary to repeated episodes of nighttime hypoxaemia and hypercapnia and sleep fragmentation (Laaban and Chailleux, 2005). Higher concentrations of serum leptin (a protein secreted by adipocytes that regulates body weight) appears to be associated with a reduced respiratory drive and a reduced hypercapnic response (López-Acevedo et al., 2009). In women, OHS has been putatively related to the impact of menopause on hormone-related respiratory drive. Since progesterone is known as a respiratory stimulant, post-menopausal status could result in a decrease of the ventilatory drive, unmasking hypoventilation in the severely obese.

Lowered chest wall compliance and a decreased strength of inspiratory muscles together with a restrictive pattern are common in patients with OHS, and are thought to be related, at least in part, to a mechanical problem induced by excessive fat accumulation in the thorax or around UAW. The most persistent PFT abnormalities in obesity are reduced expiratory reserve volume (ERV) and FRC due to alterations in chest wall mechanics, which also lead to decreased total respiratory compliance and likely a closure of some peripheral lung units (Resta et al., 2000). Obese, non-smoking individuals may also have reduced FVC, TLC, and FEV_1 at low lung volumes associated with increased residual volume (RV), RV/TLC, and airway resistance (Sahebjami and Gartside, 1996). Low MVV may result from diaphragmatic muscle weakness as well as from peripheral airway abnormalities, suggested by reduced maximum expiratory flow rates at low lung volumes and air trapping. As a result of air trapping, inspiratory muscles are placed at a mechanical disadvantage leading to lower inspiratory pressure and flow (Sahebjami and Gartside, 1996).

Clinical presentation

Despite high prevalence and mortality statistics and prior encounters with the medical system, OHS may not be recognized by healthcare providers, with the majority of these patients being formally diagnosed late in their fifth or sixth decade of life. OHS patients are more likely to have received a diagnosis of congestive heart failure (OR: 9), angina (OR: 9), and cor pulmonale (OR: 9) than obese controls (Berg et al., 2001).

OHS patients have high co-morbidity burden. There are higher rates of systemic hypertension, diabetes mellitus, hypothyroidism, asthma, and osteoarthritis. Testing of memory and concentration ability reveals lower scores in the obesity-associated hypoventilation than simple obesity (Nowbar et al., 2004). Patients may suffer from functional impairment and respiratory symptoms, but specifically from the sequels of chronic respiratory failure such as daytime sleepiness, morning headaches, and sleep disturbances.

The association of OHS plus OSAS appears to be much more frequent than OHS without OSAS. Due to the high overlap with OSA, the majority of patients have the classic symptoms of loud snoring, nocturnal choking episodes, and witnessed apnoeas. However, OHS patients appear to be heavier than non-OHS patients and display more severe OSAS and more somnolence than non-OHS patients (Akashiba et al., 2006). Prevalence of dyspnoea on exertion at the time of diagnosis may reach 100%, with progressive worsening of this condition during the past years (Kessler et al., 2001).

On laboratory investigations, haematocrit, liver, and cholesterol tests can be abnormal (Akashiba et al., 2006). OHS patients can have the most severe awake and nocturnal arterial blood gas disturbances compared to patients with OSAS or OSAS with COPD (Kessler et al., 2001). Nocturnal polysomnographic findings include a lower total sleep time (in patients with OHS and OSAS), a lower proportion of stage 3, stage 4, and also of REM sleep (similar to normocapnic OSA patients) (Kessler et al., 2001).

Complications and adverse effects on health

Patients with OHS face an increased morbidity and mortality. Those undergoing bariatric surgery have an increased risk for post-operative respiratory failure, development of pulmonary embolism, CAD, and heart failure, prompting a recommendation for preoperative CPAP and intensive care in the post-operative period (Mokhlesi et al., 2008; Yuan et al., 2009). In patients evaluated preoperatively for bariatric surgery, the most informative investigations are polysomnography and electrocardiogram (ECG) (Catheline et al., 2008). The delay in recognizing and treating this condition increases healthcare resource use and the likelihood of requiring hospitalization compared with patients who have similar degrees of obesity. In a study of 20 patients with OHS matched to 2 control groups (Berg et al., 2001), OHS patients had an increased number of hospital admissions with 70% of patients being admitted to the hospital at least once in the year prior to diagnosis, as well as being much more likely to be hospitalized than controls in the 5 years prior to diagnosis. OHS patients spent 7.2 additional days/year in the hospital and a much higher number of days in the intensive care unit (ICU) as compared with controls. Another study of 47 hospitalized OHS patients reported an increased likelihood of requiring invasive mechanical ventilation during their hospital stay as well as long-term care at discharge (Nowbar et al., 2004). Effective treatment was instituted in only 13% of patients. At 18 months, mortality was 23% among patients with obesity-associated hypoventilation compared with 9% among patients with simple obesity. Patients with obesity-associated hypoventilation had a hazard ratio for mortality of 4.0 (95% CI: 1.5–10.4). Most deaths occurred in the first 3 months following hospital discharge. In contrast, OHS patients who are adherent with therapy have an 18-month mortality of 3% and a 2-year rate of 8% (Budweiser et al., 2007b).

Effect of therapy

Use of positive pressure therapy can lead to regression of daytime hypercapnia, even in the absence of weight loss or improved ventilatory function (Han et al., 2001). Bi-level positive airway pressure (BiPAP) ventilation, introduced in the late 1980s, is the most widely used in situations of obesity-hypoventilation. More recently, VT targeting has been shown to be a potentially useful feature to improve efficacy of BiPAP ventilation (Janssens et al., 2009). OHS patients treated with non-invasive ventilation demonstrate better scores on QOL questionnaires than COPD, restrictive, or neuromuscular disease-related chronic respiratory failure (Budweiser et al., 2007a). The proportion of OHS patients having one or more hospital admissions decreased from 70% in the year prior to the initiation of treatment to 15% in the second year after initiation of treatment (Berg et al., 2001). The mean number of days spent annually in hospital decreased 68.4%.

Summary

Obesity hypoventilation syndrome is an under-recognized, but increasingly prevalent condition associated with significant adverse morbidity and mortality. It is frequently associated with OSA, but can also occur in its absence, depending on the predominant mechanism (obstructive vs. central). Positive airway pressure therapy has beneficial effects increasing QOL, reducing length of stay, and hospital admissions, as well as mortality.

Interaction of sleep with respiratory diseases

Sleep and asthma

Introduction

Asthma is a chronic disorder of the airways which poses an increasing public health burden. Its prevalence (7.7% in 2005) is rising (Fuhlbrigge et al., 2002) and up to 75% of asthmatics report nocturnal symptoms (Turner-Warwick, 1988) despite availability of effective treatments. Associated morbidity and mortality are staggering, most recently in the United States alone causing 1.8 million ER visits, 497,000 hospitalizations, and 4,055 deaths (CDC, 2005). Resulting costs strongly correlate with disease severity (Weiss and Sullivan, 2001) and amounted to $12.7 billion (2% of total health expenditures) in 1998 (Godard et al., 2002). The observations that many asthma patients report sleep disturbances and that up to 68% of asthma deaths occur at night (Cochrane and Clark, 1975; Robertson et al., 1990), underlines the importance of understanding asthma and sleep interactions.

Epidemiology of sleep disturbances in asthma

Data indicate that sleep disturbances in asthmatics are global in nature, and multi-factorial in aetiology rather than being solely the result of nocturnal asthma symptoms.

Difficulties of initiating and maintaining sleep

Compared with general population, epidemiological data regarding sleep in asthmatics shows higher prevalence of DIMS (difficulties of initiating and maintaining sleep) (e.g. 38%, with the highest prevalence [75%] for asthma co-morbid with chronic bronchitis) (Klink and Quan, 1987), falling asleep (e.g. 27%) (Mastronarde et al., 2008), maintaining sleep (e.g. 55%) (Janson et al., 1990), and early morning awakenings (e.g. 11.2%) (Janson et al., 1996). Furthermore, mild-to-moderate asthma patients recorded abnormal global scores on the Pittsburgh Sleep Quality Index (PSQI) (mean ± SD: 7.78 ± 3.76) with 79% of participants being 'poor sleepers' (PSQI ≥ 5); a diagnosis of insomnia was reported by 45% of participants (Mastronarde et al., 2008).

Although nocturnal asthma is a well-known disruptor of sleep, even clinically stable asthma may be associated with sleep disturbances. In a study of well-controlled young asthmatics, the prevalence of self-reported sleep disturbances on questionnaires was 93% (Vir et al., 1997). Sleep diaries confirmed that 90% of the asthma patients had sleep disturbances as compared with 27% of normal subjects. Most frequently reported were difficulties maintaining sleep (60% vs. none) and early morning awakenings (47% vs. none).

Little polysomnographic data are available in asthma individuals. In a study of 12 nocturnal asthma patients in stable condition compared with controls, there was a longer sleep latency and a lower amount of stage 4 sleep in asthmatics (Fitzpatrick et al., 1991). Mean daytime sleep latency did not differ between groups.

Overall, the sleep quality of asthma patients appears worse when compared to other chronic conditions such as cystic fibrosis and end-stage renal disease (Fig. 7.3) (Mastronarde et al., 2008).

Sleep duration and asthma

Individuals with asthma appear to have a shorter duration of sleep. In a community-based study of 1,478 subjects, compared to non-asthmatics, asthma subjects had a higher prevalence of 'too little sleep' (39% with 29%) and a higher risk (OR: 2) of unrefreshing sleep. After adjusting for

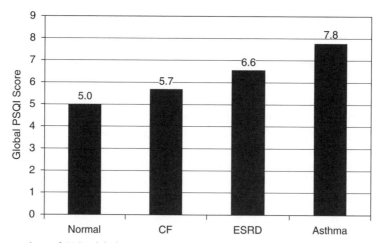

Fig 7.3 Comparison of PSQI global score in asthmatics versus people with other chronic disease. Asthma, baseline data; CF, cystic fibrosis; ESRD, end-stage renal disease
Source: Adapted from Mastronarde, J.G., Wise, R.A., Shade, D.M., et al. (2008). Sleep quality in asthma: results of a large prospective clinical trial. *J Asthma*, **45**, 183–189, with permission from Informa Healthcare, *Journal of Asthma*.

age, gender, and snoring, asthma retained an independent relationship with obtaining less hours of sleep and reporting unrefreshing sleep (Fitzpatrick et al., 1993). Similarly, in diaries, asthma subjects record shorter sleep time compared with controls (Janson et al., 1990; Vir et al., 1997).

Excessive daytime sleepiness in asthma

Excessive daytime sleepiness is more common among asthma patients. In 98 asthmatics, EDS was reported by 44% (Janson et al., 1990). Among 115 asthmatics, 55% perceived EDS and on the ESS, 47% had abnormal scores (>10) (Teodorescu et al., 2006). In 177 patients, the prevalence of EDS was 46%, and 39% recorded ESS scores >10, both significantly higher than in a control population of Internal Medicine patients (Mastronarde et al., 2008). Other studies reported 39% (Mastronarde et al., 2008) and 40% (Auckley et al., 2008) of mild-to-moderate asthma patients had an ESS score >10. The prevalence appears higher in patients with more severe disease, with moderate and severe asthma patients' ESS scores being worse than in healthy controls. In a sample of 22 difficult-to-control asthma patients, 91% reported EDS (Yigla et al., 2003).

Pathophysiology of sleep disturbances in asthma

Disturbed sleep and EDS of asthma patients are likely to be multi-factorial in aetiology. *Nocturnal asthma* represents a common feature of the disease and is an important contributor to sleep disturbance. A survey of 7,729 asthmatics reported that 74% awoke at least once per week with asthma symptoms, while 64% reported nocturnal symptoms at least three times per week and 39% experienced symptoms nightly (Turner-Warwick, 1988). In a study of 3,129 asthmatic patients who maintained a record of 1,631 acute asthma episodes, asthma was approximately 70-fold more frequent between 4:00 a.m. and 5:00 a.m. than between 2:00 p.m. and 3:00 p.m. (Dethlefsen and Repgas, 1985). Nocturnal asthma is marked by a decrease in FEV_1 of at least 15% between bedtime and waking in patients with clinical and physiological evidence of asthma (Sutherland, 2005). Among contributing mechanisms are circadian-related augmentation of airway inflammation, increased airway hyper-responsiveness, enhanced airways resistance related to decrement in lung volumes, changes in autonomic tone and 2 and glucocorticoid receptor function, and hormones such as cortisol and melatonin (Shigemitsu and Afshar, 2007). As the number of acute asthmatic attacks increases (correlating with more nocturnal breathing problems), there appears to be an increase of difficulty in maintaining sleep and nocturnal wakefulness (Janson et al., 1990). A decline in estimated sleep time and raise in nocturnal wakefulness was noted with decreasing FEV_1%. Difficulties falling asleep appear most pronounced in patients with nocturnal asthma symptoms as compared with 'morning dippers' (morning peak expiratory flow [PEF] of less than 80% of the previous evening PEF occurring three or more times/week without symptoms) and the least in stable asthmatics (Van Keimpema et al., 1997).

Asthma control scores and marginally FEV_1% correlate with global PSQI (Mastronarde et al., 2008). Conversely, improvement in PSQI is associated with better asthma control (Mastronarde et al., 2008). Objective data with actigraphy in asthma patients found that those with not well-controlled disease take longer to fall asleep, wake more often, and spend more time awake during the night (Krouse et al., 2008). Circadian PEF variation was found to be the strongest factor influencing polysomnographically (PSG) documented time spent awake at night in nocturnal asthmatics (Fitzpatrick et al., 1991).

Reports of associations of asthma control indices with sleepiness are mixed. For example, in the actigraphic study of 10 patients (Krouse et al., 2008), asthma control scores, use of rescue medications, and symptoms correlated with ESS scores, which related with total time awake during the night, longer sleep latency, and longer wake episodes at night. In contrast, in large interventional study, no significant correlation was found at baseline between asthma control and FEV_1% with ESS.

Similarly, ESS was not associated with the frequency of asthma exacerbations. Interestingly, improved asthma control, but not lung function, correlated with improvements in ESS (Mastronarde et al., 2008). These findings suggest an important contribution of asthma symptoms to sleep fragmentation. However, studies do not always clearly differentiate asthma symptom-related awakenings from awakenings due to other putative factors to sleep disturbance.

Many other conditions, more frequently occurring in asthma patients, may disturb sleep and contribute to the complaint of daytime sleepiness. *OSA*, a common and frequently unrecognized condition (Young et al., 1993, 1997), appears to be more common among asthmatics (see OSA in asthma below). Other co-morbidities, such as nasal disease (rhinitis, sinusitis), gastroesophageal reflux disease (GERD), obesity, and psychopathology (anxiety, depression, and panic disorders) (Ip et al., 2001) can disrupt sleep and are all known to be associated with daytime sleepiness (Bixler et al., 2005; Hasler et al., 2005; Janson et al., 1995, 1996). Furthermore, medications (corticosteroids, β-adrenergics, theophylline) commonly prescribed for asthma treatment tend to have stimulating or anxiety-provoking properties that could interfere with sleep quality and worsen daytime sleepiness. One recent cross-sectional study addressed the potential role of these factors in sleepiness (Teodorescu et al., 2006). Among 115 asthma patients at routine specialty clinic visits and not on treatment for SDB, ESS correlated with OSA risk scores, assessed on a validated instrument, male gender, and asthma severity step; however, in a multiple regression model, ESS was independently associated with OSA risk and male gender, but not with asthma severity step. There were no associations of ESS with age, BMI, FEV_1%, co-morbidities, or medications used to treat asthma. These data suggest that untreated OSA in outpatients with asthma may make substantial contributions to their complaint of EDS. The lack of associations with asthma severity, co-morbidities, and medications, does not exclude the possibility that in an individual asthmatic these factors could still contribute to the complaint of daytime sleepiness, as both asthma and co-morbidities were recognized, potentially reducing their contribution to sleepiness.

Obstructive sleep apnoea in asthma

Accumulating data suggest that asthma patients have an increased risk for OSA. In large epidemiological studies, asthma individuals more frequently report OSA symptoms. In the European Community Health Respiratory Survey, the prevalence of self-reported habitual snoring and apnoea were significantly higher in asthmatics as compared to non-asthmatics (14.7% vs. 9.2% and 3.8% vs. 1.2%, respectively) (Janson et al., 1996). Moreover, the associations of asthma with snoring (OR: 1.7) and apnoeas (OR: 3.7) were independent of BMI, age, gender, and smoking (Janson et al., 1996). Data from the Obstructive Lung Disease Study in Northern Sweden also revealed a higher prevalence of problem snoring in subjects with physician-diagnosed asthma (17.9 vs. 10.1). In a population-based cohort of 677 young atopic women, the prevalence of habitual snoring was 20.5% (Kalra et al., 2006). Symptomatic asthma almost doubled the risk of snoring (OR: 1.8), independent of upper respiratory tract symptoms (e.g. rhinitis), cigarette smoking, and race. A prospective study from Busselton, Australia provides the first evidence in support of a pathogenic role of asthma in OSA. After 14 years of observation, asthma emerged as an independent risk factor for development of habitual snoring (relative risk [RR]: 2.8), when adjusting for potential confounders, including BMI at baseline and BMI change during this long time interval (Knuiman et al., 2006).

Clinic-based studies of well-characterized asthma patients provide further support for this relationship. One such study (Teodorescu et al., 2006) revealed a high prevalence of self-reported snoring with any frequency (86%), habitual snoring (38%), and witnessed apnoea (31%). Furthermore, 51 (44%) of these subjects met a high OSA risk on a validated scale (Douglass et al., 1994). These symptoms were reported up to 4.4 times more often than in general populations when using similar survey methodology (Teodorescu et al., 2006). As compared to Internal Medicine clinic patients, asthmatics are more likely to report habitual snoring (18.5% vs. 8.0%) and witnessed apnoeas (11.8% vs. 6.1%) (Auckley et al., 2008). A similar OSA risk prevalence as above was found in asthma clinic patients, and significantly higher than in the Internal Medicine group (39.5% vs. 27.2%) despite similar proportions of obese subjects (Auckley et al., 2008).

Lastly, two studies with nocturnal PSG found a high prevalence of OSA in more severe asthmatics. Yigla et al. (2003) reported that 21 out of 22 (95.5%) difficult-to-control asthma patients had OSA on PSG. More recently, OSA was significantly more prevalent among those with severe (88%) compared with moderate asthma (58%), and more prevalent for both groups than controls (12%) (Julien et al., 2009). In both studies, the very high prevalence of OSA in severe asthmatics was unexpected for the degree of excess weight observed in these samples (mean BMI: 29.8 ± 1.1 and 27.8 ± 1.1 kg/m^2, respectively). Furthermore, no correlation was found between OSA severity and BMI or neck circumference (Yigla et al., 2003).

Multiple pathways may intervene in OSA pathogenesis in asthma. Among 244 asthma patients not on treatment for SDB, aside from traditional risk factors for OSA such as excess weight and nasal congestion, independent predictors of high OSA risk included asthma severity step (OR: 1.6 for the linear trend), GERD (OR: 2.7), and use of inhaled corticosteroid (ICS) (OR: 4.1), the latter in a dose-dependent fashion ($P = 0.0006$ for the linear trend) (Teodorescu et al., 2009). Women demonstrated a 2.1 times greater odds for OSA, when controlling for the above covariates (Teodorescu et al., 2009), portending that the well-recognized male gender predominance for OSA symptoms may be reversed in these patients, as other studies have also suggested (Mastronarde et al., 2008; Kalra et al., 2006). It is conceivable that asthmatics, particularly women, have a unique set of characteristics, including the disease itself and perhaps corticosteroid use, which may alter their pharyngeal UAW patency setting the stage for OSA.

Health-related outcomes related to sleep in asthma

Sleep disturbances and disorders, such as OSA, may have adverse consequences on asthma. Inverse relationships of global PSQI score and ESS with asthma-related QOL (AQOL) were reported (Mastronarde et al., 2008). Improved PSQI and ESS scores during this 6-month study correlated with improvements in asthma control and AQOL. Each full point improvement in PSQI and ESS corresponded approximately to a doubling and 46% increase, respectively, in the odds of a 'clinically significant' improvement in the AQOL measure (Mastronarde et al., 2008). ESS scores inversely correlated with AQOL symptom scale and activity limitations in the actigraphic study of 10 asthma subjects (Krouse et al., 2008). More episodes of awakening and shorter sleep time during the night resulted in lower emotional functioning and a reduced tolerance for physical activity during the daytime (Krouse et al., 2008).

The effect of chronic sleep restriction, which is increasingly more common in our society, on asthma outcomes is unknown. However, 36 hours of acute sleep deprivation in asthmatics raised the arousal threshold to induced bronchoconstriction during the ensuing recovery sleep, allowing more bronchoconstriction to occur (Ballard et al., 1990b). This observation suggests a potential important role of acute sleep deprivation in asthma control, but the effect of chronic sleep restriction needs to be studied.

Asthma subjects with nocturnal symptoms exhibit lower daytime cognitive performance, specifically concentration and attention, than age- and intellect-matched normal counterparts. In one study, a circadian peak expiratory flow rate (PEFR) variation > 20% was the only independent predictor of lower performance (Fitzpatrick et al., 1991; Weersink et al., 1997). Asthma patients recorded significantly lower sleep time but it is unknown whether this effect was independent of their degree of asthma-related sleep disruption/loss, as such adjusted analyses were not reported.

Although various interventions are effective at reducing asthma symptoms and nocturnal PEFR variation, these studies provide little if any evidence for effects on remediating daytime cognitive deficits to levels comparable to healthy individuals (Bender and Annett, 1999).

OSA appears to be linked with worse asthma outcomes. OSA was recently identified as an important risk factor (OR: 3.4) for frequent exacerbations in the prior year in 63 difficult-to-treat asthma patients (ten Brinke et al., 2005). In a population-based study which included 2,713 subjects with asthma-related symptoms, health-related QOL (measured on Medical Outcomes Survey Short Form-12 [SF-12]) was adversely related with snoring and observed apnoeas (Ekici et al., 2005). Treatment for OSA with CPAP appears to improve asthma. In nine severe nocturnal asthmatics with PSG-diagnosed OSA, CPAP therapy for 2 weeks reduced the frequency of asthma symptoms and bronchodilator use, and improved PEFRs (Chan et al., 1988). Cessation of CPAP returned PEFRs to levels prior to therapy. Two other studies in patients selected for predominantly nocturnal attacks, reported reduction in nocturnal asthma (Guilleminault et al., 1988; Ciftci et al., 2005), but no effect on $FEV_1\%$ (Ciftci et al., 2005). Furthermore, improved AQOL was reported after 6 weeks of CPAP therapy in 20 asthma patients with OSA (Lafond et al., 2007). No adverse effects linked to CPAP therapy have been reported in any of these studies.

Death in asthma patients can occur suddenly at night and in a tight time window. In a retrospective analysis of 38 deaths from asthma, 68% occurred between 12:00 a.m. and 8:00 a.m. (Cochrane and Clark, 1975). In another retrospective study of 1,169 consecutive hospital admissions for asthma, the risk of sudden death correlated with excessive diurnal variation of PEFR. Likewise, most of the acute episodes occurred between 12:00 a.m. and 6:00 a.m. (Hetzel et al., 1977). Whether this strikingly nocturnal-predominant mortality is also favoured by co-morbidities discussed above remains unknown.

Summary

Asthmatics have a globally disturbed sleep which results in prominent daytime sleepiness. Although nocturnal asthma is an important contributor to sleep disturbance, numerous other factors may add to this adverse interaction. Particularly, emerging evidence supports an unfavourable bi-directional relationship with SDB/OSA. Adverse outcomes, especially deaths, observed in these patients at night emphasize the importance of better understanding of asthma-sleep interactions as well as their mechanistic underpinning.

Sleep and COPD

Introduction

Chronic obstructive pulmonary disease is a progressive pulmonary disease characterized by chronic, progressive, and poorly reversible airflow obstruction associated with abnormal inflammatory response to noxious inhaled substances, in addition to systemic inflammation and extrapulmonary manifestations. The majority of cases are due to chronic cigarette use; however, other risk factors exist and include occupational or environmental exposures, HIV, alpha-1-antitrypsin deficiency. COPD ranks fourth among the leading causes of morbidity and mortality worldwide (WHO, 2000). The prevalence of COPD worldwide is estimated to be about 8% of the population aged 25 and greater and 10% of the population aged 40 and greater (Halbert et al., 2006). The disorder typically affects adults older than 40 years of age and is more common in males; however, the prevalence and mortality in females is increasing (CDC, 2008). Per-patient direct costs related to COPD in 2005 were estimated at $2,700–$5,900 annually, with $6,100–$6,600 excess cost for COPD patients compared to non-COPD patients annually, with the greatest costs occurring in patients with more severe COPD (Foster et al., 2006).

Indicators and associations of morbidity and mortality in COPD

The forced expiratory volume in one second (FEV_1) is the main indicator for disease severity and progression in COPD patients (GOLD, 2008); however, the combination of measures of pulmonary function (FEV_1), functional capacity (6-minute walk distance), degree of dyspnoea (Modified Medical Research Council [MMRC] dyspnoea score), and BMI as the BODE index correlates well with mortality (Celli et al., 2004) with additional predictors of mortality consisting of hypoxaemia, reduced peak flow rates, decreased exercise capacity, frequency of exacerbations, smoking status, reduced BMI, increasing age, and decreased general health-related (Medical Outcomes Survey Short Form-36 [SF-36]) (Ware et al., 1993) and respiratory-specific QOL (St. George's Respiratory Questionnaire [SGRQ]) (Jones et al., 1992).

Fatigue is the second most common complaint in COPD individuals after dyspnoea with additional symptoms of insomnia and sleep disruption. Fatigue is strongly correlated with declining lung function, exercise tolerance, and QOL (Breslin et al., 1998). In addition, dyspnoea and fatigue are strongly correlated, with dyspnoea, depression, and sleep quality explaining about 42% of the variance in fatigue as measured by the Fatigue Assessment Instrument (FAI) (Kapella et al., 2006). Thus, fatigue may be a function of sleep abnormalities in COPD.

Epidemiology of sleep disorders in COPD

The Sleep Heart Health Study was a multi-centre cohort study, comprised of 6,440 men and women over the age of 40, designed to examine the effect of SDB on the incidence of cardiovascular disease. Increasing severity of SDB, insomnia, and EDS were associated with worse health-related QOL measured by the SF-36 (Baldwin et al., 2001). To assess the impact of SDB, insomnia, and EDS on QOL, each of the eight SF-36 subscales was analyzed separately using multiple variable logistic regression adjusting for age and race. A linear association of SDB severity was shown with the vitality scale. Persons with severe SDB had significantly worse health-related QOL on several SF-36 subscales. Insomnia and EDS were associated with poorer health-related QOL after adjusting for age, gender, ethnicity, BMI, and smoking status. SF-36 score profiles in subjects with SDB were similar to those seen in other chronic disease populations suggesting that sleep symptoms are important contributors to impaired QOL.

COPD is associated with impairment in both general and respiratory-specific QOL (Jones, 1995; van Manen et al., 2003), but we would not expect that SDB would impact respiratory-specific QOL (Mermigkis et al., 2007). At least one study has shown an association with co-morbid SDB and worse respiratory-specific QOL assessed by the SGRQ. This raises an interesting question with regards to the impact of sleep disorders on morbidity in COPD as it relates to lung function, exertional capacity, and other predictors of mortality.

It is estimated that at least 50% of COPD patients suffer from sleep problems (Klink and Quan, 1987). There are many sleep disorders that occur in COPD patients, with the most frequent being insomnia affecting 30–70% of patients with most symptoms including difficulty falling asleep and early morning awakenings with morning fatigue (Bellia et al., 2003). Disruptions of sleep architecture are quite prevalent with notable increases in stage N1 sleep, decreased slow wave and REM sleep, increased sleep stage changes, reduced total sleep time with increased arousals, and reduced sleep efficiency with periods of frequent wakefulness (Fleetham et al., 1982).

Individuals with COPD have a higher prevalence of SDB-related symptoms including snoring (OR: 1.34), apnoeas (OR: 1.46), and EDS (OR: 2.04) compared to non-COPD patients (Karachaliou et al., 2007). In 87 COPD patients compared to matched controls, restless legs syndrome (RLS) was also more prevalent in COPD than controls (36.8% vs. 11%), and RLS seemed to be more severe with a greater degree of daytime sleepiness (Lo Coco et al., 2009). A retrospective study assessing periodic limb movements during sleep suggests that periodic limb movements occur more frequently in COPD patients with sleep complaints of insomnia and snoring compared to sleep apnoea patients, and the periodic leg movements with associated arousals was drastically greater in COPD patients than in patients who had periodic limb movement disorder (Charokopos et al., 2008). This increase in periodic leg movements may be reflective of nocturnal hypoxaemia as the mean oxyhaemoglobin saturation was lower in the COPD group. Alternatively, periodic limb movements may occur due to R_{UAW} syndrome, which is felt to occur at an increased prevalence in COPD (Becker et al., 1999).

The combination of COPD and OSA, or SDB, is referred to as overlap syndrome. Previous studies had suggested an increased prevalence of COPD in patients with SDB compared to the general population, with estimates near 11–14% (Bradley et al., 1986). With current, more accurate estimates of COPD prevalence in the general population being at least 10%, there does not appear to be an increased prevalence of COPD in the sleep apnoea population (Weitzenblum et al., 2008). Currently, there is conflicting evidence in the literature with regards to the prevalence of sleep apnoea in the COPD population. Some studies suggest increased prevalence of COPD (11%) in OSA (Chaouat et al., 1995) compared to reports in general population. However, Sanders et al. (2003) studied the relationship of sleep apnoea-hypopnoea (SAH) to obstructive airway disease (OAD-FEV_1/FVC < 70%) in a larger population of SHHS participants. In the subgroup of 1,132 individuals with OAD predominantly of mild severity (defined by FEV_1/FVC [63.8 ± 6.6%]), the SAH prevalence was not increased compared to non-OAD participants. However, in OAD participants without SAH, as FEV_1/FVC decreased, the odds of having >5% of sleep time with oxygen saturation <90% were increased when compared to controls (FEV_1/FVC ≥ 80%) suggesting that COPD is associated with sleep-induced hypoventilation. A more recent retrospective study of 73 patients who previously had sleep studies and pulmonary function testing revealed that although the overall severity of SDB was no different in subjects with SDB alone versus overlap syndrome, those patients with FEV_1 less than 80% predicted had higher REM-related RDI than those with higher FEV_1 (López-Acevedo et al., 2009). Within sleep literature, there have been variations in what is considered SDB between different trials. Therefore, differences in outcomes may be a result of differences in definitions of SDB events (apnoeas or hypopnoeas with 4% oxygen desaturation vs. respiratory effort-related arousal), the sensitivity of the measurement of airflow (thermistor vs. nasal cannula), and the method of classification of SDB (AHI ≥ 15 vs. AHI ≥ 10 vs. AHI ≥ 5 events per hour plus symptoms). Larger studies with more sensitive measures of airflow and in a more moderate-to-severe COPD population are needed to more accurately assess the prevalence of SDB in COPD. Based on estimates of COPD prevalence of 10%, and of SDB of 5–10% in the general population, if SDB is not increased in COPD, then the prevalence of overlap syndrome is approximately 0.5–1% of the population over the age of 40 (Weitzenblum et al., 2008).

It is known that patients with overlap syndrome have increased morbidity and mortality compared to COPD or SDB alone. The degree of nocturnal hypoxaemia is increased in overlap syndrome compared to COPD alone or sleep apnoea alone, as patients with COPD do not typically return to a normal baseline saturation level. This, in turn, results in increasing severity of pulmonary hypertension (PH) and cor pulmonale. The prevalence of cor pulmonale in patients with overlap syndrome is 80%, with 5-year survival of about 30% (Rasche et al., 2007). In addition to increased morbidity and mortality, patients with overlap syndrome have higher healthcare utilization and healthcare costs than COPD patients alone. An analysis of Maryland Medicaid COPD patients aged 40–64 years old showed that beneficiaries with overlap syndrome had a $4,155 higher medical cost compared to beneficiaries with COPD alone (Shaya et al., 2009).

Pathophysiology of sleep disturbances in COPD

Sleep fragmentation and insomnia may be related to medications; depression or anxiety; dyspnoea, cough, or other respiratory symptoms; and increased work of breathing as seen in R_{UAW} or sleep apnoea. At least one small study identified anxiety with regards to breathlessness as a factor contributing to poor sleep quality (Shackell et al., 2007). Although -agonist bronchodilators have been intermittently associated with insomnia, there has been no evidence of worsening in the sleep architecture, as assessed on polysomnography, with use of longer-acting bronchodilators, including β-agonists and anticholinergics. In fact, these medications improved nocturnal oxygen saturation nadir in COPD. ICS have not been shown to adversely affect sleep architecture; however, oral corticosteroids have known side effects of insomnia and other cognitive side effects (Roth, 2009). Hypoxaemia and increases in nocturnal carbon dioxide have been associated with increased arousals; however, hypoxaemia in itself may not necessarily be the aetiology of increased arousals during sleep in COPD (Fleetham et al., 1982). The only proven predictors for nocturnal hypoxaemia in COPD are presence of daytime hypoxemia ($PaO_2 < 65$ mmHg) and daytime hypercarbia ($PaCO_2 \geq 45$ mmHg) (Plywaczewski et al., 2000). Hypercarbia has been shown to be a better predictor of nocturnal hypoxaemia than exercise (Mulloy et al., 1995) and is associated with more severe nocturnal hypoxaemia than observed in patients without hypercarbia. During sleep, even normal individuals have a slight decrease in PaO_2 and slight increase in $PaCO_2$, with associated reductions in VT, FRC, and minute ventilation. In addition, there are reduced responses of the respiratory centres in the central nervous system to gas exchange abnormalities, as well as reduced responsiveness of the respiratory muscles (Douglas et al., 1982). Proposed mechanisms for nocturnal hypoxaemia in COPD include the above explanations taking into account the oxyhaemoglobin dissociation curve, with COPD patients having larger decreases in PaO_2 given their location on the steep portion of this curve. Increased risk for hypoxaemia occurs with further reductions in FRC as seen in REM sleep. This is a particularly vulnerable stage of sleep for the COPD patient, as many patients rely on accessory muscle usage to maintain ventilation during a hyperinflated state (Johnson and Remmers, 1984). The reclining position and changes in FRC produce alteration in ventilation and perfusion matching within the lung which may lead to significant changes in ventilation and oxygenation in patients with emphysema. There is a circadian impact of lower airway caliber with increased bronchoconstriction during the night. Moreover, loss of UAW muscle tone leads to increased R_{UAW} during sleep, which is most pronounced during REM sleep, hence the increased severity of OSA during REM sleep (Johnson and Remmers, 1984). As a result, the combination of COPD and sleep apnoea can be associated with profound oxyhaemoglobin desaturations during the night and more so during REM sleep.

One theory supporting the argument that there is no increase in sleep apnoea in COPD, is that there is reduced REM sleep in COPD patients, thereby a reduction in overall SDB events. From a physiological perspective, air trapping and hyperinflation result in larger resting lung volumes. This hyperinflation state provides traction on the UAW, thereby preventing significant UAW collapse and by altering the critical closing pressure of the airway. Other arguments would suggest that even a mild increase in R_{UAW}, such as with snoring, would increase work of breathing in an individual who is at near maximal ventilatory capacity to an extent that a slight increase in work of breathing and/or $PaCO_2$ would lead to an early arousal prior to significant oxyhaemoglobin desaturation (Fleetham et al., 1982). The changes that occur in respiratory timing indices in normal individuals who are subjected to inspiratory flow limitation is to increase inspiratory time to maintain ventilation at the risk of a decreased expiratory time. In a COPD individual requiring a prolonged expiration due to lower airways obstruction, this increase in inspiratory time may not be possible (Herpel et al., 2007). This inability to compensate for R_{UAW} loading, similar to increased work of breathing seen with exercise, may lead to the early arousal and increased sleep fragmentation seen in the COPD patient.

Clinical presentation

The clinical presentation of sleep disorders in COPD patients is typically a complaint of fatigue. Most patients will readily volunteer insomnia symptoms when asked. Patients may have snoring and nocturnal symptoms of UAW obstruction, and other associated risk factors for sleep apnoea, such as obesity, modified Mallampati score of 3 or 4, increased neck circumference, family history, co-morbidities of AF, heart failure, hypertension, diabetes, and CVD that would be indications for a polysomnogram. Additional signs of potential SDB in COPD include presence of polycythaemia and PH out of proportion to the patient's daytime PaO_2 (ATS, 2004). There are no current recommendations for an overnight screening polysomnogram in COPD in the absence of sleep apnoea symptoms. If clinical suspicion for SDB exists, the American Academy of Sleep Medicine recommends evaluation with an attended in-laboratory overnight polysomnogram, with optional addition of measures of CO_2 such as end-tidal CO_2 (Kushida et al., 2005).

Complications and health outcomes

Sleep disorders such as insomnia and sleep apnoea are associated with increased morbidity and worsening QOL. Interestingly, several studies have recognized worsening SGRQ in COPD patients with sleep apnoea compared to those without. There are little data regarding the effect of untreated sleep apnoea on the rate of decline in lung function or exacerbations in COPD. In 15 men (mean ± SD: 57 ± 3 years) with COPD ($FEV_1/FVC < 60\%$), pulmonary function testing performed after a night with and without sleep deprivation demonstrated a small but significant decrease in FEV_1 (mean ± SD: 1.06 ± 0.11 to 1.00 ± 0.09 L; $P < 0.05$) and in FVC (2.56 ± 0.20 to 2.43 ± 0.17 L; $P < 0.05$) following sleep deprivation (Phillips et al., 1987). There are accumulating data supporting the concept of increased systemic inflammatory mediators associated with both, COPD and sleep apnoea, and the possibility that untreated sleep apnoea may contribute to increased airway or systemic inflammation in COPD remains unexplored (McNicholas, 2009).

Use of non-benzodiazepine hypnotics for insomnia is considered a safe option for patients with mild-to-moderate lung disease (Roth, 2009), but there are some data to suggest that these drugs may promote apnoea, which is known to significantly exacerbate hypoxaemia in these patients. The amnestic and cognitive effects of non-benzodiazepine hypnotics make their use less attractive, particularly in this elderly COPD population already predisposed to cognitive deficits. Traditional benzodiazepines on the other hand, which are very effective for anxiety and occasionally for insomnia, can produce significant central respiratory suppression worsening nocturnal hypoventilation, hypoxaemia, and hypercarbia (Roth, 2009). Use of melatonin or melatonin receptor agonists have not shown to have similar problems with respiratory disturbances and have resulted in improved sleep duration and efficiency (Kryger et al., 2008).

Treatment with oxygen is indicated for nocturnal hypoxaemia related to alveolar hypoventilation. It is well-known that continuous oxygen therapy improves mortality in COPD (NOTT, 1980); however, the duration and severity of hypoxaemia that benefit from oxygen therapy is less clear with clinical trials designed to answer this question currently underway. Oxygen therapy in hypoxaemic patients has been shown in some studies to improve sleep quality and reduce arousal index (Calverley et al., 1982). Typical recommendations for treatment of nocturnal hypoxaemia are based on Medicare guidelines of 10 consecutive minutes of oxygen saturation <90% or 10% of total sleep time <90%. Approximately 47% of COPD patients who are hypoxaemic during the day will spend about 30% of their sleep time with oxygen saturation <90% while on continuous oxygen therapy (Plywaczewski et al., 2000). Current recommendations for nocturnal oxygen therapy is to increase the oxygen concentration by 1 L/minute above the baseline oxygen flow rate needed to maintain a saturation >90% during resting wakefulness with delivery method continuously via nasal cannula or face mask (ATS, 2004).

It is well-known that CPAP treatment improves cardiovascular and cerebrovascular outcomes for sleep apnoea patients; however, it is less clear if COPD patients require CPAP *or* BiPAP therapy as the first-line therapy for sleep apnoea/overlap syndrome. Current recommendations indicate that CPAP should be the first-line therapy for overlap syndrome. A study of 603 COPD patients requiring long-term oxygen therapy revealed that 15.7% of these patients had moderate-to-severe OSA. Mortality in COPD patients who require oxygen therapy is high, with estimates of 5-year survival in oxygen treated versus untreated being 62% versus 16%, respectively (NOTT, 1980; MRC, 1981). In hypoxaemic COPD patients with moderate-to-severe SDB, the 5-year survival was 71% versus 26% in those treated with CPAP plus oxygen versus oxygen alone, independent of baseline post-bronchodilator FEV_1 (Machado et al., 2009). There is no specific cut-off with regards to FEV_1 for prescribing PAP; in general, daytime hypercarbia or nocturnal hypoxaemia in spite of oxygen therapy is an indication for nocturnal BiPAP therapy, regardless of the presence of sleep apnoea. It is unclear whether these patients should be titrated in a sleep laboratory or in a hospital setting. It is also not known if therapy with long-term non-invasive nocturnal ventilation for COPD patients without sleep apnoea improves COPD outcomes. One study randomized 122 COPD patients hospitalized with respiratory failure to long-term oxygen therapy versus non-invasive nocturnal ventilation plus oxygen therapy. There was an improvement in health-related QOL, and reduction in length of ICU stay in the non-invasive ventilation group, but no difference in mortality or subsequent hospitalizations (Clini et al., 2002). In stable hypercarbic COPD patients, there is no clear evidence of improvement in mortality with use of nocturnal non-invasive ventilation in COPD patients without sleep apnoea in spite of evidence of improved daytime gas exchange (Gay et al., 1996; Meecham Jones et al., 1995), but additional long-term studies are needed. Lung volume reduction, a surgical procedure indicated for highly select patients with severe COPD, has been shown to reduce hyperinflation, improve nocturnal hypoxaemia, and improve total sleep time and sleep efficiency in patients without SDB (Krachman et al., 2005). More studies need to be done to determine if reduction in hyperinflation impacts SDB occurrence and sleep-related morbidity.

Sleep and pulmonary vascular disease and interstitial lung disease

Sleep and pulmonary hypertension

Pulmonary hypertension defines a heterogeneous group of disorders characterized by increased pulmonary vascular resistance. SDB is considered a chronic respiratory disorder which can cause or exacerbate PH. However, the interaction between sleep and PH is much more complex than this single causal relationship. Sleep inadequacy and fragmentation are often seen in patients with chronic respiratory conditions for a variety of reasons, and may contribute to poor daytime function, poor QOL, and progression of the PH severity.

There are data to support strongly the concept of SDB causing PH. First, there are plausible biological mechanisms for the development of PH. SDB is associated with intermittent hypoxia (Zielinski, 2005), hypercoagulability and a prothrombotic state (von Kanel et al., 2001), systemic inflammation (Vgontzas et al., 1997), left ventricular dysfunction (Golbin et al., 2008), and excessive catecholamine states, all of which can cause increases in pulmonary arterial pressures. Second, there are animal models that corroborate the theory that sleep apnoea causes PH.

When rats were exposed to 30 seconds of severe hypoxia followed by 30 seconds of normoxia for 8 hours per day for 5 weeks (to mimic OSA), their mean ($\pm$SD) pulmonary arterial pressure increased from 20.7 ± 6.8 to 31.3 ± 7.2 mmHg and pathologically they demonstrated pulmonary vascular remodeling and right ventricular hypertrophy (McGuire and Bradford, 2001). In humans, however, the direct pathogenesis of persistent PH from OSA has not been as definitively shown.

Estimates of the prevalence of PH in patients with OSA vary considerably, from 17% to 53%, based on the methodology of the study and the definition of PH used (Atwood et al., 2004). Many of these earlier studies had small sample size, varying methods to measure right heart pressures, and a referral bias to the subject selection. More recent studies have attempted to address this issue with standard right heart catheterization for defining PH and larger, generalizable patient populations. Chaouat et al. (1996) studied 220 patients with OSA. Using right heart catheterization, they found 17% of patients with OSA had a resting mean pulmonary arterial pressure (mPAP) $\geq$20 mmHg. Similarly, Shinozaki et al. (1995) studied 25 patients with OSA and found that 32% of these patients had a mPAP $\geq$20 mmHg. Both studies found that the presence of obstructive lung disease was significantly correlated with the presence of PH; the latter study also found that higher waking arterial CO_2 levels, lower waking arterial O_2 levels, and higher weight were also risk factors for PH. Interestingly, there was no correlation found between AHI or ODI and presence of PH. In order to address the confounding of chronic lung disease causing PH, some studies reported on PH among OSA patients with normal PFTs and normal arterial blood gases at rest. Among these studies, prevalence of PH ranged from 0% to 41% (Judd et al., 2003). These studies, however, varied on their diagnosis of PH and in their selection of patients. For example, studies with the higher reported prevalence of PH used Doppler echocardiography to define PH (as opposed to right heart catheterization), and selected for the sickest patients who needed to be hospitalized.

When PH is attributed to OSA alone, PH tends to be mild, with an average mPAP of <30 mmHg, and tends to affect patients who are older, heavier, and have worse lung function as compared to patients with sleep apnoea without PH (Atwood et al., 2004). The severity of PH does not seem to be associated with the severity of the SDB.

Treatment of SDB lowers the pulmonary arterial pressures, although it may not normalize them if vascular remodeling has occurred. Arias et al. (2006) studied pulmonary haemodynamics and OSA in 23 patients, and found that effective CPAP treatment for OSA significantly reduced pulmonary systolic pressure (from 28.9 to 24.0 mmHg). Those who were most likely to respond to therapy were patients with PH at baseline. There are other studies, however, that show no change in pulmonary arterial pressure after either tracheostomy (Coccagna et al., 1972) or CPAP (Chaouat et al., 1997) for treatment of OSA. Collectively, based on these data, the effect of treatment of OSA on pulmonary haemodynamics is likely to be beneficial.

Although there is good reason to believe that SDB results in mild PH, the prevalence of sleep disorders among patients with PH is less well-understood. Different aetiologies of PH may increase the risk of different sleep disorders. Left-sided heart failure predisposes to Cheyne-Stokes respiration; connective tissue diseases causing PH are frequently treated with steroids, which can increase the risk of obstructive SDB; patients with HIV may be treated with highly active anti-retroviral treatment, which has been associated with hypoventilation. The prevalence of SDB in each of these groups, however, has not been well-studied. One study addresses the prevalence and characteristics of RLS in patients with PH (Minai et al., 2008). While their patients were heterogeneous in cause of PH, they found that 43.6% of 55 patients with PH had RLS, and 54% of these had moderate-to-severe symptoms. This study concluded that patients with PH should be screened for RLS, as this disorder is easily treatable and may also improve the patient's sleep and QOL.

Summary

Pulmonary hypertension is a chronic disorder with significantly increased mortality. Although therapies exist for PH, and treatment of the underlying causes can sometimes improve pulmonary artery pressures, sleep disorders play a significant role in the progression of disease as well. SDB and its intermittent hypoxia can worsen PH. Further studies in this field should be directed towards the effects of treatment of sleep disorders on the outcomes of PH. RLS is likely prevalent in this patient population as well, but more studies are needed to determine the impact of other sleep disorders on PH.

Sleep and interstitial lung disease

Interstitial lung diseases (ILD) include a broad range of diseases unified by the common feature of inflammation and fibrosis in the lung parenchyma, causing restrictive lung disease. Knowledge of the prevalence of sleep disorders in patients with ILD is quite limited. There are many reasons to believe sleep disorders are common in ILD patients and may contribute to significant morbidity and mortality. ILD patients suffer from fatigue, reduced QOL, and increased mortality (ATS/ ERS, 2002; De Vries et al., 2001; Swigris et al., 2005), which are features shared with patients with sleep disorders.

Most of the literature addressing sleep disorders in patients with ILD focuses on disorders of sleep architecture and sleep-related breathing. The literature is largely limited to small case series or case-control studies. The available knowledge, however, demonstrates significant disruption of normal sleep physiology in these patients. In a recent study of 41 subjects with idiopathic pulmonary fibrosis who were prospectively identified, daytime sleepiness (measured by the ESS) and poor quality of sleep (measured by a modified PSQI) were reported frequently (Krishnan et al., 2008). Indices of QOL, including physical function, vitality, and role of emotions were significantly associated with sleep dysfunction. Polysomnography was not performed to verify sleep disorders in this study, but the data suggest frequent sleep disorders and the association with morbidity in ILD patients.

ILD patients suffer from significantly fragmented sleep. Perez-Padilla et al. (1985) reported the results of a case-control study of patients with and without ILD. Eleven subjects with ILD and age- and sex-matched controls underwent polysomnography, and marked sleep architecture distortion was noted in the ILD patients. Stage N1 sleep was increased (33% of TST vs. 13.5%), REM sleep (11.9% vs. 19.9%) was reduced in the ILD patients; slow wave sleep was reduced and sleep arousals/sleep transitions were more frequent as well. In a more recent study, Aydogdu et al. (2006) found similarly disrupted sleep. Using full-night polysomnography, sleep architecture of 37 patients with ILD was studied. Total sleep time, time spent in slow wave sleep, and time in REM sleep and sleep efficiency were all decreased. This study did not, however, include a control group for comparison. Nonetheless, both studies reflect significant sleep disturbance and fragmentation in patients with ILD.

A number of reasons have been presented to explain sleep disorders in patients with ILD. Chronic disease can cause significant anxiety and stress, which can contribute to sleep initiation and sleep maintenance. Therapeutic interventions for ILD include corticosteroids, which are known to disturb sleep. Limitations in oxygenation due to parenchymal lung disease make sleep hypopnoeas more likely to be diagnosed on a polysomnography. Patients with chronic restrictive lung disease may be more prone to hypoventilation during sleep, particularly in the face of UAW obstruction.

SDB is also common in patients with ILD. Midgren et al. (1987) reported on 16 patients with ILD and moderate-to-severe restrictive ventilatory defect (mean total lung capacity 66% of predicted) and evidence of hypoxaemia during rest or with exercise. Four patients had oxygen saturations <89% during nocturnal wakefulness and seven patients had an average oxygen saturation <89% during sleep. This study does not address the presence of nocturnal hypoxia in patients with ILD who do not exhibit daytime hypoxaemia. Bye et al. (1984) studied 13 patients with ILD and found evidence of significant oxygen desaturations during sleep, particularly during REM sleep. Two of four patients who snored had significant OSA, but all patients had greater than 10% falls in O_2 saturation during NREM sleep. Seven of the nine non-snoring subjects exhibited significant hypoxaemia during REM sleep. Nocturnal hypoxaemia should be considered in patients with ILD, particularly in those who exhibit hypoxaemia during wakefulness.

The prevalence of OSA in patients with ILD is not certain. Bye et al. (1984) reported evidence of inspiratory flow limitation (snoring) in 4 of 13 (31%) patients studied, and definite OSA in 15% of patients. Mermigkis et al. (2009) performed a retrospective study of 18 patients with ILD who underwent polysomnography. They found that 11 subjects (61%) had OSA and the remaining patients exhibited evidence of snoring or R_{UAW} syndrome. This study is, however, subject to a referral bias that may falsely elevate the estimation of prevalence of sleep apnoea. In a prospective study however, the reported prevalence of OSA was similar. Among 37 patients with ILD, OSA (with AHI > 5 events per hour) was diagnosed in 24 (64.9%) patients (Aydogdu et al., 2006). The presence of UAW obstruction in addition to the baseline restrictive disorder may predispose these patients to significant oxygenation and ventilatory compromise during sleep. Oxygenation during sleep would be expected to be worse than during wakefulness, due to associated hypoventilation. Hypoventilation during sleep is an expected physiological change, due to reductions in VT. In addition, patients with ILD may have altered ventilatory control, resulting in an even more rapid shallow breathing pattern with sleep than with wakefulness. There are no studies to date that address the role that OSA plays in the prognosis of ILD. Similarly, there are no data available to study the effects of treatment of OSA on prognosis and survival of patients with ILD.

There is surprisingly little information available regarding other sleep disorders in patients with ILD. RLS has been reported to be common in patients with systemic sclerosis. Thirteen of 27 patients (48%) were noted to have periodic limb movements during sleep >5/hour, and 6 patients (22%) were diagnosed with RLS (Prado et al., 2002). Although the authors do not describe in detail the presence of ILD in this population, they report that 63% of subjects reported dyspnoea and 48% had documented pulmonary function abnormalities. Other sleep disorders, including insomnia, hypersomnias, and sleep-related movement disorders, have not been studied in patients with ILD.

Summary
Sleep disorders appear common in ILD. Significant sleep fragmentation, nocturnal hypoxaemia, and OSA have been frequently reported in patients with ILD, and may contribute to the significant reduction in QOL, daytime symptoms of fatigue, and mortality seen in this patient population. Larger prospective studies of sleep in ILD patients are necessary to understand the actual impact of sleep disorders on ILD and its progression. Further directions of research should focus on the effect of treatment of sleep disorders on outcomes in ILD.

Summary box

+ Sleep has a significant impact on breathing through withdrawal of the wakefulness stimulus and alterations in reflex responses, muscular tone, lung properties, ventilatory chemosensitivity, and metabolic rate.
+ OSA and sleep-related hypoventilation are highly prevalent and frequently unrecognized sleep breathing disorders, with significant impact on health.
+ Among the many factors promoting their development, obesity represents the most important modifiable risk factor.
+ There is increased recognition that a dual interaction between sleep/sleep disorders and chronic lung disease exists. On one hand, there is increased prevalence of globally disturbed sleep, insomnia, and RLS in chronic lung disease. These patients may be more prone to sleep apnoea and/or hypoventilation during sleep. On the other hand, sleep is a vulnerable time for these patients and there are data to suggest worse respiratory outcomes and QOL in patients with coexistent sleep disorders.
+ Many gaps remain in our knowledge of the nature of these interactions, their underlying mechanisms, and implications for these already compromised populations.

References

Akashiba, T., Akahoshi, T., Kawahara, S., et al. (2006). Clinical characteristics of obesity-hypoventilation syndrome in Japan: a multi-center study. *Intern Med*, **45**, 1121–1125.

Ancoli-Israel, S., Kripke, D.F., Klauber, M.R., et al. (1991). Sleep-disordered breathing in community-dwelling elderly. *Sleep*, **14**, 486–495.

Arias, M.A., Garcia-Rio, F., Alonso-Fernandez, A., et al. (2006). Pulmonary hypertension in obstructive sleep apnoea: effects of continuous positive airway pressure: a randomized, controlled cross-over study. *Eur Heart J*, **27**, 1106–1113.

Arzt, M., Young, T., Finn, L., et al. (2006). Sleepiness and sleep in patients with both systolic heart failure and obstructive sleep apnea. *Arch Intern Med*, **166**, 1716–1722.

Aston-Jones, G. (2005). Brain structures and receptors involved in alertness. *Sleep Med*, **6**(Suppl 1), S3–S7.

ATS (2004). American Thoracic Society and European Respiratory Society. Standards for the Diagnosis and Management of Patients with COPD. Available at: http://www.thoracic.org/sections/copd/resources/copddoc.pdf (accessed August 15, 2009).

ATS/ERS (2002). American Thoracic Society/European Respiratory Society International Multidisciplinary Consensus Classification of the Idiopathic Interstitial Pneumonias. This joint statement of the American Thoracic Society (ATS), and the European Respiratory Society (ERS) was adopted by the ATS board of directors, June 2001 and by the ERS Executive Committee, June 2001. *Am J Respir Crit Care Med*, **165**, 277–304.

Atwood, C.W., Jr., McCrory, D., Garcia, J.G., et al. (2004). Pulmonary artery hypertension and sleep-disordered breathing: ACCP evidence-based clinical practice guidelines. *Chest*, **126**, 72S–77S.

Auckley, D., Moallem, M., Shaman, Z., et al. (2008). Findings of a Berlin Questionnaire survey: comparison between patients seen in an asthma clinic versus internal medicine clinic. *Sleep Med*, **9**, 494–499.

Aydogdu, M., Ciftci, B., Firat Guven, S., et al. (2006). Assessment of sleep with polysomnography in patients with interstitial lung disease. *Tuberk Toraks*, **54**, 213–221.

Baldwin, C.M., Griffith, K.A., Nieto, F.J., et al. (2001). The association of sleep-disordered breathing and sleep symptoms with quality of life in the Sleep Heart Health Study. *Sleep*, **24**, 96–105.

Ballard, R.D., Irvin, C.G., Martin, R.J., et al. (1990a). Influence of sleep on lung volume in asthmatic patients and normal subjects. *J Appl Physiol*, **68**, 2034–2041.

Ballard, R.D., Tan, W.C., Kelly, P.L., et al. (1990b). Effect of sleep and sleep deprivation on ventilatory response to bronchoconstriction. *J Appl Physiol*, **69**, 490–497.

Becker, H.F., Piper, A.J., Flynn, W.E., et al. (1999). Breathing during sleep in patients with nocturnal desaturation. *Am J Respir Crit Care Med*, **159**, 112–118.

Bellia, V., Catalano, F., Scichilone, N., et al. (2003). Sleep disorders in the elderly with and without chronic airflow obstruction: the SARA study. *Sleep*, **26**, 318–323.

Ben-Dov, I.Z., Kark, J.D., Ben-Ishay, D., et al. (2007). Predictors of all-cause mortality in clinical ambulatory monitoring: unique aspects of blood pressure during sleep. *Hypertension*, **49**, 1235–1241.

Bender, B.G. & Annett, R.D. (1999). Neuropsychological outcomes of nocturnal asthma. *Chronobiol Int*, **16**, 695–710.

Berg, G., Delaive, K., Manfreda, J., et al. (2001). The use of health-care resources in obesity-hypoventilation syndrome. *Chest*, **120**, 377–383.

Berger, K.I., Ayappa, I., Chatr-Amontri, B., et al. (2001). Obesity hypoventilation syndrome as a spectrum of respiratory disturbances during sleep. *Chest*, **120**, 1231–1238.

Bixler, E.O., Vgontzas, A.N., Ten Have, T., et al. (1998). Effects of age on sleep apnea in men: I. Prevalence and severity. *Am J Respir Crit Care Med*, **157**, 144–148.

Bixler, E.O., Vgontzas, A.N., Lin, H.M., et al. (2001). Prevalence of sleep-disordered breathing in women: effects of gender. *Am J Respir Crit Care Med*, **163**, 608–613.

Bixler, E.O., Vgontzas, A.N., Lin, H.M., et al. (2005). Excessive daytime sleepiness in a general population sample: the role of sleep apnea, age, obesity, diabetes, and depression. *J Clin Endocrinol Metab*, **90**, 4510–4515.

Bradley, T.D., Rutherford, R., Lue, F., et al. (1986). Role of diffuse airway obstruction in the hypercapnia of obstructive sleep apnea. *Am Rev Respir Dis*, **134**, 920–924.

Breslin, E., van der Schans, C., Breukink, S., et al. (1998). Perception of fatigue and quality of life in patients with COPD. *Chest*, **114**, 958–964.

Breugelmans, J.G., Ford, D.E., Smith, P.L., et al. (2004). Differences in patient and bed partner-assessed quality of life in sleep-disordered breathing. *Am J Respir Crit Care Med*, **170**, 547–552.

Budweiser, S., Hitzl, A.P., Jorres, R.A., et al. (2007a). Health-related quality of life and long-term prognosis in chronic hypercapnic respiratory failure: a prospective survival analysis. *Respir Res*, **8**, 92.

Budweiser, S., Riedl, S.G., Jorres, R.A., et al. (2007b). Mortality and prognostic factors in patients with obesity-hypoventilation syndrome undergoing noninvasive ventilation. *J Intern Med*, **261**, 375–383.

Bulow, K. (1963). Respiration and wakefulness in man. *Acta Physiol Scand Suppl*, **209**, 1–110.

Bye, P.T., Issa, F., Berthon-Jones, M., et al. (1984). Studies of oxygenation during sleep in patients with interstitial lung disease. *Am Rev Respir Dis*, **129**, 27–32.

Calverley, P.M., Brezinova, V., Douglas, N.J., et al. (1982). The effect of oxygenation on sleep quality in chronic bronchitis and emphysema. *Am Rev Respir Dis*, **126**, 206–210.

Catheline, J.M., Bihan, H., Le Quang, T., et al. (2008). Preoperative cardiac and pulmonary assessment in bariatric surgery. *Obes Surg*, **18**, 271–277.

CDC (2005). US Centers for Disease Control and Prevention. National Center for Health Statistics. Fast Stats A to Z. Asthma Prevalence, Health Care Use and Mortality, Available at: http://www.cdc.gov/nchs/products/pubs/pubd/hestats/ashtma03-05/asthma03-05.htm (accessed August 15, 2009).

CDC (2008). US Centers for Disease Control and Prevention. Deaths from chronic obstructive pulmonary disease—United States, 2000-2005. *MMWR Morb Mortal Wkly Rep*, **57**, 1229–1232.

Celli, B.R., Cote, C.G., Marin, J.M., et al. (2004). The body-mass index, airflow obstruction, dyspnea, and exercise capacity index in chronic obstructive pulmonary disease. *N Engl J Med*, **350**, 1005–1012.

Chan, C.S., Woolcock, A.J. & Sullivan, C.E. (1988). Nocturnal asthma: role of snoring and obstructive sleep apnea. *Am Rev Respir Dis*, **137**, 1502–1504.

Chaouat, A., Weitzenblum, E., Krieger, J., et al. (1995). Association of chronic obstructive pulmonary disease and sleep apnea syndrome. *Am J Respir Crit Care Med*, **151**, 82–86.

Chaouat, A., Weitzenblum, E., Krieger, J., et al. (1996). Pulmonary hemodynamics in the obstructive sleep apnea syndrome. Results in 220 consecutive patients. *Chest*, **109**, 380–386.

Chaouat, A., Weitzenblum, E., Kessler, R., et al. (1997). Five-year effects of nasal continuous positive airway pressure in obstructive sleep apnoea syndrome. *Eur Respir J*, **10**, 2578–2582.

Charokopos, N., Leotsinidis, M., Pouli, A., et al. (2008). Periodic limb movement during sleep and chronic obstructive pulmonary disease. *Sleep Breath*, **12**, 155–159.

Ciftci, T.U., Ciftci, B., Guven, S.F., et al. (2005). Effect of nasal continuous positive airway pressure in uncontrolled nocturnal asthmatic patients with obstructive sleep apnea syndrome. *Respir Med*, **99**, 529–534.

Cistulli, P.A. (1996). Craniofacial abnormalities in obstructive sleep apnoea: implications for treatment. *Respirology*, **1**, 167–174.

Clini, E., Sturani, C., Rossi, A., et al. (2002). The Italian multicentre study on noninvasive ventilation in chronic obstructive pulmonary disease patients. *Eur Respir J*, **20**, 529–538.

Coccagna, G., Mantovani, M., Brignani, F., et al. (1972). Tracheostomy in hypersomnia with periodic breathing. *Bull Physiopathol Respir (Nancy)*, **8**, 1217–1227.

Cochrane, G.M. & Clark, J.H. (1975). A survey of asthma mortality in patients between ages 35 and 64 in the Greater London hospitals in 1971. *Thorax*, **30**, 300–305.

Davies, D.P., Rodgers, H., Walshaw, D., et al. (2003). Snoring, daytime sleepiness and stroke: a case-control study of first-ever stroke. *J Sleep Res*, **12**, 313–318.

De Vries, J., Kessels, B.L. & Drent, M. (2001). Quality of life of idiopathic pulmonary fibrosis patients. *Eur Respir J*, **17**, 954–961.

Dethlefsen, U. & Repgas, R. (1985). Ein neues Therapieprinzip bei Nachtlichen Asthma. *Clin Med*, **80**, 44–47.

Douglas, N.J., White, D.P., Pickett, C.K., et al. (1982). Respiration during sleep in normal man. *Thorax*, **37**, 840–844.

Douglass, A.B., Bornstein, R., Nino-Murcia, G., et al. (1994). The Sleep Disorders Questionnaire. I: Creation and multivariate structure of SDQ. *Sleep*, **17**, 160–167.

Durán, C. (2001). Prevalence of obstructive sleep apnea-hypopnea and related clinical features in the elderly: a population-based study in the general population aged 71–100. In: World Conference. *Sleep Odyssey*, October 21–26, Montevideo, Uruguay.

Ekici, A., Ekici, M., Kurtipek, E., et al. (2005). Association of asthma-related symptoms with snoring and apnea and effect on health-related quality of life. *Chest*, **128**, 3358–3363.

Fenik, V.B., Davies, R.O. & Kubin, L. (2005). REM sleep-like atonia of hypoglossal (XII) motoneurons is caused by loss of noradrenergic and serotonergic inputs. *Am J Respir Crit Care Med*, **172**, 1322–1330.

Ferre, A., Guilleminault, C. & Lopes, M.C. (2006). Cyclic alternating pattern as a sign of brain instability during sleep. *Neurologia*, **21**, 304–311.

Fitzpatrick, M.F., Engleman, H., Whyte, K.F., et al. (1991). Morbidity in nocturnal asthma: sleep quality and daytime cognitive performance. *Thorax*, **46**, 569–573.

Fitzpatrick, M.F., Martin, K., Fossey, E., et al. (1993). Snoring, asthma and sleep disturbance in Britain: a community-based survey. *Eur Respir J*, **6**, 531–535.

Fleetham, J., West, P., Mezon, B., et al. (1982). Sleep, arousals, and oxygen desaturation in chronic obstructive pulmonary disease. The effect of oxygen therapy. *Am Rev Respir Dis*, **126**, 429–433.

Foster, T.S., Miller, J.D., Marton, J.P., et al. (2006). Assessment of the economic burden of COPD in the U.S.: a review and synthesis of the literature. *COPD*, **3**, 211–218.

Fuhlbrigge, A.L., Adams, R.J., Guilbert, T.W., et al. (2002). The burden of asthma in the United States: level and distribution are dependent on interpretation of the national asthma education and prevention program guidelines. *Am J Respir Crit Care Med*, **166**, 1044–1049.

Gay, P.C., Hubmayr, R.D. & Stroetz, R.W. (1996). Efficacy of nocturnal nasal ventilation in stable, severe chronic obstructive pulmonary disease during a 3-month controlled trial. *Mayo Clin Proc*, **71**, 533–542.

Godard, P., Chanez, P., Siraudin, L., et al. (2002). Costs of asthma are correlated with severity: a 1-yr prospective study. *Eur Respir J*, **19**, 61–67.

Golbin, J.M., Somers, V.K. & Caples, S.M. (2008). Obstructive sleep apnea, cardiovascular disease, and pulmonary hypertension. *Proc Am Thorac Soc*, **5**, 200–206.

GOLD (2008). Global Initiative for Chronic Obstructive Lung Disease (GOLD). *Global Strategy for the Diagnosis, Management, and Prevention of Chronic Obstructive Pulmonary Disease: Executive Summary Update.*

Gora, J., Kay, A., Colrain, I.M., et al. (1998). Load Available at: http://www.goldcopd.org (accessed August 11, 2009).compensation as a function of state during sleep onset. *J Appl Physiol*, **84**, 2123–2131.

Greenburg, D.L., Lettieri, C.J. & Eliasson, A.H. (2009). Effects of surgical weight loss on measures of obstructive sleep apnea: a meta-analysis. *Am J Med*, **122**, 535–542.

Guilleminault, C., Quera-Salva, M.A., Powell, N., et al. (1988). Nocturnal asthma: snoring, small pharynx and nasal CPAP. *Eur Respir J*, **1**, 902–907.

Halbert, R.J., Natoli, J.L., Gano, A., et al. (2006). Global burden of COPD: systematic review and meta-analysis. *Eur Respir J*, **28**, 523–532.

Han, F., Chen, E., Wei, H., et al. (2001). Treatment effects on carbon dioxide retention in patients with obstructive sleep apnea-hypopnea syndrome. *Chest*, **119**, 1814–1819.

Hasler, G., Buysse, D.J., Gamma, A., et al. (2005). Excessive daytime sleepiness in young adults: a 20-year prospective community study. *J Clin Psychiatry*, **66**, 521–529.

Henke, K.G., Badr, M.S., Skatrud, J.B., et al. (1992). Load compensation and respiratory muscle function during sleep. *J Appl Physiol*, **72**, 1221–1234.

Herpel, L.B., Brown, C.D., Goring, K.L., et al. (2007). COPD cannot compensate for upper airway obstruction during sleep. *Am J Respir Crit Care Med*, **175**, A71.

Hetzel, M.R., Clark, T.J. & Branthwaite, M.A. (1977). Asthma: analysis of sudden deaths and ventilatory arrests in hospital. *Br Med J*, **1**, 808–811.

Horner, R.L., Rivera, M.P., Kozar, L.F., et al. (2001). The ventilatory response to arousal from sleep is not fully explained by differences in CO(2) levels between sleep and wakefulness. *J Physiol*, **534**, 881–890.

Howard, M.E., Desai, A.V., Grunstein, R.R., et al. (2004). Sleepiness, sleep-disordered breathing, and accident risk factors in commercial vehicle drivers. *Am J Respir Crit Care Med*, **170**, 1014–1021.

Hudgel, D.W. & Devadatta, P. (1984). Decrease in functional residual capacity during sleep in normal humans. *J Appl Physiol*, **57**, 1319–1322.

Ip, M.S., Lam, B., Lauder, I.J., et al. (2001). A community study of sleep-disordered breathing in middle-aged Chinese men in Hong Kong. *Chest*, **119**, 62–69.

Janson, C., Gislason, T., Boman, G., et al. (1990). Sleep disturbances in patients with asthma. *Respir Med*, **84**, 37–42.

Janson, C., Gislason, T., De Backer, W., et al. (1995). Daytime sleepiness, snoring and gastro-oesophageal reflux amongst young adults in three European countries. *J Intern Med*, **237**, 277–285.

Janson, C., De Backer, W., Gislason, T., et al. (1996). Increased prevalence of sleep disturbances and daytime sleepiness in subjects with bronchial asthma: a population study of young adults in three European countries. *Eur Respir J*, **9**, 2132–2138.

Janssens, J.P., Metzger, M. & Sforza, E. (2009). Impact of volume targeting on efficacy of bi-level non-invasive ventilation and sleep in obesity-hypoventilation. *Respir Med*, **103**, 165–172.

Johnson, M.W. & Remmers, J.E. (1984). Accessory muscle activity during sleep in chronic obstructive pulmonary disease. *J Appl Physiol*, **57**, 1011–1017.

Jones, P.W. (1995). Issues concerning health-related quality of life in COPD. *Chest*, **107**, 187S–193S.

Jones, P.W., Quirk, F.H., Baveystock, C.M., et al. (1992). A self-complete measure of health status for chronic airflow limitation. The St. George's Respiratory Questionnaire. *Am Rev Respir Dis*, **145**, 1321–1327.

Judd, B.G., Liu, S. & Sateia, M.J. (2003). Cardiovascular abnormalities in sleep-disordered breathing. *Semin Respir Crit Care Med*, **24**, 315–322.

Julien, J.Y., Martin, J.G., Ernst, P., et al. (2009). Prevalence of obstructive sleep apnea-hypopnea in severe versus moderate asthma. *J Allergy Clin Immunol*, **124**, 371–376.

Kalra, M., Biagini, J., Bernstein, D., et al. (2006). Effect of asthma on the risk of obstructive sleep apnea syndrome in atopic women. *Ann Allergy Asthma Immunol*, **97**, 231–235.

Kapella, M.C., Larson, J.L., Patel, M.K., et al. (2006). Subjective fatigue, influencing variables, and consequences in chronic obstructive pulmonary disease. *Nurs Res*, **55**, 10–17.

Karachaliou, F., Kostikas, K., Pastaka, C., et al. (2007). Prevalence of sleep-related symptoms in a primary care population—their relation to asthma and COPD. *Prim Care Respir J*, **16**, 222–228.

Kessler, R., Chaouat, A., Schinkewitch, P., et al. (2001). The obesity-hypoventilation syndrome revisited: a prospective study of 34 consecutive cases. *Chest*, **120**, 369–376.

Kline, L.R., Hendricks, J.C., Davies, R.O., et al. (1986). Control of activity of the diaphragm in rapid-eye-movement sleep. *J Appl Physiol*, **61**, 1293–1300.

Klink, M. & Quan, S.F. (1987). Prevalence of reported sleep disturbances in a general adult population and their relationship to obstructive airways diseases. *Chest*, **91**, 540–546.

Knuiman, M., James, A., Divitini, M., et al. (2006). Longitudinal study of risk factors for habitual snoring in a general adult population: the Busselton Health Study. *Chest*, **130**, 1779–1783.

Krachman, S.L., Chatila, W., Martin, U.J., et al. (2005). Effects of lung volume reduction surgery on sleep quality and nocturnal gas exchange in patients with severe emphysema. *Chest*, **128**, 3221–3228.

Krieger, J. (2005). Respiratory physiology: breathing in normal subjects. In: Kryger, M.H., Roth, T. & Dement, W.C. *Principles and Practice of Sleep Medicine*. Fourth edition. Philadelphia, PA: WB Saunders.

Krishnan, V., McCormack, M.C., Mathai, S.C., et al. (2008). Sleep quality and health-related quality of life in idiopathic pulmonary fibrosis. *Chest*, **134**, 693–698.

Krouse, H.J., Yarandi, H., McIntosh, J., et al. (2008). Assessing sleep quality and daytime wakefulness in asthma using wrist actigraphy. *J Asthma*, **45**, 389–395.

Kryger, M.H., Wang-Weigand, S., Zhang, J., et al. (2008). Effect of ramelteon, a selective MT(1)/MT(2)-receptor agonist, on respiration during sleep in mild to moderate COPD. *Sleep Breath*, **12**, 243–250.

Kuniyoshi, F.H., Garcia-Touchard, A., Gami, A.S., et al. (2008). Day-night variation of acute myocardial infarction in obstructive sleep apnea. *J Am Coll Cardiol*, **52**, 343–346.

Kushida, C.A., Littner, M.R., Morgenthaler, T., et al. (2005). Practice parameters for the indications for polysomnography and related procedures: an update for 2005. *Sleep*, **28**, 499–521.

Laaban, J.P. & Chailleux, E. (2005). Daytime hypercapnia in adult patients with obstructive sleep apnea syndrome in France, before initiating nocturnal nasal continuous positive airway pressure therapy. *Chest*, **127**, 710–715.

Lafond, C., Series, F. & Lemiere, C. (2007). Impact of CPAP on asthmatic patients with obstructive sleep apnoea. *Eur Respir J*, **29**, 307–311.

Lavie, P., Herer, P. & Hoffstein, V. (2000). Obstructive sleep apnoea syndrome as a risk factor for hypertension: population study. *BMJ*, **320**, 479–482.

Lee, R.W., Chan, A.S., Grunstein, R.R., et al. (2009). Craniofacial phenotyping in obstructive sleep apnea—a novel quantitative photographic approach. *Sleep*, **32**, 37–45.

Lo Coco, D., Mattaliano, A., Lo Coco, A., et al. (2009). Increased frequency of restless legs syndrome in chronic obstructive pulmonary disease patients. *Sleep Med*, **10**, 572–576.

López-Acevedo, M.N., Torres-Palacios, A., Elena Ocasio-Tascón, M., et al. (2009). Overlap syndrome: an indication for sleep studies? A pilot study. *Sleep Breath*, **13**(4), 409–413.

Machado, M.C., Vollmer, W.M., Togeiro, S.M., et al. (2010). CPAP treatment and survival of patients with moderate-to-severe OSAS and hypoxemic COPD. *Eur Respir J*, **35**(1), 132–137.

Marin, J.M., Carrizo, S.J., Vicente, E., et al. (2005). Long-term cardiovascular outcomes in men with obstructive sleep apnoea-hypopnoea with or without treatment with continuous positive airway pressure: an observational study. *Lancet*, **365**, 1046–1053.

Marshall, N.S., Wong, K.K., Liu, P.Y., et al. (2008). Sleep apnea as an independent risk factor for all-cause mortality: the Busselton Health Study. *Sleep*, **31**, 1079–1085.

Mastronarde, J.G., Wise, R.A., Shade, D.M., et al. (2008). Sleep quality in asthma: results of a large prospective clinical trial. *J Asthma*, **45**, 183–189.

McGuire, M. & Bradford, A. (2001). Chronic intermittent hypercapnic hypoxia increases pulmonary arterial pressure and haematocrit in rats. *Eur Respir J*, **18**, 279–285.

McNicholas, W.T. (2009). COPD and obstructive sleep apnea: overlaps in pathophysiology, systemic inflammation and cardiovascular disease. *Am J Respir Crit Care Med*, **180**(8), 692–700.

Meecham Jones, D.J., Paul, E.A., Jones, P.W., et al. (1995). Nasal pressure support ventilation plus oxygen compared with oxygen therapy alone in hypercapnic COPD. *Am J Respir Crit Care Med*, **152**, 538–544.

Mermigkis, C., Kopanakis, A., Foldvary-Schaefer, N., et al. (2007). Health-related quality of life in patients with obstructive sleep apnoea and chronic obstructive pulmonary disease (overlap syndrome). *Int J Clin Pract*, **61**, 207–211.

Mermigkis, C., Stagaki, E., Amfilochiou, A., et al. (2009). Sleep quality and associated daytime consequences in patients with idiopathic pulmonary fibrosis. *Med Princ Pract*, **18**, 10–15.

Midgren, B., Hansson, L., Eriksson, L., et al. (1987). Oxygen desaturation during sleep and exercise in patients with interstitial lung disease. *Thorax*, **42**, 353–356.

Minai, O.A., Malik, N., Foldvary, N., et al. (2008). Prevalence and characteristics of restless legs syndrome in patients with pulmonary hypertension. *J Heart Lung Transplant*, **27**, 335–340.

Mokhlesi, B., Kryger, M.H. & Grunstein, R.R. (2008). Assessment and management of patients with obesity hypoventilation syndrome. *Proc Am Thorac Soc*, **5**, 218–225.

MRC (1981). Long term domiciliary oxygen therapy in chronic hypoxic cor pulmonale complicating chronic bronchitis and emphysema. Report of the Medical Research Council Working Party. *Lancet*, **1**, 681–686.

Mulgrew, A.T., Nasvadi, G., Butt, A., et al. (2008). Risk and severity of motor vehicle crashes in patients with obstructive sleep apnoea/hypopnoea. *Thorax*, **63**, 536–541.

Mulloy, E., Fitzpatrick, M., Bourke, S., et al. (1995). Oxygen desaturation during sleep and exercise in patients with severe chronic obstructive pulmonary disease. *Respir Med*, **89**, 193–198.

Netzer, N.C., Eliasson, A.H. & Strohl, K.P. (2003). Women with sleep apnea have lower levels of sex hormones. *Sleep Breath*, **7**, 25–29.

NOTT (1980). Continuous or nocturnal oxygen therapy in hypoxemic chronic obstructive lung disease: a clinical trial. Nocturnal Oxygen Therapy Trial Group. *Ann Intern Med*, **93**, 391–398.

Nowbar, S., Burkart, K.M., Gonzales, R., et al. (2004). Obesity-associated hypoventilation in hospitalized patients: prevalence, effects, and outcome. *Am J Med*, **116**, 1–7.

O'Connor, C., Thornley, K.S. & Hanly, P.J. (2000). Gender differences in the polysomnographic features of obstructive sleep apnea. *Am J Respir Crit Care Med*, **161**, 1465–1472.

Ogden, C.L., Carroll, M.D., Curtin, L.R., et al. (2006). Prevalence of overweight and obesity in the United States, 1999-2004. *JAMA*, **295**, 1549–1555.

Orem, J. (1980). Medullary respiratory neuron activity: relationship to tonic and phasic REM sleep. *J Appl Physiol*, **48**, 54–65.

Orem, J.M., Lovering, A.T. & Vidruk, E.H. (2005). Excitation of medullary respiratory neurons in REM sleep. *Sleep*, **28**, 801–807.

Patel, S.R. (2005). Shared genetic risk factors for obstructive sleep apnea and obesity. *J Appl Physiol*, **99**, 1600–1606.

Peker, Y., Carlson, J. & Hedner, J. (2006). Increased incidence of coronary artery disease in sleep apnoea: a long-term follow-up. *Eur Respir J*, **28**, 596–602.

Peker, Y., Glantz, H., Thunstrom, E., et al. (2009). Rationale and design of the Randomized Intervention with CPAP in Coronary Artery Disease and Sleep Apnoea—RICCADSA trial. *Scand Cardiovasc J*, 43, 24–31.

Perez-Padilla, R., West, P., Lertzman, M., et al. (1985). Breathing during sleep in patients with interstitial lung disease. *Am Rev Respir Dis*, 132, 224–229.

Phillips, B.A., Cooper, K.R. & Burke, T.V. (1987). The effect of sleep loss on breathing in chronic obstructive pulmonary disease. *Chest*, 91, 29–32.

Plywaczewski, R., Sliwinski, P., Nowinski, A., et al. (2000). Incidence of nocturnal desaturation while breathing oxygen in COPD patients undergoing long-term oxygen therapy. *Chest*, 117, 679–683.

Prado, G.F., Allen, R.P., Trevisani, V.M., et al. (2002). Sleep disruption in systemic sclerosis (scleroderma) patients: clinical and polysomnographic findings. *Sleep Med*, 3, 341–345.

Punjabi, N.M. (2008). The epidemiology of adult obstructive sleep apnea. *Proc Am Thorac Soc*, 5, 136–143.

Rasche, K., Orth, M., Kutscha, A., et al. (2007). Pulmonary diseases and heart function. *Internist (Berl)*, 48, 276–282.

Raschke, F. & Moller, K.H. (1989). The diurnal rhythm of chemosensitivity and its contribution to nocturnal disorders of respiratory control. *Pneumologie*, 43(Suppl 1), 568–571.

Redline, S., Tishler, P.V., Tosteson, T.D., et al. (1995). The familial aggregation of obstructive sleep apnea. *Am J Respir Crit Care Med*, 151, 682–687.

Redline, S., Schluchter, M.D., Larkin, E.K., et al. (2003). Predictors of longitudinal change in sleep-disordered breathing in a nonclinic population. *Sleep*, 26, 703–709.

Resta, O., Foschino-Barbaro, M.P., Bonfitto, P., et al. (2000). Prevalence and mechanisms of diurnal hypercapnia in a sample of morbidly obese subjects with obstructive sleep apnoea. *Respir Med*, 94, 240–246.

Resta, O., Foschino-Barbaro, M.P., Carpagnano, G.E., et al. (2003). Diurnal $PaCO_2$ tension in obese women: relationship with sleep disordered breathing. *Int J Obes Relat Metab Disord*, 27, 1453–1458.

Robertson, C.F., Rubinfeld, A.R. & Bowes, G. (1990). Deaths from asthma in Victoria: a 12-month survey. *Med J Aust*, 152, 511–517.

Roth, T. (2009). Hypnotic use for insomnia management in chronic obstructive pulmonary disease. *Sleep Med*, 10, 19–25.

Sahebjami, H. & Gartside, P.S. (1996). Pulmonary function in obese subjects with a normal FEV1/FVC ratio. *Chest*, 110, 1425–1429.

Sanders, M.H., Newman, A.B., Haggerty, C.L., et al. (2003). Sleep and sleep-disordered breathing in adults with predominantly mild obstructive airway disease. *Am J Respir Crit Care Med*, 167, 7–14.

Schwab, R.J., Pasirstein, M., Kaplan, L., et al. (2006). Family aggregation of upper airway soft tissue structures in normal subjects and patients with sleep apnea. *Am J Respir Crit Care Med*, 173, 453–463.

Shackell, B.S., Jones, R.C., Harding, G., et al. (2007). 'Am I going to see the next morning?' A qualitative study of patients' perspectives of sleep in COPD. *Prim Care Respir J*, 16, 378–383.

Shaya, F.T., Lin, P.J., Aljawadi, M.H., et al. (2009). Elevated economic burden in obstructive lung disease patients with concomitant sleep apnea syndrome. *Sleep Breath*, 13(4), 317–323.

Shigemitsu, H. & Afshar, K. (2007). Nocturnal asthma. *Curr Opin Pulm Med*, 13, 49–55.

Shinozaki, T., Tatsumi, K., Sakuma, T., et al. (1995). Daytime pulmonary hypertension in the obstructive sleep apnea syndrome. *Nihon Kyobu Shikkan Gakkai Zasshi*, 33, 1073–1079.

Skatrud, J.B. & Dempsey, J.A. (1983). Interaction of sleep state and chemical stimuli in sustaining rhythmic ventilation. *J Appl Physiol*, 55, 813–822.

Somers, V.K., White, D.P., Amin, R., et al. (2008). Sleep apnea and cardiovascular disease: an American Heart Association/American College of Cardiology Foundation Scientific Statement from the American Heart Association Council for High Blood Pressure Research Professional Education Committee, Council on Clinical Cardiology, Stroke Council, and Council On Cardiovascular Nursing.

In collaboration with the National Heart, Lung, and Blood Institute National Center on Sleep Disorders Research (National Institutes of Health). *Circulation*, **118**, 1080–1111.

Sorajja, D., Gami, A.S., Somers, V.K., et al. (2008). Independent association between obstructive sleep apneaapnoea and subclinical coronary artery disease. *Chest*, **133**, 927–933.

Stanchina, M.L., Malhotra, A., Fogel, R.B., et al. (2003). The influence of lung volume on pharyngeal mechanics, collapsibility, and genioglossus muscle activation during sleep. *Sleep*, **26**, 851–856.

Sutherland, E.R. (2005). Nocturnal asthma. *J Allergy Clin Immunol*, **116**, 1179–1186; quiz 1187.

Swigris, J.J., Kuschner, W.G., Jacobs, S.S., et al. (2005). Health-related quality of life in patients with idiopathic pulmonary fibrosis: a systematic review. *Thorax*, **60**, 588–594.

Tabachnik, E., Muller, N.L., Bryan, A.C., et al. (1981). Changes in ventilation and chest wall mechanics during sleep in normal adolescents. *J Appl Physiol*, **51**, 557–564.

ten Brinke, A., Sterk, P.J., Masclee, A.A., et al. (2005). Risk factors of frequent exacerbations in difficult-to-treat asthma. *Eur Respir J*, **26**, 812–818.

Teodorescu, M., Consens, F.B., Bria, W.F., et al. (2006). Correlates of daytime sleepiness in patients with asthma. *Sleep Med*, **7**, 607–613.

Teodorescu, M., Consens, F.B., Bria, W.F., et al. (2009). Predictors of habitual snoring and obstructive sleep apnea risk in patients with asthma. *Chest*, **135**, 1125–1132.

Turner-Warwick, M. (1988). Epidemiology of nocturnal asthma. *Am J Med*, **85**, 6–8.

Van Keimpema, A.R., Ariaansz, M., Tamminga, J.J., et al. (1997). Nocturnal waking and morning dip of peak expiratory flow in clinically stable asthma patients during treatment. Occurrence and patient characteristics. *Respiration*, **64**, 29–34.

van Manen, J.G., Bindels, P.J., Dekker, F.W., et al. (2003). The influence of COPD on health-related quality of life independent of the influence of comorbidity. *J Clin Epidemiol*, **56**, 1177–1184.

Vgontzas, A.N., Papanicolaou, D.A., Bixler, E.O., et al. (1997). Elevation of plasma cytokines in disorders of excessive daytime sleepiness: role of sleep disturbance and obesity. *J Clin Endocrinol Metab*, **82**, 1313–1316.

Vir, R., Bhagat, R. & Shah, A. (1997). Sleep disturbances in clinically stable young asthmatic adults. *Ann Allergy Asthma Immunol*, **79**, 251–255.

von Kanel, R., Le, D.T., Nelesen, R.A., et al. (2001). The hypercoagulable state in sleep apnea is related to comorbid hypertension. *J Hypertens*, **19**, 1445–1451.

Ware, J.E., Snow, K.K., Kosinski, M., **et al.** (1993). *SF-36 Health Survey: Manual and Interpretation Guide*. Second edition. Boston, MA: The Health Institute, New England Medical Center.

Weersink, E.J., van Zomeren, E.H., Koeter, G.H., et al. (1997). Treatment of nocturnal airway obstruction improves daytime cognitive performance in asthmatics. *Am J Respir Crit Care Med*, **156**, 1144–1150.

Weiss, K.B. & Sullivan, S.D. (2001). The health economics of asthma and rhinitis. I. Assessing the economic impact. *J Allergy Clin Immunol*, **107**, 3–8.

Weitzenblum, E., Chaouat, A., Kessler, R., et al. (2008). Overlap syndrome: obstructive sleep apnea in patients with chronic obstructive pulmonary disease. *Proc Am Thorac Soc*, **5**, 237–241.

WHO (2000). World Health Organization: *World Health Report*. Geneva. Available at: http://www.who.int/whr/2000/en/statistics.htm (accessed August 20, 2009).

Wiegand, D.A., Latz, B., Zwillich, C.W., et al. (1990). Upper airway resistance and geniohyoid muscle activity in normal men during wakefulness and sleep. *J Appl Physiol*, **69**, 1252–1261.

Worsnop, C., Kay, A., Pierce, R., et al. (1998). Activity of respiratory pump and upper airway muscles during sleep onset. *J Appl Physiol*, **85**, 908–920.

Xie, A., Wong, B., Phillipson, E.A., et al. (1994). Interaction of hyperventilation and arousal in the pathogenesis of idiopathic central sleep apnea. *Am J Respir Crit Care Med*, **150**, 489–495.

Xie, A., Rutherford, R., Rankin, F., et al. (1995). Hypocapnia and increased ventilatory responsiveness in patients with idiopathic central sleep apnea. *Am J Respir Crit Care Med*, **152**, 1950–1955.

Xie, A., Skatrud, J.B., Barczi, S.R., et al. (2009). Influence of cerebral blood flow on breathing stability. *J Appl Physiol*, **106**, 850–856.

Yigla, M., Tov, N., Solomonov, A., et al. (2003). Difficult-to-control asthma and obstructive sleep apneaapnoea. *J Asthma*, **40**, 865–871.

Yinon, D., Lowenstein, L., Suraya, S., et al. (2006). Pre-eclampsia is associated with sleep-disordered breathing and endothelial dysfunction. *Eur Respir J*, **27**, 328–333.

Young, T., Palta, M., Dempsey, J., et al. (1993). The occurrence of sleep-disordered breathing among middle-aged adults. *N Engl J Med*, **328**, 1230–1235.

Young, T., Hutton, R., Finn, L., et al. (1996). The gender bias in sleep apnea diagnosis. Are women missed because they have different symptoms? *Arch Intern Med*, **156**, 2445–2451.

Young, T., Evans, L., Finn, L., et al. (1997). Estimation of the clinically diagnosed proportion of sleep apnea syndrome in middle-aged men and women. *Sleep*, **20**, 705–706.

Young, T., Finn, L., Peppard, P.E., et al. (2008). Sleep disordered breathing and mortality: eighteen-year follow-up of the Wisconsin sleep cohort. *Sleep*, **31**, 1071–1078.

Yuan, X., Hawver, L.R., Ojo, P., et al. (2009). Bariatric surgery in Medicare patients: greater risks but substantial benefits. *Surg Obes Relat Dis*, **5**(3), 299–304.

Zielinski, J. (2005). Effects of intermittent hypoxia on pulmonary haemodynamics: animal models versus studies in humans. *Eur Respir J*, **25**, 173–180.

Chapter 8

The epidemiology of sleep and depression

S. Weich

The relationship between sleep and depression: why does it matter?

Psychiatric disorders, and depression in particular, are the most prevalent of all health conditions associated with disturbances of sleep. Perhaps because of the near ubiquity of sleep problems among those with depression, this association has been extensively researched over the past two decades. Despite this effort, disagreement persists about whether these are independent, co-morbid conditions which might predispose, precipitate, or modify the course of one another, or whether they are in fact manifestations of a common underlying pathophysiology (Staner, 2009).

Depression is a major cause of disability worldwide and is associated with physical and social morbidity, increased mortality, and vast economic cost. From a public health perspective, it is imperative that associations between these conditions are fully elucidated. There would be major public health and clinical implications—and significant potential for preventive gain—were sleep disorders proven to be modifiable risk factor in the onset, course, or outcome of depression (Franzen and Buysse, 2008).

Depressive symptoms and depressive disorder

The term 'depression' describes both symptoms and disorder. The latter is best viewed as a clinical syndrome (or perhaps syndromes) comprising several distinct symptoms, all of which (like the disorder itself) are continuously distributed. The main feature of all depressive conditions is a lowered mood which, when more severe, may be accompanied by fatigue and a lack of interest or pleasure in usual activities. Thinking becomes persistently negative and the depressed individual may feel worthless, guilty about past actions, worried about themselves, their family, their health, job or finances, pessimistic about the future, and suicidal. Other common symptoms of depression include anxiety, fatigue and lack of energy, sleep disturbance (typically insomnia, but less commonly hypersomnia), impaired concentration and memory, irritability and impaired personal relationships—often manifest as social withdrawal and avoidance of interactions with others.

Diagnostic criteria for depression are codified in ICD-10 (International Classification of Diseases, version 10) (World Health Organization, 1993) and DSM-IV (Diagnostic and Statistical Manual of Mental Disorders, fourth edition) (DSM-IV, 2000), where depression is sub-classified into (unipolar) depressive disorder and bipolar disorder. According to ICD-10, depressive episodes are either mild, moderate, or severe (according to the number and intensity of symptoms experienced); diagnosis of even a mild depressive episode requires that an individual must have experienced at least two of low mood, fatigue (feeling tired or having little energy), or anhedonia (lack of interest or enjoyment in things) for most of the day, nearly every day for a minimum of 2 weeks. In addition, two other symptoms (from a list of 10) must be present at the same time, of which three are *early morning waking*, *hypersomnia*, and *fatigue*. Remission from a depressive episode is said to occur when the criteria for a depressive episode are not met for 8 continuous weeks, and depression is said to be chronic when no remission occurs for 2 years. Those who experience significant sub-clinical depressive symptoms (without meeting diagnostic criteria for a depressive episode) are classified as suffering from dysthymia. Within DSM-IV, major depressive disorder is said to occur when five or more core symptoms are present for nearly every day for 2 weeks or longer, of which two of which are *'insomnia or hypersomnia'* and *'fatigue or loss of energy'*. Bipolar depression is diagnosed where an individual has had at least one prior episode of mania or hypomania. The latter conditions are characterized by elevated mood and/or elation, excessive energy, overactivity, disinhibition (including overspending and sexual promiscuity), and grandiosity. Sleep is often disturbed in mania, with those affected typically reporting little need for sleep (Gruber et al., 2009).

Depression (when all episode severities are combined) has a community prevalence of 10% (Singleton et al., 2001), and is associated with increased rates of mortality, physical morbidity, and social impairment (Spitzer et al., 1995; Cassano and Fava, 2002). By 2020, depression is expected to become the second highest cause of disease burden worldwide (Murray and Lopez, 1997). The annual cost of depression in England alone was estimated at £9 billion in 2000, of which 90% was attributable to an estimated 110 million lost working days (Thomas and Morris, 2003). Depression is strongly associated with socioeconomic status, particularly when this is measured according to employment status, income, education, and standard of living as opposed to occupational social class (Lorant et al., 2003). Unmet need for treatment (Singleton et al., 2001; Bebbington et al., 2000) is even more apparent when considering only cases of severe disorder (Demyttenaere et al., 2004; Wang et al., 2005). Depression is commonly co-morbid with other psychiatric disorders—most notably anxiety and personality disorders, and drug and alcohol misuse. This is particularly so in community and primary care settings (where the overwhelming majority of pathology occurs and is treated), with the term 'cothymia' being coined to describe this phenomenon (Shorter and Tyrer, 2003; Kessler et al., 2005).

Sleep problems and depression: the evidence

Studying the relationship between sleep problems and depression is particularly challenging given that the former are included in the diagnostic criteria for the latter. Sleep disturbance not only counts as a symptom of depression (and therefore contributes to the rating of depression severity), but it may also contribute to the diagnosis in indirect ways, for example by increasing tiredness, impairing daytime concentration, and adding to frustration and irritability. Time spent awake is often occupied in anxious or guilty rumination. This tautology may explain why it has proven so difficult to elucidate a clear chronology in the association between sleep and depression. Given the absence of a pathophysiological definition of depression and the magnitude of observed associations between depression and insomnia, many—with good reason—believe that these share a common underlying (or at least overlapping) pathology (Riemann et al., 2001; Staner, 2009; Mendlewicz, 2009).

Sleep disturbances are extremely common in depression (Benca and Peterson, 2008). Those with depression characteristically report difficulty initiating sleep, nocturnal awakening and early morning waking (waking more than an hour earlier than intended without being able to return to sleep), non-restorative sleep, and daytime fatigue. A minority of people with depression report hypersomnia, or problems waking. Both are often associated with fatigue, anergia, and daytime drowsiness.

Those with hypersomnia describe staying in bed for prolonged periods and/or daytime napping. Estimates from unselected populations report that around three-quarters of those with depression also report insomnia, defined as difficulty in getting to sleep or remaining asleep and/or failing to experience sleep as restorative (Liu et al., 2007; Ohayon et al., 2000). The prevalence of self-reported sleep problems is even higher in clinical settings, where these may be linked to help-seeking; one review found that 90% of those receiving care for depression complained of poor sleep quality (Tsuno et al., 2005).

In contrast to an extensive literature on insomnia and depression, there are relatively few studies of hypersomnia. Hypersomnia is much rarer than insomnia among those who are depressed (Liu et al., 2007), and is reported by around one-quarter of those affected. An early report, based on a cohort study of nearly 8,000 US community residents, confirmed that hypersomnia (defined as self-report of 'sleeping too much' for 2 weeks or longer) was less common than insomnia but was associated with psychiatric disorders to a degree that was similar to or in excess of that found for insomnia (Ford and Kamerow, 1989) (64% vs. 58% of those with hypersomnia and insomnia, respectively, met diagnostic criteria for at least one psychiatric disorder). This study found associations of similar magnitude between major depression and both hypersomnia and insomnia, cross-sectionally and over 12 months. This was also the case in the US Nurses Health Study II of 60,000 women aged 25–46 years, cross-sectional associations were reported between longer sleeping (>8 hours per day) and current depressive symptoms (odds ratio [OR] 2.9; 95% confidence interval [CI]: 2.6–3.2). By contrast, a study of 17,000 university students aged 17–30 years in 24 countries found no evidence that those who slept for >8 hours a day were at increased risk of depression (Steptoe et al., 2006) (see also Chapter 5).

Cross-sectional studies over two decades or more have found that those who report insomnia are also very likely to be depressed and *vice versa* (Staner, 2009; Mellinger et al., 1985; Ford and Kamerow, 1989; Kuppermann et al., 1995; Jansson-Fröjmark and Lindblom, 2008). A cross-sectional survey of nearly 800 US community-dwelling participants aged 20–90 years (stratified by age) found that people with self-reported insomnia (defined as being of at least 6 months' duration and characterized by significant trouble initiating or remaining asleep) were 9.8 and 17.8 times more likely than those without insomnia to have clinically significant depression and anxiety, respectively. The number and severity of sleep problems were associated with greater severity of depression and anxiety (Taylor et al., 2005). When lifetime histories of depression were considered in a sample of 21–30 years old in Michigan, the OR for major depression (ever) was 16.6 (95% CI: 9.4–29.4) among those with a lifetime history of insomnia (Breslau et al., 1996).

A recent study of nearly 16,000 adolescents found an association (with dose-response effect) between bedtime (highly correlated with sleeping time) and both depressive symptoms and suicidal thoughts (Gangwisch et al., 2010). Those with parental set bedtimes of midnight or later were at higher risk of reporting clinically significant depressive symptoms (on self-report questionnaire) (OR: 1.24; 95% CI: 1.04–1.49) and suicidal thoughts (OR: 1.20; 95% CI: 1.01–1.41, also adjusted for depression score) than those whose parents stipulated a bedtime of 10:00 p.m. or earlier after adjusting for age, sex, and socioeconomic status and perceptions of how much their parents cared about them. Neither association was statistically significant after further adjusting for participants' perceptions of whether or not they were getting enough sleep. In both sets of analyses, U-shaped associations were found with participants' reports of sleep duration.

A study of 553 children in Hungary with major depression aged 7–14 years found that almost three-quarters (72.7%) experienced clinically significant difficulty sleeping, of whom the majority (almost 90%) reported insomnia (Liu et al., 2007). In the United States, the OR for depression among adolescents aged 12–18 years (using a single question regarding the frequency of depressive feelings in the past week) was 3.18 (95% CI: 2.45–4.14) among those with insomnia (significant difficulty falling asleep or staying asleep on most nights over the past year), after adjusting for gender and previous history of depression (Roane and Taylor, 2006).

In Sweden, symptoms of depression were highly correlated with self-reported insomnia over the preceding 3 months ($P < 0.01$) among 1,188 randomly selected community residents aged 20–60 years. No estimate was reported of the OR of relative risk of depression among those with insomnia (Jansson-Fröjmark and Lindblom, 2008).

Longitudinal research

Despite (or perhaps because of) the ubiquity of co-morbidity between insomnia and depression, several longitudinal studies have looked for temporal associations between sleep problems and the later occurrence (incidence or recurrence) of depressive episodes.

Nearly, but not quite all (Neckelmann et al., 2007) of these studies reported statistically significant positive results. One of the earliest and most methodologically robust studies was a 44-year follow-up of 1,271 male Johns Hopkins medical students (Chang et al., 1997) who graduated between 1948 and 1964. Using annual surveys and survival analyses, those who reported insomnia at baseline, that is, while still at medical school (using a standardized self-report questionnaire), had a relative risk (RR) of 2.0 (95% CI: 1.2–2.7) of developing a depressive episode (ascertained using a variety of self-report indicators). Cumulative incidence data indicated that the difference in risk between groups with and without insomnia at medical school first appeared after about 15 years' follow-up, and increased sharply thereafter. This association was unaffected by adjusting for age, parental history of depression, measures of temperament, and coffee drinking. The results were also unchanged by excluding eight participants who subsequently committed suicide.

A Swedish cohort study of 1,870 community residents aged 45–65 years in 1983 measured associations between questionnaire responses about sleep and mental health over an interval of 12 years (with a follow-up rate of 78%). Insomnia at baseline predicted depression at follow-up in women only (OR: 4.1; 95% CI: 2.1–7.2) (Mallon et al., 2000). In a more recent Swedish cohort study, at 1-year follow-up the OR for depression (ascertained by self-report questionnaire) was 3.51 (95% CI: 2.11–5.83) among those reporting insomnia (by questionnaire) in 3 months prior to baseline (Jansson-Fröjmark and Lindblom, 2008). This paper also reported a similar association between depression at baseline and insomnia at follow-up (OR: 2.28; 95% CI: 1.41–3.68). In a study of 979 21–30 years old Health Maintenance Organization [HMO] patients in Michigan, those who reported insomnia nearly every night for 2 weeks or more were more likely to be depressed (both ascertained using a standardized clinical interview) 3.5 years later (OR: 2.1; 95% CI: 1.1–4.0), after adjusting for depressive symptoms at baseline (Breslau et al., 1996).

A 20-year, 6-wave follow-up study of young adults (aged 19 and 20 years) in Switzerland examined the directionality of insomnia and depression, using standardized clinical assessments and DSM-equivalent diagnoses of both conditions (Buysse et al., 2008). Despite variable intervals ranging from 2 to 6 years, clear associations were found between insomnia of at least 2 weeks' duration and depression at the next (OR: 1.9; 95% CI: 1.3–2.6) or any subsequent (OR: 1.6, 95% CI: 1.1–2.1) interview. A similar association was reported between major depression and insomnia (for 2 weeks or more) at any (OR 1.5: 95% CI: 1.1–2.1), but not the next interview to a statistically significant degree. Further exploration of the dataset revealed that mixed depression-with-insomnia accounted for most cases of either insomnia or depression that were found to be associated with either insomnia or depression, respectively, between waves. Roane and Taylor (2006) followed up 4,494 US adolescents aged 12–18 years from 1994 to 2002. Insomnia was defined as trouble falling asleep or staying asleep almost or nearly every day in the preceding 12 months. Depressive symptoms were ascertained using a single question about how often participants felt depressed in the week prior to interview. Those who reported insomnia at baseline were at significantly increased risk of having depressive symptoms at follow-up (OR: 2.20; 95% CI: 1.34–3.58).

Using in-depth clinical interviews to ascertain DSM-IV sleep and mood disorders, Johnson and his colleagues (2006) sought to date the onset of each very precisely in a sample of 1,014 adolescents who were each interviewed with a parent. Insomnia was defined using a strict duration criteria of problems lasting for 1 month or longer. Lifetime histories of anxiety and depression were elicited *excluding symptoms of insomnia*. Unlike depression, prior insomnia was not associated with the onset of anxiety disorders to a statistically significant degree. Anxiety was likely to precede the onset of insomnia (as was the case in 73% of anxiety disorders), while for depression the temporal sequence was reversed (insomnia was reported to have preceded depression in 69% of those with a lifetime history of depression).

A small number of studies have extended this research into adolescence and childhood. Notwithstanding methodological difficulties of studying mental health problems in very young children—which are manifested in different ways from adults—these studies all confirm both cross-sectional and longitudinal associations between sleep problems (chiefly insomnia) and emotional and behavioural difficulties (Chorney et al., 2008; Coulombe et al., 2009; Reid et al., 2009; Sivertsen et al., 2009). Among the most notable is a genetically informed, prospective cohort study of 250 twin pairs aged 8 years at baseline, who were followed-up 2 years later (Gregory et al., 2009). Data were gathered at ages 8 and 10 about sleep problems (using a 33-item parental questionnaire covering 8 aspects of sleeping) and depression (assessed using a 27-item self-report questionnaire completed by children). Point estimates for the cross-sectional correlations between sleep problem and depression scores were identical (and statistically significant) at both ages ($r = 0.20$). Correlations for both sleep scores and depression scores, respectively, across waves were greater for monozygotic (MZ) than dizygotic (DZ) twins. Further analysis estimated that 66% and 63% of the variability in sleep scores were explained by genetic factors at ages 8 and 10, respectively. Cross-lagged analyses found a small but statistically significant association between sleep problems at age 8 and higher depression scores at age 10 (partial regression coefficient = 0.10; 95% CI: 0.01–0.18), but *not* between depression at 8 and sleep problems at 10 (partial regression coefficient = 0.03; 95% CI: –0.03–0.10). Attempts to decompose the association between sleep problems at age 8 and depression scores at 10 were non-significant and inconclusive.

There is no evidence from epidemiological studies that the association between insomnia and depression varies with age (Franzen and Buysse, 2008). At the other end of the lifespan, a meta-analysis of five prospective studies among older adults (aged 50 and older) found a summary OR of 2.6 (95% CI: 1.9–3.7) in the association between sleep disturbance and depression (Cole and Dendukuri, 2003). Little information was presented in this review about methodological variation in the ascertainment of sleep problems or depression in primary studies, or in the duration of follow-up. In a study not included in the review by Cole and Dendukuri, Cho et al. (2008) followed 351 community-dwelling older adults aged 60 years and over for 2 years. After adjusting for prior depression, the OR for developing an onset of depression was 3.05 (95% CI: 1.07–8.75) among those reporting sleep disturbance (using the Pittsburgh Sleep Quality Index, PSQI). It was noted that this association was most evident in the 40% of participants with prior depression, and further analysis indicated that nearly all recurrences of depression in this group were preceded by sleep difficulties (Cox hazard ratio for recurrence among those with sleep problems 4.84; 95% CI: 1.4–16.7). This association was independent of medical disorders and antidepressant use.

It is worth noting the findings from the sole study that failed to find a highly significant prospective association between insomnia and depression (Neckelmann et al., 2007), particularly since this was the largest sample of any of the studies included in this review. Despite reporting significant cross-sectional associations between insomnia and anxiety and depression, a cohort study of over 25,000 community residents in Norway found an association between self-reported insomnia and anxiety—but not depression—after 11 years. The authors concluded that depression was therefore 'a state-like marker' for depression.

Demonstrating that sleep problems increasing vulnerability to other risk factors for depression would be compelling evidence of a causal link. An Australian sample of 1,033 seriously injured trauma survivors (excluding those with significant brain injury) aged 16–70 years underwent psychiatric assessment and completed a 5-item self-report sleep measure enquiring about problems in the 2 weeks before injury. At follow–up 3 months after the injury, statistically significant associations were found between sleep problems at baseline and the occurrence of a range of psychiatric disorders. On restricting analyses to participants without evidence of lifetime psychiatric disorder at baseline, and adjusting for age, gender, type of injury, and injury severity, the OR for depression at follow-up among those with sleep problems in the 2 weeks prior to injury was 3.98 (95% CI: 1.87–6.25), compared to those without sleep problems at the time (Bryant et al., 2010).

Depression treatment studies

Pharmacological studies have reported that insomnia is a common residual symptom following successful treatment for depression. There appears to be no difference in the rate of insomnia following treatment-induced remission between psychological and pharmacological treatments. One recent study found that about one in five of those who experienced remission following treatment continued to have difficulty sleeping (Carney et al., 2007).

Pigeon et al. (2008) examined the relationship between insomnia (ascertained using three self-report questions) and response to treatment in a US multi-centre randomized controlled trial of a multi-domain 'enhanced' depression treatment intervention versus usual care in a sample of 1,800 older adults (aged 60 years and over) with major depression or dysthymia. Participants with persistent insomnia during the first 3 months of treatment had significantly worse depression treatment outcomes at 6 months post-baseline (OR for unremitted depression compared with the no insomnia group 2.8; 95% CI: 1.7–4.8), though not at 12-month follow-up (OR: 1.13; 95% CI: 0.6–2.0).

Manber et al. (2008) addressed the question of whether treating co-morbid insomnia in addition to depression improved outcomes. A randomized controlled pilot trial ($n = 30$) found that participants allocated to antidepressant (escitalopram) plus seven sessions of cognitive behaviour therapy for insomnia (CBTi), which focused only on sleep, had better depression and insomnia outcomes than those receiving escitalopram plus an attentional control intervention (psychoeducation about insomnia). Remission of depression (61.5% vs. 33.3%) ($P = 0.13$) and remission of insomnia (50.0% vs. 7.7%) ($P = 0.05$) were both increased in the antidepressant plus CBTi group. Across both groups, participants whose insomnia remitted were more likely to experience remission of depression (83% vs. 39%) ($P = 0.08$) than those with unremitted insomnia.

Summary of the epidemiological evidence

This brief review of the epidemiology of depression and insomnia reveals consistent evidence that they are closely associated both cross-sectionally and longitudinally. Notwithstanding heterogeneity in methods—measures of depression and sleep, duration of follow-up, age of participants, and settings—the findings across studies appear remarkably consistent. In cross-sectional surveys, insomnia is reported by about three-quarters of those with clinically significant depression in population surveys, rising to around 90% in clinical samples. ORs for depression among those reporting significant difficulty in falling asleep or remaining asleep ranged from 3.2 among adolescents, after adjusting for prior depressive symptoms, to 9.8 in an age-stratified community sample of people aged 20–90 years old. When lifetime histories of depression or insomnia 'ever' were analyzed, an OR of almost 17 was reported in a community sample of those aged 21–30 years.

Longitudinal studies (of which there have been many) are also consistent in their findings. Only one study—albeit a very large one (Neckelmann et al., 2007)—failed to find a highly significant and positive prospective association between insomnia and subsequent depression. These studies varied in the ages of participants (from adolescence to old age) and in the duration of follow-up (from 1 to 12 years). With one or two notable exceptions (Buysse et al., 2008), most employed questionnaire-based self-report measures of both insomnia and depression. These studies typically reported that those with insomnia at baseline were between two and five times more likely than those without insomnia to report depression at follow-up. It is notable that that the study with the most rigorous ascertainment of insomnia and depression (Buysse et al., 2008) reported one of the lowest effect sizes (though still statistically significant) for the association in question. Smaller effect sizes were also observed in studies with the longest follow-up intervals. There was no evidence in the studies reviewed above that the association between insomnia and depression varied with age.

Fewer studies have assessed the reverse association (depression leading to insomnia) prospectively; those that have done have reported mixed results (Jansson-Fröjmark and Lindblom, 2008; Gregory et al., 2009). One study that used detailed clinical interviews to ascertain the timing of lifetime episodes of insomnia and psychiatric disorder in adolescents reported that insomnia was twice as likely to begin before depression as the other way around.

A number of recent studies using different designs support the view that insomnia is a risk factor for depression, including evidence that this modifies the psychological impact of trauma (Bryant et al., 2010). There is growing evidence that insomnia may persist even after other depressive symptoms have remitted (Carney et al., 2007), which may have consequences for relapse and even response to future treatment. At least one prospective study found that insomnia may be a particularly potent risk factor for relapse among those with a previous history of depression (Cho et al., 2008). Another recent study reported, intriguingly, that insomnia assessed at the start of treatment predicted a worse response to treatment for depression (Pigeon et al., 2008).

Neurobiological studies

One major limitation of the epidemiological research which has sought to understand and explicate the relationship between depression and sleep disturbance has been the dearth of validated phenotypes (Ford and Cooper-Patrick, 2001). Most studies to date have classified insomnia on the basis of survey responses to a small number of questions about problems initiating or maintaining sleep. These are unlikely to accurately capture changes in underlying physiological processes. Although a full consideration of the neurobiology of sleep and depression are beyond the scope of this chapter, several studies of direct relevance to understanding their association will be considered.

By contrast, neurobiological studies have highlighted the different physiological (and pathological) processes which characterize sleep disturbance in depression. Sleep electroencephalography (EEG) has shown consistently that people with depression have increased sleep latency (they take longer to fall asleep), reduced sleep time, increased sleep fragmentation (more awakenings), shorter rapid eye movement (REM) latency, greater REM density in the earlier sleep phases, and less slow wave sleep (Benca and Peterson, 2008; Benca et al., 1992). These changes appear to be associated with the severity of depression, with those who are most depressed experiencing the greatest deviation from normal sleep architecture. This corresponds to epidemiological evidence of a correlation between sleep disturbance and depression severity (Liu et al., 2007).

Neurobiological research has also revealed associations between depression and localized persistence in metabolic activity in regions of the fronto-parietal cortex and thalamus on moving from wakefulness to non-rapid eye movement (NREM) (Germain et al., 2004; Nofzinger et al., 2005). These correspond to the common lament among many patients with depression who 'can't switch off' their thoughts when trying to sleep at night. Reduced serotonergic transmission, increased pontine cholinergic activity, and/or an excess of noradrenaline and corticotropin-releasing hormone (CRH) have all been suggested as possible neuroendocrine mechanisms to explain these phenomena (Thase, 1998).

A small study compared 48 adolescents at high risk of depression (by virtue of a parental history of depression) with a similar number of community controls (Rao et al., 2009). Sleep EEGs and measures of hypothalamo-pituitary axis (HPA) function were undertaken at baseline and participants followed up at six monthly intervals for 5 years. Statistically significant differences were found at baseline (in the expected direction) in the amount of REM sleep and REM latency, and in nocturnal urinary free cortisol after adjusting for differences in (sub-clinical) depressive symptoms. All three variables were associated with the subsequent onset of depression and, taken together, predicted this outcome with 57% specificity and 99% sensitivity. These results support the view that physiological differences in sleep architecture and HPA activation predate the onset of major depression and may mediate the risk of developing this disorder, at least in adolescents with a family history of depression.

Another piece of this puzzle comes in the form of a study of genetic linkages (Utge et al., 2009) (see also Chapter 12). In keeping with recent neurobiological studies, investigators in Finland examined DNA from 1,654 adult participants in a population-based survey. This study tested the hypothesis that different phenotypes would also be genotypically distinct, and found some evidence to support this view when comparing individuals with depression only, depression with fatigue, and depression with early morning waking. This was the first candidate gene study of its type, and these results require replication.

Conclusion

There is abundant evidence that both sleep problems and depression are highly prevalent, distressing, disabling, and costly problems that impact significantly on the public health.

Tautology or true co-morbidity?

It has proven remarkably difficult to establish causality in the relationship between insomnia and depression (Taylor, 2008), and opinion continues to be divided about the degree of commonality between these conditions. The answer of course is that both camps are right, with caveats.

There are strong arguments for viewing insomnia as integral to depression, particularly when the latter is constructed as a categorical, syndromal phenotype based on descriptive phenomenology, as enshrined within DSM-IV and ICD-10. In short, the notion that these are truly independent conditions lacks face validity when the direct (difficulty falling asleep and remaining asleep, non-restorative sleep) and indirect (fatigue, impaired concentration) manifestations of insomnia are also diagnostic criteria for depression. And although it has been argued that insomnia as classified within DSM-IV excludes disturbances of sleep due to depression (Staner, 2009), this distinction is rarely—if ever—imposed in population-based studies, which rely most often on self-report of difficulties in falling asleep or remaining asleep, and checklists of depressive symptoms.

Cross-sectional studies have shown consistently that insomnia and depression are highly correlated when these are assessed using self-report checklists of symptoms, and they co-occur more often than either occurs on its own. And they also co-occur far more often than predicted by chance if they were in fact independent conditions. Taken together, these findings confirm the near-ubiquity of insomnia among those who are depressed, an aspect of depression that is well recognized by those who have ever suffered from this condition. And neurobiological evidence also suggests that the same processes are involved in the regulation—and dysregulation—of both mood and sleep (Thase, 2006; Mendlewicz, 2009).

On the other hand, epidemiological evidence from several prospective, longitudinal studies indicates that insomnia frequently (but not always) precedes the onset of depression, in all settings and across all age groups. Insomnia also appears to modify the effects of other risk factors and treatments for depression. And insomnia often persists when other depressive symptoms have remitted. Finally, recent studies have shown that the association between (self-reported) sleep duration and the number of (other) depressive symptoms is U-shaped (see also Chapters 4 and 5).

So should this be taken as definitive evidence of independence and 'bi-directionalilty' in the association between insomnia (and/or hypersomnia) and depression (Jansson-Fröjmark and Lindblom, 2008; Mendlewicz, 2009; Taylor, 2008)? Perhaps not. The evidence reviewed in this chapter should be seen as necessary but not sufficient for true independence of sleep problems and depression. The studies considered here highlight the limitations of traditional epidemiological approaches as applied to this question, and gaps in our knowledge. It could be argued that existing evidence is equally consistent with the view that sleep disturbances are 'merely' the most prominent prodromal symptoms of depression, and equally robust indicators of residual symptoms during the recovery phase. It is also possible that insomnia and/or hypersomnia are indicative of the (greater) severity of depressive episodes. This would in turn explain why those with insomnia are more susceptible to the depressogenic effects of traumatic life events, as well as being prone to the relapse of depressive episodes. The possibility also remains that associations identified between insomnia and depression might be confounded by other, co-morbid psychiatric disorders (especially anxiety).

Implications for future research and practice

Newer methodologies—and phenotypes—are needed to advance our understanding of the relationship between sleep and depression, and future studies should be informed by findings emerging from neurobiological research. Research has to acknowledge and embrace the phenomenological heterogeneity within the syndrome currently identified as 'depression', as well as extensive co-morbidity between depressive and other psychiatric symptoms (including drug and alcohol misuse) (Kessler et al., 2005).

Future research needs to go beyond the estimation of associations between 'black box' syndromes to test hypotheses that are based on models of underlying pathophysiology. Studies are therefore needed that make use of what we know about specific depressive symptoms (for instance, low mood, anxiety, and fatigue) and the physiological changes in sleep which have been so consistently identified up till now in people with depression (namely increased REM sleep latency and density and reduction in slow wave sleep). Future studies need to explore newer ways of recording physiological sleep data in population samples, and to test for associations between specific sleep parameters and individual depressive symptoms after controlling for psychiatric co-morbidity. Findings from research of this kind will ultimately facilitate genetically informed as well as interventional studies.

But why does this matter? Why is it worth investing limited resources in further study of the relationship between disturbances of sleep and depression? The merit and utility of further research in this area lies in the prospect for primary, secondary, and/or tertiary prevention of depression, insomnia, or suicide (Ağargün et al., 1997). It is imperative to establish whether insomnia (or indeed hypersomnia) is a 'true' (unconfounded) risk factor for depression, the onset (Perlis et al., 2006) or relapse of (Jindal et al., 2002; Cho et al., 2008; Pigeon et al., 2008) depression, or for suicide among those who are, or who are at high risk of becoming, depressed. It is also possible that insomnia (and/or hypersomnia) is not a risk factor (as we understand this) but 'merely' a very visible marker of a 'true' depressive phenotype. Utility here might come from greater recognition of depression (Rao et al., 2009) in a manner that would enhance case detection in universal or targeted screening. Further breakthroughs will therefore also require interventional and other applied health services research. An important empirical question remains untested: do interventions for insomnia (including hypnotics as well as the recently developed CBTi (Manber et al., 2008) prevent the future occurrence (or recurrence) of depression in those not currently depressed? Until this is shown to be the case, it cannot be asserted that insomnia is a risk factor for depression. Further studies are also needed to confirm and quantify improved depressive outcomes in those receiving simultaneous treatment for depression and insomnia. Studies are needed that assess functional as well as symptomatic outcomes (e.g. impacts on employment, absence from work, and other measures of social functioning), as well as quality of life (QOL) and drug and alcohol misuse.

Quantitative and qualitative studies are needed that explore the user experience. The voice of those who have experienced depression is silent in current evidence regarding the role and impact of insomnia (and hypersomnia). Depression continues to carry a heavy burden of stigma and exclusion, not least in interactions with healthcare professionals. Many people with depression avoid seeking help for this condition for fear of being labelled, and many of those who do seek help report the sense of not being listened to. Sleep problems are extremely prevalent, and may indeed represent a common presenting complaint in depression; reluctance of GPs in particular to prescribe hypnotics (and perhaps an over-readiness to prescribe antidepressants) can lead to conflict and lack of therapeutic concordance. Further research is needed to understand these processes, and to enhance the content and mode of delivery of future interventions for the very large number of people with depression and problems sleeping.

Summary box

- Disturbances of sleep (and insomnia in particular) are extremely common in depression and *vice versa*. These conditions co-occur more often than each occurs on its own.
- Insomnia, hypersomnia, and fatigue are also diagnostic criteria for depressive disorders. Concerns remain therefore as to whether these can be considered as independent conditions.
- Longitudinal studies have demonstrated that sleep disturbances often begin before the onset of other depressive symptoms. Insomnia may (adversely) affect the response to treatment of depression and, if residual, predict depressive relapse. Insomnia might also modify the effects of other risk factors for depression, thereby increasing vulnerability. Early evidence suggests that persistent insomnia may increase the risk of suicide among people who are depressed.
- Interventions for insomnia are worthy of evaluation as a means of preventing the onset of depression (primary prevention) or reducing the severity or duration of co-occurring depressive disorders (secondary prevention).
- Even if not causally related to depression, better methods for recognizing sleep disturbance in populations might assist in the early detection of depression, or in identifying those at high risk of suicide.

References

Ağargün, M.Y., Kara, H. & Solmaz, M. (1997). Subjective sleep quality and suicidality in patients with major depression. *J Psychiatr Res*, **31**, 377–381.

American Psychiatric Association Task Force on DSM-IV (2000). *Diagnostic and Statistical Manual of Mental Disorders: DSM-IV-TR, Fourth Edition (Text Review)*. Washington, DC: American Psychiatric Association.

Bebbington, P.E., Brugha, T.S., Meltzer, H., et al. (2000). Neurotic disorders and the receipt of psychiatric treatment. *Psychol Med*, **30**, 1369–1376.

Benca, R.M., Obermeyer, W.H., Thisted, R.A. & Gillin, J.C. (1992). Sleep and psychiatric disorders. A meta-analysis. *Arch Gen Psychiatry*, **49**, 651–668.

Benca, R.M. & Peterson, M.J. (2008). Insomnia and depression. *Sleep Med*, 9(Suppl 1), S3–S9.

Breslau, N., Roth, T., Rosenthal, L. & Andreski, P. (1996). Sleep disturbance and psychiatric disorders: a longitudinal epidemiological study of young adults. *Biol Psychiatry*, **39**, 411–418.

Bryant, R.A., Creamer, M., O'Donnell, M., Silove, D. & McFarlane, A.C. (2010). Sleep disturbance immediately prior to trauma predicts subsequent psychiatric disorder. *Sleep*, **33**, 69–74.

Buysse, D.J., Angst, J., Gamma, A., Ajdacic, V., Eich, D. & Rössler, W. (2008). Prevalence, course, and comorbidity of insomnia and depression in young adults. *Sleep*, **31**, 473–480.

Carney, C.E., Segal, Z.V., Edinger, J.D. & Krystal, A.D. (2007). A comparison of rates of residual insomnia symptoms following pharmacotherapy or cognitive-behavioral therapy for major depressive disorder. *J Clin Psychiatry*, **68**, 254–260.

Cassano, P. & Fava, M. (2002). Depression and public health. An overview. *J Psychosom Res*, **53**, 849–857.

Chang, P.P., Ford, D.E., Mead, L.A., Cooper-Patrick, L. & Klag, M.J. (1997). Insomnia in young men and subsequent depression. The Johns Hopkins Precursors Study. *Am J Epidemiol*, **146**, 105–114.

Cho, H.J., Lavretsky, H., Olmstead, R., Levin, M.J., Oxman, M.N. & Irwin, M.R. (2008). Sleep disturbance and depression recurrence in community-dwelling older adults: a prospective study. *Am J Psychiatry*, **165**, 1543–1550.

Chorney, D.B., Detweiler, M.F., Morris, T.L. & Kuhn, B.R. (2008). The interplay of sleep disturbance, anxiety, and depression in children. *J Pediatr Psychol*, **33**, 339–348.

Cole, M.G. & Dendukuri, N. (2003). Risk factors for depression among elderly community subjects: a systematic review and meta-analysis. *Am J Psychiatry*, **160**, 1147–1156.

Coulombe, J.A., Reid, G.J., Boyle, M.H. & Racine, Y. (2009). Concurrent associations among sleep problems, indicators of inadequate sleep, psychopathology, and shared risk factors in a population-based sample of healthy Ontario children. *J Pediatr Psychol* [Epub ahead of print].

Demyttenaere, K., Bruffaerts, R., Posada-Villa, J., et al. (2004). Prevalence, severity and unmet need for treatment of mental disorders in the World Health Organization World Mental Health Surveys. *JAMA*, **291**, 2581–2590.

Ford, D.E. & Kamerow, D.B. (1989). Epidemiologic study of sleep disturbances and psychiatric disorders. An opportunity for prevention? *JAMA*, **262**, 1479–1484.

Ford, D.E. & Cooper-Patrick, L. (2001). Sleep disturbances and mood disorders: an epidemiologic perspective. *Depress Anxiety*, **14**, 3–6.

Franzen, P.L. & Buysse, D.J. (2008). Sleep disturbances and depression: risk relationships for subsequent depression and therapeutic implications. *Dialogues Clin Neurosci*, **10**, 473–481.

Gangwisch, J.E., Babiss, L.A., Malaspina, D., Turner, J.B., Zammit, G.K. & Posner, K. (2010). Earlier parental set bedtimes as a protective factor against depression and suicidal ideation. *Sleep*, **33**, 97–106.

Germain, A., Nofzinger, E.A., Kupfer, D.J. & Buysse, D.J. (2004). Neurobiology of non-REM sleep in depression: further evidence for hypofrontality and thalamic dysregulation. *Am J Psychiatry*, **161**, 1856–1863.

Gregory, A.M., Rijsdijk, F.V., Lau, J.Y., Dahl, R.E. & Eley, T.C. (2009). The direction of longitudinal associations between sleep problems and depression symptoms: a study of twins aged 8 and 10 years. *Sleep*, **32**, 189–199.

Gruber, J., Harvey, A.G., Wang, P.W., et al. (2009). Sleep functioning in relation to mood, function, and quality of life at entry to the Systematic Treatment Enhancement Program for Bipolar Disorder (STEP-BD). *J Affect Disord*, **114**, 41–49.

Jansson-Fröjmark, M. & Lindblom, K. (2008). A bidirectional relationship between anxiety and depression, and insomnia? A prospective study in the general population. *J Psychosom Res*, **64**, 443–449.

Jindal, R.D., Thase, M.E., Fasiczka, A.L., et al. (2002). Electroencephalographic sleep profiles in single-episode and recurrent unipolar forms of major depression: II. Comparison during remission. *Biol Psychiatry*, **51**, 230–236.

Johnson, E.O., Roth, T., & Breslau, N. (2006). The association of insomnia with anxiety disorders and depression: exploration of the direction of risk. *J Psychiatr Res*, **40**, 700–708

Kessler, R.C., Chiu, W.T., Demler, O. & Walters, E.E. (2005). Prevalence, severity, and comorbidity of 12-month DSM-IV disorders in the National Comorbidity Survey replication. *Arch Gen Psychiatry*, **62**, 617–627.

Kuppermann, M., Lubeck, D.P., Mazonson, P.D., et al. (1995). Sleep problems and their correlates in a working population. *J Gen Intern Med*, **10**, 25–32.

Liu, X., Buysse, D.J., Gentzler, A.L., et al. (2007). Insomnia and hypersomnia associated with depressive phenomenology and comorbidity in childhood depression. *Sleep*, **30**, 83–90.

Lorant, V., Deliège, D., Eaton, W., Robert, A., Philipott, P. & Ansseau, M. (2003). Socio-economic inequalities in depression: a meta-analysis. *Am J Epidemiol*, **157**, 98–112.

Mallon, L., Broman, J.E. & Hetta, J. (2000). Relationship between insomnia, depression, and mortality: a 12-year follow-up of older adults in the community. *Int Psychogeriatr*, **12**, 295–306.

Manber, R., Edinger, J.D., Gress, J.L., San Pedro-Salcedo, M.G., Kuo, T.F. & Kalista, T. (2008). Cognitive behavioral therapy for insomnia enhances depression outcome in patients with comorbid major depressive disorder and insomnia. *Sleep*, **31**, 489–495.

Mellinger, G.D., Balter, M.B. & Uhlenhuth, E.H. (1985). Insomnia and its treatment. Prevalence and correlates. *Arch Gen Psychiatry*, **42**, 225–232.

Mendlewicz, J. (2009). Sleep disturbances: core symptoms of major depressive disorder rather than associated or comorbid disorders. *World J Biol Psychiatry*, 1–7 [Epub ahead of print].

Murray, C.J.L. & Lopez, A.D. (1997). Alternative projections of mortality and disability by cause 1990-2020: Global Burden of Disease Study. *Lancet*, **349**, 1498–1504.

Neckelmann, D., Mykletun, A. & Dahl, A.A. (2007). Chronic insomnia as a risk factor for developing anxiety and depression. *Sleep*, **30**, 873–880.

Nofzinger, E.A., Buysse, D.J., Germain, A., et al. (2005). Alterations in regional cerebral glucose metabolism across waking and non-rapid eye movement sleep in depression. *Arch Gen Psychiatry*, **62**, 387–396.

Ohayon, M.M., Shapiro, C.M. & Kennedy, S.H. (2000). Differentiating DSM-IV anxiety and depressive disorders in the general population: comorbidity and treatment consequences. *Can J Psychiatry*, **45**, 166–172.

Perlis, M.L., Smith, L.J., Lyness, J.M., et al. (2006). Insomnia as a risk factor for onset of depression in the elderly. *Behav Sleep Med*, **4**, 104–113.

Pigeon, W.R., Hegel, M., Unützer, J., et al. (2008). Is insomnia a perpetuating factor for late-life depression in the IMPACT cohort? *Sleep*, **31**, 481–488.

Rao, U., Hammen, C.L. & Poland, R.E. (2009). Risk markers for depression in adolescents: sleep and HPA measures. *Neuropsychopharmacology*, **34**, 1936–1945.

Reid, G.J., Hong, R.Y. & Wade, T.J. (2009). The relation between common sleep problems and emotional and behavioral problems among 2- and 3-year-olds in the context of known risk factors for psychopathology. *J Sleep Res*, **18**, 49–59.

Riemann, D., Berger, M. & Voderholzer, U. (2001). Sleep and depression—results from psychobiological studies: an overview. *Biol Psychol*, **57**, 67–103.

Roane, B.M. & Taylor, D.J. (2006). Adolescent insomnia as a risk factor for early adult depression and substance abuse. *Sleep*, **31**, 1351–1356.

Shorter, E. & Tyrer, P. (2003). Separation of anxiety and depressive disorders: blind alley in psychopharmacology and classification of disease. *Br Med J*, **327**, 158–160.

Singleton, N., Bumpstead, R., O'Brien, M., Lee, A. & Meltzer, H. (2001). *Psychiatric morbidity among adults living in private households, 2000*. London: The Stationery Office.

Sivertsen, B., Hysing, M., Elgen, I., Stormark, K.M. & Lundervold, A.J. (2009). Chronicity of sleep problems in children with chronic illness: a longitudinal population-based study. *Child Adolesc Psychiatry Ment Health*, **3**, 22.

Spitzer, R.L., Kroenke, K., Linzer, M., et al. (1995). Health-related quality of life in primary care patients with mental disorders. *JAMA*, **274**, 1511–1517.

Staner, L. (2009). Comorbidity of insomnia and depression. *Sleep Med Rev* [Epub ahead of print].

Steptoe, A., Peacey, V. & Wardle, J. (2006). Sleep duration and health in young adults. *Arch Intern Med*, **166**, 1689–1692.

Taylor, D.J. (2008). Commentary: insomnia and depression. *Sleep*, **31**, 447–448.

Taylor, D.J., Lichstein, K.L., Durrence, H.H., Reidel, B.W. & Bush, A.J. (2005). Epidemiology of insomnia, depression, and anxiety. *Sleep*, **28**, 1457–1464.

Thase, M.E. (1998). Depression, sleep, and antidepressants. *J Clin Psychiatry*, **59**(S4), 55–65.

Thase, M.E. (2006). Depression and sleep: pathophysiology and treatment. *Dialogues Clin Neurosci*, **8**, 217–226.

Thomas, C.M. & Morris, S. (2003). Cost of depression among adults in England in 2000. *Br J Psychiatry*, **183**, 514–519.

Tsuno, N., Besset, A. & Ritchie, K. (2005). Sleep and depression. *J Clin Psychiatry*, **66**, 1254–1269.

Utge, S., Soronen, P., Partonen, T., et al. (2010). A population-based association study of candidate genes for depression and sleep disturbance. *Am J Med Genet B Neuropsychiatr Genet*, **153**, 468–476.

Wang, P.S., Lane, M., Olfson, M., Pincus, H.A., Wells, K.B. & Kessler, R.C. (2005). Twelve-month use of mental health services in the United States. *Arch Gen Psychiatry*, **62**, 629–640.

World Health Organization (1993). *The ICD-10 Classification of Mental and Behavioural Disorders: Diagnostic Criteria for Research*. Geneva: WHO.

Chapter 9

Sleep and neurological disorders

D.A. Cohen and A. Roy

Introduction

Sleep states are associated with physiological changes that affect the functioning of multiple organ systems, but sleep is fundamentally a nervous system process (Hobson, 2005). Mutually inhibitory sleep and arousal regions of the brain interact so that sleep and wakefulness 'switch' on and off in a coordinated fashion (Saper et al., 2005). Endogenous circadian rhythms that regulate the timing of sleep and wakefulness are controlled by pacemaker activity in the suprachiasmatic nucleus (SCN) of the hypothalamus (Reppert and Weaver, 2002). Respiratory patterns in sleep, a topic of considerable importance in relationship to sleep disorders, are driven by brainstem mechanisms that integrate information about carbon dioxide and oxygen exchange at the lungs (Afifi and Bergman, 2005); the mechanics of breathing itself is a product of reflex mechanisms that affect upper dilator muscles and the powering of respiratory muscles to promote ventilation. Sensorimotor processing in the nervous system remains necessary for normal movements during sleep, for example to prevent crush injury to a peripheral nerve from a prolonged position, or to maintain some level of vigilance to the environment, for example to awaken from a physical threat such as a fire. Diseases of the nervous system can disrupt these processes at multiple levels and cause sleep disorders (Fig. 9.1). In turn, sleep disorders may disrupt processes critical for neuronal reorganization and repair (Savage and West, 2007) and may therefore negatively impact the underlying neurological disorders.

Neurodegenerative diseases

Neurodegenerative diseases are a heterogeneous collection of conditions associated with progressive cognitive and motor disability. Abnormal folding and aggregation of several disease-related proteins preferentially target specific neuronal populations, leading to recognizable clinical phenotypes (Seeley et al., 2009). The correlation of post-mortem pathological findings with sleep disorders in these populations has helped refine our understanding of the mechanisms underlying the sleep disorders and increase our understanding of the functional neuroanatomy of sleep-wake regulation. The largest focus on sleep in neurodegenerative conditions has been studies in Alzheimer's disease and Parkinson's disease.

Alzheimer's disease

Alzheimer's disease (AD) is the most common neurodegenerative disease, with a prevalence of roughly 3% between 70 and 79 years old and increasing exponentially with age (Rocca et al., 1991). The hallmark feature is a primary memory storage deficit, and neuropathological findings include amyloid plaques and neurofibrillary tangles. The prevalence of any sleep disturbance is reported to be as low as 27% (Lyketsos et al., 2002; Tractenberg et al., 2005) and as high as 43–54% (Chen et al., 2000; Hart et al., 2003; Craig et al., 2006), compared to 18% in age-matched controls

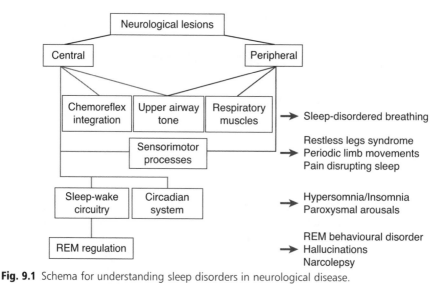

Fig. 9.1 Schema for understanding sleep disorders in neurological disease.
The nervous system is generally divided into the CNS (brain and spinal cord) and the peripheral nervous system (nerves and muscles). Lesions at any level may disrupt multiple sleep regulatory processes and lead to several sleep disorders. A special note should be made for spinal cord disease; although it is a CNS structure, damage at the level of the anterior horn cells in the ventral grey matter of the cord produces similar 'lower motor neuron' findings as peripheral lesions. Damage to the descending pathways above this level produces central, 'upper motor neuron' findings. Some diseases, such as amyotrophic lateral sclerosis, cause dysfunction at both levels.

(Tractenberg et al., 2005). The prevalence of sleep disorders generally parallels the severity of cognitive impairment (McCurry et al., 1999). In a community-based sample of 205 AD patients, 24% woke family members at night, and 70% of these caregivers found it moderately to severely distressing (McCurry et al., 1999). In fact, sleep disruption is a significant factor leading to institutionalization in a long-term care facility (Bianchetti et al., 1995). Daytime napping is common, with a prevalence of 71% compared to 24% of elderly controls (Ohadinia et al., 2004). Higher sleep propensity has been objectively shown with multiple sleep latency test (MSLT), with a 2- to 4-minute reduction of mean sleep latency (Bonanni et al., 2005). However, independent of the association with cognitive decline, excessive sleepiness in AD is linked to decreased functional status (Lee et al., 2007). In addition, the relationship of sleep disorders and the neurodegenerative process may be bi-directional. For example, the accumulation of toxic extracellular amyloid-β, part of the pathogenic process in AD, is increased by chronic sleep restriction (Kang et al., 2009).

Abnormalities in the waking and sleep electroencephalogram (EEG) have been demonstrated in AD including: slowing of the posterior dominant rhythm, reduced stage N3 sleep, and reduced rapid eye movement (REM) (Prinz et al., 1982; Montplaisir et al., 1995, 1998); a reduction in fast spindle activity (Rauchs et al., 2008); and higher proportions of delta and theta slowing in waking and sleep (Montplaisir et al., 1995, 1998). The increased sleep delta activity does not have the same physiological characteristics of normal slow wave sleep (SWS) (Crowley et al., 2005). Collectively, these EEG changes imply that the disease causes fundamental change in sleep-wake circuitry.

Circadian abnormalities have been found in AD. These include: reduced melatonin secretion with lower amplitude and more variable circadian rhythms (Mishima et al., 1999); a fivefold reduction in cerebrospinal fluid (CSF) melatonin concentration (Liu et al., 1999); phase delay of the core body temperature rhythms in proportion to the burden of AD pathology (Harper et al., 2004, 2005); and an abnormal phase relationship between the circadian rhythm and the sleep-wake cycle (Lee et al., 2004), with more disorganization of the circadian sleep-wake rhythm as the disease worsens (Werth et al., 2002). Circadian disruption in AD has been postulated to contribute to an evening increase in agitation, or 'sundowning' (Martin et al., 2000; Volicer et al., 2001). Intrinsic sleep disorders, such as sleep-disordered breathing (SDB), can increase morning confusion and agitation (Bliwise et al., 1989; Gehrman et al., 2003).

Parkinson's disease and dementia with Lewy bodies

Parkinson's disease (PD) and dementia with Lewy bodies (DLB) are neuropathologically related conditions in which abnormal accumulation of alpha-synuclein protein forms neuronal Lewy bodies. The distribution of Lewy bodies determines the clinical phenotype along a spectrum in terms of the degree of motor symptoms (stiffness, slowness, tremor, and poor balance) or cognitive symptoms (visual hallucinations, visuospatial impairment, fluctuating level of arousal and attention) (Press, 2004). In a community-based sample, 60% of patients with PD reported a sleep compliant compared to 33% of age-matched controls (Tandberg et al., 1998). In a longitudinal study spanning 8 years, more than half of patients with PD reported insomnia; difficultly turning in bed and nightmares became more prevalent with disease progression (Gjerstad et al., 2007).

Excessive daytime sleepiness has received the most attention compared to other sleep-related complaints in these patients. Subjective excessive daytime sleepiness is present in up to 50% of PD patients, and one study demonstrated a pathologically short mean sleep latency (<8 minutes) on the MSLT in 8/9 patients with idiopathic PD; one of these patients had 4/4 sleep onset REM periods and a mean sleep latency of 2.6 minutes (Baumann et al., 2005), which would satisfy criteria for narcolepsy secondary to a medical condition. Subjective impairment in sleep quality and excessive daytime sleepiness, napping, or fluctuating attention are more frequent in PD and DLB than in AD (Boddy et al., 2007; Grace et al., 2000; Ferman et al., 2004). It should be noted that dopaminergic therapies used for motor features of Parkinsonism may directly cause excessive sleepiness, even in young healthy volunteers (Micallef et al., 2009).

Restless legs syndrome (RLS) is more common in PD than age-matched controls. In a recent case-control study of 200 PD patients, the prevalence of RLS was 3% compared to 0.5% of controls (Loo and Tan, 2008). There is also a threefold increase in the number of periodic limb movements of sleep (PLMS) in PD (Diederich et al., 2005). These conditions all may share an underlying central dopamine deficit.

Abnormal regulation of REM sleep may cause REM behavioural disorder (RBD), characterized by excessive, potentially injurious behaviours occurring during REM sleep that may correspond to the contents of a dream. RBD has been linked to PD and other disorders with abnormal alpha-synuclein accumulation (synucleinopathies), such as multiple system atrophy (MSA). In fact, RBD has been linked to a synucleinopathy in 97% of cases in a recent review, with the highest prevalence in MSA (up to 95%), followed by DLB (up to 80%), and then PD (up to 60%) (Boeve et al., 2007). RBD increases the risk of injury to both patients and their bed partners, for example secondary to punching and kicking movements that may correspond to a fighting them of a dream. In addition, abnormal REM regulation with the inappropriate release of REM sleep dream-like imagery intruding into wakefulness may be a cause of visual hallucinations (Manni et al., 2002; Whitehead et al., 2008; Sinforiani et al., 2007).

Mechanisms in neurodegenerative disease

Neurodegenerative diseases are associated with injury or functional disruption of the sleep-wake circuitry, including serotonin (Aletrino et al., 1992; Kish et al., 2008), norepinephrine

(Chan-Palay, 1990), acetylcholine (Mufson et al., 1988; Hirsch et al., 1987), and orexin/hypocretin (Fronczek et al., 2007) systems. The degree of sleep-wake disruption may reflect a predilection for certain types of degenerative processes to affect different components of these systems. For example, Lewy body pathology may have a particular predilection for sleep-wake regulatory circuits compared to AD (Harper et al., 2004).

The circadian system may be damaged in neurodegenerative disease, including primary degeneration of the SCN (Wu and Swaab, 2005), disruption of the molecular circadian clock in the SCN (Morton et al., 2005), or a functional disconnection between SCN pacemaker activity and the rhythmic expression of circadian clock genes in the pineal gland (Wu et al., 2006) or other targets. In addition, patients with neurodegenerative diseases are at a higher risk of reduced exposure to environmental time cues to entrain the circadian system; for example, patients with AD living at home are exposed to significantly less bright light than controls (Campbell et al., 1988).

Treatment

The main emphasis of treatment studies in patients with neurodegenerative conditions is based on targeting the circadian system, predominantly with light and melatonin. Bright light exposure (2,000–10,000 lux) for 45 minutes to 2 hours may reduce restlessness, sundowning, and agitation behaviour (Satlin et al., 1992; Lovell et al., 1995; Koyama et al., 1999; Haffmans et al., 2001; Dowling et al., 2007; Skjerve et al., 2004) and improve sleep-wake patterns (Ito et al., 2001; Yamadera et al., 2000; Van Someren et al., 1997; Sloane et al., 2007; Fetveit et al., 2003; Ancoli-Israel et al., 2003; Mishima et al., 1998; McCurry et al., 2005), although some light therapy trials failed to find such benefits (Lyketsos et al., 1999; Colenda et al., 1997; Ancoli-Israel et al., 2002; Dowling et al., 2005; Skjerve et al., 2004). Melatonin 2.5–3 mg may improve sleep-wake patterns, either alone or in combination with light therapy (Medeiros et al., 2007; Asayama et al., 2003; Riemersma-van der Lek et al., 2008; Dowling et al., 2008), but several studies have failed to find such benefits (Haffmans et al., 2001; Serfaty et al., 2002; Gehrman et al., 2009; Singer et al., 2003).

Neurodevelopmental disorders

Neurodevelopmental disorders (NDD) encompass a wide variety of conditions affecting the number, distribution, morphology, and connectivity of neurons. Abnormal nervous system development can stem from a wide array of mechanisms, including genetic, metabolic, immunologic, toxic, traumatic, and vascular mechanisms. The underlying mechanisms of sleep disorders in these conditions are often not well-understood, but abnormal development of the sleep-wake and circadian systems, visual impairment (affecting circadian entrainment), pain, motor disability, and behavioural disturbances may play a role depending on the disorder.

Insomnia and hypersomnia

In a 6-month longitudinal study of pre-school-aged children with normal development, autism, or developmental delay, the incidence of parent-reported sleep disturbances in their children was 14–33% of those with normal development and 35–48% in both neurodevelopmentally disordered groups (Goodlin-Jones et al., 2009). The childhood sleep disorder impacts the caregivers, for example parents of children with autism report reduced sleep quality (Meltzer and Moore, 2008). Some disorders are associated with daytime sleepiness, for example subjective sleepiness is reported in 77% of young adults with Williams syndrome, despite 9 hours time in bed and 7.5 hours of actigraphy estimated sleep per night (Goldman et al., 2009). Some disorders are more frequently associated with insomnia, for example as frequent as 75–90% of patients with Asperger syndrome (Tani et al., 2003). Spectral analysis of sleep EEG data in this population has demonstrated reduced delta power and increased theta in sleep, similar to other populations with insomnia (Tani et al., 2004). Children with cerebral palsy have approximately a fourfold increase in sleep problems compared to normal developing children, including more problems with difficulty initiating or maintaining sleep and more sleep-wake transitions (Newman et al., 2006).

Sleep, inattention, and hyperactivity

Sleep disruption in childhood causes restlessness, irritability, and poor concentration more so than sleepiness (Chervin et al., 1997). Therefore, a primary sleep disorder may cause symptoms that are diagnosed as attention deficit hyperactivity disorder (ADHD). In addition, stimulant treatment used to improve concentration and hyperactivity can impair sleep (Corkum et al., 2008). Therefore, the associations of sleep disorders and ADHD or its treatment may have a bi-directional relationship. In addition, arousal and attentional networks share overlapping neural circuitry, and a common developmental abnormality may cause both cognitive and sleep symptoms. A recent meta-analysis reviewing studies of ADHD patients compared to controls found increased rates of SDB, excessive daytime sleepiness, bedtime resistance, difficulty with both sleep onset and morning awakenings, and fragmented nocturnal sleep (Cortese et al., 2009). In ADHD, the prevalence of SDB may be as high as 50% compared to 22% in controls (Golan et al., 2004). Treatment of OSA by adenotonsillectomy in an ADHD population with an apnoea-hypopnoea index (AHI) range of 1–5 events per hour can improve the ADHD symptoms equally or greater than methylphenidate (Huang et al., 2007). These data indicate that for many of these patients, the sleep disorder may have been the primary cause of cognitive and behavioural symptoms rather than impaired neural development of attentional networks. Recent data also link ADHD with a 15% prevalence of periodic limb movement disorder (PLMD) (Golan et al., 2004) and a 44% prevalence of RLS (Cortese et al., 2005), which are substantially higher than the general population. Iron therapy, which is commonly a treatment for RLS/PLMD, improved ADHD symptoms in a randomized, double-blind, placebo-controlled study (Konofal et al., 2007). It is possible that these conditions have overlapping pathophysiology such as central dopamine dysfunction, but for some individuals the sleep disorder may be the primary problem causing inattention.

Sleep-disordered breathing

There are several mechanisms in which the NDD may cause SDB. In cerebral palsy, one mechanism may involve abnormal excessive muscle tone (spasticity) in respiratory muscles (McCarty et al., 2001). Cranial-facial abnormalities in NDD also contribute to an increased risk of OSA, for example in 54.6% of children with Down syndrome having significant OSA (de Miguel-Diez et al., 2003). Malformation or mechanical compression of medullary structures can cause central sleep apnoea from impaired respiratory pattern generation or impairment of chemoreflex integration of blood gases. For example, surgical decompression of the medulla in the setting of a Chiari malformation can improve central sleep apnoea (Van den Broek et al., 2009). SDB may be more prevalent in children with autism spectrum disorders (Liu et al., 2006), but the underlying mechanism is unknown.

Sleep and neuroplasticity

In recent years, there is a growing body of literature linking sleep to processes of neuroplasticity, the experience-dependent changes that occur at a synaptic level (Maquet, 2001). Processes of neuroplasticity shape the functional connections between neural networks that become specialized for different types of information processing. Conceivably, in the developing brain sleep disorders may impair these processes leading to cognitive and emotional disorders (Dang-Vu et al., 2006). For example, a prospective 5-year longitudinal study demonstrated a significantly higher chance of developing ADHD by 5.5 years of age for infants 6–12 months old who have severe sleep difficulties, particularly sleep initiation problems (Thunstrom, 2002). It is possible that the sleep difficulties in this study were a marker for impaired neuronal development, but a sleep disorder during critical periods may potentially causally affect neurodevelopment. Such a framework would predict that treating sleep disorders in early childhood might be a vital component of minimizing future neurological disability.

Treatment

Carefully designed treatment trials for children with NDD are seldom found in the medical literature (Owens and Palermo, 2008). In clinical practice, melatonin is commonly used in this population. A systematic review of randomized controlled trials including a total of 35 patients with NDD and melatonin doses 0.5–7.5 mg suggested an improvement in sleep latency, with increased efficacy in those with greater baseline sleep disturbance (Phillips and Appleton, 2004). In a more recent randomized, placebo-controlled trial in patients with NDD, melatonin 5 mg (1 mg immediate release, 4 mg sustained release) improved sleep latency and total sleep time by approximately 30 minutes (Wasdell et al., 2008). In preparation for a new melatonin trial for children with NDD, it has been shown that melatonin remains stable when mixed in water, orange juice, milk, yogurt, and jam, common ways parents administer melatonin to children with NDD (Shah et al., 2008). Clonidine, an alpha 2-receptor agonist, qualitatively improved behaviour around bedtime, reduced sleep fragmentation, and extended sleep time in six children with NDD (Ingrassia and Turk, 2005). Clearly, more studies are greatly needed to determine safe and effective treatments for sleep disorders in this population.

Cerebrovascular disease

The most studied relationship between cerebrovascular disease and sleep disorders is the strong association between cerebrovascular disease and SDB (Partinen and Palomaki, 1985). Approximately 70% of patients with stroke have SDB, and their disease tends to be severe (Dyken et al., 1996; Bassetti et al., 1996). It is possible that this relationship may be partly explained by common risk factors such as obesity, but several lines of evidence suggest causal associations.

Stroke as a cause of sleep-disordered breathing

Stroke may cause SDB. One study found that patients with sleep apnoea following stroke generally did not have historical features such as snoring, obesity, or daytime sleepiness to suggest sleep apnoea prior to the stroke (Mohsenin and Valor, 1995). SDB improves from the acute phase to sub-acute phase of a stroke, particularly central sleep apnoea, but residual obstructive SDB is present in at least half of the patients (Harbison et al., 2002; Parra et al., 2000). Stroke may increase the risk of central SDB by damaging brainstem structures involved with respiratory pattern generation and chemoreflex control of breathing (Lyons, 1971; Devereaux et al., 1973) or obstructive sleep apnoea (OSA) from brainstem or hemispheric lesions that impair coordination of upper airway muscles (Urban et al., 2002).

Sleep-disordered breathing as a cause of stroke

Sleep-disordered breathing may also be part of the causal pathway for stroke, particularly with an AHI of 20 events per hour or more (Arzt et al., 2005; Munoz et al., 2006; Valham et al., 2008).

An argument for this direction of causality is that the prevalence of sleep apnoea does not differ based on the type of stroke (ischaemic vs. haemorrhagic), lesion location, or even if there is no permanent tissue damage (transient ischaemic attack) (Dyken et al., 1996; Parra et al., 2000). This association may be mediated by several mechanisms. OSA is associated with increased intracranial pressure, blood pressure instability, hypertension, increased sympathetic activity and catecholamine levels, increased blood viscosity, and platelet activation, predisposing to vasculopathy (Hornyak et al., 1991; Klingelhofer et al., 1992; Bassetti et al., 2006; Young et al., 1997; Lloyd-Jones et al., 2009; Peppard et al., 2000). In fact, sleep apnoea patients have increased intima-media thickness of the carotid artery (Silvestrini et al., 2002), a marker of atherosclerosis. Sleep apnoea may also increase the risk of cardioembolic stroke, mediated by atrial fibrillation or right-to-left intracardiac shunting through a patent foramen ovale and paradoxical embolization secondary to the intrathoracic pressure changes associated with apnoeas (Gami et al., 2004; Beelke et al., 2002).

Functional recovery following stroke

Following brain injury from a stroke, the presence of SDB may worsen functional outcome (Good et al., 1996) or increase the risk of death (Sahlin et al., 2008). In the setting of stroke, there may be tissue that has been damaged but that may potentially recover if sufficient blood flow is restored. Presumably, changes in cerebral oxygenation or blood flow secondary to SDB impair this potential recovery, extending the size of permanent injury. In addition, functional recovery depends on processes of neuroplasticity, which may be impaired in the context of a sleep disorder. Therefore, addressing SDB in particular and sleep disorders in general early in the course of stroke may become a vital component of stroke care.

Neuromuscular disorders

Neuromuscular disorders (NMD) include disorders that affect the alpha motor neurons in the spinal cord, nerve roots, peripheral nerves, neuromuscular junction, and muscles. These disorders predominantly cause muscle weakness and/or sensory symptoms. Daytime symptoms related to disturbed sleep are common in this population, including: fatigue (83%), sleepiness (63%), restless legs (54%), and morning headaches (45%) (Labanowski et al., 1996). Primary mechanisms of sleep disruption include SDB, RLS/PLMS, and pain.

Sleep-disordered breathing

The prevalence of SDB across several studies of patients with NMD was estimated to be approximately 70% (Van Lunteren and Kaminski, 1999). SDB in this population may come in two primary forms: (1) OSA and (2) hypercapneic hypoventilation. Depending on the disease, there may be an evolution in the type of SDB. For example, in a study of children with Duchenne muscular dystrophy, upper airway obstruction developed about 5 years prior to hypoventilation (Suresh et al., 2005).

Coordinated neuromuscular recruitment of upper airway muscles is essential to maintain airway patency in the face of negative intraluminal upper airway pressures during inspiration (Patil et al., 2007). NMD can affect the recruitment of pharyngeal dilator muscles or reduce the amount of force they generate, promoting upper airway collapsibility and OSA (Dziewas et al., 2008; Aboussouan et al., 2007). Even if the muscle force generation is preserved, damage to autonomic fibres may interfere with upper airway reflex responses to mechanical forces. For example, in patients with diabetic autonomic neuropathy, obstructive events last longer and there is greater degrees of hypoxaemia compared to those with spared autonomic function (Bottini et al., 2008). In addition, functioning of the vocal cords can be affected in some disorders, and obstruction at the level of the larynx has also been associated with OSA in populations such as those with post-polio syndrome (Steljes et al., 1990). Steroid treatment in disorders such as myasthenia gravis (MG), an autoimmune condition affecting the neuromuscular junction, may cause myopathy of the upper airway muscles and weight gain, which may be additional factors that may increase the risk of OSA (Amino et al., 1998).

Respiratory failure with hypercapnia and hypoxia is one of the leading causes of death and disability in patients with significant neuromuscular impairment, and respiratory insufficiency generally begins during sleep (Benditt, 2009). Ventilation falls during normal sleep, particularly during REM sleep in which tone to accessory respiratory muscles is reduced and the diaphragm drives ventilation in relative isolation. Nocturnal ventilation in NMD falls in parallel to declining respiratory muscle strength (Bye et al., 1990); daytime pulmonary function tests may be useful to predict nocturnal hypoventilation (Bye et al., 1990; Ragette et al., 2002), but they are not always reliable predictors (Labanowski et al., 1996). Therefore, a high index of suspicion is warranted with a low threshold for obtaining nocturnal polysomnography (PSG). Complications of hypoventilation include: hypoxia, pulmonary hypertension, and right-sided heart failure (Krachman et al., 2003). In one study of 31 patients with NMD, oxygen levels during sleep fell below 85% saturation in more than 75% of patients (Weinberg et al., 2003). Chronic nocturnal hypoventilation may result in blunted sensitivity of chemoreflex ventilatory control mechanisms, leading to central apnoeas (Alves et al., 2009); evidence for this is that nocturnal positive pressure ventilation can improve the ventilatory responses to hypercarbia in these patients (Annane et al., 1999).

Treatment of the underlying disorder, when possible, should be the primary goal for addressing SDB in patients with neuromuscular disease. For example, medically stable patients with MG do not seem to have higher levels of SDB than the general population (Prudlo et al., 2007), and thymectomy, a treatment for MG, may significantly decrease OSA in these patients (Amino et al., 1998). In the past, when assistance with ventilation was necessary, invasive mechanical ventilation at night with tracheostomy (Sivak and Streib, 1980) or negative pressure ventilation (with a so called 'iron lung') was often used. Negative pressure ventilators can actually increase upper airway obstruction and worsen OSA secondary to the lowered intraluminal pressure (Ellis et al., 1987). Bi-level non-invasive positive pressure ventilation (NIPPV) through a mask interface has now become the standard approach to treating these patients. NIPPV can improve both upper airway obstruction and hypoventilation, reducing objective measures of daytime sleepiness (Guilleminault et al., 1998); waking blood oxygen and carbon dioxide levels (Kerby et al., 1987; Heckmatt et al., 1990; Ellis et al., 1987); and headache, insomnia, and cognitive abilities (Kerby et al., 1987) in patients with NMD. The use of NIPPV, primarily overnight during sleep, prolonged survival by 205 days and improved quality of life (QOL) in patients with amyotrophic lateral sclerosis who had moderate-to-good facial muscle strength (Bourke et al., 2006). Severe weakness of facial muscles may hinder the ability to form a good seal with mask ventilation, and more invasive methods may be necessary.

Pain

Patients with painful neuropathy have a twofold increase in reported sleep disturbance and sleepiness compared to the general population (Zelman et al., 2006). Treatment of neuropathic pain can substantially reduce sleep disruption by as much as 30%, using agents such as pregabalin, gabapentin, tramadol, oxcarbezapine, lidocaine patch, and others (Freeman et al., 2007, 2008; Backonja et al., 1998; Erdemoglu and Varlibas, 2006; White et al., 2003). Painful leg cramps may also cause secondary insomnia (Rubinsztein et al., 1998).

Restless legs syndrome

The prevalence of RLS in peripheral neuropathy has been found to be 5%, roughly 5–10 times higher than the general population (Rutkove et al., 1996). Others have found a much higher prevalence of 54%, arguing that lower reported estimates relate to RLS being overlooked in this population given other sensory complaints from the neuropathy (Nineb et al., 2007). RLS may be more likely to occur when the pathology to peripheral nerves is axonal in nature rather than demyelinating (Iannaccone et al., 1995).

Paroxysmal disorders

Epilepsy

Epilepsy, defined as a propensity for unprovoked seizures, is one of the most common disorders in neurology. Individual seizures reflect abnormal, excessive, synchronized discharges in a population of neurons, and the clinical manifestations depend on the specific neural networks that are involved. The seizure threshold is influenced by sleep-wake state, and many seizures occur predominantly during sleep, particularly non-rapid eye movement (NREM) sleep (Steriade et al., 1994; Sammaritano et al., 1991; Bazil et al., 2000). In fact, the probability of detecting abnormal EEG activity that is diagnostic of epilepsy changes from approximately 8–28% during wakefulness to 72–98% during sleep (Rocamora et al., 2008). It is well-established that sleep disruption can provoke seizure activity (Hauser et al., 1993; Foldvary-Schaefer and Grigg-Damberger, 2009; Mendez and Radtke, 2001) and seizures can cause arousals and interfere with sleep (Hoeppner et al., 1984). Therefore, there is a bi-directional relationship between epilepsy and sleep disorders.

Patients with epilepsy have altered quality and amount of sleep (Abad-Alegria et al., 1997). Excessive daytime sleepiness is reported in 25–50% of patients (Weintraub et al., 2005; Malow et al., 1997a), with MSLT evidence of pathological sleep propensity (mean sleep latency < 5 minutes) in 10% of patients (Drake et al., 1994). Antiepileptic medication causes relaxation of the upper airway, and weight gain from these medications or limited activity in this population increase the risk of SDB (Foldvary-Schaefer and Grigg-Damberger, 2009). The prevalence of SDB in epilepsy has been reported to be 10–33% and twice as common in men compared to women (Young et al., 1993; Malow et al., 2000). The prevalence of RLS or PLMS in epilepsy is not well-established (Foldvary-Schaefer, 2002), but one study found that 36% of patients with epilepsy had PLMS (Malow et al., 1997b). Finally, patients with epilepsy commonly have poor sleep habits (Foldvary-Schaefer and Grigg-Damberger, 2009).

Paroxysmal seizure phenomena during sleep can be difficult to distinguish from parasomnias (Pedley, 1983). A brief frontal lobe seizure may appear similar to a confusional arousal (Provini et al., 1999). Episodic nocturnal wanderings are a manifestation of frontal lobe epilepsy that can be indistinguishable from sleepwalking (Plazzi et al., 1995). Adding to the difficulty distinguishing seizures from parasomnias, EEG is often normal during frontal lobe seizures, and there is often normal awareness without confusion immediately following the event (Zucconi et al., 1997). Seizures are often abrupt in onset, with explosive activity, but the key distinguishing feature of seizures is the stereotyped nature of the spells. In fact, recurrent and stereotyped dreams are also a well-defined manifestation of seizures (Epstein, 1964).

Treatment of a primary sleep disorder improves seizure control. Positive airway pressure treatment for SDB can improve seizure control in 40–86% of adult patients (Foldvary-Schaefer, 2002; Devinsky et al., 1994) and reduce the number of epileptic discharges on EEG (Oliveira et al., 2000). In addition, reduction of PLMS may also reduce seizures by improving sleep continuity (Mendez and Radtke, 2001). It is also possible that antiepileptic drugs can improve seizure frequency by stabilizing sleep, independent of the direct effects of the medications on seizure mechanisms.

Headache

Headache is a common neurological disorder, with 33% of the population affected by tension-type headaches, 14% with migraines, and 4% with chronic daily headache (Sheffield, 1998). The relationship between headaches and sleep is clinically important in certain headache patients. Early observations noted that certain headaches would occur exclusively during sleep, particularly REM sleep (Dexter, 1979), and other headaches would be triggered by insufficient sleep or by too much sleep and that sleep could relieve some headaches (Sahota and Dexter, 1990; Blau, 1990; Rains and Poceta, 2005). Changes in sleep during the prior one to three nights is the best predictor of headache (Rains and Poceta, 2005). Therefore, a brief sleep history should be incorporated into the evaluation of all headache patients.

Detailed epidemiological data linking specific sleep disorders and defined headache syndromes are generally lacking. Patients with cluster headache have an increased incidence of SDB (Chervin et al., 2000). Snoring, a marker for OSA, has been associated with all types of headache (Jennum and Sjol, 1994), particularly morning headaches (Ulfberg et al., 1996). Morning headaches have also been associated with insomnia, reduced sleep efficiency or REM duration, circadian rhythm disorders, PLMS, and nightmares (Ohayon, 2004; Aldrich and Chauncey, 1990; Poceta and Dalessio, 1995). A sleep disorder that required treatment was found in approximately 10% of patients with headache, and treatment of the sleep disorder substantially improved headache frequency in the majority of these patients (Paiva et al., 1997).

Potential mechanism for the relationship between SDB and headache may relate to intermittent hypoxaemia, blood pressure surges, and increased intracranial pressure during obstructive apnoeas. These physiological changes may be particularly important in vascular headaches, with resultant activation of the trigeminal nucleus and the genesis of headache (Welch, 2003). Sleep deprivation can lower pain thresholds (Onen et al., 2001), and therefore sleep disruption or deprivation from a variety of causes can increase headache. Migraine in particular has been linked to serotonin signalling (Dodick et al., 2003), and the modulation of neurotransmitter tone secondary to sleep-wake state changes may trigger some headaches.

Multiple sclerosis

Multiple sclerosis (MS) is an autoimmune disorder with predominantly demyelinating pathology in the central nervous system (CNS). In most patients, at least early in the disease course, there are discrete attacks with neurological deficits lasting days to weeks followed by periods of remission and relative recovery. The prevalence of moderate-to-severe sleep disturbances in MS has been estimated to be 51.5% in a population-based survey with 1,062 MS patient respondents (Bamer et al., 2008). These include both complaints of sleep initiation and maintenance insomnia as well as excessive daytime sleepiness. Poor sleep in MS is an independent predictor for reduced QOL (Merlino et al., 2009), and sleep disturbances may be one mechanism for the common symptom of fatigue in these patients (Kaynak et al., 2006). In a large, multi-centre trial including 861 patients with MS, the prevalence of RLS was 19% compared to 4% in age- and sex-matched controls (Manconi et al., 2008a). Damage to descending dopaminergic pathways to the spinal cord, particularly with cervical spinal cord dysfunction, may play a role in the pathophysiology of RLS in this population (Manconi et al., 2008a, b). Cases of RBD have been reported from MS lesions in the pons (Gomez-Choco et al., 2007; Tippmann-Peikert et al., 2006), and MS can also cause narcolepsy (Nishino and Kanbayashi, 2005). In one case, MSLT showed a 2.8-minute mean sleep latency and 5/5 sleep onset REM periods, undetectable CSF orexin levels, and bilateral hypothalamic demyelinating lesions on brain magnetic resonance imaging (MRI). Several months later, the clinical symptoms, MSLT findings, and CSF orexin levels normalized, paralleling MRI improvement of the hypothalamic lesions (Oka et al., 2004). The central control of breathing may be impaired from demyelination affecting the brainstem respiratory control centres (Auer et al., 1996; Rizvi et al., 1974), but whether MS is associated with a higher prevalence of OSA remains unclear (Brass et al., 2010). Spasticity, muscle spasms, and pain are additional factors that disrupt sleep in these patients, and medications to reduce these symptoms can improve sleep quality (Bensmail et al., 2006; Solaro et al., 2000). Since insufficient sleep can trigger changes in the immune system and inflammatory processes (Frey et al., 2007), it is possible that sleep disorders can exacerbate the tendency for MS flares.

Trauma

Traumatic brain injury

In the acute setting, 36% of patients with traumatic brain injury (TBI) have SDB, and the majority of apnoeas are central in nature (Webster et al., 2001). In one study, 70% of patients admitted to a rehabilitation unit for closed head TBI had disrupted nighttime sleep (Makley et al., 2008). The resumption of organized sleep-wake cycles, sleep efficiency, and the duration of REM sleep parallel cognitive improvement (Ron et al., 1980; Makley et al., 2009). Early sleep disturbances may be a marker for the severity of neuronal injury, but sleep disturbances may also influence recovery. In the chronic setting, those with persistent sleep disorders have worse sustained attention (Bloomfield et al., 2009; Wilde et al., 2007). Several sleep disorders persist 3–6 months following the injury, including: SDB (23–30%), post-traumatic hypersomnia (3–52%), insomnia (5–33%), post-traumatic narcolepsy (5–15%), and RBD (13%) (Baumann et al., 2007; Castriotta et al., 2009; Verma et al., 2007). Traumatic injury to the hypothalamus, causing a reduction in the number of orexin neuron and CSF orexin levels (Baumann et al., 2007, 2009) may play a causal role in the sleep-wake disturbances. Circadian rhythm sleep disorders, including delayed sleep-phase and irregular sleep-wake types, have also been found in the setting of TBI (Quinto et al., 2000; Ayalon et al., 2007; Nagtegaal et al., 1997; Patten and Lauderdale, 1992). Consistent with these reports, abnormalities in serum melatonin profiles have been found in the acute setting of TBI (Paparrigopoulos et al., 2006).

Spinal cord injury

Central pain is a common problem in spinal cord injury (SCI) and is a significant factor that disrupts sleep (Norrbrink, 2009). Medications used to reduce neuropathic pain, such as pregabalin, can improve sleep quality in these patients (Siddall et al., 2006). The circadian regulation of melatonin release from the pineal gland depends on the integrity of descending sympathetic fibres to the superior cervical ganglion, and complete cervical cord transection can abolish nocturnal melatonin production (Zeitzer et al., 2000) and reduced sleep efficiency (Scheer et al., 2006). These data suggest that impaired circadian regulation of sleep may be a factor contributing to sleep disturbances in this population. SDB is common in SCI, with a prevalence as high as 69% acutely that may decrease over time (Tran et al., 2010). Factors relevant to SDB in this population include: respiratory muscle weakness, influence of medications on upper airway tone, supine sleep posture, weight gain, and increased neck circumference in this population (Tran et al., 2010).

Tumours

Depending on the location, tumours of the CNS can cause a variety of sleep disorders. Most of the literature in this population stems from individual case reports. For example, a patient with a thalamic tumour developed adult-onset sleep terrors, with documented sudden arousal from SWS (Di Gennaro et al., 2004). A reduction of sleep spindles on the side of the lesion was interpreted as evidence that thalamocortical mechanisms for sleep regulation were impaired. Other sleep disorders with focal tumours include: secondary narcolepsy from hypothalamic tumours (Marcus et al., 2002), RBD from tumours in the pons (De Barros-Ferreira et al., 1975; Zambelis et al., 2002), and OSA (Greenough et al., 1999) and central sleep apnoea (Ito et al., 1996) from brainstem tumours. Sleep disorders may also be related to treatment of a brain tumour; brain irradiation has been associated with the somnolence syndrome, which may reflect demyelination of arousal regions; however, somnolence syndrome in the setting of focal irradiation to the pineal region has been reported (Kelsey and Marks, 2006) conceivably by disrupting circadian regulation of arousal. Finally, the nervous system response to a non-CNS tumour, a paraneoplastic reaction, can result in brainstem inflammation and sleep apnoea (Lee et al., 2006).

Conclusion

Damage to the nervous system or impaired neural development can cause a wide array of sleep disorders, and in turn sleep disruption may impair neuroplastic processes that are important for functional recovery after nervous system insults. Sleep disorders in patients with neurological disease can negatively affect QOL for both the patients and the caregivers. In addition, cardiovascular, metabolic, and immune process changes associated with sleep disorders may exacerbate the underlying neuropathological changes in neurological disease. This framework suggests that early intervention for sleep disorders in these patients may substantially improve neurological outcomes. Scientific investigation of the relationships between sleep and neurological disorders is at a relatively early stage, and more randomized, controlled treatment trials will ultimately help determine the optimal timing and treatment modalities for the sleep disorders in these patients.

Summary box

- Sleep-related processes are disturbed by neurological illnesses at multiple levels of the nervous system.
- Abnormal sleep may worsen neurological disease by disrupting normal processes of neuroplasticity and immune, endothelial, and metabolic function.
- Circadian disruption is a cause of sundowning in dementia.
- Bright light and melatonin therapy may improve sleep and wakefulness in neurodegenerative diseases, but the optimal dose and timing need more study.
- Sleep disorders in children often present as ADHD, and treatment of OSA and RLS/PLMD substantially improves ADHD symptoms in many children.
- Stroke worsens SDB, particularly in the acute phase, and OSA is emerging as a risk factor for developing cerebrovascular disease.
- Nocturnal NIPPV in patients with neuromuscular disease improves waking blood oxygen and carbon dioxide levels.

Summary box *(continued)*

- Treatment of painful peripheral neuropathy can substantially improve sleep quality.
- Treatment of primary sleep disorders, particularly OSA, improves seizure and headache control.
- Focal hypothalamic lesions from MS or brain tumours can cause narcolepsy and pontine lesions can cause REM behavioural disorder.
- Hypersomnia following TBI, at least in some individuals, may be mediated by transient functional disruption of the orexin-signalling pathways.

References

Aabad-Alegria, F., Lopez-Mallen, M.E. & De Francisco-Maqueda, P. (1997). Insomnia and somnolence in epilepsy. *Rev Neurol*, **25**, 1171–1172.

Aboussouan, L.S., Lewis, R.A. & Shy, M.E. (2007). Disorders of pulmonary function, sleep, and the upper airway in Charcot-Marie-Tooth disease. *Lung*, **185**, 1–7.

Afifi, A.K. & Bergman, R.A. (2005). *Functional Neuroanatomy: Text and Atlas*. New York, NY: Lange Medical Books.

Aldrich, M.S. & Chauncey, J.B. (1990). Are morning headaches part of obstructive sleep apnea syndrome? *Arch Intern Med*, **150**, 1265–1267.

Aletrino, M.A., Vogels, O.J., Van Domburg, P.H. & Ten Donkelaar, H.J. (1992). Cell loss in the nucleus raphes dorsalis in Alzheimer's disease. *Neurobiol Aging*, **13**, 461–468.

Alves, R.S., Resende, M.B., Skomro, R.P., Souza, F.J. & Reed, U.C. (2009). Sleep and neuromuscular disorders in children. *Sleep Med Rev*, **13**, 133–148.

Amino, A., Shiozawa, Z., Nagasaka, T., et al. (1998). Sleep apnoea in well-controlled myasthenia gravis and the effect of thymectomy. *J Neurol*, **245**, 77–80.

Ancoli-Israel, S., Martin, J.L., Kripke, D.F., Marler, M. & Klauber, M.R. (2002). Effect of light treatment on sleep and circadian rhythms in demented nursing home patients. *J Am Geriatr Soc*, **50**, 282–289.

Ancoli-Israel, S., Gehrman, P., Martin, J.L., et al. (2003). Increased light exposure consolidates sleep and strengthens circadian rhythms in severe Alzheimer's disease patients. *Behav Sleep Med*, **1**, 22–36.

Annane, D., Quera-Salva, M.A., Lofaso, F., et al. (1999). Mechanisms underlying effects of nocturnal ventilation on daytime blood gases in neuromuscular diseases. *Eur Respir J*, **13**, 157–162.

Arzt, M., Young, T., Finn, L., Skatrud, J.B. & Bradley, T.D. (2005). Association of sleep-disordered breathing and the occurrence of stroke. *Am J Respir Crit Care Med*, **172**, 1447–1451.

Asayama, K., Yamadera, H., Ito, T., Suzuki, H., Kudo, Y. & Endo, S. (2003). Double blind study of melatonin effects on the sleep-wake rhythm, cognitive and non-cognitive functions in Alzheimer type dementia. *J Nippon Med Sch*, **70**, 334–341.

Auer, R.N., Rowlands, C.G., Perry, S.F. & Remmers, J.E. (1996). Multiple sclerosis with medullary plaques and fatal sleep apnea (Ondine's curse). *Clin Neuropathol*, **15**, 101–105.

Ayalon, L., Borodkin, K., Dishon, L., Kanety, H. & Dagan, Y. (2007). Circadian rhythm sleep disorders following mild traumatic brain injury. *Neurology*, **68**, 1136–1140.

Backonja, M., Beydoun, A., Edwards, K.R., et al. (1998). Gabapentin for the symptomatic treatment of painful neuropathy in patients with diabetes mellitus: a randomized controlled trial. *JAMA*, **280**, 1831–1836.

Bamer, A.M., Johnson, K.L., Amtmann, D. & Kraft, G.H. (2008). Prevalence of sleep problems in individuals with multiple sclerosis. *Mult Scler*, **14**, 1127–1130.

Bassetti, C., Aldrich, M.S., Chervin, R.D. & Quint, D. (1996). Sleep apnea in patients with transient ischemic attack and stroke: a prospective study of 59 patients. *Neurology*, **47**, 1167–1173.

Bassetti, C.L., Milanova, M. & Gugger, M. (2006). Sleep-disordered breathing and acute ischemic stroke: diagnosis, risk factors, treatment, evolution, and long-term clinical outcome. *Stroke*, **37**, 967–972.

Baumann, C., Ferini-Strambi, L., Waldvogel, D., Werth, E. & Bassetti, C.L. (2005). Parkinsonism with excessive daytime sleepiness—a narcolepsy-like disorder? *J Neurol*, **252**, 139–145.

Baumann, C.R., Werth, E., Stocker, R., Ludwig, S. & Bassetti, C.L. (2007). Sleep-wake disturbances 6 months after traumatic brain injury: a prospective study. *Brain*, **130**, 1873–1883.

Baumann, C.R., Bassetti, C.L., Valko, P.O., et al. (2009). Loss of hypocretin (orexin) neurons with traumatic brain injury. *Ann Neurol*, **66**, 555–559.

Bazil, C.W., Castro, L.H. & Walczak, T.S. (2000). Reduction of rapid eye movement sleep by diurnal and nocturnal seizures in temporal lobe epilepsy. *Arch Neurol*, **57**, 363–368.

Beelke, M., Angeli, S., Del Sette, M., et al. (2002). Obstructive sleep apnea can be provocative for right-to-left shunting through a patent foramen ovale. *Sleep*, **25**, 856–862.

Benditt, J.O. (2009). Initiating noninvasive management of respiratory insufficiency in neuromuscular disease. *Pediatrics*, **123**(Suppl 4), S236–S238.

Bensmail, D., Quera Salva, M.A., Roche, N., et al. (2006). Effect of intrathecal baclofen on sleep and respiratory function in patients with spasticity. *Neurology*, **67**, 1432–1436.

Bianchetti, A., Scuratti, A., Zanetti, O., et al. (1995). Predictors of mortality and institutionalization in Alzheimer disease patients 1 year after discharge from an Alzheimer dementia unit. *Dementia*, **6**, 108–112.

Blau, J.N. (1990). Sleep deprivation headache. *Cephalalgia*, **10**, 157–160.

Bliwise, D.L., Yesavage, J.A., Tinklenberg, J.R. & Dement, W.C. (1989). Sleep apnea in Alzheimer's disease. *Neurobiol Aging*, **10**, 343–346.

Bloomfield, I.L., Espie, C.A. & Evans, J.J. (2009). Do sleep difficulties exacerbate deficits in sustained attention following traumatic brain injury? *J Int Neuropsychol, Soc*, **16**, 17–25.

Boddy, F., Rowan, E.N., Lett, D., O'Brien, J.T., McKeith, I.G. & Burn, D.J. (2007). Subjectively reported sleep quality and excessive daytime somnolence in Parkinson's disease with and without dementia, dementia with Lewy bodies and Alzheimer's disease. *Int J Geriatr Psychiatry*, **22**, 529–535.

Boeve, B.F., Silber, M.H., Saper, C.B., et al. (2007). Pathophysiology of REM sleep behaviour disorder and relevance to neurodegenerative disease. *Brain*, **130**, 2770–2788.

Bonanni, E., Maestri, M., Tognoni, G., et al. (2005). Daytime sleepiness in mild and moderate Alzheimer's disease and its relationship with cognitive impairment. *J Sleep Res*, **14**, 311–317.

Bottini, P., Redolfi, S., Dottorini, M.L. & Tantucci, C. (2008). Autonomic neuropathy increases the risk of obstructive sleep apnea in obese diabetics. *Respiration*, **75**, 265–271.

Bourke, S.C., Tomlinson, M., Williams, T.L., Bullock, R.E., Shaw, P.J. & Gibson, G.J. (2006). Effects of non-invasive ventilation on survival and quality of life in patients with amyotrophic lateral sclerosis: a randomised controlled trial. *Lancet Neurol*, **5**, 140–147.

Brass, S.D., Duquette, P., Proulx-Therrien, J. & Auerbach, S. (2010). Sleep disorders in patients with multiple sclerosis. *Sleep Med Rev*, **14**, 121–129.

Bye, P.T., Ellis, E.R., Issa, F.G., Donnelly, P.M. & Sullivan, C.E. (1990). Respiratory failure and sleep in neuromuscular disease. *Thorax*, **45**, 241–247.

Campbell, S.S., Kripke, D.F., Gillin, J.C. & Hrubovcak, J.C. (1988). Exposure to light in healthy elderly subjects and Alzheimer's patients. *Physiol Behav*, **42**, 141–144.

Castriotta, R.J., Atanasov, S., Wilde, M.C., Masel, B.E., Lai, J.M. & Kuna, S.T. (2009). Treatment of sleep disorders after traumatic brain injury. *J Clin Sleep Med*, **5**, 137–144.

Chan-Palay, V. (1990). Neuronal communication breakdown in neurotransmitter systems in Alzheimer's and Parkinson's dementias. *J Neurocytol*, **19**, 802–806.

Chen, J.C., Borson, S. & Scanlan, J.M. (2000). Stage-specific prevalence of behavioral symptoms in Alzheimer's disease in a multi-ethnic community sample. *Am J Geriatr Psychiatry*, **8**, 123–133.

Chervin, R.D., Dillon, J.E., Bassetti, C., Ganoczy, D.A. & Pituch, K.J. (1997). Symptoms of sleep disorders, inattention, and hyperactivity in children. *Sleep*, **20**, 1185–1192.

Chervin, R.D., Zallek, S.N., Lin, X., Hall, J.M., Sharma, N. & Hedger, K.M. (2000). Sleep disordered breathing in patients with cluster headache. *Neurology*, **54**, 2302–2306.

Colenda, C.C., Cohen, W., McCall, W.V. & Rosenquist, P.B. (1997). Phototherapy for patients with Alzheimer disease with disturbed sleep patterns: results of a community-based pilot study. *Alzheimer Dis Assoc Disord*, **11**, 175–178.

Corkum, P., Panton, R., Ironside, S., MacPherson, M. & Williams, T. (2008). Acute impact of immediate release methylphenidate administered three times a day on sleep in children with attention-deficit/hyperactivity disorder. *J Pediatr Psychol*, **33**, 368–379.

Cortese, S., Konofal, E., Lecendreux, M., et al. (2005). Restless legs syndrome and attention-deficit/hyperactivity disorder: a review of the literature. *Sleep*, **28**, 1007–1013.

Cortese, S., Faraone, S.V., Konofal, E. & Lecendreux, M. (2009). Sleep in children with attention-deficit/hyperactivity disorder: meta-analysis of subjective and objective studies. *J Am Acad Child Adolesc Psychiatry*, **48**, 894–908.

Craig, D., Hart, D.J. & Passmore, A.P. (2006). Genetically increased risk of sleep disruption in Alzheimer's disease. *Sleep*, **29**, 1003–1007.

Crowley, K., Sullivan, E.V., Adalsteinsson, E., Pfefferbaum, A. & Colrain, I.M. (2005). Differentiating pathologic delta from healthy physiologic delta in patients with Alzheimer disease. *Sleep*, **28**, 865–870.

Dang-Vu, T.T., Desseilles, M., Peigneux, P. & Maquet, P. (2006). A role for sleep in brain plasticity. *Pediatr Rehabil*, **9**, 98–118.

De Barros-Ferreira, M., Chodkiewicz, J.P., Lairy, G.C. & Salzarulo, P. (1975). Disorganized relations of tonic and phasic events of REM sleep in a case of brain-stem tumour. *Electroencephalogr Clin Neurophysiol*, **38**, 203–207.

de Miguel-Diez, J., Villa-Asensi, J.R. & Alvarez-Sala, J.L. (2003). Prevalence of sleep-disordered breathing in children with Down syndrome: polygraphic findings in 108 children. *Sleep*, **26**, 1006–1009.

Devereaux, M.W., Keane, J.R. & Davis, R.L. (1973). Automatic respiratory failure associated with infarction of the medulla. Report of two cases with pathologic study of one. *Arch Neurol*, **29**, 46–52.

Devinsky, O., Ehrenberg, B., Barthlen, G.M., Abramson, H.S. & Luciano, D. (1994). Epilepsy and sleep apnea syndrome. *Neurology*, **44**, 2060–2064.

Dexter, J.D. (1979). The relationship between stage III + IV + REM sleep and arousals with migraine. *Headache*, **19**, 364–369.

Di Gennaro, G., Autret, A., Mascia, A., Onorati, P., Sebastiano, F. & Paolo Quarato, P. (2004). Night terrors associated with thalamic lesion. *Clin Neurophysiol*, **115**, 2489–2492.

Diederich, N.J., Vaillant, M., Leischen, M., et al. (2005). Sleep apnea syndrome in Parkinson's disease. A case-control study in 49 patients. *Mov Disord*, **20**, 1413–1418.

Dodick, D.W., Eross, E.J., Parish, J.M. & Silber, M. (2003). Clinical, anatomical, and physiologic relationship between sleep and headache. *Headache*, **43**, 282–292.

Dowling, G.A., Mastick, J., Hubbard, E.M., Luxenberg, J.S. & Burr, R.L. (2005). Effect of timed bright light treatment for rest-activity disruption in institutionalized patients with Alzheimer's disease. *Int J Geriatr Psychiatry*, **20**, 738–743.

Dowling, G.A., Graf, C.L., Hubbard, E.M. & Luxenberg, J.S. (2007). Light treatment for neuropsychiatric behaviors in Alzheimer's disease. *West J Nurs Res*, **29**, 961–975.

Dowling, G.A., Burr, R.L., Van Someren, E.J., et al. (2008). Melatonin and bright-light treatment for rest-activity disruption in institutionalized patients with Alzheimer's disease. *J Am Geriatr Soc*, **56**, 239–246.

Drake, M.E., Jr., Weate, S.J., Newell, S.A., Padamadan, H. & Pakalnis, A. (1994). Multiple sleep latency tests in epilepsy. *Clin Electroencephalogr*, **25**, 59–62.

Dyken, M.E., Somers, V.K., Yamada, T., Ren, Z.Y. & Zimmerman, M.B. (1996). Investigating the relationship between stroke and obstructive sleep apnea. *Stroke*, **27**, 401–407.

Dziewas, R., Waldmann, N., Bontert, M., et al. (2008). Increased prevalence of obstructive sleep apnoea in patients with Charcot-Marie-Tooth disease: a case control study. *J Neurol Neurosurg Psychiatry*, **79**, 829–831.

Ellis, E.R., Bye, P.T., Bruderer, J.W. & Sullivan, C.E. (1987). Treatment of respiratory failure during sleep in patients with neuromuscular disease. Positive-pressure ventilation through a nose mask. *Am Rev Respir Dis*, **135**, 148–152.

Epstein, A.W. (1964). Recurrent dreams; their relationship to temporal lobe seizures. *Arch Gen Psychiatry*, **10**, 25–30.

Erdemoglu, A.K. & Varlibas, A. (2006). Effectiveness of oxcarbazepine in symptomatic treatment of painful diabetic neuropathy. *Neurol India*, **54**, 173–177; discussion 177.

Ferman, T.J., Smith, G.E., Boeve, B.F., et al. (2004). DLB fluctuations: specific features that reliably differentiate DLB from AD and normal aging. *Neurology*, **62**, 181–187.

Fetveit, A., Skjerve, A. & Bjorvatn, B. (2003). Bright light treatment improves sleep in institutionalised elderly—an open trial. *Int J Geriatr Psychiatry*, **18**, 520–526.

Foldvary-Schaefer, N. (2002). Sleep complaints and epilepsy: the role of seizures, antiepileptic drugs and sleep disorders. *J Clin Neurophysiol*, **19**, 514–521.

Foldvary-Schaefer, N. & Grigg-Damberger, M. (2009). Sleep and epilepsy. *Semin Neurol*, **29**, 419–428.

Freeman, R., Raskin, P., Hewitt, D.J., et al. (2007). Randomized study of tramadol/acetaminophen versus placebo in painful diabetic peripheral neuropathy. *Curr Med Res Opin*, **23**, 147–161.

Freeman, R., Durso-Decruz, E. & Emir, B. (2008). Efficacy, safety, and tolerability of pregabalin treatment for painful diabetic peripheral neuropathy: findings from seven randomized, controlled trials across a range of doses. *Diabetes Care*, **31**, 1448–1454.

Frey, D.J., Fleshner, M. & Wright, K.P., Jr. (2007). The effects of 40 hours of total sleep deprivation on inflammatory markers in healthy young adults. *Brain Behav Immun*, **21**, 1050–1057.

Fronczek, R., Overeem, S., Lee, S.Y., et al. (2007). Hypocretin (orexin) loss in Parkinson's disease. *Brain*, **130**, 1577–1585.

Gami, A.S., Pressman, G., Caples, S.M., et al. (2004). Association of atrial fibrillation and obstructive sleep apnea. *Circulation*, **110**, 364–367.

Gehrman, P.R., Martin, J.L., Shochat, T., Nolan, S., Corey-Bloom, J. & Ancoli-Israel, S. (2003). Sleep-disordered breathing and agitation in institutionalized adults with Alzheimer disease. *Am J Geriatr Psychiatry*, **11**, 426–433.

Gehrman, P.R., Connor, D.J., Martin, J.L., Shochat, T., Corey-Bloom, J. & Ancoli-Israel, S. (2009). Melatonin fails to improve sleep or agitation in double-blind randomized placebo-controlled trial of institutionalized patients with Alzheimer disease. *Am J Geriatr Psychiatry*, **17**, 166–169.

Gjerstad, M.D., Wentzel-Larsen, T., Aarsland, D. & Larsen, J.P. (2007). Insomnia in Parkinson's disease: frequency and progression over time. *J Neurol Neurosurg Psychiatry*, **78**, 476–479.

Golan, N., Shahar, E., Ravid, S. & Pillar, G. (2004). Sleep disorders and daytime sleepiness in children with attention-deficit/hyperactive disorder. *Sleep*, **27**, 261–266.

Goldman, S.E., Malow, B.A., Newman, K.D., Roof, E. & Dykens, E.M. (2009). Sleep patterns and daytime sleepiness in adolescents and young adults with Williams syndrome. *J Intellect Disabil Res*, **53**, 182–188.

Gomez-Choco, M.J., Iranzo, A., Blanco, Y., Graus, F., Santamaria, J. & Saiz, A. (2007). Prevalence of restless legs syndrome and REM sleep behavior disorder in multiple sclerosis. *Mult Scler*, **13**, 805–808.

Good, D.C., Henkle, J.Q., Gelber, D., Welsh, J. & Verhulst, S. (1996). Sleep-disordered breathing and poor functional outcome after stroke. *Stroke*, **27**, 252–259.

Goodlin-Jones, B., Schwichtenberg, A.J., Iosif, A.M., Tang, K., Liu, J. & Anders, T.F. (2009). Six-month persistence of sleep problems in young children with autism, developmental delay, and typical development. *J Am Acad Child Adolesc Psychiatry*, **48**, 847–854.

Grace, J.B., Walker, M.P. & McKeith, I.G. (2000). A comparison of sleep profiles in patients with dementia with Lewy bodies and Alzheimer's disease. *Int J Geriatr Psychiatry*, **15**, 1028–1033.

Greenough, G., Sateia, M. & Fadul, C.E. (1999). Obstructive sleep apnea syndrome in a patient with medulloblastoma. *Neuro Oncol*, **1**, 289–291.

Guilleminault, C., Philip, P. & Robinson, A. (1998). Sleep and neuromuscular disease: bilevel positive airway pressure by nasal mask as a treatment for sleep disordered breathing in patients with neuromuscular disease. *J Neurol Neurosurg Psychiatry*, **65**, 225–232.

Haffmans, P.M., Sival, R.C., Lucius, S.A., Cats, Q. & Van Gelder, L. (2001). Bright light therapy and melatonin in motor restless behaviour in dementia: a placebo-controlled study. *Int J Geriatr Psychiatry*, **16**, 106–110.

Harbison, J., Ford, G.A., James, O.F. & Gibson, G.J. (2002). Sleep-disordered breathing following acute stroke. *QJM*, **95**, 741–747.

Harper, D.G., Stopa, E.G., McKee, A.C., Satlin, A., Fish, D. & Volicer, L. (2004). Dementia severity and Lewy bodies affect circadian rhythms in Alzheimer disease. *Neurobiol Aging*, **25**, 771–781.

Harper, D.G., Volicer, L., Stopa, E.G., McKee, A.C., Nitta, M. & Satlin, A. (2005). Disturbance of endogenous circadian rhythm in aging and Alzheimer disease. *Am J Geriatr Psychiatry*, **13**, 359–368.

Hart, D.J., Craig, D., Compton, S.A., et al. (2003). A retrospective study of the behavioural and psychological symptoms of mid and late phase Alzheimer's disease. *Int J Geriatr Psychiatry*, **18**, 1037–1042.

Hauser, W.A., Annegers, J.F. & Kurland, L.T. (1993). Incidence of epilepsy and unprovoked seizures in Rochester, Minnesota: 1935-1984. *Epilepsia*, **34**, 453–468.

Heckmatt, J.Z., Loh, L. & Dubowitz, V. (1990). Night-time nasal ventilation in neuromuscular disease. *Lancet*, **335**, 579–582.

Hirsch, E.C., Graybiel, A.M., Duyckaerts, C. & Javoy-Agid, F. (1987). Neuronal loss in the pedunculopontine tegmental nucleus in Parkinson disease and in progressive supranuclear palsy. *Proc Natl Acad Sci U S A*, **84**, 5976–5980.

Hobson, J.A. (2005). Sleep is of the brain, by the brain and for the brain. *Nature*, **437**, 1254–1256.

Hoeppner, J.B., Garron, D.C. & Cartwright, R.D. (1984). Self-reported sleep disorder symptoms in epilepsy. *Epilepsia*, **25**, 434–437.

Hornyak, M., Cejnar, M., Elam, M., Matousek, M. & Wallin, B.G. (1991). Sympathetic muscle nerve activity during sleep in man. *Brain*, **114**(Pt 3), 1281–1295.

Huang, Y.S., Guilleminault, C., Li, H.Y., Yang, C.M., Wu, Y.Y. & Chen, N.H. (2007). Attention-deficit/hyperactivity disorder with obstructive sleep apnea: a treatment outcome study. *Sleep Med*, **8**, 18–30.

Iannaccone, S., Zucconi, M., Marchettini, P., et al. (1995). Evidence of peripheral axonal neuropathy in primary restless legs syndrome. *Mov Disord*, **10**, 2–9.

Ingrassia, A. & Turk, J. (2005). The use of clonidine for severe and intractable sleep problems in children with neurodevelopmental disorders—a case series. *Eur Child Adolesc Psychiatry*, **14**, 34–40.

Ito, K., Murofushi, T., Mizuno, M. & Semba, T. (1996). Pediatric brain stem gliomas with the predominant symptom of sleep apnea. *Int J Pediatr Otorhinolaryngol*, **37**, 53–64.

Ito, T., Yamadera, H., Ito, R., Suzuki, H., Asayama, K. & Endo, S. (2001). Effects of vitamin B12 on bright light on cognitive and sleep-wake rhythm in Alzheimer-type dementia. *Psychiatry Clin Neurosci*, **55**, 281–282.

Jennum, P. & Sjol, A. (1994). Self-assessed cognitive function in snorers and sleep apneics. An epidemiological study of 1,504 females and males aged 30-60 years: the Dan-MONICA II Study. *Eur Neurol*, **34**, 204–208.

Kang, J.E., Lim, M.M., Bateman, R.J., et al. (2009). Amyloid-{beta} dynamics are regulated by orexin and the sleep-wake cycle. *Science*, **326**, 1005–1007.

Kaynak, H., Altintas, A., Kaynak, D., et al. (2006). Fatigue and sleep disturbance in multiple sclerosis. *Eur J Neurol*, **13**, 1333–1339.

Kelsey, C.R. & Marks, L.B. (2006). Somnolence syndrome after focal radiation therapy to the pineal region: case report and review of the literature. *J Neurooncol*, **78**, 153–156.

Kerby, G.R., Mayer, L.S. & Pingleton, S.K. (1987). Nocturnal positive pressure ventilation via nasal mask. *Am Rev Respir Dis*, **135**, 738–740.

Kish, S.J., Tong, J., Hornykiewicz, O., et al. (2008). Preferential loss of serotonin markers in caudate versus putamen in Parkinson's disease. *Brain*, **131**, 120–131.

Klingelhofer, J., Hajak, G., Sander, D., Schulz-Varszegi, M., Ruther, E. & Conrad, B. (1992). Assessment of intracranial hemodynamics in sleep apnea syndrome. *Stroke*, **23**, 1427–1433.

Konofal, E., Cortese, S., Marchand, M., Mouren, M.C., Arnulf, I. & Lecendreux, M. (2007). Impact of restless legs syndrome and iron deficiency on attention-deficit/hyperactivity disorder in children. *Sleep Med*, **8**, 711–715.

Koyama, E., Matsubara, H. & Nakano, T. (1999). Bright light treatment for sleep-wake disturbances in aged individuals with dementia. *Psychiatry Clin Neurosci*, **53**, 227–229.

Krachman, S.L., Criner, G.J. & Chatila, W. (2003). Cor pulmonale and sleep-disordered breathing in patients with restrictive lung disease and neuromuscular disorders. *Semin Respir Crit Care Med*, **24**, 297–306.

Labanowski, M., Schmidt-Nowara, W. & Guilleminault, C. (1996). Sleep and neuromuscular disease: frequency of sleep-disordered breathing in a neuromuscular disease clinic population. *Neurology*, **47**, 1173–1180.

Lee, J.H., Friedland, R., Whitehouse, P.J. & Woo, J.I. (2004). Twenty-four-hour rhythms of sleep-wake cycle and temperature in Alzheimer's disease. *J Neuropsychiatry Clin Neurosci*, **16**, 192–198.

Lee, J.H., Bliwise, D.L., Ansari, F.P., et al. (2007). Daytime sleepiness and functional impairment in Alzheimer disease. *Am J Geriatr Psychiatry*, **15**, 620–626.

Lee, K.S., Higgins, M.J., Patel, B.M., Larson, J.S. & Rady, M.Y. (2006). Paraneoplastic coma and acquired central alveolar hypoventilation as a manifestation of brainstem encephalitis in a patient with ANNA-1 antibody and small-cell lung cancer. *Neurocrit Care*, **4**, 137–139.

Liu, R.Y., Zhou, J.N., Van Heerikhuize, J., Hofman, M.A. & Swaab, D.F. (1999). Decreased melatonin levels in postmortem cerebrospinal fluid in relation to aging, Alzheimer's disease, and apolipoprotein E-epsilon4/4 genotype. *J Clin Endocrinol Metab*, **84**, 323–327.

Liu, X., Hubbard, J.A., Fabes, R.A. & Adam, J.B. (2006). Sleep disturbances and correlates of children with autism spectrum disorders. *Child Psychiatry Hum Dev*, **37**, 179–191.

Lloyd-Jones, D., Adams, R., Carnethon, M., et al. (2009). Heart disease and stroke statistics—2009 update: a report from the American Heart Association Statistics Committee and Stroke Statistics Subcommittee. *Circulation*, **119**, 480–486.

Loo, H.V. & Tan, E.K. (2008). Case-control study of restless legs syndrome and quality of sleep in Parkinson's disease. *J Neurol Sci*, **266**, 145–149.

Lovell, B.B., Ancoli-Israel, S. & Gevirtz, R. (1995). Effect of bright light treatment on agitated behavior in institutionalized elderly subjects. *Psychiatry Res*, **57**, 7–12.

Lyketsos, C.G., Lindell Veiel, L., Baker, A. & Steele, C. (1999). A randomized, controlled trial of bright light therapy for agitated behaviors in dementia patients residing in long-term care. *Int J Geriatr Psychiatry*, **14**, 520–525.

Lyketsos, C.G., Lopez, O., Jones, B., Fitzpatrick, A.L., Breitner, J. & Dekosky, S. (2002). Prevalence of neuropsychiatric symptoms in dementia and mild cognitive impairment: results from the cardiovascular health study. *JAMA*, **288**, 1475–1483.

Lyons, H.A. (1971). Another curse of Ondine. *Chest*, **59**, 590–591.

Makley, M.J., English, J.B., Drubach, D.A., Kreuz, A.J., Celnik, P.A. & Tarwater, P.M. (2008). Prevalence of sleep disturbance in closed head injury patients in a rehabilitation unit. *Neurorehabil Neural Repair*, **22**, 341–347.

Makley, M.J., Johnson-Greene, L., Tarwater, P.M., et al. (2009). Return of memory and sleep efficiency following moderate to severe closed head injury. *Neurorehabil Neural Repair*, **23**, 320–326.

Malow, B.A., Bowes, R.J. & Lin, X. (1997a). Predictors of sleepiness in epilepsy patients. *Sleep*, **20**, 1105–1110.

Malow, B.A., Fromes, G.A. & Aldrich, M.S. (1997b). Usefulness of polysomnography in epilepsy patients. *Neurology*, **48**, 1389–1394.

Malow, B.A., Levy, K., Maturen, K. & Bowes, R. (2000). Obstructive sleep apnea is common in medically refractory epilepsy patients. *Neurology*, **55**, 1002–1007.

Manconi, M., Ferini-Strambi, L., Filippi, M., et al. (2008a). Multicenter case-control study on restless legs syndrome in multiple sclerosis: the REMS study. *Sleep*, **31**, 944–952.

Manconi, M., Rocca, M.A., Ferini-Strambi, L., et al. (2008b). Restless legs syndrome is a common finding in multiple sclerosis and correlates with cervical cord damage. *Mult Scler*, **14**, 86–93.

Manni, R., Pacchetti, C., Terzaghi, M., Sartori, I., Mancini, F. & Nappi, G. (2002). Hallucinations and sleep-wake cycle in PD: a 24-hour continuous polysomnographic study. *Neurology*, **59**, 1979–1981.

Maquet, P. (2001). The role of sleep in learning and memory. *Science*, **294**, 1048–1052.

Marcus, C.L., Trescher, W.H., Halbower, A.C. & Lutz, J. (2002). Secondary narcolepsy in children with brain tumors. *Sleep*, **25**, 435–439.

Martin, J., Marler, M., Shochat, T. & Ancoli-Israel, S. (2000). Circadian rhythms of agitation in institutionalized patients with Alzheimer's disease. *Chronobiol Int*, **17**, 405–418.

McCarty, S.F., Gaebler-Spira, D. & Harvey, R.L. (2001). Improvement of sleep apnea in a patient with cerebral palsy. *Am J Phys Med Rehabil*, **80**, 540–542.

McCurry, S.M., Logsdon, R.G., Teri, L., et al. (1999). Characteristics of sleep disturbance in community-dwelling Alzheimer's disease patients. *J Geriatr Psychiatry Neurol*, **12**, 53–59.

McCurry, S.M., Gibbons, L.E., Logsdon, R.G., Vitiello, M.V. & Teri, L. (2005). Nighttime insomnia treatment and education for Alzheimer's disease: a randomized, controlled trial. *J Am Geriatr Soc*, **53**, 793–802.

Medeiros, C.A., Carvalhedo De Bruin, P.F., Lopes, L.A., et al. (2007). Effect of exogenous melatonin on sleep and motor dysfunction in Parkinson's disease. A randomized, double blind, placebo-controlled study. *J Neurol*, **254**, 459–464.

Meltzer, L.J. & Moore, M. (2008). Sleep disruptions in parents of children and adolescents with chronic illnesses: prevalence, causes, and consequences. *J Pediatr Psychol*, **33**, 279–291.

Mendez, M. & Radtke, R.A. (2001). Interactions between sleep and epilepsy. *J Clin Neurophysiol*, **18**, 106–127.

Merlino, G., Fratticci, L., Lenchig, C., et al. (2009). Prevalence of 'poor sleep' among patients with multiple sclerosis: an independent predictor of mental and physical status. *Sleep Med*, **10**, 26–34.

Micallef, J., Rey, M., Eusebio, A., et al. (2009). Antiparkinsonian drug-induced sleepiness: a double-blind placebo-controlled study of L-dopa, bromocriptine and pramipexole in healthy subjects. *Br J Clin Pharmacol*, **67**, 333–340.

Mishima, K., Hishikawa, Y. & Okawa, M. (1998). Randomized, dim light controlled, crossover test of morning bright light therapy for rest-activity rhythm disorders in patients with vascular dementia and dementia of Alzheimer's type. *Chronobiol Int*, **15**, 647–654.

Mishima, K., Tozawa, T., Satoh, K., Matsumoto, Y., Hishikawa, Y. & Okawa, M. (1999). Melatonin secretion rhythm disorders in patients with senile dementia of Alzheimer's type with disturbed sleep-waking. *Biol Psychiatry*, **45**, 417–421.

Mohsenin, V. & Valor, R. (1995). Sleep apnea in patients with hemispheric stroke. *Arch Phys Med Rehabil*, **76**, 71–76.

Montplaisir, J., Petit, D., Lorrain, D., Gauthier, S. & Nielsen, T. (1995). Sleep in Alzheimer's disease: further considerations on the role of brainstem and forebrain cholinergic populations in sleep-wake mechanisms. *Sleep*, **18**, 145–148.

Montplaisir, J., Petit, D., Gauthier, S., Gaudreau, H. & Decary, A. (1998). Sleep disturbances and EEG slowing in Alzheimer's disease. *Sleep Res Online*, **1**, 147–151.

Morton, A.J., Wood, N.I., Hastings, M.H., Hurelbrink, C., Barker, R.A. & Maywood, E.S. (2005). Disintegration of the sleep-wake cycle and circadian timing in Huntington's disease. *J Neurosci*, **25**, 157–163.

Mufson, E.J., Mash, D.C. & Hersh, L.B. (1988). Neurofibrillary tangles in cholinergic pedunculopontine neurons in Alzheimer's disease. *Ann Neurol*, **24**, 623–629.

Munoz, R., Duran-Cantolla, J., Martinez-Vila, E., et al. (2006). Severe sleep apnea and risk of ischemic stroke in the elderly. *Stroke*, **37**, 2317–2321.

Nagtegaal, J.E., Kerkhof, G.A., Smits, M.G., Swart, A.C. & Van Der Meer, Y.G. (1997). Traumatic brain injury-associated delayed sleep phase syndrome. *Funct Neurol*, **12**, 345–348.

Newman, C.J., O'Regan, M. & Hensey, O. (2006). Sleep disorders in children with cerebral palsy. *Dev Med Child Neurol*, **48**, 564–568.

Nineb, A., Rosso, C., Dumurgier, J., Nordine, T., Lefaucheur, J.P. & Creange, A. (2007). Restless legs syndrome is frequently overlooked in patients being evaluated for polyneuropathies. *Eur J Neurol*, **14**, 788–792.

Nishino, S. & Kanbayashi, T. (2005). Symptomatic narcolepsy, cataplexy and hypersomnia, and their implications in the hypothalamic hypocretin/orexin system. *Sleep Med Rev*, **9**, 269–310.

Norrbrink, C. (2009). Transcutaneous electrical nerve stimulation for treatment of spinal cord injury neuropathic pain. *J Rehabil Res Dev*, **46**, 85–93.

Ohadinia, S., Noroozian, M., Shahsavand, S. & Saghafi, S. (2004). Evaluation of insomnia and daytime napping in Iranian Alzheimer disease patients: relationship with severity of dementia and comparison with normal adults. *Am J Geriatr Psychiatry*, **12**, 517–522.

Ohayon, M.M. (2004). Prevalence and risk factors of morning headaches in the general population. *Arch Intern Med*, **164**, 97–102.

Oka, Y., Kanbayashi, T., Mezaki, T., et al. (2004). Low CSF hypocretin-1/orexin-A associated with hypersomnia secondary to hypothalamic lesion in a case of multiple sclerosis. *J Neurol*, **251**, 885–886.

Oliveira, A.J., Zamagni, M., Dolso, P., Bassetti, M.A. & Gigli, G.L. (2000). Respiratory disorders during sleep in patients with epilepsy: effect of ventilatory therapy on EEG interictal epileptiform discharges. *Clin Neurophysiol*, **111**(Suppl 2), S141–S145.

Onen, S.H., Alloui, A., Gross, A., Eschallier, A. & Dubray, C. (2001). The effects of total sleep deprivation, selective sleep interruption and sleep recovery on pain tolerance thresholds in healthy subjects. *J Sleep Res*, **10**, 35–42.

Owens, J. & Palermo, T. (2008). Introduction to the special issue: sleep in children with neurodevelopmental and psychiatric disorders. *J Pediatr Psychol*, **33**, 335–338.

Paiva, T., Farinha, A., Martins, A., Batista, A. & Guilleminault, C. (1997). Chronic headaches and sleep disorders. *Arch Intern Med*, **157**, 1701–1705.

Paparrigopoulos, T., Melissaki, A., Tsekou, H., et al. (2006). Melatonin secretion after head injury: a pilot study. *Brain Inj*, **20**, 873–878.

Parra, O., Arboix, A., Bechich, S., et al. (2000). Time course of sleep-related breathing disorders in first-ever stroke or transient ischemic attack. *Am J Respir Crit Care Med*, **161**, 375–380.

Partinen, M. & Palomaki, H. (1985). Snoring and cerebral infarction. *Lancet*, **2**, 1325–1326.

Patil, S.P., Schneider, H., Marx, J.J., Gladmon, E., Schwartz, A.R. & Smith, P.L. (2007). Neuromechanical control of upper airway patency during sleep. *J Appl Physiol*, **102**, 547–556.

Patten, S.B. & Lauderdale, W.M. (1992). Delayed sleep phase disorder after traumatic brain injury. *J Am Acad Child Adolesc Psychiatry*, **31**, 100–102.

Pedley, T.A. (1983). Differential diagnosis of episodic symptoms. *Epilepsia*, **24**(Suppl 1), S31–S44.

Peppard, P.E., Young, T., Palta, M. & Skatrud, J. (2000). Prospective study of the association between sleep-disordered breathing and hypertension. *N Engl J Med*, **342**, 1378–1384.

Phillips, L. & Appleton, R.E. (2004). Systematic review of melatonin treatment in children with neurodevelopmental disabilities and sleep impairment. *Dev Med Child Neurol*, **46**, 771–775.

Plazzi, G., Tinuper, P., Montagna, P., Provini, F. & Lugaresi, E. (1995). Epileptic nocturnal wanderings. *Sleep*, **18**, 749–756.

Poceta, J.S. & Dalessio, D.J. (1995). Identification and treatment of sleep apnea in patients with chronic headache. *Headache*, **35**, 586–589.

Press, D.Z. (2004). Parkinson's disease dementia—a first step? *N Engl J Med*, **351**, 2547–2549.

Prinz, P.N., Vitaliano, P.P., Vitiello, M.V., et al. (1982). Sleep, EEG and mental function changes in senile dementia of the Alzheimer's type. *Neurobiol Aging*, **3**, 361–370.

Provini, F., Plazzi, G., Tinuper, P., Vandi, S., Lugaresi, E. & Montagna, P. (1999). Nocturnal frontal lobe epilepsy. A clinical and polygraphic overview of 100 consecutive cases. *Brain*, **122**(Pt 6), 1017–1031.

Prudlo, J., Koenig, J., Ermert, S. & Juhasz, J. (2007). Sleep disordered breathing in medically stable patients with myasthenia gravis. *Eur J Neurol*, **14**, 321–326.

Quinto, C., Gellido, C., Chokroverty, S. & Masdeu, J. (2000). Posttraumatic delayed sleep phase syndrome. *Neurology*, **54**, 250–252.

Ragette, R., Mellies, U., Schwake, C., Voit, T. & Teschler, H. (2002). Patterns and predictors of sleep disordered breathing in primary myopathies. *Thorax*, **57**, 724–728.

Rains, J.C. & Poceta, J.S. (2005). Sleep-related headache syndromes. *Semin Neurol*, **25**, 69–80.

Rauchs, G., Schabus, M., Parapatics, S., et al. (2008). Is there a link between sleep changes and memory in Alzheimer's disease? *Neuroreport*, **19**, 1159–1162.

Reppert, S.M. & Weaver, D.R. (2002). Coordination of circadian timing in mammals. *Nature*, **418**, 935–941.

Riemersma-van der Lek, R.F., Swaab, D.F., Twisk, J., Hol, E.M., Hoogendijk, W.J. & Van Someren, E.J. (2008). Effect of bright light and melatonin on cognitive and noncognitive function in elderly residents of group care facilities: a randomized controlled trial. *JAMA*, **299**, 2642–2655.

Rizvi, S.S., Ishikawa, S., Faling, L.J., Schlessinger, L., Satia, J. & Seckel, B. (1974). Defect in automatic respiration in a case of multiple sclerosis. *Am J Med*, **56**, 433–436.

Rocamora, R., Sanchez-Alvarez, J.C. & Salas-Puig, J. (2008). The relationship between sleep and epilepsy. *Neurologist*, **14**, S35–S43.

Rocca, W.A., Hofman, A., Brayne, C., et al. (1991). Frequency and distribution of Alzheimer's disease in Europe: a collaborative study of 1980-1990 prevalence findings. The EURODEM-Prevalence Research Group. *Ann Neurol*, **30**, 381–390.

Ron, S., Algom, D., Hary, D. & Cohen, M. (1980). Time-related changes in the distribution of sleep stages in brain injured patients. *Electroencephalogr Clin Neurophysiol*, **48**, 432–441.

Rubinsztein, J.S., Rubinsztein, D.C., Goodburn, S. & Holland, A.J. (1998). Apathy and hypersomnia are common features of myotonic dystrophy. *J Neurol Neurosurg Psychiatry*, **64**, 510–515.

Rutkove, S.B., Matheson, J.K. & Logigian, E.L. (1996). Restless legs syndrome in patients with polyneuropathy. *Muscle Nerve*, **19**, 670–672.

Sahlin, C., Sandberg, O., Gustafson, Y., et al. (2008). Obstructive sleep apnea is a risk factor for death in patients with stroke: a 10–year follow-up. *Arch Intern Med*, **168**, 297–301.

Sahota, P.K. & Dexter, J.D. (1990). Sleep and headache syndromes: a clinical review. *Headache*, **30**, 80–84.

Sammaritano, M., Gigli, G.L. & Gotman, J. (1991). Interictal spiking during wakefulness and sleep and the localization of foci in temporal lobe epilepsy. *Neurology*, **41**, 290–297.

Saper, C.B., Scammell, T.E. & Lu, J. (2005). Hypothalamic regulation of sleep and circadian rhythms. *Nature*, **437**, 1257–1263.

Satlin, A., Volicer, L., Ross, V., Herz, L. & Campbell, S. (1992). Bright light treatment of behavioral and sleep disturbances in patients with Alzheimer's disease. *Am J Psychiatry*, **149**, 1028–1032.

Savage, V.M. & West, G.B. (2007). A quantitative, theoretical framework for understanding mammalian sleep. *Proc Natl Acad Sci USA*, **104**, 1051–1056.

Scheer, F.A., Zeitzer, J.M., Ayas, N.T., Brown, R., Czeisler, C.A. & Shea, S.A. (2006). Reduced sleep efficiency in cervical spinal cord injury; association with abolished night time melatonin secretion. *Spinal Cord*, **44**, 78–81.

Seeley, W.W., Crawford, R.K., Zhou, J., Miller, B.L. & Greicius, M.D. (2009). Neurodegenerative diseases target large-scale human brain networks. *Neuron*, **62**, 42–52.

Serfaty, M., Kennell-Webb, S., Warner, J., Blizard, R. & Raven, P. (2002). Double blind randomised placebo controlled trial of low dose melatonin for sleep disorders in dementia. *Int J Geriatr Psychiatry*, **17**, 1120–1127.

Shah, T., Tse, A., Gill, H., et al. (2008). Administration of melatonin mixed with soft food and liquids for children with neurodevelopmental difficulties. *Dev Med Child Neurol*, **50**, 845–849.

Sheffield, R.E. (1998). Migraine prevalence: a literature review. *Headache*, **38**, 595–601.

Siddall, P.J., Cousins, M.J., Otte, A., Griesing, T., Chambers, R. & Murphy, T.K. (2006). Pregabalin in central neuropathic pain associated with spinal cord injury: a placebo-controlled trial. *Neurology*, **67**, 1792–1800.

Silvestrini, M., Rizzato, B., Placidi, F., Baruffaldi, R., Bianconi, A. & Diomedi, M. (2002). Carotid artery wall thickness in patients with obstructive sleep apnea syndrome. *Stroke*, **33**, 1782–1785.

Sinforiani, E., Terzaghi, M., Pasotti, C., Zucchella, C., Zambrelli, E. & Manni, R. (2007). Hallucinations and sleep-wake cycle in Alzheimer's disease: a questionnaire-based study in 218 patients. *Neurol Sci*, **28**, 96–99.

Singer, C., Tractenberg, R.E., Kaye, J., et al. (2003). A multicenter, placebo-controlled trial of melatonin for sleep disturbance in Alzheimer's disease. *Sleep*, **26**, 893–901.

Sivak, E.D. & Streib, E.W. (1980). Management of hypoventilation in motor neuron disease presenting with respiratory insufficiency. *Ann Neurol*, **7**, 188–191.

Skjerve, A., Holsten, F., Aarsland, D., Bjorvatn, B., Nygaard, H.A. & Johansen, I.M. (2004). Improvement in behavioral symptoms and advance of activity acrophase after short-term bright light treatment in severe dementia. *Psychiatry Clin Neurosci*, **58**, 343–347.

Sloane, P.D., Williams, C.S., Mitchell, C.M., et al. (2007). High-intensity environmental light in dementia: effect on sleep and activity. *J Am Geriatr Soc*, **55**, 1524–1533.

Solaro, C., Uccelli, M.M., Guglieri, P., Uccelli, A. & Mancardi, G.L. (2000). Gabapentin is effective in treating nocturnal painful spasms in multiple sclerosis. *Mult Scler*, **6**, 192–193.

Steljes, D.G., Kryger, M.H., Kirk, B.W. & Millar, T.W. (1990). Sleep in postpolio syndrome. *Chest*, **98**, 133–140.

Steriade, M., Contreras, D. & Amzica, F. (1994). Synchronized sleep oscillations and their paroxysmal developments. *Trends Neurosci*, **17**, 199–208.

Suresh, S., Wales, P., Dakin, C., Harris, M.A. & Cooper, D.G. (2005). Sleep-related breathing disorder in Duchenne muscular dystrophy: disease spectrum in the paediatric population. *J Paediatr Child Health*, **41**, 500–503.

Tandberg, E., Larsen, J.P. & Karlsen, K. (1998). A community-based study of sleep disorders in patients with Parkinson's disease. *Mov Disord*, **13**, 895–899.

Tani, P., Lindberg, N., Nieminen-Von Wendt, T., et al. (2003). Insomnia is a frequent finding in adults with Asperger syndrome. *BMC Psychiatry*, **3**, 12.

Tani, P., Lindberg, N., Nieminen-Von Wendt, T., et al. (2004). Sleep in young adults with Asperger syndrome. *Neuropsychobiology*, **50**, 147–152.

Thunstrom, M. (2002). Severe sleep problems in infancy associated with subsequent development of attention-deficit/hyperactivity disorder at 5.5 years of age. *Acta Paediatr*, **91**, 584–592.

Tippmann-Peikert, M., Boeve, B.F. & Keegan, B.M. (2006). REM sleep behavior disorder initiated by acute brainstem multiple sclerosis. *Neurology*, **66**, 1277–1279.

Tractenberg, R.E., Singer, C.M. & Kaye, J.A. (2005). Symptoms of sleep disturbance in persons with Alzheimer's disease and normal elderly. *J Sleep Res*, **14**, 177–185.

Tran, K., Hukins, C., Geraghty, T., Eckert, B. & Fraser, L. (2010). Sleep-disordered breathing in spinal cord-injured patients: a short-term longitudinal study. *Respirology*, 15, 272–276.

Ulfberg, J., Carter, N., Talback, M. & Edling, C. (1996). Headache, snoring and sleep apnoea. *J Neurol*, 243, 621–625.

Urban, P.P., Morgenstern, M., Brause, K., et al. (2002). Distribution and course of cortico-respiratory projections for voluntary activation in man. A transcranial magnetic stimulation study in healthy subjects and patients with cerebral ischemia. *J Neurol*, 249, 735–744.

Valham, F., Mooe, T., Rabben, T., Stenlund, H., Wiklund, U. & Franklin, K.A. (2008). Increased risk of stroke in patients with coronary artery disease and sleep apnea: a 10-year follow-up. *Circulation*, 118, 955–960.

Van den Broek, M.J., Arbues, A.S., Chalard, F., et al. (2009). Chiari type I malformation causing central apnoeas in a 4-month-old boy. *Eur J Paediatr Neurol*, 13, 463–465.

Van Lunteren, E. & Kaminski, H.J. (1999). Disorders of sleep and breathing during sleep in neuromuscular disease. *Sleep Breath*, 3, 23–30.

Van Someren, E.J., Kessler, A., Mirmiran, M. & Swaab, D.F. (1997). Indirect bright light improves circadian rest-activity rhythm disturbances in demented patients. *Biol Psychiatry*, 41, 955–963.

Verma, A., Anand, V. & Verma, N.P. (2007). Sleep disorders in chronic traumatic brain injury. *J Clin Sleep Med*, 3, 357–362.

Volicer, L., Harper, D.G., Manning, B.C., Goldstein, R. & Satlin, A. (2001). Sundowning and circadian rhythms in Alzheimer's disease. *Am J Psychiatry*, 158, 704–711.

Wasdell, M.B., Jan, J.E., Bomben, M.M., et al. (2008). A randomized, placebo-controlled trial of controlled release melatonin treatment of delayed sleep phase syndrome and impaired sleep maintenance in children with neurodevelopmental disabilities. *J Pineal Res*, 44, 57–64.

Webster, J.B., Bell, K.R., Hussey, J.D., Natale, T.K. & Lakshminarayan, S. (2001). Sleep apnea in adults with traumatic brain injury: a preliminary investigation. *Arch Phys Med Rehabil*, 82, 316–321.

Weinberg, J., Klefbeck, B., Borg, J. & Svanborg, E. (2003). Polysomnography in chronic neuromuscular disease. *Respiration*, 70, 349–354.

Weintraub, D., Buchsbaum, R., Resor, S.R., Jr. & Hirsch, L.J. (2005). Effect of antiepileptic drug comedication on lamotrigine clearance. *Arch Neurol*, 62, 1432–1436.

Welch, K.M. (2003). Contemporary concepts of migraine pathogenesis. *Neurology*, 61, S2–S8.

Werth, E., Savaskan, E., Knoblauch, V., et al. (2002). Decline in long-term circadian rest-activity cycle organization in a patient with dementia. *J Geriatr Psychiatry Neurol*, 15, 55–59.

White, W.T., Patel, N., Drass, M. & Nalamachu, S. (2003). Lidocaine patch 5% with systemic analgesics such as gabapentin: a rational polypharmacy approach for the treatment of chronic pain. *Pain Med*, 4, 321–330.

Whitehead, D.L., Davies, A.D., Playfer, J.R. & Turnbull, C.J. (2008). Circadian rest-activity rhythm is altered in Parkinson's disease patients with hallucinations. *Mov Disord*, 23, 1137–1145.

Wilde, M.C., Castriotta, R.J., Lai, J.M., Atanasov, S., Masel, B.E. & Kuna, S.T. (2007). Cognitive impairment in patients with traumatic brain injury and obstructive sleep apnea. *Arch Phys Med Rehabil*, 88, 1284–1288.

Wu, Y.H. & Swaab, D.F. (2005). The human pineal gland and melatonin in aging and Alzheimer's disease. *J Pineal Res*, 38, 145–152.

Wu, Y.H., Fischer, D.F., Kalsbeek, A., et al. (2006). Pineal clock gene oscillation is disturbed in Alzheimer's disease, due to functional disconnection from the "master clock". *FASEB J*, 20, 1874–1876.

Yamadera, H., Ito, T., Suzuki, H., Asayama, K., Ito, R. & Endo, S. (2000). Effects of bright light on cognitive and sleep-wake (circadian) rhythm disturbances in Alzheimer-type dementia. *Psychiatry Clin Neurosci*, 54, 352–353.

Young, T., Palta, M., Dempsey, J., Skatrud, J., Weber, S. & Badr, S. (1993). The occurrence of sleep-disordered breathing among middle-aged adults. *N Engl J Med*, 328, 1230–1235.

Young, T., Peppard, P., Palta, M., et al. (1997). Population-based study of sleep-disordered breathing as a risk factor for hypertension. *Arch Intern Med*, **157**, 1746–1752.

Zambelis, T., Paparrigopoulos, T. & Soldatos, C.R. (2002). REM sleep behaviour disorder associated with a neurinoma of the left pontocerebellar angle. *J Neurol Neurosurg Psychiatry*, **72**, 821–822.

Zeitzer, J.M., Ayas, N.T., Shea, S.A., Brown, R. & Czeisler, C.A. (2000). Absence of detectable melatonin and preservation of cortisol and thyrotropin rhythms in tetraplegia. *J Clin Endocrinol Metab*, **85**, 2189–2196.

Zelman, D.C., Brandenburg, N.A. & Gore, M. (2006). Sleep impairment in patients with painful diabetic peripheral neuropathy. *Clin J Pain*, **22**, 681–685.

Zucconi, M., Oldani, A., Ferini-Strambi, L., Bizzozero, D. & Smirne, S. (1997). Nocturnal paroxysmal arousals with motor behaviors during sleep: frontal lobe epilepsy or parasomnia? *J Clin Neurophysiol*, **14**, 513–522.

Chapter 10

Sleep in children: the evolving challenge of catching enough and quality Zzz's

K. Spruyt and D. Gozal

If sleep doesn't serve an absolutely vital function, it is the biggest mistake evolution ever made.
Alan Rechtschaffen, PhD, The University of Chicago

Sleep duration: the sleeping child

Studies have clearly shown (National Sleep Foundation, 2004, 2006; Sadeh et al., 2000; Knutson and Lauderdale, 2009; Dollman et al., 2007; Yang et al., 2005; Warner et al., 2008) that children in our society are very unlikely to obtain sufficient sleep on a stable and regular schedule. For example, the 'Sleep in America' poll (National Sleep Foundation, 2004) surveyed parents about their children's sleep habits, behaviour, problems, and disorders in association with their daily schedules, and 2 years later the same approach was pursued in teens and adolescents (National Sleep Foundation, 2006). Both polls indicated that we actually overestimate the amount our children sleep, and that our children sleep much less than what we thought was appropriate for their stage of development. In fact, it is said that we sleep ~1 hour less than what we used to sleep one century ago. Lately, increasingly more studies have been published on sleep duration in children, with most of these studies aiming to evaluate the potentially adverse impact of poor sleep on health outcomes. To picture the complexity in documenting the sleep duration in children, a synopsis of published surveys (note few of these publications actually applied objective measurements of sleep or inquired about differences in sleep during week or weekend) on such sleep-wake patterns is provided in Table 10.1. However, even to the naked eye, it is readily apparent that although these studies are methodologically heterogeneous, they reflect marked changes taking place in our rapidly evolving 24/7 society. Table 10.1 and Fig. 10.1 further provoke critical reflection, and more importantly lead to a call for national longitudinal studies on sleep-wake patterns in children, particularly if we want to address the impact on health from a valid ecological standpoint. Indeed, few longitudinal studies that have primarily focused on sleep-wake patterns in children (e.g. Thorleifsdottir et al., 2002; Dollman et al., 2007; Knutson and Lauderdale, 2009; Iglowstein et al., 2003; Klackenberg, 1982) have been performed. Furthermore, only a number of studies have investigated sleep behaviours (e.g. Iglowstein et al., 2006; Jenni et al., 2005). As such, what constitutes normal sleep patterns during childhood, and even what constitutes normal sleep behaviour remain open questions. This absence of reliable data is all the more surprising considering that a child engages in sleeping activities more than in any other activity during the 24-hour cycle, and parents and health professionals have meticulously delineated, observed, and quantified normal patterns of activities such as eating or playing, and yet not done so for

Table 10.1 Sleep duration

First author (year*) Country	n	Age (years) Respondent	M†	Time frame	Bedtime‡			
					A	B	C	D
Hertel (1840) Denmark	4352	6–16 Parent	Q					9:03§
Bernhard (1884) Germany	6551	6–14						
Ravenhil (1884) England	6180	6–14						
Terman (1911–1912) US	2692	6–20						
Gulliford (1990) England and Scotland	9913	5–11	S		Schooldays			20:47
		Parent (1980s)			Weekend			21:32
Meijer (2000) The Netherlands	449	9.5–14.5 Self-report	Q		Schooldays			20:56
					Weekend			22:06
Iglowstein (2003) Switzerland	280	Birth–16 Parent (in 1978–1993)						
National Sleep Foundation (2004) US	1473	≤ 10 Parent	TI		Weeknights	21:11	20:42	20:55	21:07
Gaina (2005) Japan	91	13–14	A	7 days	Weekday			22:51§
					Weekend			23:02§
National Sleep Foundation (2006) US	1602	11–17 Parent & self-report	TI		Weeknights			
El-Sheik (2007) US	2454	5.5–19.1	TD	2 days randomly	1 Weekday			21:09
		Self-report			1 Weekend day			21:25
Dollman (2007) Australia	390	10–15 Self-report (in 1985)	Q		Sunday to Thursday nights			21:47
	510	11–15 Self-report (in 2004)	Q		Sunday to Thursday nights			22:12
Jenni (2007) Switzerland	305	<10 Parent	SSRI					

| | Total sleep time[‡] | | | | | | Rise time[‡] | | | | | |
F	A	B	C	D	E	F	A	B	C	D	E	F
49[§]				9.8[§]	8.9[§]							
				8.9								
				9.2								
				10.1	8.8	8.5						
				10						7:33		
				10.8						8:20		
				10.3						7:11		
				—						—		
	11.3	11.5	11.2	10.1	8.6	8.1						
	9	9.8	9.6	9.4			7:14	7:29	7:23	7:05		
				6.5						6:34		
				7.4						7:40		
:38	10:39				8.2	7.2					6:32	
2:24				9.3	9.2					6:58	7:02	
2:48				10.3	10.1					8:12	9:04	
				9.2						7:01		
				8.7						6:57		
	14.4	13.4	11.9	10.7								

(Continued)

Table 10.1 (continued) Sleep duration

First author (year*) Country	n	Age (years) Respondent	M†	Time frame		Bedtime‡ A	B	C	D
Warner (2008) Australia	310	15–18	Sleep log	School term	Week				
		Self-report			Weekday				
					Weekend				
				Holiday	Week				
					Weekday				
					Weekend				
Gillian (2008) New Zealand	519	7.26	A	24 hours	Week				20:15
					Weekend¶				20:42
El-Sheikh (2008) US	64	7.17–11	A	1 week					21:18
Xiao-na (2009) China	1278	≤5 Caregiver & significant other	Q	Past month					
Knutson (2009) US	130 (in 1981)	15–17	TD	24 hours	Schooldays = day taking class				
		Self-report			Non-schooldays				
	2978 (in 2003–2006)	15–17	TD	24 hours	Schooldays = day taking class				
		Self-report			Non-schooldays				

*Year of publication may coincide with year of study, note this is not always the case.

†Method (M): Q: questionnaire, S: survey, TI: telephone interview, A: actigraphy, TD: time-diary, SSRI: structured sleep-related interview.

‡A: infants; B: toddlers; C: preschoolers; D: school-aged; E: middle school-aged (6th to 8th grade); F: high school adolescents (9th to 12th grade).

§Pooled averages.

¶Friday and Saturday.

		Total sleep time‡						Rise time‡					
E	F	A	B	C	D	E	F	A	B	C	D	E	F
						8.2							
22:47						7.9				7:04			
00:47						8.9				9:22			
						9.1							
24:00						9.2				09:38			
00:46						8.9				10:04			
					10.9						7:08		
					10.5						7:17		
					7						5.59		
		9.4	9.8	9.5									
22:21						8.3						6:32	
23:01						9.6						8:58	
22:21						8.1						6:26	
22:45						9.9						9:33	

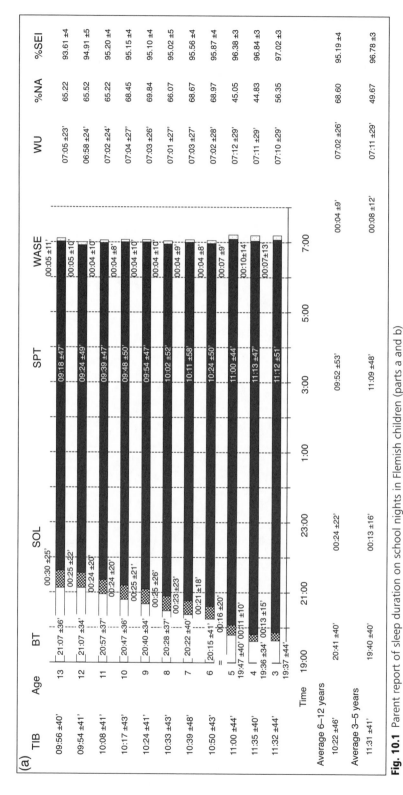

Fig. 10.1 Parent report of sleep duration on school nights in Flemish children (parts a and b)
During weekend BT shifts on average 1 hour, SOL is shorter, WU shifts also ~1 hour, yet children slept only ~30 minutes more. In spite of an extra hour, the majority of children still needed to be awakened during weekend. Furthermore, 1 in 12 children has an irregular sleep-wake pattern.

Abbreviations: TIB, time in bed; BT, bedtime; SOL, sleep onset latency; SPT, sleep period time; WASE, wakefulness after sleep end; WU, wake-up time; %NA, % children not spontaneously awake; %SEI, sleep efficiency index in %. More information on school-aged children can be found in Spruyt, K. (2007).

Source: Reproduced from Spruyt, K. (2007). *Slaapproblemen bij kinderen. Basisgids voor ouders en hulpverleners.* Tielt, Belgium, Lannoo; Spruyt, K., O'Brien, L.M., Cluydts, R., Verleye, G.B. & Ferri, R. (2005). Odds, prevalence and predictors of sleep problems in school-age normal children. *J Sleep Res*, **14**, 163–176, with permission.

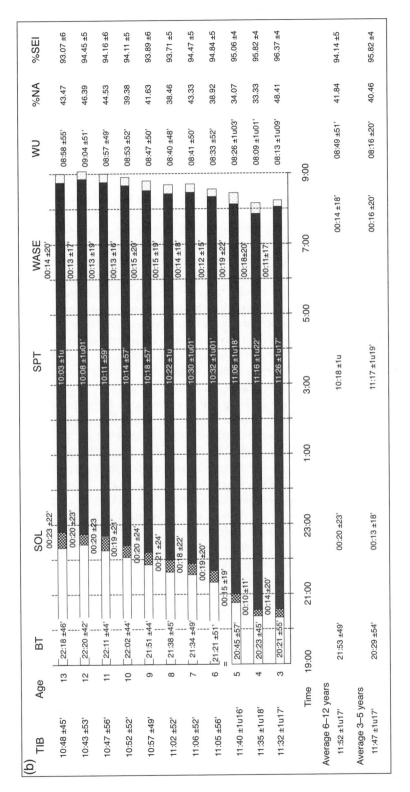

Fig. 10.1 (continued)

sleeping patterns. Therefore, the most forgotten, overlooked, or even actively ignored behaviour of this century is undoubtedly childhood sleep. However, trends aiming to reduce sleep in children have emerged, and regrettably continue to gain momentum.

Acknowledging both parents and professionals working with children take particular pleasure and pride at their accomplishments, such as the first steps, the first words, the good grades, extra-curricular activities, and so forth; it becomes apparent that our society places most emphasis on daytime functioning, and, in doing so, all too often we forget the critically important role of sleep in this context. It is now quite well-established that sleep plays a vital role in brain maturation, somatic growth, information processing, memory consolidation, learning, and other important cognitive functions. Since sleep subserves so many aspects of overall well-being, it likewise can exert multi-organ impact on functioning as will become clear throughout this book. A multitude of environmental factors and daytime activities tend to intrude into our life, and potentially rob children of their sleep needs. For example, 43% of school-aged children and 57% of adolescents have a TV in their bedroom (National Sleep Foundation, 2004, 2006; Spruyt, 2007). As many as 42% have a mobile phone in their bedroom and many other electronic devices, such as computers, video games, and others are pre-eminently and frequently present in children's bedrooms (Li et al., 2007; Spruyt, 2007). Denigration of the night and the dark as an adverse period has also become pervasively communicated to children, such that 60–72% of children routinely have a nightlight in their bedroom (National Sleep Foundation, 2004). Moreover, continued urge for sustained uninterrupted social e-contact is increasingly observed in youngsters, and at lower and lower ages. In summary, historical trends point to increasing reductions in the opportunity for sleep in children and also to the 'pollution' of that sleep opportunity by a variety of intrusionary elements that may further lead to reduced sleep duration.

If an ephemeral lifestyle emerges as the irremediable consequence of modern society, how well do children adapt? Associations between poor sleep and stress levels are increasingly being reported, and, likewise, findings on the associations between environmental and societal changes and sleep are also accumulating (National Sleep Foundation, 2004; El-Sheikh et al., 2008; Rona et al., 1998; Brand et al., 2009). Not in the least, since the familial context is rapidly changing in our society, the potential associations between family structure and function and sleep in children have led to several important studies, all of which suggest that family life changes impose major changes in sleep habits and duration in children (Simard et al., 2008; Brand et al., 2009). Although such findings clearly raise a red flag, further assessment and intervention studies are needed before we can formulate and implement adequate guidelines.

The collective evidence that hopefully will be collected in the forthcoming years will reveal the multi-directional relationships between poor sleep and health in our current society worldwide. Notwithstanding, surveys already indicate the prevalence of sleep complaints in children as ranging between 20% and 60% (e.g. bedtime resistance, excessive daytime somnolence, co-sleeping, delayed sleep onset, bedtime anxiety, snoring, enuresis, night terrors) (Spruyt et al., 2005; Owens, 2008). Since sleep behaviour and sleep duration are unmistakably interrelated, the need for more empirical evidence is pressing. Although it is not the scope of this chapter to review in detail each possible sleep complaint, we should emphasize that over 50 different sleep disorders are described in the book *Principles and Practice of Pediatric Sleep Medicine* (Sheldon et al., 2005), and three important aspects are apparent: (1) sleep, and its problems in children is different from adults; (2) sleep complaints, problems, and disorders can be grouped into psychological or physical; and (3) misdiagnosis, and possibly under-diagnosis, of most sleep problems is commonplace (see Chapter 14). Of special interest in the realm of this chapter are disorders of excessive somnolence, which are becoming a major societal concern. The difficulty here is how to disentangle daytime sleepiness and somnolence. On the one hand, the definition of the two is problematic in children and on the other hand, both subjective and objective findings of sleepiness may not always converge in children. Indeed, somnolence can be expressed using physiological dimensions such as those comprising the inclination to sleep or sleep propensity, that is, a sleep drive, often assessed by the multiple sleep latency test. Conversely, how we subjectively experience sleepiness, or how it feels to be somnolent forms the subjective dimension, and, how somnolence is expressed and thus observed and reported by others is the behavioural dimension. In a developing child, the somnolence phenotype can be quite challenging to unravel, since it may encompass externalizing and internalizing behaviours. Furthermore, these three dimensions of somnolence are often interchanged, and are interchangeable. Nonetheless, more explicit and systematic use of these measures should serve as a guide to the diagnostic process of sleep duration and behaviour problems in the child. In fact, sleepiness and alertness are perceived as correlates of the sleep-wake system. However, the variety of causes and pathways leading to low quantity and poor quality of sleep in children may co-exist, and therefore pose a formidable challenge to their recognition and treatment (Spruyt et al., 2005).

In contrast with such assumptions, our practice has shown that parental and child education on appropriate sleep and hygiene, and small modifications to the bedroom environment are accompanied with a relatively high degree of success in improving many of the presenting complaints. A valuable rule of thumb regarding optimal amount of sleep has been: more than 12 hours for preschoolers, about 12 hours for the school-aged children, and about 9 hours thereafter. More specifically, when school 'learning load' increases, that is, at age 6, the child should sleep at least 11 hours and from then onwards ~15 minutes less per subsequent birthday.

It is clear from the data compiled in Tables 10.1 and 10.2 that sleep in children is rarely if ever optimal, and that bedtime has especially shifted to later hours, which converges with presenting complaints by parents, such as bedtime reluctance and excessive daytime fatigue, tiredness, lack of energy, poor attention span, irritability, mood swings, and somnolence. Moreover, findings in some of those sleep duration or behaviour studies suggest that especially those children raised in

Table 10.2 Percentage of children not awakening spontaneously after a normal night sleep*

Age (years)	Percentage (%)
6	21.2
7	19
8	23.3
9	19.1
10	22.8
11	20.3
12	23.6
13	24.7
14	26
15	31.6
16	38.7
17	39.9
18	47.7

*Note the persistent increase with age, particularly during adolescence.
Source: Adapted from Terman, L.M. & Hocking, A. (1913). The sleep of school children, its distribution according to age, and its relation to physical and mental efficiency. *J Educ Psychol*, **4**, 138–147.

disadvantageous situations are at increased risk of chronic poor sleep. In his textbook, Professor Gregory Stores (2001) assigned a role to the caregiver in the majority of sleep problems in children by stating that 'the caregiver(s) play a role in *defining, causing, or maintaining* their child's sleep problems'. Indeed, poor sleep is one of the most reported complaints by caregivers, but children seldom if ever complain about their own sleep. As such, in research and in clinical practice, one needs to be conscious of the different perceptions on sleep by the complainant, the sufferer, and the observer (e.g. clinician or teacher). From aforementioned considerations, it becomes apparent why poor sleep remains a very common and yet markedly under-recognized health problem.

Animal studies consistently suggest an adverse impact on health by sustained sleep loss; for instance, sleep loss may trigger generalized inflammatory and stress responses in the brain. Although substantive causative relationships between sleep loss and end-organ dysfunction are missing in children, it is widely assumed that when sleep is reduced either acutely or chronically, it is not without changes in brain and behaviour (Cirelli, 2006; Pilcher and Huffcutt, 1996). Collective evidence increasingly points to disruptions of endocrine and metabolic functions as well as lower self-esteem, mood symptoms, and somnolence and inattentiveness at school, and more recently suggests a link between insufficient or short sleep and obesity. Therefore, studies on the impact of poor or insufficient sleep in a developing child in the context of our highly media overloaded life where time of sleep is abused are critically needed. Hence, defining in a first stage what normal sleep behaviour and habits are in a child is the first step of the process. The delineation of normative sleep should encompass the wide range of normal development, physical and maturational changes across childhood, as well as cultural, environmental, and social influences, finally leading to the determination and characterization of potential sleep phenotypes. This approach subsequently summates the multitude of relationships with sleep duration. Schematically, findings discussed in this chapter potentially reflect five variables that may vary with respect to sleep (see Fig. 10.2):

1. Bedtime
2. Sleep time, which can be shortened or fragmented/disrupted by endogenous or exogenous factors
3. Rise time
4. Occurrence of the sleep phase within the circadian rhythm
5. Variability of the sleep phase within the circadian rhythm for weekdays and weekend days (irregular sleep)

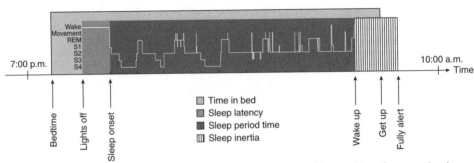

Fig. 10.2 The construct of sleep duration: five variables that would be pertinent for screening in primary care settings.

What was already hypothesized as early as during 1884 is now becoming supported by the cumulative evidence: 'In childhood the growth of the brain is very rapid, and its natural activity is very great; during this period of intense mental energy there is danger that the immature brain will be taxed beyond the proper limit, and be nourished at the expense of other tissues; for mental activity requires a large expenditure of vital force, and if the brain is compelled to work beyond its powers, it will draw upon other organs of the body for its support, depriving them of their necessary nourishment, and causing various disorders in consequence'. (Baker, 1884)

Practice points

- Inquire about sleep quantity and quality
- Evaluate sleep environment and hygiene (habits, potential disruptors), and determine regularity
- Critically reflect on behavioural signs (e.g. physical complaints, learning difficulties, somnolence, emotional difficulty) in realm of poor or insufficient sleep
- Embed poor or insufficient sleep in context (e.g. exam, stress, anxiety, traumatic experience, depression, ruminating, cultural setting, parenting)
- Compare subjective and objective measures from several respondents in the child's environment (parents, siblings and friends, teachers, other)
- Establish sleep duration needs and formulate realistic expectations to correct sleep-related deficiencies

Bedtime is an extremely crucial and daily turning point in many families. It is rather apparent that many if not most children will do their best to postpone their bedtime with varying degrees of success, the latter depending for instance on parenting style (Spruyt, 2007). Unequivocally, shifts in bedtime will also affect total sleep times, since during school weekdays, rise time is quite rigid due to the standard and rather consistent school start times. During weekends, both bedtime and rise time can shift drastically, and this can be either sporadically or assume a more chronic and consistent pattern. Shifts are much more likely to arise in adolescence, and during weekends the sleep phase rhythm can be seriously disrupted. Of importance to the changes in bedtime is the interrelation between bedtime and the other variables, such that it becomes very arbitrary when a certain degree of irregularity in bedtime leads to changes in sleep and wake that are considered dysfunctional. Conversely, for example when comparing Table 10.2 versus Fig. 10.1, a potentially forgotten marker of poor sleep is spontaneous awakening despite the 'mandatory' rise time, that is, increasingly more children are awakened and do not arisen spontaneously!

Questions a healthcare provider readily can ask

- What is the usual bedtime?
- How many times is bedtime later than this usual bedtime? How much later?
- How long does it usually take to fall asleep?
- Are there night awakenings? How often? And how long does it take to return to sleep?
- What is the usual rise time?
- How many times is rise time later than the usual rise time? How much later?
- Is awakening occurring spontaneously or does the child need to be awakened?

A difficulty regarding interpreting results emanating from research on sleep deprivation and disruption in children is that laboratory and naturalistic environment conditions may differ substantially regarding these five variables, and this problem therefore impedes generalization of findings. Research is furthermore hampered by the ongoing search for accurate ways to objectively collect sleep-wake pattern data in the home environment, by the lack of clear definitions for sleep problems and disorders in childhood as to what is normal or pathological pertaining to certain developmental ages, and finally the research is further challenged by the confounding factors related to baseline sleep duration. Notwithstanding, complaints of poor sleep being voiced by parents should be taken seriously and attempts to quantify them should be undertaken, despite these methodological issues. As mentioned above, a promising research field is the impact of family functioning on sleep (Meltzer and Mindell, 2007; Brand et al., 2009), such that discerning the common threads linking family environment and its adverse impact on sleep, and therefore the impact of poor sleep on children, should generate clusters of aggregate data that enable formulation of initial strategies regarding effective management of poor sleep in children. Hence, in the future, we will have to incorporate measures of familial functioning and of the fast changing community functioning to the evaluation of sleep in children, particularly on parameters such as bedtime and variability of sleep phase. Since societal and family behaviours are undoubtedly important modifiers and critical determinants of sleep habits in children, tools to quantify such aspects of sleep will have to be developed.

The scant findings to date in other areas of sleep in children will restrict our focus on three major areas linked to poor sleep, namely impairment of cognitive performance, affect, and health.

Effects on cognition: the learning child

Prior to discussing the effects of sleep and poor sleep on cognition, some potential limitations need to be highlighted. The construct of 'school or academic performance' has been variously defined and measured (e.g. a low grade is not necessarily the same everywhere or perceived similarly by everyone). Similar issues apply to intelligence and intellectual ability (i.e. results need to be interpreted based on the theoretical paradigm of the instrument). Furthermore, the vast majority of studies are within (young) adolescent populations, and only a minority of such studies has been conducted in younger children. These prescriptive limitations are presumably the result of the well-known observation that in naturalistic environments adolescents show irregular sleep durations, and shifts in bedtime and rise time are not uncommon.

We should note that absence of objective documentation of preceding sleep while testing cognitive abilities may create biased findings; in addition, other confounding variables such as drugs, social activities, mood, and puberty, to name a few, need to be considered when interpreting some of the results not only on cognition, but also on affect (see section 'Effects on affect: the happy child'). For instance, in surveys social desirability or with respect to teens 'un'desirability, since it is considered 'unpopular to sleep', needs to be examined. Finally, studies often limit their design frame such that the day of testing follows immediately after the sleep duration manipulation. It would be interesting to look at the cumulative effect of irregular sleep durations over more extended periods of time, since these experimental protocols may better mimic real-life conditions. A similar comment can be made regarding time of experimental testing the following day (e.g. sleep inertia and circadian rhythm effects) (see Fig. 10.2).

Several studies on experimental manipulation of sleep duration and its impact on performance in adolescents have been performed, usually consisting of one night's sleep deprivation, and have revealed reduced performance (Carskadon et al., 1981). More interestingly, the researchers noticed the presence of sleepiness during testing, and significant associations between sleepiness and decreased performance on an additional task and word memory task were found. Randazzo et al. (1998) discussed earlier studies from the 1970s as suggestive of decreased psychomotor function after total sleep deprivation, but not partial deprivation. Based on such literature, they invoked the differences that should be operational between acute and chronic loss of sleep as well as the differing interactions of cognitive functioning with total and partial deprivation. These investigators have subsequently implemented an acute sleep restriction design in the laboratory by allowing 16 children (mean age 11.6 years) only 5 hours in bed and this acute sleep restriction was achieved by postponing bedtime to 3:00 a.m. and rise time prescribed at 8:00 a.m., the latter being similar to the control group. Sleep-restricted children performed worse on areas of verbal fluency and originality and exhibited greater physiological sleepiness, but no differences were found on the other 'low cognitive load'. It was suggested that the repetitive nature of the tasks might be the basis for the absence of statistical significance for some of the functions, even though verbal and creativity components were significantly affected in the sleep-restricted children. The authors proposed that sleep restriction elicits executive dysfunction. This important study sets the stage for any future sleep duration studies in children, by delineating which experimental condition is the most sensitive and specific, and which cognitive function is most likely affected. Indeed, subsequent experimental designs by investigators have used this initial construct in an attempt to characterize the neurobehavioural vulnerability to severity of sleep deprivation or restriction. For example, Fallone et al. (2001) included an objective five-night baseline actigraphic sleep recording prior to a randomly assigned optimized (10 hours) or restricted (4 hours) laboratory sleep with next day testing. The 8–15 years old in the restriction sleep group exhibited shorter daytime sleep latency, more subjective sleepiness, and inattentiveness, whereas the optimized sleep group tended to make more commission errors on the continuous performance test. It is noteworthy that in the restricted sleep group results showed no fewer errors of commission or more errors of omission. Meritorious aspects of this study include the multi-methodological approach to performance (i.e. cognition and emotion, several tests for each), as well as the objective baseline sleep assessment. Interestingly, the investigators also conducted direct observations while the child was in the laboratory and noticed the disparity in how the 'sleepy child' is being perceived by different responders, that is, sleep laboratory personnel. This fits well with the difficulty in conducting objective evaluations, particularly regarding the various daytime sleepiness dimensions. In their conclusions, Fallone et al. questioned the validity of the hypothesized prefrontal impairment associated with sleep restriction, but it was not clear if the authors controlled for age in their analyses considering the age-range of their sample, particularly since this brain region is known to develop substantially in the transition to adolescence. In 2005, the same team of investigators (Fallone et al., 2005) implemented a home-based within-subject design entailing three week-long sleep schedules (counterbalanced: baseline—optimized and restricted) in school-aged children and investigated teacher ratings of academic performance and behaviour. They found empirical evidence of reduced academic performance as illustrated by difficulties in the classroom and school-related attention problems characterized by 'sluggish cognitive tempo' when sleep was restricted. These children were slower to process information and more forgetful. Sadeh et al. (2000) also performed a series of studies with respect to objectively measured sleep duration. In one study, they assessed daytime functioning in relation to five nights of actigraphic sleep. Of the second to sixth grade students included in this study, 18% had a sleep percentage lower than 90 and three or more waking per night on average, defined by the authors as 'poor sleep'. Older children especially expressed sleepiness, which was confirmed by the parental report of unplanned daytime sleep episodes. In a subsequent study, Sadeh et al. (2002) found that fragmented sleep in children was associated with lower performance on more complex tasks, such as continuous performance test and a symbol-digit substitution test (both computerized tests). Subsequently, the investigators (Sadeh et al., 2003) experimentally implemented a sleep restriction or extension design by shifting bedtime by 1 hour for three consecutive nights in a subset of children from the previous sample. Of particular interest was the reluctance of parents from the youngest group to participate in a 1-hour restriction experiment, and in only about 60% extension or restriction by an average of 30 minutes was effectively accomplished, whereas in the remainder of the cohort, the experimental condition was unsuccessfully implemented. With respect to sleep, the authors found that children in the restricted condition had better sleep quality by increased sleep percentage and quiet sleep and reduced number of awakenings, thereby in concordance with theories of compensatory physiological mechanisms that regulate sleep. The delayed shift created also increased evening fatigue and shorter sleep latency. The children in the sleep-extension group showed the opposite trend. With respect to cognitive performance, extension of sleep improved performance on digit forward memory test, in continuous performance test reaction time. Overall performance of the children in the restriction and the unsuccessful condition did not change, except that reaction times deteriorated, and this is in concurrence with the 'sluggish cognitive tempo' noted by Fallone et al. (2005). The research paradigm by Sadeh and his group deserves mention, because of the naturalistic aspect of their studies in young children. However, it would have been interesting to characterize in greater detail the sleep habits among the restriction and unsuccessful groups, since they were a subgroup of an earlier study sample. It is conceivable that some of the restricted children were already chronically deprived, or for the unsuccessful group that familial factors interfered, or that some children are more sensitive to bedtime shifts. This type of observation may be very informative for future study design, and, as such, they should increase the ecological validity of the findings. Notwithstanding, the findings of both Fallone et al. and Sadeh et al. are suggestive of impaired processing speed and memory when sleep in children is restricted.

In adolescents reduced total sleep time, irregular sleep schedules, and increased sleep onset latencies showed clear associations with poorer academic achievement (Wolfson and Carskadon, 2003; Curcio et al., 2006; Lamberg, 2009; Warner et al., 2008). Adolescents with C or lower grades, in comparison to those with As and Bs reported lower total sleep time, later bedtimes on school- and weekend nights, and later weekend rise times. However, the sleep characteristics were all based on self-reports. Others have found associations between subjective sleepiness and executive dysfunction, and have accordingly speculated on this issue, especially among adolescents raised in a disadvantageous environment (Anderson et al., 2009; Curcio et al., 2006). Moreover, the irregularity of sleep duration and concomitant reported fatigue may further promote school failure, though one should be cautious and not draw too hasty conclusions (e.g. motivational factors or other factors may likely contribute). More recently, Beebe et al. (2009) suggested an increased brain-load when sleep was restricted. Although these studies included only a very small sample size, the functional magnetic resonance imaging (fMRI) study results suggested that increased activity of brain regions was present among those regions normally active with the working memory task, whereas increased suppression of brain regions normally suppressed during this task occurred as well. Thus, chronic sleep restriction may create a more polarized brain network activity pattern aiming to sustain optimal performance. Future studies should reveal the mechanisms, limits, and developmental processes behind this compensatory cerebral response. Indeed, incorporating developmental neuropsychology models may additionally increase our understanding of the impact of sleep restriction on the developing brain. For example, attention-deficit disorder (ADD) type without hyperactivity could share parallel features of the sleepy phenotype. Indeed, attention studies within the field of developmental neuropsychology suggest that besides prefrontal and orbitofrontal cortices, the posterior parietal mechanisms are additionally involved and are known as being primarily associated with sluggishness, withdrawal, passivity, failure to engage, or with deficits in sustained attention. These brain activities only become apparent when tested in a sensitive and specific matter, such as imaging, such that respondents and evaluators of a field survey may perceive and interpret these aspects in a very different fashion.

Thus far, we have primarily focused on changes in bedtime. However, the issue of delayed school start times has received intense media coverage in recent years. Similar to grading school performance, school times and even schooldays may vary substantially among studies, and among geographical regions. Again, the interrelations with environment and in broader sense the interdependencies in society need to be incorporated, especially among those adolescents who are prone to develop delayed sleep onset and who are confronted with early school start times. Indeed, these children will be more likely to exhibit increased daytime sleepiness, frequently fall asleep in class, and manifest inattentiveness, all of which can lead to decreased school perform-ance (Wolfson and Carskadon, 2003; Wolfson et al., 2007; Warner et al., 2008). Shifting school start times has proven to increase total sleep time on average by ~50 minutes, and despite the modest increases in sleep duration, it seems to have a beneficial effect. However, how well these manipulations can be globalized needs to be determined, with some reflections on other potential modifiable factors being necessary, such as: vicinity to school, transport to school, subsequent shift to later hours of the extra-curricular activities, co-parenting where a child alternates weeks between parents. One may even ponder if we should consider shorter schooldays but more schooldays? Furthermore, how is this shift in bedtime versus in rise time affecting sleep architec-ture, since both rapid eye movement (REM) and non-rapid eye movement (NREM) sleep play distinct roles in learning and memory consolidation. Indeed, in the future the five variables need to be critically examined in relation to sleep duration.

Studies within populations with cognitive deficits and the relation to their sleep have also been of interest. In this context, we would like to touch upon some intriguing findings with respect to sleep in children with cognitive deficits. More hypnagogic hypersynchrony characteristic of drow-siness and stage 1 sleep was found in children with learning disabilities in comparison to controls (de Alba et al., 2003). Similarly, reading disabled children have altered sleep architecture with more stage 4 sleep, less REM, and longer REM onset latency allowing the authors to associate this to chronic sleep deprivation and maturational delay (Mercier et al., 1993). Such sleep architecture findings alone or in relation to other factors could underlie the outcome of impaired information processing and cognitive dysfunction. To overcome reading difficulties, dyslexic subjects exces-sively activate thalamocortical and hippocampal circuitry to transfer information between corti-cal posterior and anterior areas (Bruni et al., 2009).

In summary, sleepiness or increased homeostatic drive is seen in children and adolescents undergoing sleep restriction by primarily shifting bedtime designs. Age and sleepiness are impor-tant variables to study or control for in sleep duration studies, especially since findings in adult populations have started to focus on individual susceptibility, which might be a reflection of inherited susceptibility or vulnerable genes (Gottlieb et al., 2007). However, societal factors are also likely to be important contributors. This issue brings us back to the question of how well do we adapt to sleep restriction as a child, and Darwin's school of environmentally driven genetic changes (i.e. epigenetics) in a fast evolving and poorly sleeping society. Though most studies are still confronted with many methodological difficulties, disentangling the degree of sleepiness versus the degree of sleep loss through careful study design and explaining findings by applying pertinent statistical analyses will be required if we wish to progress in this area.

Effects on affect: the happy child

The relation between affect and sleep is very complex and highly intriguing because of the puta-tive role of sleep in psychopathology, and hence the possibility of spurious associations between psychiatric diagnosis and sleep behaviours. Since particular phenotypes of sleep behaviour in childhood are yet to be well-characterized, developmental differences, severity, duration, and impact as well as response to intervention or environmental factors will be extremely important informational components in our aim to evaluate poor sleep as being transient or persistent throughout the lifespan. As is said in 1884, by L.W. Baker, 'Sleep is the rest of the brain, and is never more essential to mental integrity than during the formative period of life'. Longitudinal studies are clearly needed to further delineate: (a) the sleep problems characteristic among child-hood psychiatric disorders, (b) how often children with a sleep complaints (e.g. difficulty initiating and maintaining sleep) meet criteria of mental health diagnosis, and (c) if early poor sleep predicts later development of emotional and behavioural problems. In short, *sleep as the window on emotion*.

The disruption of sleep and emotional regulation has received some interest and attention, especially in early childhood. Indeed, studies have focused on temperament of the child and sleep, as well as explored relationships on the synergy between sleep and maternal well-being, and parenting. Taken together, poor sleep is associated with difficult temperament and *vice versa*. The multi-directionality of the relationships between disrupted infant or toddler sleep, temperament, and parenting makes conclusive results difficult. For example, sleep time issues need to be examined not only in the context of learned inappropriate sleep onset associations such as bottle feeding or TV viewing, but also in the context of individual cultural and home environment influences, such as when co-sleeping is culturally common. Furthermore, actigraphic sleep assessments or other objective sleep assessment techniques need to be incorporated into the research in this area to further validate the putative relationships that emerge from subjective parental sleep reporting.

The impact of sleep on emotion is not only unmistakable, and likely more profound than on cognition (Pilcher and Huffcutt, 1996), but also potentially more challenging to investigate. Inattentiveness in relation to poor sleep is probably the most commonly discussed association, based on the consistent observation that increased homeostatic sleep drive in the child can become manifest as behaviours resembling attention-deficit hyperactivity disorder (ADHD) symptoms. Additionally, experimental findings on the impact of sleep deprivation or restriction on mood and affect regulation in children are scant, apart from disrupted sleep in the context of underlying health issues. The vast majority of literature relating to emotion and behaviour focuses on disrupted sleep in the case of a physical or mental health problem, or in clinical samples. Thus, to date the spectrum of affective dysfunction in relation to poor sleep in the otherwise healthy child remains unexplored, and the existing findings are not always conclusive and not in the least confirmed. Nonetheless, the link between sleep problems, low quantity, and poor quality of sleep with psychopathological signs has been clearly made (Dahl, 1996; Alfano and Gamble, 2009), and therefore needs to be incorporated into the assessment when examining the emotional development of the child.

Before discussing findings on poor sleep in the context of psychopathological symptomatology, we will review some studies in which the sleep deprivation or restriction designs, which are not always ethically or 'parentally' permissible in children, attempted to include some 'affective' functioning. Noteworthy, studies in adolescents by default contain cognitive, behavioural, social, and emotional 'dys'functioning due to their developmental progress (i.e. puberty). In this population, the bedroom becomes the 'this is my life' room, with TV, music, food, and other entertainment, potentially promoting the sleepy adolescent. Extrapolation from these studies in adolescence to childhood might therefore not be applicable. In the process of experimental manipulation of bedtime, adolescents showed increases in inattentiveness, oppositional behaviour, irritability, behavioural dysregulation, and mood difficulties (i.e. signs of depression, anxiety) as expressed via self-report (Wolfson and Carskadon, 2003). In younger school-aged children, more frequent and more severe behavioural problems, but not necessarily hyperactive-impulsive problems (Fallone et al., 2005) were suggested. Despite few empirical studies, survey results in youth suggest likewise correlations between poor sleep and increased overall behavioural problems, delinquent behaviour, thought problems, and negative mood (Sadeh et al., 2002; Wolfson and Carskadon, 2003). The paucity of experimentally conducted studies only allows us to date to conclude there is clearly 'an adverse impact' of poor sleep on affect. However, extended sleep is also being related to lower sleep quality, and restricting sleep has been proven clinically therapeutic in depressed children. Thus, the question remains: how much sleep is optimal to feel well?

The brain regions believed to be particularly vulnerable to poor sleep are the prefrontal cortices, which develop well into adolescence. Given that brain maturation entails brain plasticity, neurobehavioural compounds of the developing frontostriatal system might be sensitive to this suboptimal sleep-wake state. In fact, Tourette syndrome, obsessive-compulsive disorder, ADHD, schizophrenia, autism, and depression all closely (but not exclusively) relate to the basal ganglia and the wider frontostriatal system, and, indeed, signs of these neurodevelopmental disorders are noted in correlational studies questioning sleep duration and behaviour in children. Conversely, sleep problems (such as parasomnias), low sleep quantity, and poor quality are not uncommon in these disorders. Given that co-morbidity of sleep and psychopathology is frequent, the field of paediatric sleep will have to better incorporate a neurodevelopmental paradigm in order to increase knowledge on individual susceptibility as well as vulnerability at young ages. Sleep in children, and duration of sleep should ideally be questioned in *any* history-taking and systematically documented using appropriate tools.

The high prevalence of sleep complaints in childhood psychiatric disorders has been recently reviewed (Alfano and Gamble, 2009). Up to 20% of children exhibit anxiety disorders, such as separation anxiety, generalized anxiety, or post-traumatic anxiety disorders (i.e. excluding the developmentally appropriate childhood fears). These children for the vast majority show increased number of nighttime awakenings (hence, fragmented sleep) and delay of bedtimes (hence, shorter total sleep time). Sleep problems in children with obsessive-compulsive disorder tend to indicate a more severe form of the disorder, which is not the case with post-traumatic stress disorder. Yet, trouble sleeping (i.e. difficulty initiating, excessive arousal, nightmares) and daytime tiredness are not uncommon in both. Interestingly, similar signs can be seen in relation to transient stress. A history of trauma or abuse also clearly disturbs sleep, as such; assessment of sleep in these cases should be the standard of care (cf. in 1970 reports of psychosocial dwarfism, likelihood of abuse during night or when child is in bed). Again, we like to draw attention to the potential multi-directional relationships and aspects of environment such as over-involved parenting or inadequate parenting, but also the influence of pharmacological interventions in the realm of psychopathological symptoms and disorders, potentially masking correlational findings. The psychopathological disorders or environmental factors (e.g. psychopathology of parent), might further promote ill-timing of sleep. More objective studies in these disorders are encouraged. Lately, pervasive developmental disorders gained substantial attention in which sleep problems are highly prevalent (i.e. 50–80%). Irregular sleep-wake patterns, delayed sleep onset, and overall inadequate sleep are typical complaints and findings. Moreover it is suggested that the worse the sleep, the worse the pervasive developmental deficits. Equally, some correlation findings suggest that daytime sleepiness additionally hampers social interactions or interpersonal contacts. The last two psychopathological disorders, depressive and ADHD, are increasingly related to the next section, namely to health issues. Mostly insomnia, but also hypersomnia leading to and resulting from poor sleep quality can be frequently found in depressed children. Additionally, a positive correlation with severity and relapse is suggested, that is, between significant sleep disruption (inability to sleep, hypersomnia, excessive daytime sleepiness) and longer and more severe depressive episodes, especially when exhibiting early in life sleep complaints (early morning awakenings, sleep onset, and maintaining problems). In health care, outcome and co-morbidity of depression in childhood and adolescence is known to be unfavourable on the psychosocial, psychiatric, and medical domain, and therefore sleep problems should be examined as early as possible. In the case of bipolar disorder, the mania phase will be characterized by drastic decreases in need for sleep. Especially in these 'depressive' cases (objective) sleep and circadian rhythm regulation remain unexplored. Noteworthy, objective findings do not always converge with the subjective reports. Although ADHD has an estimated prevalence of 2–17% in the population, the role of sleep problems herein has its own peculiar history (cf. inclusion/exclusion of sleep problems in Diagnostic and Statistical Manual). Sleep symptoms and complaints in children with ADHD are highly prevalent. Furthermore, co-occurring sleep problems with ADHD include periodic limb movement disorder and restless legs syndrome, as well as sleep-disordered breathing (SDB). There is a wealth of publications dealing with ADHD and sleep that is beyond the scope of this chapter, and includes not only subjective and objective studies on the unmedicated child with ADHD, but also on whether medications used to treat these disorders may adversely impact sleep.

Other aspects of sleep that merit attention include the emotional load surrounding sleep problems, for example enuresis, somnambulism, night terrors, narcolepsy, etc., which are not always addressed by the primary care physician or by researchers. Likewise with respect to environmental factors that might influence the amount of sleep a child actually gets, for example marital discussions, or bullying in school. An intriguing example are findings of sleep in juvenile offenders. The imposed routine and environment of prison would suggest a potential beneficial impact on sleep. However, apart from likely psychopathological symptoms, initiating and maintaining sleep problems are frequent occurrences in prison. Furthermore, interesting case studies discussing clinical observations with respect to the interrelation of affect and poor sleep can also be found. For example, treating the sleep problem relieved affective or behavioural problems (like increase in self-injury with disruption of sleep duration, reduced aggression, and violent behaviour after treatment of sleep apnoea).

In summary, the suggested role of dopaminergic systems and the frontostriatal networks with respect to the commonalities and disparities between sleep (neuro)behaviour and psychopathological (neuro)behaviour remains largely unexplored in children. Most findings have emerged from correlational studies that have not always controlled for potential confounding factors. Especially with respect to sleep neurobehaviour and psychopathological neurobehaviour, the sometimes unclear distinction between clinical relevance versus statistical significance, or observation/interpretation and fact, underscores the need for additional empirical data. As a result, poor sleep in clinical samples has been the drive behind most emotional and behavioural findings in children. Within a neurodevelopmental context, the question 'What are the cumulative effects of diminished or unrefreshing sleep?' remains unanswered.

Effects on health: the active child

In health psychology, theories have underlined the concerted importance of cognition and emotions associated to motivation towards health. Namely, the way we think or feel will influence what we do and *vice versa*, and eventually will result in who we are. In other words, do we eat high energy food because we feel fatigued, do we feel fatigued because we eat low-quality food, do we eat more because we are awake longer and food is available, or does the non-stop availability of 'energy-boost food' prevent us from sleeping? Since food is easily available do we 'exercise' less, do we feel too fatigued to engage in physical activity, and so forth. In short, emphasis on one functional domain would be an imperfect reflection of human functioning or as A. Damasio argues: Descartes' Error (Damasio, 1994).

The vast amount of studies with respect to the impact of poor sleep on health focuses on fragmented sleep, which is often seen as a resembling partial sleep deprivation and to a lesser extent as total sleep deprivation. Fragmented sleep often represents a state of cumulatively short sleep, and is frequently seen in SDB. Lately, a vast amount of literature can be found on the commonalities and disparities of SDB and obesity. Both of these conditions are linked to shortened sleep duration, and it remains unclear whether short sleep duration plays a causative and mechanistic role in the context of obesity, the epidemic disease of the twenty-first century.

SDB is characterized by repeated events of partial or complete upper airway obstruction during sleep, resulting in disruption of normal ventilation, hypoxaemia, and sleep fragmentation, with its primary symptom being snoring. As a result, habitual snoring, that is, primary snoring without alterations in sleep architecture, alveolar ventilation, and oxygenation is regarded as the less severe form of SDB, whereas in obstructive sleep apnoea (OSA) sleep is clearly disrupted. This spectrum of disease severity ranging from snoring to apnoea affects 12–20% of children, with OSA affecting 1–3%. In children, SDB has been associated with complex clinical presentations and SDB encompasses substantial and diverse end-organ morbidities (Gozal, 2008). Indeed, SDB in children can lead to behavioural disturbances and learning deficits, cardiovascular morbidity, and compromised somatic growth as well as decreased quality of life (QOL) and depression. Compelling evidence to support a causative association between SDB and hyperactivity and inattentive behaviours in children has emerged in the last two decades. In addition, daytime sleepiness, hyperactivity, and aggressive behaviours have all been documented in children who snore, even in the absence of OSA. In children, there are few published studies that have thus far examined the interrelations between SDB, obesity, and the metabolic syndrome. In a large cohort of snoring children, we have recently shown that both insulin resistance and lipid dysregulation are primarily determined by the degree of adiposity, and that SDB plays a minimal, if any role in the occurrence of insulin resistance in non-obese children. In another study conducted in obese children with SDB, insulin resistance was found to correlate with the severity of the respiratory disease independently of the degree of obesity (Gozal et al., 2007). As a corollary to those morbidity findings, improvements in learning and behaviour have been reported following treatment for SDB in children, and suggest that the neurocognitive and behavioural deficits are at least partially reversible. However, the exact mechanisms by which SDB elicits and treatment resolves these morbidities remain unknown.

Children with a body mass index (BMI) in the 85 to >95th percentile for age and sex are diagnosed as being overweight to obese. The prevalence of overweight children in the United States (US) is ~10.4% among toddlers, ~15.3% among school-aged children, and ~15.5% among adolescents, with an increased prevalence in low income families and among Mexican American and non-Hispanic Black adolescents (Ogden et al., 2002). Both SDB and obesity are associated with ethnicity, are clustered in affected families, and lead to depression and reduced QOL, decreased physical activity, and disturbed or insufficient sleep. In the management of obesity, assessments of the 'obesogenic' lifestyle, such as dietary and physical activity patterns are needed, as well as evaluation of the quality of sleep and the co-existence of SDB. However, food choices and physical activity levels are modified by numerous factors, such that unhealthy food intake and activity habits have been associated with deprivation, family structure, ethnicity, parental perception and/or education, and societal changes. Conversely, analysis of the systems controlling appetite and body weight suggests the presence of multiple key determinants, such as orexigenic hormones (Zheng and Berthoud, 2008). Although being associated with modification in neurotransmitter systems of the central nervous system, the biological adaptation to hunger (or the 24/7 availability of food) may either correspond to a 'state' or to a 'trait' (Duchesne et al., 2004) underlying a difficulty in the capability of controlling impulses. The moderating effect of executive dysfunctions with respect to food intake as well as to sleep is an infrequently addressed question in children, but of great relevance considering the impact of poor sleep on cognition and emotion. It has been suggested that watching 8 or more hours television at age 3 is related to obesity, and this association is also true for sleeping less than 10.5 hours (Reilly et al., 2005). Although few studies had a longitudinal design, adequate sleep at younger age seems 'protective' against obesity (Agras et al., 2004; Landhuis et al., 2008). The influence of gender might confound the relative risk for being overweight when sleep duration is short, that is, boys being at an increased risk (Knutson, 2005; Cole, 2006), especially with puberty onset. Lower socioeconomic status (Puder and Kriemler, 2008; Lobstein et al., 2004) increases the vulnerability to poor diet and limited opportunities for physical activity, and subsequently limits the resources that foster health (Lobstein et al., 2004; Flynn et al., 2006). Family structure is not only important with respect to sleep-wake pattern, but also to food eating patterns in the developing child, such that parental overweight is more likely to lead to childhood obesity (Cole, 2006). All these factors likely contour the health behaviour (e.g. inactivity) and health status (e.g. depression) (Lobstein et al., 2004; Adam et al., 2007) of a developing child. We would go as far as to pose the following question: *Is the obese, sleepy child a reflection of our twenty-first century?*

Other health conditions may affect the sleep duration of a child or lead to symptoms of disrupted sleep duration (e.g. somnolence). Sleep architecture and daytime alertness can be influenced by seizures and antiepileptic medications (Kotagal et al., 1994). Under-researched themes include the impact of chronic physical illness, where pain or nocturnal discomfort may disrupt the sleep of the child, and in many other medical disorders of childhood. Regrettably, few studies exist on sleep and specific disorders, despite the potential beneficial effect that good sleep can have on the underlying disease itself, or, conversely, the effect the disease can have on sleep, and therefore on many of the issues discussed heretofore (e.g. Bandla and Splaingard, 2004). In summary, description and identification of potential mechanisms implicated in health morbidities that either directly or indirectly are associated with poor sleep emerges as a mandatory priority for investigation. It would be important also to take advantage of the obesity epidemic and promote increased awareness among healthcare providers about the importance of sleep as well as the importance of sleep in health and disease.

Conclusion

The impact of poor sleep in the developing child is tremendously underrated and virtually unexplored. The normative, age-appropriate sleep needs during development remain undefined to a large extent. Furthermore, it remains crucial to realize that relations between sleep duration and cognition, effect, and health, are all multi-directional. The most consistent result from insufficient or disrupted sleep is increased daytime somnolence, which can become manifest in multiple and diverse ways in the developing child. Therefore, sleep in the child might serve not only as a reliable reporter of multiple settings, such as parental characteristics, psychopathology, education, and parenting skills, as well as psychosocial stress and trauma, cultural and social demands, but also ultimately lead to increased health-related burden. Consequently, each healthcare provider should monitor periodically any condition that may affect the amount of sleep in a developing child. Thorough sleep history-taking by the healthcare provider and use of objective sleep assessments are potential first steps and should include the five sleep variables, namely bedtime, rise time, total sleep duration, variability of sleep over time, and alignment of sleep with other circadian factors. Fine attunement between the social rhythms to the biological rhythm throughout lifespan should be a priority, and this principle applies to sleep. Incorporation of sleep as an important component of many research studies should be done *a priori* rather than as an afterthought.

We need to continue exploring the beneficial effects of healthy sleep and also how disrupted, shortened, or insufficient sleep may be adversely impacting on our children cognitive and affective functioning, may be compromising their health, and therefore may be imposing a heavy price on our socioeconomic structure. If we aim for successful society and economy where individual productivity is fostered and encouraged, then we need to preserve and promote sleep, so that dreams can be fulfilled. For our children, for our future, we should all campaign for 2010 as the beginning of the *'Decade of Sleep'*!

Summary box

- Sleep and why we sleep has long intrigued mankind. Although in the past we took for granted that sleep was inherently preserved and optimal in children, it is only in the last decade that the importance of sleep duration with respect to children's emotions, cognition, and health or overall development is being realized. Thus, sleep in a child is a public health issue of utmost importance.
- Given that two 'epidemics' are reciprocally evolving, namely decreases in sleep duration and increases in obesity rates, chronic inadequate sleep of the child may contribute to a wide range of not only specific health issues but also to neurobehavioural problems (i.e. cognitive and emotional). As such, have we overlooked or misinterpreted the evolving signs or should we take a preemptive role to prevent another 'epidemic'?
- Neurocognitively a child may appear 'sluggish', whereas behaviourally he or she may appear 'inattentive'. However, because sleep duration is determined by several factors namely, bedtime, adequate sleep time, rise time, occurrence of sleep time within the circadian rhythm,variability of sleep time within the circadian rhythm, as well as by individual (developmental) characteristics, adequate characterization of sleep phenotype can be quite challenging. Therefore, child healthcare providers should *always reflect on adequate sleep, not just on sleep duration.*
- Demographic status (i.e. age, gender, race/ethnicity), socioeconomic status (i.e. parental education, employment), as well as family structure contour the health behaviour and health status of the developing child. Given that parents generally overestimate the amount of sleep the child actually gets, and that increasingly more children obtain inadequate sleep, the need to embed the concerted impact of social and contextual determinants on sleep, and the need to take into consideration the outcome of poor sleep on social and contextual environments is apparent.
- Ultimately, societal productivity is fostered, cultured, and encouraged, and to enhance such targets it is critically important to optimize sleep.

References

Adam, E.K., Snell, E.K. & Pendry, P. (2007). Sleep timing and quantity in ecological and family context: a nationally representative time-diary study. *J Fam Psychol*, **21**, 4–19.

Agras, W.S., Hammer, L.D., McNicholas, F. & Kraemer, H.C. (2004). Risk factors for childhood overweight: a prospective study from birth to 9.5 years. *J Pediatr*, **145**, 20–25.

Alfano, C.A. & Gamble, A.L. (2009). The role of sleep in childhood psychiatric disorders. *Child Youth Care Forum*, **38**, 327–340.

Anderson, B., Storfer-Isser, A., Taylor, H.G., Rosen, C.L. & Redline, S. (2009). Associations of executive function with sleepiness and sleep duration in adolescents. *Pediatrics*, **123**(4), e701–e707.

Baker, L.W. (1884). SLEEP. *J Educ*, **20**, 2393–2293.

Bandla, H. & Splaingard, M. (2004). Sleep problems in children with common medical disorders. *Pediatr Clin North Am*, **51**, 203–227, viii.

Beebe, D.W., Difrancesco, M.W., Tlustos, S.J., McNally, K.A. & Holland, S.K. (2009). Preliminary fMRI findings in experimentally sleep-restricted adolescents engaged in a working memory task. *Behav Brain Funct*, **5**, 9.

Brand, S., Gerber, M., Hatzinger, M., Beck, J. & Holsboer-Trachsler, E. (2009). Evidence for similarities between adolescents and parents in sleep patterns. *Sleep Med*, **10**(10), 1124–1131.

Bruni, O., Ferri, R., Novelli, L., et al. (2009). Slow EEG amplitude oscillations during NREM sleep and reading disabilities in children with dyslexia. *Dev Neuropsychol*, **34**, 539–551.

Carskadon, M.A., Harvey, K. & Dement, W.C. (1981). Sleep loss in young adolescents. *Sleep*, **4**, 299–312.

Cirelli, C. (2006). Cellular consequences of sleep deprivation in the brain. *Sleep Med Rev*, **10**, 307–321.

Cole, T.J. (2006). The international growth standard for preadolescent and adolescent children: statistical considerations. *Food Nutr Bull*, **27**, S237–S243.

Curcio, G., Ferrara, M. & De Gennaro, L. (2006). Sleep loss, learning capacity and academic performance. *Sleep Med Rev*, **10**, 323–337.

Dahl, R.E. (1996). The regulation of sleep and arousal: development and psychopathology. *Dev Psychopathol*, **8**, 3–27.

Damasio, A.R. (1994). *Descartes' Error: Emotion, Reason, and the Human Brain*. New York, NY: Putnam Publishing.

de Alba, G.O.G., Fraire-Martãnez, M.I. & Valenzuela-Romero, R. (2003). Clinical correlation of hypnagogic hypersynchrony during sleep in normal children and those with learning disability. *Rev Neurol*, **36**, 720–723.

Dollman, J., Ridley, K., Olds, T. & Lowe, E. (2007). Trends in the duration of school-day sleep among 10- to 15-year-old South Australians between 1985 and 2004. *Acta Paediatr*, **96**, 1011–1014.

Duchesne, M., Mattos, P., Fontelle, L.F., Veiga, H., Rizo, L. & Appolinario, J.C. (2004). Neuropsychology of eating disorders: a systematic review.

El-Sheikh, M., Buckhalt, J.A., Keller, P.S. & Granger, D.A. (2008). Children's objective and subjective sleep disruptions: links with afternoon cortisol levels. *Health Psychol*, **27**, 26–33.

Fallone, G., Acebo, C., Arnedt, J.T., Seifer, R. & Carskadon, M.A. (2001). Effects of acute sleep restriction on behaviour, sustained attention, and response inhibition in children. *Percept Mot Skills*, **93**, 213–229.

Fallone, G., Acebo, C., Seifer, R. & Carskadon, M.A. (2005). Experimental restriction of sleep opportunity in children: effects on teacher ratings. *Sleep*, **28**, 1561–1567.

Flynn, M.A., McNeil, D.A., Maloff, B., et al. (2006). Reducing obesity and related chronic disease risk in children and youth: a synthesis of evidence with 'best practice' recommendations. *Obes Rev*, **7**(Suppl 1), 7–66.

Gottlieb, D.J., O'Connor, G.T. & Wil, J.B. (2007). Genome-wide association of sleep and circadian phenotypes. *BMC Med Genet*, **8**(Suppl 1), S9.

Gozal, D. (2008). Obstructive sleep apnea in children: implications for the developing central nervous system. *Semin Pediatr Neurol*, **15**, 100–106.

Gozal, D., Capdevila, O.S., Kheirandish-Gozal, L. & Crabtree, V.M. (2007). APOE epsilon 4 allele, cognitive dysfunction, and obstructive sleep apnea in children. *Neurology*, **69**, 243–249.

Iglowstein, I., Jenni, O.G., Molinari, L. & Largo, R.H. (2003). Sleep duration from infancy to adolescence: reference values and generational trends. *Pediatrics*, **111**, 302–307.

Iglowstein, I., Latal Hajnal, B., Molinari, L., Largo, R.H. & Jenni, O.G. (2006). Sleep behaviour in preterm children from birth to age 10 years: a longitudinal study. *Acta Paediatr*, **95**, 1691–1693.

Jenni, O.G., Fuhrer, H.Z., Iglowstein, I., Molinari, L. & Largo, R.H. (2005). A longitudinal study of bed sharing and sleep problems among Swiss children in the first 10 years of life. *Pediatrics*, **115**, 233–240.

Klackenberg, G. (1982). Somnambulism in childhood—prevalence, course and behavioural correlations. A prospective longitudinal study (6–16 years). *Acta Paediatr Scand*, **71**, 495–499.

Knutson, K.L. (2005). Sex differences in the association between sleep and body mass index in adolescents. *J Pediatr*, **147**, 830–834.

Knutson, K.L. & Lauderdale, D.S. (2009). Sociodemographic and behavioural predictors of bed time and wake time among US adolescents aged 15 to 17 years. *J Pediatr*, **154**, 426–430.

Kotagal, S., Gibbons, V.P. & Stith, J.A. (1994). Sleep abnormalities in patients with severe cerebral palsy. *Dev Med Child Neurol*, **36**, 304–311.

Lamberg, L. (2009). High schools find later start time helps students' health and performance. *JAMA*, **301**, 2200–2201.

Landhuis, C.E., Poulton, R., Welch, D. & Hancox, R.J. (2008). Childhood sleep time and long-term risk for obesity: a 32-year prospective birth cohort study. *Pediatrics*, **122**, 955–960.

Li, S., Jin, X., Wu, S., Jiang, F., Yan, C. & Shen, X. (2007). The impact of media use on sleep patterns and sleep disorders among school-aged children in China. *Sleep*, **30**, 361–367.

Lobstein, T., Baur, L. & Uauy, R. (2004). Obesity in children and young people: a crisis in public health. *Obes Rev*, **5**, 4–104.

Meltzer, L.J. & Mindell, J.A. (2007). Relationship between child sleep disturbances and maternal sleep, mood, and parenting stress: a pilot study. *J Fam Psychol*, **21**, 67–73.

Mercier, L., Pivik, R.T. & Busby, K. (1993). Sleep patterns in reading disabled children. *Sleep*, **16**, 207–215.

National Sleep Foundation (2004). *Sleep in America Poll—Sleep in Children Survey*. Available at: http://www.sleepfoundation.org/article/sleep-america-polls/2004-children-and-sleep. Accessed April 29th, 2010

National Sleep Foundation (2006). *Sleep in America Poll—Teens and Sleep*. Available at: http://www.sleepfoundation.org/article/sleep-america-polls/2006-teens-and-sleep. Accessed April 29th, 2010

Ogden, C.L., Flegal, K.M., Carroll, M.D. & Johnson, C.L. (2002). Prevalence and trends in overweight among US children and adolescents, 1999-2000. *JAMA*, **288**, 1728–1732.

Owens, J. (2008). Classification and epidemiology of childhood sleep disorders. *Prim Care*, **35**, 533–546, vii.

Pilcher, J.J. & Huffcutt, A.I. (1996). Effects of sleep deprivation on performance: a meta-analysis. *Sleep*, **19**, 318–326.

Puder, J.J. & Kriemler, S. (2008). Can we stop the epidemic of childhood obesity? *Praxis (Bern 1994)*, **97**, 17–23.

Randazzo, A.C., Muehlbach, M.J., Schweitzer, P.K. & Walsh, J.K. (1998). Cognitive function following acute sleep restriction in children ages 10–14. *Sleep*, **21**, 861–868.

Reilly, J.J., Armstrong, J., Dorosty, A.R., et al. (2005). Early life risk factors for obesity in childhood: cohort study. *BMJ*, **330**, 1357.

Rona, R.J., Li, L., Gulliford, M.C. & Chinn, S. (1998). Disturbed sleep: effects of sociocultural factors and illness. *Arch Dis Child*, **78**, 20–25.

Sadeh, A., Raviv, A. & Gruber, R. (2000). Sleep patterns and sleep disruptions in school-age children. *Dev Psychol*, **36**, 291–301.

Sadeh, A., Gruber, R. & Raviv, A. (2002). Sleep, neurobehavioural functioning, and behaviour problems in school-age children. *Child Dev*, **73**, 405–417.

Sadeh, A., Gruber, R. & Raviv, A. (2003). The effects of sleep restriction and extension on school-age children: what a difference an hour makes. *Child Dev*, **74**, 444–455.

Sheldon, S., Ferber, R. & Kryger, M. (2005). *Principles and Practice of Pediatric Sleep Medicine*. USA: Elsevier Saunders.

Simard, V., Nielsen, T.A., Tremblay, R.E., Boivin, M. & Montplaisir, J.Y. (2008). Longitudinal study of preschool sleep disturbance: the predictive role of maladaptive parental behaviours, early sleep problems, and child/mother psychological factors. *Arch Pediatr Adolesc Med*, **162**, 360–367.

Spruyt, K. (2007). *Slaapproblemen bij kinderen. Basisgids voor ouders en hulpverleners.* Tielt, Belgium, Lannoo.

Spruyt, K., O'Brien, L.M., Cluydts, R., Verleye, G.B. & Ferri, R. (2005). Odds, prevalence and predictors of sleep problems in school-age normal children. *J Sleep Res*, **14**, 163–176.

Stores, G. (2001). *A Clinical Guide to Sleep Disorders in Children and Adolescents.* New York, NY: Cambridge University Press.

Terman, L.M. & Hocking, A. (1913). The sleep of school children, its districbution according to age, and its relation to physical and mental efficiency. *J Educ Psychol*, **4**, 138–147.

Thorleifsdottir, B., Bjornsson, J.K., Benediktsdottir, B., Gislason, T. & Kristbjarnarson, H. (2002). Sleep and sleep habits from childhood to young adulthood over a 10-year period. *J Psychosom Res*, **53**, 529–537.

Warner, S., Murray, G. & Meyer, D. (2008). Holiday and school-term sleep patterns of Australian adolescents. *J Adolesc*, **31**, 595–608.

Wolfson, A.R. & Carskadon, M.A. (2003). Understanding adolescents' sleep patterns and school performance: a critical appraisal. *Sleep Med Rev*, **7**, 491–506.

Wolfson, A.R., Spaulding, N.L., Dandrow, C. & Baroni, E.M. (2007). Middle school start times: the importance of a good night's sleep for young adolescents. *Behav Sleep Med*, **5**, 194–209.

Yang, C.K., Kim, J.K., Patel, S.R. & Lee, J.H. (2005). Age-related changes in sleep/wake patterns among Korean teenagers. *Pediatrics*, **115**, 250–256.

Zheng, H. & Berthoud, H.R. (2008). Neural systems controlling the drive to eat: mind versus metabolism. *Physiology*, **23**, 75–83.

Chapter 11

Sleep, inflammation, and disease

M.A. Miller and F.P. Cappuccio

Introduction

This chapter briefly examines normal sleep behaviour and changes in sleeping patterns before examining some of the mechanisms and pathways that may be responsible for the observed associations between sleep duration and disease. The chapter focuses mainly on the possible role of inflammatory mechanisms, as pathways and mechanisms involving obesity and body fat distribution, appetite and satiety, insulin resistance and glucose homeostasis are discussed in Chapter 6. Despite decades of research, our knowledge of the function of sleep is still very minimal. It is commonly accepted that sleep is restorative and has a role in immune function, memory processing, and energy control. Evidence is emerging that disturbances in sleep and sleep disorders play a role in the morbidity of chronic conditions including obesity and hypertension as well as on all-cause mortality. It has been suggested that sleep may have an important effect on the cardiovascular system and the development of associated disease as it has an effect on many of the underlying mechanisms. However, the relationship between sleep processes and disease development, disease progression, and disease management is often unclear or understudied and numerous common medical conditions including diabetes and arthritis can have an effect on sleep quality.

Evidence suggests that there is an interaction between sleep (both quantity and quality) and parameters of cardiovascular risk (see also Chapter 5). The hypothesis that a lack of sleep may adversely affect inflammatory processes which lead to an increase in cardiovascular disease (CVD) is explored. The development and progression of such disease states are examined to see if it is possible to determine whether the sleep effect merely reflects disease progression or whether it may be in some way causally related. Possible effects of age, gender, ethnicity, and genetic make up on the relation between sleep and disease progression are also be examined. The relationship between known sleep disorders and cardiovascular risk, along with the role of inflammation in the development of obstructive sleep apnoea (OSA) is discussed. Finally, the effect of established and novel treatments for these conditions and their effect on the underlying inflammation is explored.

Specifically, the aim is to review the evidence regarding the impact of sleep on the immune processes and subsequent disease development with particular regard to the development of CVD and its complications.

Normal sleep behaviour

Sleep is a fundamental and natural process and yet the exact purpose of sleep and its effect on health and disease remains to be elucidated fully. It appears to be crucial for the maintenance and restoration of homeostasis through the regulation of energy, repair, and infection control. Moreover, it may be important in the programming of the brain (Irwin, 2002; Majde and Krueger, 2005; Siegel, 2005).

Sleep states

Physiological and pathological sleep is divided into two states: non-rapid eye movement (NREM) sleep and rapid eye movement (REM) sleep (Siegel, 2005) (see also Chapter 2). Furthermore, NREM sleep is classically sub-divided into four stages (stages 1–4). A quiet period of sleep known as slow wave sleep (SWS) occurs during NREM. During this time arterial pressure and heart rate tend to decrease, the respiratory rate is low, and vagal nerve activity predominates. By contrast, REM periods are characterized by periods of relative hypertension and tachycardia and a relative increase in sympathetic activity. During the night there is a continuous cycling between the NREM and REM phases, with the consequent cardiovascular autonomic changes (Legramante and Galante, 2005). Dreaming occurs in the REM phase which becomes increasingly longer as sleep progresses. Different hormonal changes occur during these periods. In NREM, growth hormone (GH) secretion occurs, while in REM there is an increase in prolactin and glucocorticoids. Sleep parameters are, however, known to change with age and time spent in SWS decreases in adults (Guilleminault et al., 2004).

Changes in sleeping habits

Sleeping habits within our society have been changing over the last 100 years, partly as a result of a decreased dependency on daylight hours along with an increase in shift-work and changes in lifestyle and home environments (Horrocks and Pounder, 2006; National Sleep Foundation, 2005). In the United States, statistics from the National Sleep Foundation in America suggest that approximately one-third of Americans sleep 6.5 hours a night or less (National Sleep Foundation, 2005). It is therefore crucially important that we understand the importance of sleep and understand its impact on health and disease.

Sleep and inflammation

Sleep and the immune system appear to have a reciprocal relationship. Sleep may modulate the immune system but conversely activation of the immune system and production of inflammatory cytokines may affect sleep. Anecdotally, sleep is reported to be an early response to acute infections such as the cold and influenza virus. Indeed, early Greek writings noted that sleepiness often accompanied infection. NREM and especially SWS is thought to provide more physiological restoration than other stages of sleep. However, sleep, sleep duration, and sleep quality may affect both one's susceptibility to and one's ability to fight off infection (Lange et al., 2006).

Sleep and immune response to viral challenge and vaccination

Viral diseases such as rabies that affect the central nervous system can have an effect on sleep. The influenza virus which is a negative-sense single-stranded ribonucleic acid (RNA) virus has been associated with large increases in NREM sleep. On infection of the host, the positive-sense RNA strand is formed which can anneal to the negative-sense strand to form double-stranded (ds) viral RNA. Inflammatory cytokines including interleukin-1 (IL-1) appear to be induced by this ds viral RNA. Viral pathogenic mechanisms have also been implicated in a number of conditions that involve sleep disorders including chronic fatigue syndrome and sudden infant death syndrome (Krueger and Majde, 1994).

There is evidence to suggest that sleep deprivation can alter the immune response to a viral challenge. In young healthy adults, the antibody response to the hepatitis A vaccination is much lower in those who had been sleep deprived compared to those who had a normal night's sleep (Lange et al., 2003).

Sleep and bacterial infection

The NREM sleep response to gram-negative bacteria is biphasic. In the initial phase, NREM sleep increases in intensity and duration, whereas REM sleep is inhibited. In the second phase, REM is still inhibited but the duration of NREM progressively decreases (Krueger and Majde, 1994). However, it has been noted that the route of administration as well as bacterial species involved can alter the timing of the sleep response. It is of interest to note that both killed bacteria and components of the bacterial cell wall can induce the NREM sleep changes. Moreover, some components of the bacterial cell wall including muramyl peptides are somnogenic and some of these, as well as other bacterial cell wall components, are effective stimulants of the host defence systems (Krueger and Majde, 1994).

At present there are no known synthetic pathways for muramyl peptides in mammals but these peptides are readily available to mammals via the breakdown of bacteria in the intestinal lumen. Another bacterial product which may be important in the sleep responses is the lipopolysaccharide (LPS) component of gram-negative bacterial cell walls known as endotoxin. Raised circulating levels of endotoxin have been associated with an increased risk of CVD (Miller et al., 2009b). The somnogenic dose range of endotoxin is much narrower than that for muramyl peptides and small increases above the somnogenic threshold can induce shock (Krueger and Majde, 1994). The process by which diverse microbial agents activate the host defence systems involves a complex signalling pathway which is part of the innate immune system.

Innate immunity

The innate immune system is the evolutionary conserved system which allows the body to respond to, and rapidly isolate, invading pathogens or foreign particles including tumours or transplanted material. It is related to, but distinct from, the acquired immune system. One of the key components of the innate immune system is the Toll-like receptors (TLRs), which are activated by a diverse array of microbial factors. These receptors in turn activate the nuclear factor-Kappa B (NF-κB) pathway, leading to the expression of cellular adhesion molecules and cytokines. Activation of the host defence mechanisms and immune system not only leads to an increase in inflammatory cytokines, but also leads to an increase in body temperature and longer periods of SWS and reduced wakefulness. However, in advanced stages of inflammation, the sleep promoting effects are diminished and reduced NREM and increased wakefulness may result (Mullington et al., 2001).

Activation of innate immune system pathways also appears to be important in the development of both CVD and coronary heart disease (CHD). Endothelial dysfunction may precede the development of atherosclerosis and underlies these disease processes. Accumulation of macrophages and low-density lipoproteins (LDL) activates TLRs and subsequent pathways which leads to the expression of cellular adhesion molecules and cytokines which are important in atheromatous plaque formation. Accumulating evidence suggests that there are important interactions between this innate immune system and both CVD and sleep (Majde and Krueger, 2005).

Toll-like receptors

Sleep deprivation induced activation of cytokine production can occur through stimulation of the TLR pathways which are part of the innate immune system. These pathways are also activated by the outer LPS component of bacterial cell membranes (Rosenfeld and Shai, 2006) as shown in Fig. 11.1. A recent study demonstrated that following a night of sleep loss, LPS activation of Toll-like receptor-4 (TLR-4) was greater than following a night of uninterrupted sleep (Irwin et al., 2006). There was also an increase in tumour necrosis factor-alpha

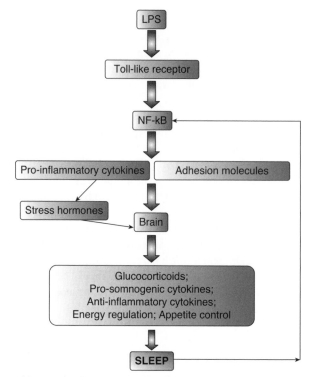

Fig. 11.1 Proposed interaction between the innate immune system and sleep regulation.
Source: Reproduced from Miller, M.A. & Cappuccio, F.P. (2007). Inflammation, sleep, obesity and cardiovascular disease. *Curr Vasc Pharmacol*, **5**(2), 93–102, with permission.

(TNF-α) transcription, enhanced expression of the circadian clock gene period 1 (Per1), and activation of multiple signal transcription pathways including the NF-κB inflammatory signalling system. One study which investigated the effect of prolonged physical activity with concomitant energy and sleep deprivation on leukocyte function, demonstrated that leukocytes responded with an increasing release of LPS-induced inflammatory cytokines as the study progressed. Multi-factorial stress can therefore activate immune cells and prime their response to a microbial challenge (Gundersen et al., 2006). Bacterial LPS can also have direct effect on sleep leading to an increase in NREM sleep and a reduction in REM sleep in rabbits (Majde and Krueger, 2005).

TLR activity is abnormal in Crohn's disease, arthritis, and heart failure (Irwin et al., 2006) and it remains to be elucidated whether long-term sleep deprivation can have similar effects on the immune system which may lead to or make one more susceptible to disease.

Nuclear factor-Kappa B signalling

Nuclear factor-Kappa B is a transcription factor which can induce the transcription of more than 200 genes including those which are involved in the production of cytokines and inflammatory markers. NF-κB exists in an inhibitor-bound inactive cytosolic form. The inhibitor (IκB) can be removed by a number of different stimuli which include bacteria and viruses as well as oxidants, cytokines, and hypoxia. On activation, NF-κB is translocated to the nucleus where on binding to DNA it activates transcription. NF-κB binding domains have been found in the promoter region of the genes of many substances thought to be involved in sleep regulation. These include the adenosine A1 receptor, cyclooxygenase-2 (Cox-2), and nitric oxide synthase (NOS) which suggests that these may all be up-regulated by NF-κB (Krueger et al., 2001). Two of the cytokines that induce NF-κB transcription are IL-1 and TNF-α. However, the presence of a positive feedback loop means that these two cytokines are also up-regulated by NF-κB. In turn, there are many substances that can dampen this positive feedback loop. These pathways, which are discussed in detail in the review by Kruegar et al. (2001), clearly demonstrate the tight regulation of somnogenic and pro-somnogenic pathways.

Sleep regulation of Type 1 and Type 2 immune response

Defence-mediated, pro-inflammatory immune response are mediated by the response of Type 1 leukocytes and include the secretion of IL-2, interferon-gamma (IFN-γ), and IL-12, whereas the action of the Type 2 response is to moderate the action of the Type 1 leukocytes by the section of anti-inflammatory cytokines including IL-4 and IL-10. An excess of the former leads to inflammation and tissue damage, whereas an excess Type 2 response leads to a susceptibility to infection and allergy. Sleep regulates the balance between Type 1 and Type 2 activity and sleep deprivation shifts the balance in favour of Type 2 activity (Lange et al., 2006) and conversely pro-inflammatory cytokines increase SWS and anti-inflammatory cytokines inhibit sleep (Majde and Krueger, 2005).

Sleep, the hypothalamic pituitary adrenocortical axis, cortisol, and growth hormone

The hypothalamic-pituitary-adrenal axis (HPA axis) is part of the neuroendocrine system that regulates interactions and feedback loops between the hypothalamus, the pituitary gland, and the adrenal glands. It regulates the body's response to stress and many body processes including digestion and immune function. The hypothalamus secretes vasopressin and corticotropin-releasing hormone (CRH). These two peptides have an effect on the pituitary gland and stimulate secretion of adrenocorticotropic hormone (ACTH), which in turn act on the adrenal cortex and affect the production of glucocorticoids. Stress, blood cortisol levels, and the sleep-wake cycle all have an effect on the release of CRH from the hypothalamus. Increased bodily stress and inflammation stimulates the HPA axis to produce the anti-inflammatory hormone cortisol so as to reduce the immune response.

In normal healthy individuals, on awakening there is a rise in cortisol levels. The time of awakening and stress are thought to influence the magnitude of the cortisol awakening response (CAR) (Williams et al., 2005). A recent study which examined men and women London Underground shift-workers suggested that early waking stress early in the day and associated cortisol levels often coincide with sleep disturbance (Williams et al., 2005). In a recent pilot study, which examined the sleep and the stress-induced cortisol response in children and adolescents, there were significant associations between the self-reported sleep quality but not quantity and the cortisol response (Capaldi Ii et al., 2005).

Sleep, and in particular deep sleep, has an inhibitory influence on the HPA axis, whereas activation of the HPA axis leads to arousal (Buckley and Schatzberg, 2005). Dysfunction of the HPA axis at any level (CRH receptor, glucocorticoid receptor, or mineralocorticoid receptor) can also disrupt sleep (Buckley and Schatzberg, 2005). Inhibition of CRH enhances NREM sleep.

It has been suggested that growth hormone releasing hormone (GHRH) may modulate sleep in a reciprocal manner and that the somnogenic activities of both GHRH as well as that of IL-1 may be related to a shared CRH feedback signal (Ranjbaran et al., 2007).

Sleep cytokines and nitric oxide

Investigators have now developed lists of criteria that need to be met before a substance can be identified as a sleep regulatory substance (SRS). These include: (i) the substance should enhance sleep if injected; (ii) if the substance is inhibited, sleep should be reduced; (iii) the level of the substance in the brain should vary with sleep propensity; (iv) the substance should act on sleep regulatory circuits; (v) the substance should be altered in pathological states that are associated with enhanced sleepiness (Krueger, 2008).

Nitric oxide (NO) fulfils the requirements of a SRS for the regulation of REMs. The mechanism of action of NO however is very complex. NO may signal through a number of different pathways including cyclic guanosine monophosphate (cGMP)/protein kinase G (PKG) or through S-nitrosylation and may modulate a number of neuronal pathways. Its release can be inhibited by IL-10 and IL-4 (Krueger, 2008). NO production is regulated by the enzyme NOS which in turn is up-regulated by NF-κB. Arginine analogs can be used to block NOS and hence production of NO and although this blocks the IL-1-induced sleep responses, it does not effect the IL-1-induced fever (Krueger et al., 2001).

Immune modulation of sleep

Fatigue and increased sleepiness are typical manifestations of inflammatory disorders such as arthritis. In these conditions, there is an immune-mediated acute phase response (APR) associated with activation of various inflammatory cells and an increase in circulating inflammatory cytokines. Animal studies have shown that injection of two of these cytokines interleukin-1beta (IL-1β) and TNF-α leads to an increase in NREM sleep. Moreover, if the effect of these cytokines is blocked, the spontaneous sleep and sleep rebound that normally occurs after sleep deprivation is blocked (Krueger et al., 2001). The role of cytokines in sleep regulation has been recently reviewed and, as indicated in this review, there are now a large number of cytokines which are known to have an effect on NREM sleep. At present, however, only IL-1 and TNF-α fulfil the criteria of an SRS (Krueger, 2008).

The precise mechanisms by which cytokines exert their effects on sleep are yet to be elucidated, but are thought to involve many biochemical intermediates including NO, GHRH, prostaglandins, CRH, and NF-κB. As well as inducing sleep, cytokines are also capable of inhibiting sleep (e.g. IL-10 and IL-4), however it is not clear if these cytokines have direct effects on sleep or whether they inhibit sleep by antagonizing the effect of IL-1β and TNF-α.

Sleep, inflammation, and risk factors for disease

Markers of inflammation are independently associated with a number of well-known risk factors for disease. These include risk factors for CVD, for example age and body mass index (BMI) (Miller and Cappuccio, 2007).

Sleep, inflammation, and age

Age is associated with changes in the length and quality of sleep, and sleep problems increase with age (Prinz, 2004). Increasing age is also a risk factor for CVD and the number of elderly individuals in the population as well as the number of individuals with chronic illnesses is increasing. Furthermore, there is an increasing body of evidence to suggest that the ageing process, sleep, and the inflammatory processes are related (Hak et al., 2001; Meier-Ewert et al., 2004; Roubenoff et al., 2003). It is important that not only are sleep regulatory mechanisms studied, but the effect of ageing on these processes is also determined. It is important that the boundaries between normal and abnormal age-related changes in sleep behaviour are understood to allow the development of intervention guidelines. Moreover, the exact nature of relationships and causality between sleep, age, and inflammation remain to be elucidated. Increased inflammatory marker levels have been observed in elderly population, for example high sensitivity C-reactive protein (hs-CRP) and IL-6 increase with age (Hak et al., 2001; Roubenoff et al., 2003).

Sleep, inflammation, gender, and ethnicity

Sleep-disordered breathing (SDB) is the term used to describe a group of disorders which are characterized by abnormalities of respiratory pattern (pauses in breathing) or the quantity of ventilation during sleep. The most common of such disorders is OSA. This is characterized by the complete or partial collapse of the pharyngeal airway during sleep. Sleep disruption then occurs as the individual needs to be aroused to resume ventilation. OSA is associated with an increased CVD risk and men are at increased risk of CVD. It is not clear whether this gender difference is associated with differences in patterns of sleep, although men are twice as likely to develop OSA when compared to women. Women, however, increase their risk if they are overweight. It has also been suggested that the menopause may be a risk for SDB (Resta et al., 2004). There are gender differences in the level of many circulating inflammatory markers (Miller et al., 2003). The hs-CRP levels were higher in post-menopausal women compared to pre-menopausal women. Furthermore, although the use of hormone replacement therapy (HRT) amongst post-menopausal women did not affect the level of hs-CRP, lower values were detected in pre-menopausal women not taking the oral contraceptive pill (OCP) compared to those taking OCP. With IL-6 the levels were higher in post-menopausal women compared to pre-menopausal women, irrespective of use of HRT amongst post-menopausal women or use of OCP in pre-menopausal women (Miller et al., 2009a). Ethnic differences in inflammatory markers have been observed which in part are associated with ethnic differences in cardiovascular risk (Miller et al., 2003).

Sleep, inflammation, and smoking

Smoking has an effect on the level of circulating inflammatory markers (Miller et al., 2003) and this may play a part in the development and progression of disease. The prevalence of OSA is higher in smokers than that in non-smokers, which may be the result of an increase in the amount of inflammation and also fluid retention in the upper airway. The risk of developing OSA declines after smoking cessation and there is a synergistic effect between cigarette smoking and sleep apnoea on some of the biochemical cardiovascular risk markers (Lavie and Lavie, 2008).

Sleep, inflammation, and exercise

Within the literature there is conflicting evidence with regard to the effect of exercise on sleep. This in part is due to the different methodologies, the different types and intensity of the exercise, the fitness of the individuals themselves, as well as the time of day at which the exercise is performed. There is some evidence to suggest that exercise performed in the morning may improve sleep as opposed to that which is performed in the evening (Santos et al., 2007).

Notwithstanding these uncertainties, the American Sleep Disorders Association considers physical exercise as a non-pharmacological treatment for sleep disorders.

The mechanisms by which physical exercise promotes changes in sleep architecture remain to be fully elucidated, however data suggest that cytokines are important in the regulation of sleep and sleep-wake behaviour. The relationship between IL-1, IL-6, and TNF-α, exercise, and sleep has been discussed in a recent review (Santos et al., 2007). It was proposed that exercise-induced sleep is mediated by cytokines, which increase the NREM sleep phase and thus stimulate the regenerative characteristics of sleep. The beneficial effects, however, of exercise on sleep appear to be true only for moderate exercise, which is carried out early in the day.

Sleep, inflammation and lipids

A recent study of 155 men with OSA and 39 men without demonstrated that a key enzyme involved in triglyceride hydrolysis, lipoprotein lipase (LPL) was reduced in OSA patients. Continuous positive airway pressure (CPAP) is used to treat OSA and the activity of this enzyme was increased following CPAP therapy. There was also a decrease in hs-CRP concentrations in these individuals. This suggests that the cardiovascular benefits associated with CPAP treatment may include improved lipid metabolism as well as effects on inflammation (Iesato et al., 2007). Hypoxia induced by OSA may also lead to the generation of reactive oxygen species (ROS) and subsequent lipid peroxidation.

Sleep, inflammation, and social economic status

Low social economic status (SES) is frequently associated with short sleep (Stranges et al., 2008b), a diminished opportunity to obtain sufficient sleep, or poor sleep quality (Van Cauter and Spiegel, 1999). There are many possible mechanisms by which SES may have an effect on health. These include mechanisms involving short sleep, but further studies are required to see if this may be mediated by an effect on inflammation.

Sleep, inflammation, and alcohol

Alcohol has a short-lived sedating effect and then there is a rebound-wakefulness as the alcohol level approaches zero. In alcohol dependency, inflammatory markers including TNF-α are associated with increased REM sleep. Alcoholic patients show profound alterations in sleep patterns and following sleep loss exhibit abnormal homeostatic recovery. Moreover, these effects are particularly pronounced in African American alcoholics (Irwin et al., 2004). There is some inconsistency in the literature, but in general it is accepted that moderate-to-large quantities of alcohol are capable of aggravating airway diseases including OSA. A recent study demonstrated that alcohol up-regulates TLRs leading to an increased production of inflammatory cytokines, which may in part explain the increased severity of airway disease in alcoholics (Bailey et al., 2009).

Inter-relationships between alcoholism, sleep loss, and ethnicity may also operate in a bi-directional manner (Irwin et al., 2004). Following sleep deprivation, African American alcoholics showed greater nocturnal levels of IL-6 and greater increases in TNF-α compared to matched controls. The increased circulating pro-inflammatory cytokines may have a negative effect on sleep initiation as pre-sleep IL-6 levels were found to be associated with sleep latency (Irwin et al., 2004). Disturbed sleep patterns affect hormonal, autonomic nervous system, and immune function and might contribute to the increased mortality rate observed in African American alcoholics (Irwin et al., 2004).

Sleep, inflammation, and genetic factors

The sleep-wake cycle in the brain is regulated by the central circadian oscillator in the hypothalamic suprachiasmatic nuclei (SCN). This oscillator is composed of many genes and proteins which interact together. Genetic factors may interact with environmental factors to influence the set-point at which a given individual's neuroendocrine stress responses and production of cytokines occur in response to different pathogens or antigens. Genetic determinants of sleep acting on the inflammatory and oxidative pathways may also contribute to the cardiovascular risk associated with sleep disruption (see also Chapter 12).

Sleep deprivation and inflammation

Following a period of sleep deprivation the body tries to recover lost sleep. This sleep 'rebound' phenomenon suggests that sleep is not a passive activity. Sleep deprivation has a profound effect on the immune system. Although it is possible that small amounts of sleep loss may help promote the host defence system, prolonged sleep loss may have devastating consequences. Moreover, althoughit is important to establish on a population basis what the optimum amount of sleep required to remain healthy and safe is, it is also important to establish what factors determined the right amount of sleep. There is also a need to establish whether all individuals require the same amount of sleep, especially as the inter-individual variability in sleep, circadian rhythm, and the response to sleep deprivation is wide.

Circadian rhythms and inflammation

Sleep regulation is extremely closely linked to the regulation of circadian rhythm. Studies have demonstrated that in mice the expression of several hundred genes in the liver may vary in a cyclical pattern over the course of the day (Majde and Krueger, 2005). Although diurnal rhythms have been reported for various cytokines in normal individuals, these variations are often related to the sleep-wake cycle (Irwin, 2002; Lange et al., 2006). SWS sleep has been reported to be associated with increases in circulating IL-1 concentrations followed by an increase in IL-2 (Irwin, 2002). Circulating IL-6 levels also demonstrate marked cyclical changes in levels. Typically, values are low during the daytime and increase to a maximum at night (Irwin, 2002). Although good sleep is associated with decreased daytime secretion of IL-6, disturbed nighttime sleep or sleep deprivation is associated with increased daytime IL-6 levels (Krueger et al., 2001). This may indicate that IL-6 expression is related to sleep-dependent rather than circadian rhythms.

A recent study, however, has demonstrated that the level of both soluble receptors for TNF (sTNF-R p55 and sTNF-R p75) shows clear-cut diurnal variations. Peak values were observed in the early morning and these variations were not significantly affected by a single night of sleep deprivation. By contrast the soluble interleukin receptor (IL-2R) did not vary systematically across the day (Haack et al., 2004). The diurnal variations in the sTNF receptors were characterized by a single cosine curve, the peak of which occurred around 6:00 hours on average. It was demonstrated that this peak occurred before the morning rise in cortisol and fluctuated inversely with the diurnal rhythm of temperature.

Experimental short-term sleep deprivation studies and inflammatory mediators

Experimental studies of sleep restriction offer the chance to observe these effects under controlled conditions. However, these studies are time consuming, logistically difficult, and costly, they are therefore often only conducted for short periods of time and on small numbers of individuals.

Studies have reported that sleep deprivation leads to an increase in circulating white blood cells (WBC) and in particular granulocytes and monocytes, as well as to an increase in the activity of natural killer cells which are a major source of inflammatory cytokines (Ranjbaran et al., 2007).

In animal studies, prolonged sleep deprivation has been shown to lead to the death of the animal possibly as a result of the failure of the host defence mechanisms. However, due to a lack of available data and the fact that studies in humans are normally short term and performed on young volunteers, there is still some controversy as to whether sleep deprivation leaves an individual more susceptible to infection.

Alterations in immune responses and increased levels of circulating cytokines such as IL-6, TNF-α, and hs-CRP have been found in experimental sleep deprivation studies (Irwin et al., 2006; Meier-Ewert et al., 2004; Vgontzas et al., 2004). The former study found that hs-CRP concentrations increased following 88 hours of total sleep deprivation as well as following 10 consecutive days of partial sleep deprivation (4.2 hours). In the second study, Irwin et al. (2008) showed that in the morning following one night's sleep loss monocyte production of IL-6 and TNF-α was significantly greater than when following a night of uninterrupted sleep. They also demonstrated that the sleep loss was associated with increased transcription of messenger RNA for both IL-6 (greater than threefold) and TNF-α (twofold). Their data suggested that this response was mediated by NF-κB. In the latter study, modest sleep restriction in healthy young subjects from 8 hours down to 6 hours per night for 1 week was associated with an increase in the total secretion of IL-6 over 24 hours. However, TNF-α levels were only found to be increased in men (Vgontzas et al., 2004). It was also noted that although the peak cortisol secretion was lower following sleep restriction than at baseline, this effect was only significant in men compared to women. This highlights the possibility that the inflammatory responses to sleep restriction may be gender specific. Further evidence to support this suggestion was found in the recent study by Irwin et al. (2008). Fourteen healthy adults were subjected to partial sleep deprivation. It was found that although sleep loss led to a rapid induction of NF-κB, this effect was mainly observed in females not males. However, as only seven men and women were studied, it is important that further studies are performed to verify these results.

In another study of young healthy adults, 40 hours sleep deprivation induced a significant increase in the cellular adhesion molecules E-selectin and intercellular adhesion molecule-1 (ICAM-1) as well as a significant increase in the inflammatory cytokines, IL-1β, and IL-1r. However, there was no change in vascular cellular adhesion molecule-1 (VCAM-1) and, unlike in the previous studies, hs-CRP and IL-6 were reduced. This adds to the evidence to suggest that the duration and type of sleep deprivation may have different effects on the immune system and that sleep deprivation may stimulate both pro- and anti-inflammatory mechanisms (Frey et al., 2007). Moreover, as IL-6 has dualistic pro- and anti-inflammatory role, it is possible that the activation of IL-6 by sleep deprivation could reflect compensatory mechanisms leading to activation of anti-inflammatory cytokines (Irwin et al., 2008).

Data from these and a number of subsequent laboratory studies have led to the view that sleep deprivation leads to enhanced levels of IL-1β and TNF-α. Increased levels of these cytokines have also been related to many of the symptoms associated with sleep deprivation including effects on memory, cognitive function, depression, sleepiness, and fatigue (Krueger, 2008).

Chronic sleep deprivation (short sleep) and inflammation

Chronic sleep restriction may arise due to work, social, and domestic demands and responsibilities and lifestyle, or arise due to the presence of a medical or sleep disorder.

Evidence is accumulating to suggest that chronic restriction of sleep below 7 hours per night leads to significant cognitive dysfunction (Banks and Dinges, 2007), increased mortality (Ferrie et al., 2007), and increased CVD risk (Cappuccio et al., 2007; Ferrie et al., 2007; Stranges et al., 2008a, b). Data from such studies are however largely based on self-reported recording of sleep duration and more longitudinal data are required to establish a causal role for reduced sleep on many of the adverse health outcomes.

To date the potential impact of chronic sleep deprivation on the inflammatory system and immune responses has not been extensively investigated. One study failed to demonstrate any significant association between hs-CRP levels and sleep duration in a combined study of men and women (Taheri et al., 2007). By contrast, in participants from the Cleveland family Study, Patel et al. (2009) have demonstrated that increased habitual sleep duration, based on self-reported sleep questionnaire data, was associated with an increase in both hs-CRP ($P < 0.004$) and IL-6 ($P < 0.0003$). In the same study, however, sleep duration, as determined by polysomnography (PSG) on the night prior to blood sampling, was inversely associated with TNF-α ($P < 0.02$).

In a separate study, Suarez (2008) demonstrated that indices of sleep disturbance were associated with greater psychosocial distress, higher fasting insulin, fibrinogen, and inflammatory biomarkers but only in women. Moreover, these findings were independent of menstrual cycle phase in pre-menopausal women.

On examination of over 4,000 individuals from the Whitehall II Study, we have demonstrated marked gender differences in the relationship between self-reported sleep and markers of inflammation. The results showed that although in men there was no association between hs-CRP and sleep in women, there was a significant non-linear association (Miller et al., 2009a). In contrast to Patel et al. (2009), in our study the level of hs-CRP was significantly higher in short sleepers (5 hours or less) after multiple adjustments ($P = 0.04$) (interaction $P < 0.05$) and as shown in Fig. 11.2. The hs-CRP did appear to be higher in those women who slept more than 8 hours as

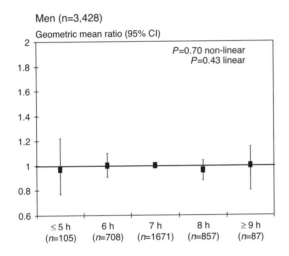

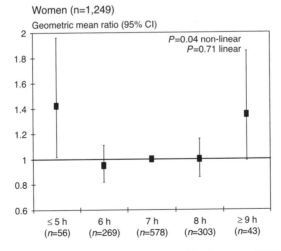

Adjusted for age, marital status, BMI, smoking, systolic blood pressure (SPB), and triglycerides

Fig. 11.2 Cross-sectional relationship between hs-CRP and duration of sleep.

compared to those sleeping 7 hours the difference was not significant (Miller et al., 2009a). This gender-specific observation is, however, consistent with the finding of Suarez (2008).

In the Cleveland Family Study, Patel et al. (2009) demonstrated that increasing sleep was associated with an increase in IL-6, while in the Whitehall II Study, following multiple adjustments there were no overall linear or non-linear trends between sleep duration and IL-6. However, in women but not men (interaction $P < 0.05$), levels of IL-6 tended to be lower in individuals who slept 8 hours (11%; 95% confidence interval [CI]: 4–17) as compared to 7 hours (Miller et al., 2009a).

It is possible that the gender interactions in the relationship between sleep and inflammation may account for some of the observed differences between studies. Taheri et al. (2007) may have failed to find an association between sleep and markers of inflammation as the number of females in their study was much smaller, and a gender-adjusted analysis, as opposed to a sex-stratified analysis, was used. Longitudinal studies are required to fully investigate possible temporal relationships between short sleep and markers of inflammation in both male and female individuals.

Serious health problems occur more often in women who suffer violence than in their non-abused counterparts (Kendall-Tackett, 2007). In a recent article Kendall-Tackett explored the possibility that this may in part be the result of the associated sleep disturbance as well as the depression and hostility suffered by such individuals (Kendall-Tackett, 2007). It has been demonstrated that the effect of the sleep disturbance is independent of depression. Although the exact mechanisms for these associations are unclear, they may be mediated through systems which affect metabolic and neuroendocrine functions and lead to activation of the HPA axis) as well as to activation of inflammatory pathways and, as such, anti-inflammatory agents may be a useful adjunct to the existing treatment regimes (Kendall-Tackett, 2007).

Sleep, inflammation, and disease

Disruption of sleep can lead to disruption of immune function. Many chronic conditions have an underlying inflammatory component, and it is therefore not surprising that evidence is accumulating which suggests that sleep deprivation may be important in the development and progression of such conditions. Evidence suggests that 'healthy' individuals who do not get enough sleep might be at risk of poor health in the future (Cappuccio et al., 2007; Ferrie et al., 2007; Gangwisch et al., 2006; Meisinger et al., 2005; Stranges et al., 2008a) and sleep disturbances may be an important determinant of both disease morbidity and mortality (Ferrie et al., 2007).

In this section, the possible mechanisms that link sleep and inflammation in these diseases will be examined with particular regard to the development of CVD. The potential mechanisms underlying the relationships between sleep and metabolic disease and in particular diabetes will only be briefly discussed as they have been examined in more detail in Chapter 6.

Sleep, inflammation, and cardiovascular disease

Inflammatory processes are important in the development of CVD. The level of circulating inflammatory cytokines can be altered by sleep (Irwin, 2002; Kokturk et al., 2005; Majde and Krueger, 2005; Miller and Cappuccio, 2007; Prinz, 2004), which in part might account for the increased all-cause mortality and CVD risk observed in short sleepers (Ferrie et al., 2007), the relationship between sleep and hypertension (Cappuccio et al., 2007), diabetes (Meisinger et al., 2005), and obesity (Stranges et al., 2008a), and the association observed with coronary events in short and long sleepers in the Nurses Health Study (Ayas et al., 2003). There is an increased risk of heart attacks and strokes during the early morning and it is possible that sleep has an effect on the endothelial function of blood vessels (Strike and Steptoe, 2003). Although such associations are evident, the need to establish causality and the temporal sequence of events that

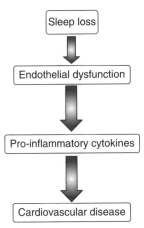

Fig. 11.3 Sleep loss, inflammation, and cardiovascular disease.
Source: Re-drawn with permission from Miller, M.A. & Cappuccio, F.P. (2007). Inflammation, sleep, obesity and cardiovascular disease. *Curr Vasc Pharmacol*, **5**(2) 93–102.

leads to morbidity and mortality remains to be clearly established. Most studies to date have examined only the effect of the number of hours of sleep on cardiovascular risk but a recent study has demonstrated that, in young women, poor sleep quality and continuity as opposed to sleep duration was associated with higher levels of hs-CRP but not IL-6 or TNF-α (Okun et al., 2009).

Sleep and ethnicity and gender differences in disease risk

The risk of CVD is higher in South Asians than Whites, and individuals of African origin appear to be protected from CHD (Balarajan, 1995). Ethnic differences in inflammatory markers have been observed (Miller et al., 2003), which in part are associated with ethnic differences in cardiovascular risk. The prevalence of insomnia is increased in African Americans compared with Whites, which may in part be attributable to ethnic differences in associated risk factors, such as obesity (Scharf et al., 2004). It is important that future studies investigate whether ethnic differences in CVD may in part be related to ethnic differences in sleep-related inflammatory processes.

Evidence from large epidemiological cohorts has suggested that short sleep duration and poor sleep quality may be more strongly associated with adverse outcomes in women rather than men (Cappuccio et al., 2007; Stranges et al., 2008b; Suarez, 2008). We have demonstrated a marked gender difference in the relationship between short sleep and blood pressure, in that the relationship was only apparent in female individuals (Cappuccio et al., 2007). However, Knutson (2005) demonstrated that while short sleep may have an effect on BMI in young men this does not appear to be the case in young women. Age may therefore be an important determinant in this association.

Gender differences in inflammatory-linked CVD risk may be related to the menstrual cycle and menopausal status. In a recent study, we have found that sleep is related to hypertension but mainly in pre-menopausal women (Stranges et al., 2009). One study has reported that although the menstrual phase does not appear to influence sleep, the use of OCP has an effect on hs-CRP levels (Okun et al., 2009).

Other pathways that may be important in explaining the gender disparities include gender-related differences in neurotransmitter pathways. Serotonin (5-HT), for example, may have effects on sleep, sleep onset, and mood regulation. Likewise, there may be gender differences in the effect of sleep on appetite control.

Sleep, inflammation, and obesity

Obesity is becoming a global epidemic in both adults and children and is associated with an increased risk of morbidity and mortality as well as reduced life expectancy (Poirier et al., 2006). It is clear that obesity may have its effect on CVD through a number of different known and possibly as yet unknown mechanisms. Moreover sleep may have an effect on these mechanisms. These include dyslipidaemia, hypertension, glucose intolerance, inflammation, OSA/hypoventilation, and the prothrombotic state (Poirier et al., 2006). Obesity leads to a change in an individual's metabolic profile and an accumulation of adipose tissue (fat) which is composed of connective tissue and adipocytes. Adipose tissue is an important endocrine organ which produces inflammatory cytokines and hormones such as resistin and leptin. Leptin plays a key role in regulating energy intake and expenditure. It has an important role in appetite regulation, and recent evidence suggests that it also has profound inflammatory effects.

In the first randomized cross-over clinical trial of short-term sleep deprivation, Spiegel et al. (2004) demonstrated that sleep deprivation was associated with decreased leptin and increased ghrelin levels. This in turn would lead to a concomitant increase in hunger and appetite, increased insulin resistance, and accumulation of fat and decreased carbohydrate metabolism (Fig. 11.4). The individuals in this study were subjected to an extreme acute sleep deprivation (<4 hours per night) for 2 days and compared with 2 days with 10 hours of sleep. A constant glucose infusion provided the individuals with their caloric intake. Following sleep restriction there was a decrease in leptin and increase in ghrelin and the change in ghrelin to leptin ratio was associated with a positive change in hunger suggesting that if the individuals had had access to food they may have increased their food intake (see also Chapter 6).

Further studies are required to determine the effects of more modest sleep deprivation (<5 hours per night) on these hormones, especially in the long-term (Spiegel et al., 2004). A study of 422 children (boys and girls aged 5–10 years) has demonstrated an association between sleep duration and the risk to develop childhood overweight/obesity (Chaput et al., 2006).

Paradoxically, obese individuals have high leptin levels and therefore should have a reduced appetite. This has led to the development of the 'leptin resistance' concept. Although the underlying

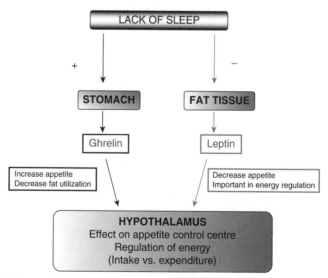

Fig. 11.4 Effect of the lack of sleep on energy regulating hormones.

mechanisms are unclear, it has been proposed that leptin may bind to circulating hs-CRP, resulting in an attenuation of its physiological effects (Knutson et al., 2007). This is of interest as sleep deprivation has been associated with an increase in hs-CRP (Meier-Ewert et al., 2004; Miller et al., 2009a; Patel et al., 2009).

In a cross-sectional study of more than 5,000 White male civil servants from the Whitehall II Study, we demonstrated that both short and long sleep duration are associated with an increased BMI and an increased odds ratio for obesity (Stranges et al., 2008a). Although these associations were highly significant, further prospective analysis failed to show any effect of sleep duration on BMI or any increased risk of obesity (Stranges et al., 2008a). In a recent review, Patel and Hu (2008) concluded that short sleep appears to be independently associated with weight gain, particularly in the younger age groups. Likewise in a recent meta-analysis we concluded that evidence from cross-sectional studies in children and adults suggests that there is an increased risk of obesity amongst short sleepers (Cappuccio et al., 2008). Further prospective studies, however, are required to establish the temporal sequence of events and to study potential underlying inflammatory mechanisms (Cappuccio et al., 2008). It is of interest that although the Nurses Health Study also demonstrated that short sleep duration leads to an increase in weight with time, there was no evidence to suggest that this resulted from an increase in appetite (Ayas et al., 2003).

The findings from the Nurses Health Study suggest that perhaps the effects of sleep on obesity occur as a result of a change in energy metabolism. Total energy expenditure (TEE) is made up of three components. The first is the resting metabolic rate (RMR), which is the energy an individual expends at rest, the second is the thermic effect of meals (TEM), which is the energy used in the process of consuming and storing a meal, and the third component is the activity-related energy expenditure (AEE), which is the energy used in all volitional and non-volitional activities (Ayas et al., 2003). The possibility of whether sleep loss has an impact on TEE has been discussed in a recent comprehensive review by Knutson et al. (2007). It has been suggested that individuals with sleep problems may have a reduction in their energy expenditure, but it is not yet clear whether this is true for all short sleepers. One mechanism that may be important is that involving the uncoupling proteins. These proteins uncouple proton exchange and adenosine triphosphate (ATP) production and their expression is affected by leptin.

The secretion of inflammatory cytokines by adipose tissue may underlie the effect of sleep on weight gain (Trayhurn et al., 2006). Lack of sleep acting via the regulatory hormones may lead to an increased fat accumulation and increased secretion of pro-inflammatory cytokines. A 2% increase in circulating soluble E-selectin (sE-selectin) level has been associated with a one unit higher BMI and a 0.01 unit greater waist-hip ratio (WHR) (Miller and Cappuccio, 2006).

Sleep, inflammation, glucose and insulin regulation, and diabetes

The relationship between sleep and glucose regulation is only briefly mentioned here, as it is discussed in detail in Chapter 6. There is a bi-directional relationship between glucose homeostasis and sleep. Diabetes can lead to the development of sleep abnormalities and short sleep can lead to a decrease in glucose tolerance. Findings from the Sleep Heart Health Study indicated that diabetes is associated with periodic breathing, a respiratory abnormality associated with changes in the central control of ventilation (Resnick et al., 2003). In normal, healthy individuals glucose tolerance is at its minimum in the middle of the night. This reduced glucose tolerance is partly due to a nighttime reduction in the insulin response to glucose, but it is also dependent on sleep, with glucose metabolism being slowest in the first half of the night when SWS predominates.

Laboratory studies demonstrated that recurrent partial sleep restriction in healthy young adults was associated with alterations in glucose metabolism, including a decrease in glucose tolerance and insulin sensitivity along with a change in appetite control (Spiegel et al., 2005a). The level of the anorexigenic hormone leptin was decreased and the level of the orexigenic factor ghrelin was increased, resulting in an increase in hunger (see Fig. 11.4). Over a long period this may lead to weight gain, insulin resistance, type 2 diabetes (T2DM), and associated inflammation (Spiegel et al., 2005a).

The hormonal effects of acute total sleep deprivation and recurrent partial sleep deprivation may differ. Furthermore, these may be different from those that arise following long-term chronic partial sleep loss as seen on a population basis (Spiegel et al., 2005b). The MONICA (Multinational **MONI**toring of trends and determinants in **CA**rdiovascular disease) study, however, demonstrated in both women and men the difficulty in maintaining sleep as opposed to the difficulty in initiating sleep was associated with a higher risk of T2DM during the subsequent mean follow-up period of 7.5 years (Meisinger et al., 2005).

The exact causal pathways linking sleep and diabetes remain to be elucidated. Sleep debt, arising either through behavioural sleep restriction or the presence of OSA may be associated with a decrease in glucose tolerance, a higher evening cortisol level, and an increased sympathetic activity, leading to increased weight, which in turn may be associated with an increased risk of sleep disorders (Spiegel et al., 2005a, b).

It remains to be seen if the diabetic complications associated with sleep disturbances have an underlying independent inflammatory component, and longitudinal studies are required to investigate whether sleep loss can predict changes in glucose metabolism or *vice versa*.

Sleep, inflammation, blood pressure, and hypertension

Normally, blood pressure has a nocturnal dip of about 10% (Mallion et al., 1999). Individuals who do not drop their blood pressure at night (non-dippers) are at increased risk of CVD. African Americans tend to display more non-dipping characteristics compared to Whites and this is associated with an increase in SDB (Pickering and Kario, 2001). The severity of SDB was recently shown to be independently associated with the level of neopterin, a marker of macrophage activation (Punjabi et al., 2007).

Acute deprivation of sleep in healthy subjects leads to an increase in blood pressure and SNS activation (Narkiewicz et al., 2005). A recent longitudinal study demonstrated that short sleep duration (≤5 hours per night) was associated with a significantly increased risk of hypertension (hazard ratio [HR]: 2.10; 95% CI: 1.58–2.79) in subjects between the ages of 32 and 59 years. Adjustment for confounding factors such as obesity and diabetes only partially attenuated this relationship, but the outcome was based on self-reported diagnosis of incident hypertension and no gender-specific analyses were included (Gangwisch et al., 2006). More recently, in a cross-sectional analysis, we have demonstrated that short sleep duration is associated with a higher risk of hypertension but only in women. This is attenuated in prospective analyses after multivariate adjustment (Cappuccio et al., 2007). Potential causal pathways linking blood pressure and sleep remain to be examined in more detail. Markers of inflammation are related to sleep and blood pressure (Miller and Cappuccio, 2007) and changes in inflammatory mediators including hs-CRP, fibrinogen, and plasminogen activator inhibitor, which are important in the development of hypertension and CVD, have also been observed in OSA patients (Kasasbeh et al., 2006). There is growing evidence to suggest that there is a causal relationship between OSA syndrome and hypertension. Patients with OSA exhibit increased resting heart rate, decreased time duration between two consecutive R waves of the electrocardiogram (RR interval) variability, and increased blood pressure variability (Kasasbeh et al., 2006).

Long-term CPAP treatment, which may have an effect on inflammation, improves daytime and nocturnal blood pressure control especially in patients with severe sleep apnoea (Pepperell et al., 2002). The Seventh Report of the Joint National Committee (JNC 7) on Prevention, Detection, Evaluation, and Treatment of High Blood Pressure has recommended not only that OSA be considered in all resistant hypertensive patients, but also that all hypertensive patients with a BMI in excess of 27 kg/m^2 should be examined for the presence of sleeping disorders (Chobanian et al., 2003).

Sleep, inflammation, and metabolic syndrome

Metabolic syndrome (MetS) is characterized by a clustering of cardiovascular and metabolic risk factors in a given individual. These include central obesity, an adverse lipid profile (high triacyglycerols and low high-density lipoprotein-cholesterol [HDL-cholesterol]), raised blood pressure, and insulin resistance or glucose intolerance. There may also be an increased pro-inflammatory state (Vega, 2004). Vgontzas et al. (2005) clearly demonstrated that inflammatory cytokines are increased in individuals with OSA and they proposed that these cytokines were the mediators of excessive daytime sleepiness (EDS). They demonstrated the importance of visceral fat in OSA syndrome and suggested that OSA and sleepiness in obese patients may be manifestations of the MetS. Data from the Third National Health and Nutrition Examination Survey (1988–1994) have also shown that in the US population the prevalence of the MetS parallels the prevalence of symptomatic OSA in general random samples (Vgontzas et al., 2005) and an increased prevalence of MetS has been observed is OSA patients compared to controls with an odds ratio of 9.1 (Coughlin et al., 2004). In a recent review of this topic, Lam and Ip (2007) concluded that although the confounding effect of obesity made it difficult to examine the associations clearly, evidence is accumulating to suggest that there may be an independent association between OSA and MetS or its components. Peled et al. (2007) demonstrated that OSA was independently associated to a number of MetS components and that it was correlated with insulin resistance and hs-CRP.

Sleep, inflammation, and depression

Depressed patients have a significant nocturnal increase in circulating IL-6 and sICAM (soluble intercellular adhesion molecule) as compared with controls (Motivala et al., 2005). Furthermore, both sleep latency and REM density are associated with these inflammatory markers (Motivala et al., 2005). It is of interest to note that in patients with depression, total sleep deprivation leads to an increase in renin secretion and a concomitant trend for a decrease in HPA axis activity in the recovery night (Murck et al., 2006). It has been suggested that these changes could be a 'fingerprint' of a rapidly anti-depressive treatment (Murck et al., 2006).

The complex inter-relationship between sleep and depression was further highlighted in a recent study of sleep factors in coronary artery disease (CAD) patients. The study demonstrated that women with stable CAD were at risk of experiencing poor sleep quality and may be more at risk of having a depressed mood compared to male stable CAD patients. These differences were still observed when adjustment was made for the effect of inflammation inhibitors on sleep quality (Edell-Gustafsson et al., 2006).

Sleep, inflammation, and arthritis

Sleep disturbances are common in arthritis patients (Ranjbaran et al., 2007), but some studies in patients with rheumatoid arthritis (RA) have revealed patterns of sleep disturbances that are not associated with the concomitant pain. Moreover, recent studies using TNF-α antagonists to treat joint inflammation in arthritis patients have reported a concomitant reduction in the daytime sleepiness reported in these individuals (Ranjbaran et al., 2007; Vgontzas, 2008). Sleep disorders are more prevalent in individuals with RA and low back pain than in individuals with just low back pain suggesting that the inflammatory component associated with RA may be important (Ranjbaran et al., 2007).

Individuals who have inflammatory conditions such as systemic lupus erythematosus are at increased cardiovascular risk (Chogle and Chakravarty, 2007; van Leuven et al., 2005) and often report sleep problems (Ranjbaran et al., 2007). The possible effect of sleep on the inflammatory pathways in these individuals needs to be investigated.

Sleep, inflammation, and asthma

Emergency departments report that most asthma attacks occur at night and sleep disorders exacerbate asthma (Majde and Krueger, 2005). This may in part be due to the role inflammatory cytokines play in asthma. These cytokines have a circadian rhythm; levels of serum IL-4 and IFN-γ, for example, are higher in asthmatics than controls at 4:00 a.m. and 4:00 p.m. Asthma also has an effect on sleep and sleep quality. Many asthmatics report being awakened by sleeping difficulties.

Sleep disorders, inflammation, and cardiovascular risk

The prevalence of OSA in the population is relatively high. It affects at least 1–5% of middle-aged individuals from many ethnic populations although men are twice as likely to have OSA as women (Lam and Ip, 2007).

Obstructive sleep apnoea, inflammation, and cardiovascular disease risk

Obstructive sleep apnoea is caused by a physical obstruction of the airway and is characterized by disrupted breathing during sleep. The link between sleep disorders such as OSA and serious health problems including CVD is well-established although the underlying mechanisms are not entirely understood (Bradley and Floras, 2009; Kasasbeh et al., 2006; Lam and Ip, 2007; Narkiewicz et al., 2005). In individuals with OSA, the cardiovascular system is exposed to cycles of hypoxia, exaggerated intrathoracic pressure, and arousals (Bradley and Floras, 2009). NREM sleep is normally accompanied by a decrease in metabolic rate, sympathetic nerve activity, and heart rate. This pattern of cardiovascular quiescence is interrupted by OSA which triggers a cascade of acute haemodynamic, autonomic, chemical, metabolic, and inflammatory effects. Long-term exposures to such effects are capable of leading to the development or exacerbation of existing CVD.

OSA is a risk factor for CAD and is an independent risk factor for arterial hypertension. Indeed, over 50% of the individuals with OSA have hypertension (Chobanian et al., 2003). Evidence suggests that although OSA and hypertension may be causally related mainly through activation of the sympathetic system, other mechanisms may also be important. These include inflammation, activation of the renin angiotensin system, and endothelial dysfunction (Wolf et al., 2007). OSA is also associated with ischaemic ST-segment changes, ventricular arrhythmias, and sudden cardiac death (Luthje and Andreas, 2008). The underlying mechanisms for these associations are complex and include neural, hormonal factors, inflammatory and oxidative stress mechanisms, as well as haemodynamic and mechanical effects. The latter two arise as a result of the recurrent negative intrathoracic pressure changes which occur when the airway is occluded. Increases in haematocrit, blood viscosity, and fibrinogen have also been demonstrated in OSA

(Luthje and Andreas, 2008). Neural effects occur as a result of sympathetic activation and auto-nomic imbalance is a key risk factor for CVD (Brook and Julius, 2000). Intermittent hypoxia (IH) may activate inflammatory pathways that impair vascular endothelial function and induce oxy-gen-free radical production (Bradley and Floras, 2009). Hormonal factors that may be important include changes in the appetite suppressant leptin, the levels of which are higher in OSA patients compared with matched obese controls (Phillips et al., 2000). Furthermore, leptin resistance may lead to a further increase in weight in OSA patients. Oxidative stress and a decreased anti-oxidant capacity may also be important in this condition (Luthje and Andreas, 2008). As well being asso-ciated with an increased CHD risk, OSA has also been associated with an increased incidence of stroke and an increase in prothrombotic process.

HPA axis hyperactivity may be a consequence of OSA and may indeed contribute to secondary pathologies such as hypertension and insulin resistance (Buckley and Schatzberg, 2005). Indeed, it is expected that nocturnal hypoxia, continuous electrocephalographic arousals, and sleep frag-mentation that is associated with OSA would lead to both activation of the systemic sympathetic adrenomedullary and HPA axis. There are, however, very few studies, which have investigated HPA activity in OSA patients and results have often been inconsistent.

The accumulating evidence which suggests that obesity and its accompanying metabolic abnor-malities play an important role in the development of OSA has been recently reviewed (Vgontzas, 2008). Obesity appears to be one of the most important reversible risk factors for OSA. Obese individuals who are not psychologically distressed and who have normal sleeping habits have unexpectedly low cortisol secretion compared with non-obese controls. However, cortisol levels are slightly elevated in matched obese individuals with OSA. Furthermore, these values are reduced on treatment with CPAP (Vgontzas, 2008). It is possible that in these obese patients the presence of low cortisol levels may predispose the individuals to the development of OSA through a mechanism involving increased CRH secretion. Studies have demonstrated that waist circum-ference is a better predictor of OSA than BMI. It is therefore possible that visceral fat and possibly the associated inflammatory cyokines produced therein, as opposed to obesity, *per se* may be of greater importance in the development of OSA (Vgontzas, 2008).

A recent review clearly presents evidence from a number of studies indicating that inflamma-tory responses are increased in OSA individuals (Gozal and Kheirandish-Gozal, 2008). These responses include an enhanced release of superoxide from stimulated polymorphonuclear neutrophils, changes in T-cells activation, and an increase in Type 2 cytokine dominance with associated increase in IL-4 expression. Although some studies have demonstrated an increase in TNF-α and hs-CRP levels in OSA patients others have not (Gozal and Kheirandish-Gozal, 2008; Guilleminault et al., 2004; Taheri et al., 2007). It is possible that this may be due to the presence or absence of concurrent risk factors such as obesity and smoking.

Studies have indicated that other inflammatory mediators including cellular adhesion mole-cules, NF-κB activity, IL-6, and monocyte chemoattractant protein-1 levels are also significantly elevated in patients with OSA compared with control subjects (Greenberg et al., 2006; Teramoto et al., 2003; Vgontzas et al., 1997). The role of these and other inflammatory biomarkers as risk factors for OSA has been recently reviewed (McNicholas, 2009). Activation of cellular adhesion molecules and other inflammatory components may arise as a result of endothelial dysfunction, but as yet it is not clear if the endothelial dysfunction that is observed in OSA is present due to presence of other co-morbidities such as obesity and hypertension or whether OSA is an inde-pendent risk factor for its development. Increased erythrocyte adhesion and aggregation has also been demonstrated (Peled et al., 2008) and the link between the innate immune system and sleep is discussed in a recent review (Majde and Krueger, 2005).

Sleep, obstructive sleep apnoea, inflammation, and paediatrics

Evidence from studies in children is of particular interest as the results in children are less likely to be confounded by the presence of co-morbidities. Children with SDB have higher hs-CRP levels than children who do not (Tauman et al., 2004). Furthermore, 94% of the children studied who had elevated hs-CRP levels also reported EDS or learning difficulties as compared to 62% of children who had hs-CRP levels in the normal range (Tauman et al., 2004).

OSA is a common disorder in children. Non-obese children with OSA aged 4–9 years have higher IL-6 and lower IL-10 levels than aged, gender ethnicity, and BMI-matched children without OSA. Furthermore, these levels returned to the level of the controls following adenotensillectomy in the OSA children (Gozal et al., 2008). These are important as they indicate that, even in the absence of obesity, perturbations in the inflammatory mechanisms occur in very young OSA patients and in turn this may lead to activation of further downstream pathways, which may lead to an increased risk of end-organ damage. It remains to be investigated, however, whether anti-inflammatory agents might be useful in the treatment of this condition as opposed to surgery.

Sleep, obstructive sleep apnoea, inflammation, and continuous positive airway pressure treatment

The current gold standard for the treatment of moderate-to-severe OSA is nasal CPAP, which acts as a pneumatic splint to prevent the collapse of the pharyngeal airway. Although it is accepted that treatment of OSA with CPAP not only improves the symptoms of this condition and decreases the risk of cardiovascular events, it is very difficult to perform true double-blind randomized controlled trials (RCTs) to validate the effect of this treatment on various outcome measures. CPAP treatment is normally associated with a decrease in apnoeas and snoring which makes it very difficult to blind the patient to treatment, likewise unlike pharmaceutical trials involving placebo tablets it is very difficult to blind therapists and doctors involved in any study to the treatment regime. Monitoring patient compliance with CPAP treatment is also very difficult. Many early studies have therefore been simply observational in nature.

Early data from observational studies have shown that CPAP therapy can have an effect on inflammatory markers (see Table 11.1). TNF-α levels were significantly elevated in male OSA patients compared with matched controls, but the levels were normalized to that of controls following 6 weeks of CPAP treatment (Ryan et al., 2005). Likewise, in separate studies, TNF-α levels were reduced in patients with OSA following 8 weeks (Dorkova et al., 2008) and 6 months of CPAP treatment (Steiropoulos et al., 2009).

In two studies, hs-CRP levels were reduced following 3 months (Burioka et al., 2008) and only 1 month of CPAP therapy (Yokoe et al., 2003). In another study, hs-CRP was reduced following 6 months of CPAP treatment but only in those individuals who showed good compliance (Steiropoulos et al., 2007). In two other studies however, there was no significant effect on hs-CRP levels following shorter periods of CPAP treatment (Dorkova et al., 2008; Ryan et al., 2007).

Homocysteine levels were reduced in one study following 6 months of CPAP treatment (Steiropoulos et al., 2007). A separate study, however, reported no significant difference in homocysteine levels following CPAP treatment (Ryan et al., 2007). One possible explanation for this, is that in the former study the levels were measured before and after 6 months of CPAP, whereas in the latter study only 6 weeks of CPAP treatment was used.

Differing effects on IL-6 have also been reported. Three studies have reported no effect (Dorkova et al., 2008; Steiropoulos et al., 2007; Vgontzas et al., 2008), whereas one study reported

Table 11.1 Effect of CPAP treatment on inflammatory markers: results from observational studies

Reference	Intervention	Subject	Effect on inflammatory markers		
Observational studies					
			Hs-CRP	IL-6 (circulating)	IL-6 (monocytes)
Yokoe (2003)	1 month CPAP	30 OSA vs. 14 obese controls	Sig. decrease ($P < 0.0001$)	Sig. decrease ($P < 0.01$)	Sig. decrease ($P < 0.001$)
					TNF-α
Ryan (2005)	6 weeks CPAP	19 male OSA vs. 17 matched controls			Sig. decrease (2.56 pg/mL; IQR, 2.01–3.42 pg/mL vs. 1.24 pg/mL; IQR, 0.78 to 2.35 pg/mL; $P = 0.002$)
			Hs-CRP	Homocysteine	
Steiropoulos (2007)	6 months CPAP (good compliance)	16 male, 4 female OSA	Sig. decrease ($P < 0.03$)	Sig. decrease ($P < 0.005$)	
			Hs-CRP	Homocysteine	
Ryan (2007)	6 weeks CPAP	49 males OSA	No sig. difference	No sig. difference	
			Hs-CRP	IL-6	
Burioka (2008)	3 month CPAP	8 subjects OSA vs. 8 matched controls	Sig. decrease (1061 ± 188 vs. 465 ± 82 ng/mL; $P < 0.05$)	Sig. decrease (6.7 ± 1.2 vs. 3.6 ± 0.6 pg/mL; $P < 0.005$)	
			Hs-CRP	IL-6	TNF-α
Dorkova (2008)	8 weeks CPAP	15 males, 1 female OSA	No sig. difference	No sig. difference	Sig. difference (2.13 ± 0.98 vs. 1.79 ± 0.69 pg/mL; $P = 0.037$)
				IL-6	TNF-α
Steiropoulus (2009)	6 months CPAP (good compliance)	32 males with OSA		No sig. difference	Sig. decrease (8.41 ± 5.7 vs. 5.72 ± 4.91 pg/mL; $P = 0.001$)
			IL-6	TNF-α	Adiponectin
Vgontzas (2008)	3 months CPAP	16 obese males with OSA, 13 non-apnoeic obese controls, 15 non-obese controls	No sig. difference	No sig. difference	No sig. difference · No sig. difference

a significant decrease in IL-6 following 3 months CPAP therapy (Burioka et al., 2008). A separate study also reported that the level of IL-6 both in the circulation and produced by monocytes were also reduced following treatment (Yokoe et al., 2003).

Other studies have shown that CPAP treatment can lead to changes in IL-6, ICAM-1, and IL-8 levels (Harsch et al., 2004; Ohga et al., 2003). In a recent study, it is of interest to note that although withdrawal of CPAP treatment in moderate-to-severe OSA patients resulted in a return of their OSA and a marked increase in sympathetic activity, no concomitant elevation of vascular inflammatory markers (hs-CRP, hs-IL-6, hs-TNF-α, vascular endothelial growth factor [VEGF]) was observed in this time period (Phillips et al., 2007).

Results from the few RCTs performed to date have been less consistent in their findings with regards to the use of CPAP and the effects of inflammatory markers (see Table 11.2). Both West et al. (2007) and Kohler et al. (2009) failed to find significant difference in hs-CRP or adiponectin following CPAP treatment. In normotensive middle-aged men with severe OSA, Drager et al. (2007) demonstrated that 4 months of effective CPAP treatment led to a significant improvement of markers of atherosclerosis. In addition, they found that in the absence of any change in weight or serum lipid levels there was a significant decrease in plasma catecholamines and hs-CRP. The duration of CPAP treatment was the longest in the study which demonstrated the significant decrease in inflammatory markers; moreover, Kohler et al. (2009) compared a therapeutic with a sub-therapeutic level of CPAP.

Further prospective studies to look at the relationship between OSA and inflammation and to address causality are needed. Such longitudinal studies are also required to observe the effect of CPAP treatment on these parameters. Moreover, to date most studies have only been performed

Table 11.2 Effect of CPAP treatment on inflammatory markers: results from RCTs

Reference	Intervention	Subject	Effect on inflammatory markers			
Randomized controlled trials						
			hs-CRP			
Drager (2007)	RCT 4 months CPAP vs. no treatment group	24 pts Severe male OSA CPAP (n = 12) vs. no Rx (n = 12)	Sig. decreases on rx (3.7 ± 1.8 vs. 2.0 ± 1.2 mg/L; P < 0.001)			
			Hs-CRP	Adiponectin		
West (2007)	RCT 3 months CPAP vs. placebo group	42 T2DM males with OSA CPAP (n = 20) vs. placebo (n = 22)	No sig. difference	No sig. difference		
			Hs-CRP	Adiponectin	IL-1	IFN–γ
Kohler (2008)	RCT 4 weeks CPAP therapeutic vs. sub-therapeutic control group	100 men moderate-to-severe OSA CPAP (n = 51) vs. sub-therapeutic dose (n = 49)	No sig. difference	No sig. difference	No sig. difference	No sig. difference

on male subjects, and possible gender and ethnic differences in the underlying inflammatory mechanisms in OSA and the response to treatment have not been investigated. Disease duration may also be an important confounder in the response to treatment.

Obstructive sleep apnoea, sleep-disordered breathing, and anti-inflammatory treatment regimes

The previous sections have highlighted that OSA is a significant risk factor for the development of CVD and that it has been associated with hypertension, T2DM, CAD, and cerebrovascular disease, and may lead to significant impairments in quality of life. It has been proposed that inflammatory mechanisms may play a key role in the development and progression of this disease.

There are a number of characteristics that are associated with OSA and these include awakening with choking, intense snoring, a large neck circumference, male gender, obesity, hypertension, and daytime sleepiness. Many of these characteristics are addressed by the treatment with CPAP which maintains the airway during sleep and maintains the oxygen supply to the brain. CPAP therapy has also been associated with a marked decrease in IL-6 and hs-CRP (Yokoe et al., 2003). However, in some individuals the daytime sleepiness associated with OSA and other sleep disorders is not always eliminated by this treatment. It is therefore important that other possible treatment regimes for this disorder are considered, including those which address the underlying inflammatory component.

Weight reduction

Evidence has accumulated to support the idea that obesity acting via a number of mechanisms including inflammation, insulin resistance, and central neural mechanisms play an important role in the pathogenesis of OSA, SDS, and the associated cardiovascular co-morbidities (Vgontzas, 2008). Obesity leads to an increase in adipose tissue and increased levels of circulating inflammatory mediators. Evidence suggests that surgical weight loss (treatment with intragastric balloon) improves the OSA symptoms in morbidly obese patients. Furthermore, even modest weight reduction results in clinically significant improvements in the cardiovascular risk profile of OSA individuals (Vgontzas, 2008).

Exercise

Exercise improves insulin resistance and adiposity independently of body weight and is associated with an improvement of OSA symptoms which may be the result of a decrease in inflammatory cytokine production (Vgontzas, 2008).

Anti-inflammatory agents and anti-oxidants

Since the cardiovascular consequences of poor sleep may arise due to its effect on the inflammatory and oxidative pathway, it is possible that the pharmacological management of sleep disorders may need to include anti-inflammatory and antioxidant agents as well. Results from a pilot study in eight male individuals have indicated that treatment with etanercept, which neutralizes TNF-α, leads to an improvement in sleep latency and reduces the number of apnoeas in a given time period (Vgontzas, 2008). This suggests that pro-inflammatory cytokines contribute to the pathogenesis of OSA and sleepiness and indicates that anti-inflammatory medications may be beneficial.

IH is a characteristic of SDB and can lead to end-organ damage in the brain. Polyphenolic compounds which are found in a variety of food items, including wine fruits and vegetables and tea have been extensively investigated and their known anti-oxidant properties investigated. Green tea contains a number of these biologically active substances. In a recent animal study, it was demonstrated that oral supplements of green tea-derived catechin polyphenols are capable of attenuating IH-induced neurobehavioural deficits in rats. Oral supplementation was accompanied by a reduction in nicotinamide adenine dinucleotide phosphate-oxidase (NADPH-oxidase) expression, lipid peroxidation, and inflammation suggesting that inhibition of these mechanisms is important for the prevention of IH-induced end-organ damage (Burckhardt et al., 2008).

It is important that large randomized trials, with sufficient follow-up periods, are conducted to determine causal relationships and the possible treatment benefits associated with anti-inflammatory and anti-oxidants in the treatment of OSA and with particular regard to the effect of these agents on the OSA-associated cardiovascular risk.

Summary

Sleep is a fundamental requirement for living individuals. In this chapter, the possibility that the relationship between sleep and CVD may be mediated by inflammatory mechanisms has been discussed. The association between sleep disorders and cardiovascular risk suggests that early identification of adverse metabolic risk factors in these individuals would have a clear clinical benefit.

Sleep and sleep disorders have a major impact on our health and well-being and need to be researched thoroughly. It is important that our understanding of the biological basis of sleep; the biochemical mechanisms involved in both health and disease; and the gender-associated differences in, for example, the association between sleep and CVD risk are understood.

Summary box

- Evidence is accumulating to suggest that sleeping 7 or 8 hours per night appears to be optimal for health, but prospective studies are needed to confirm this concept. Evidence from randomized controlled studies in healthy individuals also indicates that the temporal relationship between acute and short- term chronic deprivation and disease may in part, be mediated by inflammation. Further work is required to investigate these mechanisms more fully in large longitudinal epidemiological cohorts. Furthermore, it may be necessary to improve the measurement of sleep quality and duration in such studies either by use of PSG or by improving the self-assessment of long-term exposure by taking repeated measures of self-reported sleep duration.

- Inflammation plays an important underlying role in the development of many diseases such as diabetes, obesity, hypertension, and MetS. Recent figures have stated that the prevalence of diabetes in the United Kingdom has risen by 74% just in the last decade. Similar dramatic rises have been seen in the United States, where the prevalence of known diabetes was reported as 8% in 2007. In the United Kingdom, 24% of men and women are now obese. Data from the US National Center for Chronic Disease Prevention and Health Promotion stated that, in 2007, only one US state had a prevalence of obesity less than 20% and the prevalence has continued to increase. The number of children with obesity and diabetes is also increasing dramatically worldwide. Sleep-curtailment may lead to an increase in the inflammatory processes underlying these diseases. It remains to be determined, however, as to whether biologically restorative sleep can reverse or halt such disease progression. Future research is required to address some of these issues and to elucidate the role of sleep in public health, which may be of particular importance in the prevention of disease development and progression in children.

References

Ayas, N.T., White, D.P., Manson, J.E., et al. (2003). A prospective study of sleep duration and coronary heart disease in women. *Arch Intern Med*, **163**(2), 205–209.

Bailey, K.L., Wyatt, T.A., Romberger, D.J. & Sisson, J.H. (2009). Alcohol functionally upregulates Toll-like receptor 2 in airway epithelial cells. *Alcohol Clin Exp Res*, **33**(3), 499–504.

Balarajan, R. (1995). Ethnicity and variations in the nation's health. *Health Trends*, **27**(4), 114–119.

Banks, S. & Dinges, D.F. (2007). Behavioral and physiological consequences of sleep restriction. *J Clin Sleep Med*, **3**(5), 519–528.

Bradley, T.D. & Floras, J.S. (2009). Obstructive sleep apnoea and its cardiovascular consequences. *Lancet*, **373**(9657), 82–93.

Brook, R.D. & Julius, S. (2000). Autonomic imbalance, hypertension, and cardiovascular risk. *Am J Hypertens*, **13**(6 Pt 2), 112S–122S.

Buckley, T.M. & Schatzberg, A.F. (2005). On the interactions of the hypothalamic-pituitary-adrenal (HPA) axis and sleep: normal HPA axis activity and circadian rhythm, exemplary sleep disorders. *J Clin Endocrinol Metab*, **90**(5), 3106–3114.

Burckhardt, I.C., Gozal, D., Dayyat, E., et al. (2008). Green tea catechin polyphenols attenuate behavioral and oxidative responses to intermittent hypoxia. *Am J Respir Crit Care Med*, **177**(10), 1135–1141.

Burioka, N., Koyanagi, S., Endo, M., et al. (2008). Clock gene dysfunction in patients with obstructive sleep apnoea syndrome. *Eur Respir J*, **32**(1), 105–112.

Capaldi Ii, V.F., Handwerger, K., Richardson, E. & Stroud, L.R. (2005). Associations between sleep and cortisol responses to stress in children and adolescents: a pilot study. *Behav Sleep Med*, **3**(4), 177–192.

Cappuccio, F.P., Stranges, S., Kandala, N.B., et al. (2007). Gender-specific associations of short sleep duration with prevalent and incident hypertension: the Whitehall II Study. *Hypertension*, **50**(4), 693–700.

Cappuccio, F.P., Taggart, F.M., Kandala, N.B., et al. (2008). Meta-analysis of short sleep duration and obesity in children and adults. *Sleep*, **31**(5), 619–626.

Chaput, J.P., Brunet, M. & Tremblay, A. (2006). Relationship between short sleeping hours and childhood overweight/obesity: results from the 'Quebec en Forme' Project. *Int J Obes (Lond)*, **30**(7), 1080–1085.

Chobanian, A.V., Bakris, G.L., Black, H.R., et al. (2003). Seventh report of the Joint National Committee on Prevention, Detection, Evaluation, and Treatment of High Blood Pressure. *Hypertension*, **42**(6), 1206–1252.

Chogle, A.R. & Chakravarty, A. (2007). Cardiovascular events in systemic lupus erythematosus and rheumatoid arthritis: emerging concepts, early diagnosis and management. *J Assoc Physicians India*, **55**, 32–40.

Coughlin, S.R., Mawdsley, L., Mugarza, J.A., Calverley, P.M. & Wilding, J.P. (2004). Obstructive sleep apnoea is independently associated with an increased prevalence of metabolic syndrome. *Eur Heart J*, **25**(9), 735–741.

Dorkova, Z., Petrasova, D., Molcanyiova, A., Popovnakova, M. & Tkacova, R. (2008). Effects of continuous positive airway pressure on cardiovascular risk profile in patients with severe obstructive sleep apnea and metabolic syndrome. *Chest*, **134**(4), 686–692.

Drager, L.F., Bortolotto, L.A., Figueiredo, A.C., Krieger, E.M. & Lorenzi, G.F. (2007). Effects of continuous positive airway pressure on early signs of atherosclerosis in obstructive sleep apnea. *Am J Respir Crit Care Med*, **176**(7), 706–712.

Edell-Gustafsson, U., Svanborg, E. & Swahn, E. (2006). A gender perspective on sleeplessness behavior, effects of sleep loss, and coping resources in patients with stable coronary artery disease. *Heart Lung*, **35**(2), 75–89.

Ferrie, J.E., Shipley, M.J., Cappuccio, F.P., et al. (2007). A prospective study of change in sleep duration: associations with mortality in the Whitehall II cohort. *Sleep*, **30**(12), 1659–1666.

Frey, D.J., Fleshner, M. & Wright, K.P., Jr. (2007). The effects of 40 hours of total sleep deprivation on inflammatory markers in healthy young adults. *Brain Behav Immun*, **21**(8), 1050–1057.

Gangwisch, J.E., Heymsfield, S.B., Boden-Albala, B., et al. (2006). Short sleep duration as a risk factor for hypertension: analyses of the first National Health and Nutrition Examination Survey. *Hypertension*, 47(5), 833–839.

Gozal, D. & Kheirandish-Gozal, L. (2008). Cardiovascular morbidity in obstructive sleep apnea: oxidative stress, inflammation, and much more. *Am J Respir Crit Care Med*, 177(4), 369–375.

Gozal, D., Serpero, L.D., Sans, C.O. & Kheirandish-Gozal, L. (2008). Systemic inflammation in non-obese children with obstructive sleep apnea. *Sleep Med*, 9(3), 254–259.

Greenberg, H., Ye, X., Wilson, D., Htoo, A.K., Hendersen, T. & Liu, S.F. (2006). Chronic intermittent hypoxia activates nuclear factor-kappaB in cardiovascular tissues in vivo. *Biochem Biophys Res Commun*, 343(2), 591–596.

Guilleminault, C., Kirisoglu, C. & Ohayon, M.M. (2004). C-reactive protein and sleep-disordered breathing. *Sleep*, 27(8), 1507–1511.

Gundersen, Y., Opstad, P.K., Reistad, T., Thrane, I. & Vaagenes, P. (2006). Seven days' around the clock exhaustive physical exertion combined with energy depletion and sleep deprivation primes circulating leukocytes. *Eur J Appl Physiol*, 97(2), 151–157.

Haack, M., Pollmacher, T. & Mullington, J.M. (2004). Diurnal and sleep-wake dependent variations of soluble TNF- and IL-2 receptors in healthy volunteers. *Brain Behav Immun*, 18(4), 361–367.

Hak, A.E., Pols, H.A., Stehouwer, C.D., et al. (2001). Markers of inflammation and cellular adhesion molecules in relation to insulin resistance in nondiabetic elderly: the Rotterdam study. *J Clin Endocrinol Metab*, 86(9), 4398–4405.

Harsch, I.A., Koebnick, C., Wallaschofski, H., et al. (2004). Resistin levels in patients with obstructive sleep apnoea syndrome—the link to subclinical inflammation? *Med Sci Monit*, 10, CR510–CR515.

Horrocks, N. & Pounder, R. (2006). Working the night shift: preparation, survival and recovery—a guide for junior doctors. *Clin Med*, 6(1), 61–67.

Iesato, K., Tatsumi, K., Saibara, T., et al. (2007). Decreased lipoprotein lipase in obstructive sleep apnea syndrome. *Circ J*, 71(8), 1293–1298.

Irwin, M. (2002). Effects of sleep and sleep loss on immunity and cytokines. *Brain Behav Immun*, 16(5), 503–512.

Irwin, M., Rinetti, G., Redwine, L., Motivala, S., Dang, J. & Ehlers, C. (2004). Nocturnal proinflammatory cytokine-associated sleep disturbances in abstinent African American alcoholics. *Brain Behav Immun*, 18(4), 349–360.

Irwin, M.R., Wang, M., Campomayor, C.O., Collado-Hidalgo, A. & Cole, S. (2006). Sleep deprivation and activation of morning levels of cellular and genomic markers of inflammation. *Arch Intern Med*, 166(16), 1756–1762.

Irwin, M.R., Wang, M., Ribeiro, D., et al. (2008). Sleep loss activates cellular inflammatory signaling. *Biol Psychiatry*, 64(6), 538–540.

Kasasbeh, E., Chi, D.S. & Krishnaswamy, G. (2006). Inflammatory aspects of sleep apnea and their cardiovascular consequences. *South Med J*, 99(1), 58–67.

Kendall-Tackett, K.A. (2007). Inflammation, cardiovascular disease, and metabolic syndrome as sequelae of violence against women: the role of depression, hostility, and sleep disturbance. *Trauma Violence Abuse*, 8(2), 117–126.

Knutson, K.L. (2005). Sex differences in the association between sleep and body mass index in adolescents. *J Pediatr*, 147(6), 830–834.

Knutson, K.L., Spiegel, K., Penev, P. & Van, C.E. (2007). The metabolic consequences of sleep deprivation. *Sleep Med Rev*, 11(3), 163–178.

Kohler, M., Ayers, L., Pepperell, J.C., et al. (2009). Effects of continuous positive airway pressure on systemic inflammation in patients with moderate to severe obstructive sleep apnoea: a randomised controlled trial. *Thorax*, 64(1), 67–73.

Kokturk, O., Ciftci, T.U., Mollarecep, E. & Ciftci, B. (2005). Elevated C-reactive protein levels and increased cardiovascular risk in patients with obstructive sleep apnea syndrome. *Int Heart J*, **46**(5), 801–809.

Krueger, J.M. (2008). The role of cytokines in sleep regulation. *Curr Pharm Des*, **14**(32), 3408–3416.

Krueger, J.M. & Majde, J.A. (1994). Microbial products and cytokines in sleep and fever regulation. *Crit Rev Immunol*, **14**(3–4), 355–379.

Krueger, J.M., Obal, F.J., Fang, J., Kubota, T. & Taishi, P. (2001). The role of cytokines in physiological sleep regulation. *Ann N Y Acad Sci*, **933**, 211–221.

Lam, J.C. & Ip, M.S. (2007). An update on obstructive sleep apnea and the metabolic syndrome. *Curr Opin Pulm Med*, **13**(6), 484–489.

Lange, T., Dimitrov, S., Fehm, H.L., Westermann, J. & Born, J. (2006). Shift of monocyte function toward cellular immunity during sleep. *Arch Intern Med*, **166**(16), 1695–1700.

Lange, T., Perras, B., Fehm, H.L. & Born, J. (2003). Sleep enhances the human antibody response to hepatitis A vaccination. *Psychosom Med*, **65**(5), 831–835.

Lavie, L. & Lavie, P. (2008). Smoking interacts with sleep apnea to increase cardiovascular risk. *Sleep Med*, **9**(3), 247–253.

Legramante, J.M. & Galante, A. (2005). Sleep and hypertension: a challenge for the autonomic regulation of the cardiovascular system. *Circulation*, **112**(6), 786–788.

Luthje, L. & Andreas, S. (2008). Obstructive sleep apnea and coronary artery disease. *Sleep Med Rev*, **12**(1), 19–31.

Majde, J.A. & Krueger, J.M. (2005). Links between the innate immune system and sleep. *J Allergy Clin Immunol*, **116**(6), 1188–1198.

Mallion, J.M., Baguet, J.P., Siche, J.P., Tremel, F. & De, G.R. (1999). Clinical value of ambulatory blood pressure monitoring. *J Hypertens*, **17**(5), 585–595.

McNicholas, W.T. (2009). Obstructive sleep apnea and inflammation. *Prog.Cardiovasc Dis*, **51**(5), 392–399.

Meier-Ewert, H.K., Ridker, P.M., Rifai, N., et al. (2004). Effect of sleep loss on C-reactive protein, an inflammatory marker of cardiovascular risk. *J Am Coll Cardiol*, **43**(4), 678–683.

Meisinger, C., Heier, M. & Loewel, H. (2005). Sleep disturbance as a predictor of type 2 diabetes mellitus in men and women from the general population. *Diabetologia*, **48**(2), 235–241.

Miller, M.A. & Cappuccio, F.P. (2006). Cellular adhesion molecules and their relationship with measures of obesity and metabolic syndrome in a multiethnic population. *Int J Obes (Lond)*, **30**(8), 1176–1182.

Miller, M.A. & Cappuccio, F.P. (2007). Inflammation, sleep, obesity and cardiovascular disease. *Curr Vasc Pharmacol*, **5**(2), 93–102.

Miller, M.A., Kandala, N.B., Kivimaki, M., et al. (2009a). Gender differences in the cross-sectional relationships between sleep duration and markers of inflammation: Whitehall II study. *Sleep*, **32**(7), 857–864.

Miller, M.A., McTernan, P.G., Harte, A.L., et al. (2009b). Ethnic and sex differences in circulating endotoxin levels: a novel marker of atherosclerotic and cardiovascular risk in a British multi-ethnic population. *Atherosclerosis*, **203**(2), 494–502.

Miller, M.A., Sagnella, G.A., Kerry, S.M., Strazzullo, P., Cook, D.G. & Cappuccio, F.P. (2003). Ethnic differences in circulating soluble adhesion molecules: the Wandsworth Heart and Stroke Study. *Clin Sci (Lond)*, **104**(6), 591–598.

Motivala, S.J., Sarfatti, A., Olmos, L. & Irwin, M.R. (2005). Inflammatory markers and sleep disturbance in major depression. *Psychosom Med*, **67**(2), 187–194.

Mullington, J.M., Hinze-Selch, D. & Pollmacher, T. (2001). Mediators of inflammation and their interaction with sleep: relevance for chronic fatigue syndrome and related conditions. *Ann N Y Acad Sci*, **933**, 201–210.

Murck, H., Uhr, M., Ziegenbein, M., et al. (2006). Renin-angiotensin-aldosterone system, HPA-axis and sleep-EEG changes in unmedicated patients with depression after total sleep deprivation. *Pharmacopsychiatry*, **39**(1), 23–29.

Narkiewicz, K., Wolf, J., Lopez-Jimenez, F. & Somers, V.K. (2005). Obstructive sleep apnea and hypertension. *Curr Cardiol Rep*, **7**(6), 435–440.

National Sleep Foundation (2005). *Sleep in America Poll: Summary of Findings*. Washington, DC: National Sleep Foundation. Available at: http://www.sleepfoundation.org/sites/default/files/2005_summary_of_findings.pdf, accessed on 30.04.10.

Ohga, E., Tomita, T., Wada, H., Yamamoto, H., Nagase, T. & Ouchi, Y. (2003). Effects of obstructive sleep apnea on circulating ICAM-1, IL-8, and MCP-1. *J Appl Physiol*, **94**(1), 179–184.

Okun, M.L., Coussons-Read, M. & Hall, M. (2009). Disturbed sleep is associated with increased C-reactive protein in young women. *Brain Behav Immun*, **23**(3), 351–354.

Patel, S.R. & Hu, F.B. (2008). Short sleep duration and weight gain: a systematic review. *Obesity (Silver Spring)*, **16**(3), 643–653.

Patel, S.R., Zhu, X., Storfer-Isser, A., et al. (2009). Sleep duration and biomarkers of inflammation. *Sleep*, **32**(2), 200–204.

Peled, N., Kassirer, M., Kramer, M.R., et al. (2008). Increased erythrocyte adhesiveness and aggregation in obstructive sleep apnea syndrome. *Thromb Res*, **121**(5), 631–636.

Peled, N., Kassirer, M., Shitrit, D., et al. (2007). The association of OSA with insulin resistance, inflammation and metabolic syndrome. *Respir Med*, **101**(8), 1696–1701.

Pepperell, J.C., Ramdassingh-Dow, S., Crosthwaite, N., et al. (2002). Ambulatory blood pressure after therapeutic and subtherapeutic nasal continuous positive airway pressure for obstructive sleep apnoea: a randomised parallel trial. *Lancet*, **359**(9302), 204–210.

Phillips, B.G., Kato, M., Narkiewicz, K., Choe, I. & Somers, V.K. (2000). Increases in leptin levels, sympathetic drive, and weight gain in obstructive sleep apnea. *Am J Physiol Heart Circ Physiol*, **279**(1), H234–H237.

Phillips, C.L., Yang, Q., Williams, A., et al. (2007). The effect of short-term withdrawal from continuous positive airway pressure therapy on sympathetic activity and markers of vascular inflammation in subjects with obstructive sleep apnoea. *J Sleep Res*, **16**(2), 217–225.

Pickering, T.G. & Kario, K. (2001). Nocturnal non-dipping: what does it augur? *Curr Opin Nephrol Hypertens*, **10**(5), 611–616.

Poirier, P., Giles, T.D., Bray, G.A., et al. (2006). Obesity and cardiovascular disease: pathophysiology, evaluation, and effect of weight loss: an update of the 1997 American Heart Association Scientific Statement on Obesity and Heart Disease from the Obesity Committee of the Council on Nutrition, Physical Activity, and Metabolism. *Circulation*, **113**(6), 898–918.

Prinz, P.N. (2004). Age impairments in sleep, metabolic and immune functions. *Exp Gerontol*, **39**(11–12), 1739–1743.

Punjabi, N.M., Beamer, B.A., Jain, A., Spencer, M.E. & Fedarko, N. (2007). Elevated levels of neopterin in sleep-disordered breathing. *Chest*, **132**(4), 1124–1130.

Ranjbaran, Z., Keefer, L., Stepanski, E., Farhadi, A. & Keshavarzian, A. (2007). The relevance of sleep abnormalities to chronic inflammatory conditions. *Inflamm Res*, **56**(2), 51–57.

Resnick, H.E., Redline, S., Shahar, E., et al. (2003). Diabetes and sleep disturbances: findings from the Sleep Heart Health Study. *Diabetes Care*, **26**(3), 702–709.

Resta, O., Bonfitto, P., Sabato, R., De, P.G. & Barbaro, M.P. (2004). Prevalence of obstructive sleep apnoea in a sample of obese women: effect of menopause. *Diabetes Nutr Metab*, **17**(5), 296–303.

Rosenfeld, Y. & Shai, Y. (2006). Lipopolysaccharide (Endotoxin)-host defense antibacterial peptides interactions: role in bacterial resistance and prevention of sepsis. *Biochim Biophys Acta*, **1758**(9), 1513–1522.

Roubenoff, R., Parise, H., Payette, H.A., et al. (2003). Cytokines, insulin-like growth factor 1, sarcopenia, and mortality in very old community-dwelling men and women: the Framingham Heart Study. *Am J Med*, **115**(6), 429–435.

Ryan, S., Nolan, G.M., Hannigan, E., Cunningham, S., Taylor, C. & McNicholas, W.T. (2007). Cardiovascular risk markers in obstructive sleep apnoea syndrome and correlation with obesity. *Thorax*, **62**(6), 509–514.

Ryan, S., Taylor, C.T. & McNicholas, W.T. (2005). Selective activation of inflammatory pathways by intermittent hypoxia in obstructive sleep apnea syndrome. *Circulation*, **112**(17), 2660–2667.

Santos, R.V., Tufik, S. & de Mello, M.T. (2007). Exercise, sleep and cytokines: is there a relation? *Sleep Med Rev*, **11**(3), 231–239.

Scharf, S.M., Seiden, L., DeMore, J. & Carter-Pokras, O. (2004). Racial differences in clinical presentation of patients with sleep-disordered breathing. *Sleep Breath*, **8**(4), 173–183.

Siegel, J.M. (2005). Clues to the functions of mammalian sleep. *Nature*, **437**(7063), 1264–1271.

Spiegel, K., Knutson, K., Leproult, R., Tasali, E. & Van, C.E. (2005a). Sleep loss: a novel risk factor for insulin resistance and Type 2 diabetes. *J Appl Physiol*, **99**(5), 2008–2019.

Spiegel, K., Leproult, R., Van Cauter, E. (2005b). Metabolic and endocrine changes. In: Kushida, C. (ed.), *Sleep Deprivation: Basic Science, Physiology, and Behaviour*, vol. 192. New York, NY: Marcel Dekker, pp. 293–318.

Spiegel, K., Tasali, E., Penev, P. & Van, C.E. (2004). Brief communication: sleep curtailment in healthy young men is associated with decreased leptin levels, elevated ghrelin levels, and increased hunger and appetite. *Ann Intern Med*, **141**(11), 846–850.

Steiropoulos, P., Kotsianidis, I., Nena, E., et al. (2009). Long-term effect of continuous positive airway pressure therapy on inflammation markers of patients with obstructive sleep apnea syndrome. *Sleep*, **32**(4), 537–543.

Steiropoulos, P., Tsara, V., Nena, E., et al. (2007). Effect of continuous positive airway pressure treatment on serum cardiovascular risk factors in patients with obstructive sleep apnea-hypopnea syndrome. *Chest*, **132**(3), 843–851.

Stranges, S., Cappuccio, F.P., Kandala, N.B., et al. (2008a). Cross-sectional versus prospective associations of sleep duration with changes in relative weight and body fat distribution: the Whitehall II Study. *Am J Epidemiol*, **167**(3), 321–329.

Stranges S, Dorn JM, Cappuccio FP, et al. (2009). A population-based study of reduced sleep duration and hypertension: the strongest association may be in premenopausal women. *J Hypertens* [Epub ahead of print].

Stranges, S., Dorn, J.M., Shipley, M.J., et al. (2008b). Correlates of short and long sleep duration: a cross-cultural comparison between the United Kingdom and the United States: the Whitehall II Study and the Western New York Health Study. *Am J Epidemiol*, **168**(12), 1353–1364.

Strike, P.C. & Steptoe, A. (2003). New insights into the mechanisms of temporal variation in the incidence of acute coronary syndromes. *Clin Cardiol*, **26**(11), 495–499.

Suarez, E.C. (2008). Self-reported symptoms of sleep disturbance and inflammation, coagulation, insulin resistance and psychosocial distress: evidence for gender disparity. *Brain Behav Immun*, **22**(6), 960–968.

Taheri, S., Austin, D., Lin, L., Nieto, F.J., Young, T. & Mignot, E. (2007). Correlates of serum C-reactive protein (CRP)—no association with sleep duration or sleep disordered breathing. *Sleep*, **30**(8), 991–996.

Tauman, R., Ivanenko, A., O'Brien, L.M. & Gozal, D. (2004). Plasma C-reactive protein levels among children with sleep-disordered breathing. *Pediatrics*, **113**(6), e564–e569.

Teramoto, S., Yamamoto, H. & Ouchi, Y. (2003). Increased C-reactive protein and increased plasma interleukin-6 may synergistically affect the progression of coronary atherosclerosis in obstructive sleep apnea syndrome. *Circulation*, **107**(5), E40.

Trayhurn, P., Bing, C. & Wood, I.S. (2006). Adipose tissue and adipokines—energy regulation from the human perspective. *J Nutr*, **136**(7 Suppl), 1935S–1939S.

van Leuven, S.I., Kastelein, J.J., Hayden, M.R., d'Cruz, D., Hughes, G.R. & Stroes, E.S. (2005). Cardiovascular disease in systemic lupus erythematosus: has the time for action come? *Curr Opin Lipidol*, **16**(5), 501–506.

Van Cauter, E. & Spiegel, K. (1999). Sleep as a mediator of the relationship between socioeconomic status and health: a hypothesis. *Ann N Y Acad Sci*, **896**, 254–261.

Vega, G.L. (2004). Obesity and the metabolic syndrome. *Minerva Endocrinol*, **29**(2), 47–54.

Vgontzas, A.N. (2008). Does obesity play a major role in the pathogenesis of sleep apnoea and its associated manifestations via inflammation, visceral adiposity, and insulin resistance? *Arch Physiol Biochem*, **114**(4), 211–223.

Vgontzas, A.N., Bixler, E.O. & Chrousos, G.P. (2005). Sleep apnea is a manifestation of the metabolic syndrome. *Sleep Med Rev*, **9**(3), 211–224.

Vgontzas, A.N., Papanicolaou, D.A., Bixler, E.O., Kales, A., Tyson, K. & Chrousos, G.P. (1997). Elevation of plasma cytokines in disorders of excessive daytime sleepiness: role of sleep disturbance and obesity. *J Clin Endocrinol Metab*, **82**(5), 1313–1316.

Vgontzas, A.N., Zoumakis, E., Bixler, E.O., et al. (2008). Selective effects of CPAP on sleep apnoea-associated manifestations. *Eur J Clin Invest*, **38**(8), 585–595.

Vgontzas, A.N., Zoumakis, E., Bixler, E.O., et al. (2004). Adverse effects of modest sleep restriction on sleepiness, performance, and inflammatory cytokines. *J Clin Endocrinol Metab*, **89**(5), 2119–2126.

West, S.D., Nicoll, D.J., Wallace, T.M., Matthews, D.R. & Stradling, J.R. (2007). Effect of CPAP on insulin resistance and HbA1c in men with obstructive sleep apnoea and type 2 diabetes. *Thorax*, **62**(11), 969–974.

Williams, E., Magid, K. & Steptoe, A. (2005). The impact of time of waking and concurrent subjective stress on the cortisol response to awakening. *Psychoneuroendocrinology*, **30**(2), 139–148.

Wolf, J., Lewicka, J. & Narkiewicz, K. (2007). Obstructive sleep apnea: an update on mechanisms and cardiovascular consequences. *Nutr Metab Cardiovasc Dis*, **17**(3), 233–240.

Yokoe, T., Minoguchi, K., Matsuo, H., et al. (2003). Elevated levels of C-reactive protein and interleukin-6 in patients with obstructive sleep apnea syndrome are decreased by nasal continuous positive airway pressure. *Circulation*, **107**(8), 1129–1134.

Chapter 12

Genetics and sleep

M.A. Miller

Introduction

Sleep is a complex phenotype and as such it is possible that there are numerous genes which may each have a number of effects that control an individual's sleep pattern. Moreover, an individual's sleep duration and quality may be influenced by the interaction of their genes with the environment.

Animal studies, using inbred mice, have demonstrated that the amount, distribution, and rebound of sleep are genetically controlled (Franken et al., 1999; Tafti and Franken, 2002). Twin studies, in humans, have also demonstrated that there is a substantial heritability for sleep patterns (Heath et al., 1990; Partinen et al., 1983). Partinen et al. (1983) looked at sleep duration and quality in 2,238 monozygotic and 4,545 dizygotic adult twins and estimated that the heritability of sleep was around 44%. A similar finding was obtained from a study which investigated the genetic and environmental influences on sleep in nearly 4,000 Australian adult twins. The latter study estimated that approximately half of the variation in sleep could be attributed to genetic factors (Heath et al., 1990). To date, however, an underlying genetic basis for only a few sleep disorders has been established. This in part may be due to the complex interactions between environmental conditions and an individual's underlying genetic composition. Nevertheless, new genetic techniques may aid this search and should lead to a greater understanding of the disease pathogenesis and progression, which will aid the development of new drug therapies and a more personalized medicine approach to treatment.

Genes, normal sleep regulation, and circadian rhythm

Many biological processes exhibit a circadian rhythm which is a roughly 24-hour cycle in the biochemical, physiological, or behavioural processes. In mammals, the sleep-wake cycle is regulated by the sleep homeostat (a measure of an individual's time awake vs. time asleep) and by the central circadian clock or circadian oscillator which is located in the hypothalamic suprachiasmatic nucleus (SCN) (see also Chapter 2). This oscillator is composed of many genes and proteins which interact together and have both positive and negative feedback loops (Leloup and Goldbeter, 2004).

Although circadian rhythms are endogenously generated, they can also be entrained by external cues such as daylight or feeding. Amongst healthy living people there are individuals who prefer to sleep and wake early; these are sometimes referred to as 'larks' or 'morning people' and equally there are individuals who prefer to go to sleep later and to wake up at later times during the day who are referred to as 'owls' or 'evening people'. Research in this area is ongoing but a number of genes, including the Period (Per) genes, have been identified as being important in sleep-wake regulation. Among others, the CLOCK and BMAL1 elements promote the expression of the Per1, 2. and 3 and Crytochrome (CRY 1 and 2) genes. Polymorphic variation in some of these genes has been demonstrated. For example, a variable tandem repeat polymorphism in Per3 affects human sleep structure (Viola et al., 2007). Further investigation has demonstrated that individuals with the Per3[5/5] genotype are more likely to show morning preference (larks) as opposed to Per3[4/4] individuals who are evening or owl types (Dijk and Archer, 2009). Although these studies are of interest, there have been some inconsistencies reported. Moreover, the importance of homeostatic pressure as well as circadian phase needs to be considered (see also Chapter 2). It is anticipated that newer techniques will further contribute to the understanding of the genes involved in normal sleep and circadian biology.

The importance of genetic variation in such genes in the development of sleep disorders will be discussed in the following sections. It is expected that the utilization of new genetic techniques, including genome wide scans (GWS), will bring about further breakthrough in this area or research.

Genes and sleep disorders

Much of the early research regarding sleep and genes was to understand the genetic basis of circadian rhythms and was mainly examined using Drosophila and rodent models. However, larger studies are now being conducted in large human populations including the CoLaus Study which is aiming to phenotype a large adult population and to study genes involved in both normal sleep regulation as well as those that may be of importance in the development of sleep disorders (Firmann et al., 2008). Most sleep disorders arise from the result of complex interactions between an individual's genetic composition and environmental factors. It would be interesting to identify and study possible genes and gene products which may contribute to sleep disorders in children, as well as adults, as the former are less likely to be influenced by age-associated co-morbidities which are present in the adult populations. However, sleep disorders do exist in some children, and these would need to be excluded or diagnosed in such studies.

Sleep phase disorders

Some individuals suffer from disorders of their circadian rhythm. In some circumstances, this may result from extrinsic factors such as shift-work sleep disorder, which affects people who work nights or rotating shifts. However, in other individuals there appears to be an intrinsic disorder. These individuals appear to have a much later timing of their sleep onset and have a peak period of alertness in the middle of the night. This is known as delayed sleep phase syndrome (DSPS), while other individuals suffer from advanced sleep phase syndrome (ASPS), which causes difficulty staying awake in the evening and staying asleep in the morning. A study has shown that mutations in the human Per2 gene are responsible for an autosomal dominant form of familial ASPS (Toh et al., 2001).

Obstructive sleep apnoea

Obstructive sleep apnoea (OSA) is the most common sleep disorder and affects both adults and children. Complete or partial obstruction of the upper airway results in a number of symptoms including snoring, sleep fragmentation, transient hypoxia, and excessive daytime sleepiness. It has been shown to have multiple effects on the body including effects on the cardiovascular system. Many of the risk factors for OSA have a large heritable component. The apnoea-hypopnea index (AHI) is one of the key diagnostic factors for OSA and one study has suggested that 40% of variance may be explained by familial factors (Redline and Tishler, 2000). Patients with OSA syndrome have elevated TNF-alpha levels (Krueger and Majde, 2003). The -308A TNF-alpha gene polymorphism is responsible for increased TNF-alpha production. Individuals with OSA syndrome and their siblings are more likely to carry this polymorphism than population controls (Riha et al., 2005). Positive associations between OSA and polymorphic variants in other candidate genes, including the apolipoprotein E4 (ApoE4) gene and the leptin receptor gene polymorphism (GLN223 ARG) have also be reported (Dauvilliers and Tafti, 2008).

Narcolepsy

A number of sleep disorders, including narcolepsy, have been associated with the human leukocyte antigen (HLA) on chromosome 6. Narcolepsy is a disabling sleep condition and although it is believed to be genetically complex, evidence also suggests that there may be important environmental factors as well (Tafti, 2009). Furthermore, although evidence from different populations has highlighted the importance of various HLA loci and combinations of different HLA alleles in determining narcolepsy susceptibility (Tafti, 2009), more recent, genome-wide linkage, analysis has identified other chromosomal regions that are linked to narcolepsy which are not HLA-related genes. One such atypical HLA negative case was for a particularly severe from of narcolepsy with a very young onset and which was seen to result from a mutation in the prepro-hypocretin gene (Peyron et al., 2000). Animal studies have also led to the discovery that orexin is of great importance in human narcolepsy (Taheri and Mignot, 2002).

Kleine-Levin syndrome

Kleine-Levin syndrome (KLS) is a rare disorder which mainly occurs in adult males. It is characterized by recurrent hypersomnia and various behavioural abnormalities including compulsive hyperphagia. However, the individuals normally present as entirely normal between episodes. Although the underlying aetiology of this disorder is not known, some familial clustering has been observed (Dauvilliers and Tafti, 2008). One study, which investigated a particular family using extensive HLA typing to characterize them, reported that six of the affected family members were homozygous for DQB1*02. However, two out of six of the unaffected family members were also homozygous for the same variant (BaHammam et al., 2008).

Insomnia

Four sleep disorders so far have been shown to arise from a single gene mutation. These include familial advanced sleep-phase syndrome (see also Chapter 14) and a severe from of narcolepsy (see also Chapter 14). The other two single-gene mutation disorders that have been characterized are forms of insomnia. Fatal familial insomnia (FFI) is believed to arise from a mutation in a proton prion gene (Goldfarb et al., 1992) and is characterized by an inability to sleep and rapidly leads to death. Although a number of factors may lead to chronic primary insomnia, evidence from a family study suggests that it may also arise as a result of a single gene mutation, which occurs in the GABRB3 gene (Buhr et al., 2002). Further longitudinal family studies are however required to determine if other genetic and environmental factors may be important in this condition in the general population. See the recent review for more details (Dauvilliers and Tafti, 2008).

Parasomnias

Sleep disorders that involve abnormal movements, emotions, and behaviours that occur when an individual is either entering into sleep, is sleeping, is between sleep stages, or is awaking from sleep, are generally characterized as parasomnias.

Sleepwalking

Sleepwalking often has a strong family history which suggests that there may be an underlying genetic susceptibility which may be triggered by precipitating factors including conditions which increase slow wave sleep. A recent study suggested that there may be an association between a particular HLA subtype DQB1*05 and sleepwalking (Lecendreux et al., 2003).

Primary nocturnal enuresis

Primary nocturnal enuresis (PNE) is defined in a child aged 7 years or over who has never been dry at night. There is often a strong family history in PNE and genetic linkage studies have identified a number of different chromosomal loci which may be of importance in this condition. These suggest the presence of genetic heterogeneity and polygenetic inheritance patterns within PNE families (Dauvilliers and Tafti, 2008).

Restless legs syndrome

Restless legs syndrome (RLS) is a common sleep disorder, which is characterized by the urge to move the legs. It is often accompanied by an unpleasant sensation in the legs as well. A number of genetic studies of this condition have been conducted (Dauvilliers and Tafti, 2008). It has been concluded that although there is substantial evidence to support a genetic component for this disorder, it is equally apparent that there is a large degree of heterogeneity within this condition. It is likely to be a polygenic disorder and may involve different sets of genes in different families or populations.

Sleep, genes, and cardiovascular risk

Evidence for a link between short sleep and cardiovascular risk and potential underlying biochemical mechanisms is increasing (Ferrie et al., 2007; Miller et al., 2009). Diurnal rhythms have a large influence on normal cardiovascular physiology. Normal blood pressure across the diurnal cycle exhibits a 10% dip at night and has an increase around the awakening time. Cardiovascular incidents, such as myocardial infarcts, are approximately three times more likely to occur in the early morning than late at night (Martino and Sole, 2009). Plasminogen activator inhibitor (PAI)-1 is a primary regulator in the fibrinolytic cascade. The level of this activator displays circadian variation, with the level peaking in the morning. This variation is believed to be under the control of the Per2 gene and its regulatory elements CLOCK and BMAL (Martino and Sole, 2009).

A number of sleep conditions including OSA are associated with an increase in cardiovascular disease (CVD) (Vgontzas et al., 2003). Sleep conditions and CVD may share common genetic pathways. Further work is required to investigate the possibility that genetic determinants of sleep, acting, for example, on the oxidative and immune pathways, may be an important determinant of an individual's cardiovascular risk. The effect of potential diurnal variation on gene expression and the level of possible biomarkers for disease, for example CVD needs to be fully appreciated, understood, and adjusted for where possible (Miller et al., 2009). This is of particular importance in studies focused on the search for new disease biomarkers.

Summary

The genetic regulation of normal sleep and sleep disorders is complex and often shows strong environmental interactions. This is a relatively new and rapidly expanding area of research and the number of sleep conditions with established underlying genetic components is growing. At present, the public health benefits are limited but will increase as the identification and understanding of such genetic causes for sleep conditions improves. This in turn may lead to new diagnostic and treatment options including genetic counselling, improved therapeutic regimes, and new drug treatments.

Summary box

- The genetic regulation of normal sleep and sleep disorders is complex and often shows strong environmental interactions. There has been an increased awareness of the contribution of genetic components to the pathology of sleep disorders. Research in this field is expanding rapidly and the number of sleep conditions with known underlying genetic components is growing. Large, extensively phenotyped and well-characterized, population studies are necessary to investigate this area of research. Techniques may include the use of genome-wide scanning, utilization of sleep manipulation, and the use of well-characterized families and twin studies to investigate underlying familial components.
- Genetic studies of sleep need to focus not just on understanding the intrinsic biology of sleep regulation but also need to be able to characterize and observe other possible phenotypic associations which may be associated with sleep. For example, to investigate in more detail the association between sleep and CVD as well as allowing speculative investigation between sleep and other health outcomes including sleep and cancer and sleep and mood disorders.
- Proper family investigation in the rare but heritable fatal sleep conditions, such as FFI, is of paramount importance. Sleep conditions are observed in children as well as adults. Obesity is a major risk factor for OSA, the prevalence of which may increase in children with the observed population increase in obesity amongst children.
- Future research therefore needs to be carefully designed to facilitate the identification of the risk factors for sleep-related conditions. The important public health implications of sleep need to be acknowledged and further research is required to improve the understanding of the underlying genetic causes which may improve diagnosis, treatment, and therapeutic regimes in both adults and children.

References

BaHammam, A.S., GadElRab, M.O., Owais, S.M., Alswat, K. & Hamam, K.D. (2008). Clinical characteristics and HLA typing of a family with Kleine-Levin syndrome. *Sleep Med*, 9(5), 575–578.

Buhr, A., Bianchi, M.T., Baur, R., et al. (2002). Functional characterization of the new human GABA(A) receptor mutation beta3(R192H). *Hum Genet*, 111(2), 154–160.

Dauvilliers, Y. & Tafti, M. (2008). The genetic basis of sleep disorders. *Curr Pharm Des*, 14(32), 3386–3395.

Dijk, D.J. & Archer, S.N. (2009). PERIOD3, circadian phenotypes, and sleep homeostasis. *Sleep Med Rev*.

Ferrie, J.E., Shipley, M.J., Cappuccio, F.P., et al. (2007). A prospective study of change in sleep duration: associations with mortality in the Whitehall II cohort. *Sleep*, 30(12), 1659–1666.

Firmann, M., Mayor, V., Vidal, P.M., et al. (2008). The CoLaus study: a population-based study to investigate the epidemiology and genetic determinants of cardiovascular risk factors and metabolic syndrome. *BMC Cardiovasc Disord*, 8, 6.

Franken, P., Malafosse, A. & Tafti, M. (1999). Genetic determinants of sleep regulation in inbred mice. *Sleep*, 22(2), 155–169.

Goldfarb, L.G., Petersen, R.B., Tabaton, M., et al. (1992). Fatal familial insomnia and familial Creutzfeldt-Jakob disease: disease phenotype determined by a DNA polymorphism. *Science*, 258(5083), 806–808.

Heath, A.C., Kendler, K.S., Eaves, L.J. & Martin, N.G. (1990). Evidence for genetic influences on sleep disturbance and sleep pattern in twins. *Sleep*, 13(4), 318–335.

Krueger, J.M. & Majde, J.A. (2003). Humoral links between sleep and the immune system: research issues. *Ann N Y Acad Sci*, 992, 9–20.

Lecendreux, M., Bassetti, C., Dauvilliers, Y., Mayer, G., Neidhart, E. & Tafti, M. (2003). HLA and genetic susceptibility to sleepwalking. *Mol Psychiatry*, **8**(1), 114–117.

Leloup, J.C. & Goldbeter, A. (2004). Modeling the mammalian circadian clock: sensitivity analysis and multiplicity of oscillatory mechanisms. *J Theor Biol*, **230**(4), 541–562.

Martino, T.A. & Sole, M.J. (2009). Molecular time: an often overlooked dimension to cardiovascular disease. *Circ Res*, **105**(11), 1047–1061.

Miller, M.A., Kandala, N.B., Kivimaki, M., et al. (2009). Gender differences in the cross-sectional relationships between sleep duration and markers of inflammation: Whitehall II study. *Sleep*, **32**(7), 857–864.

Partinen, M., Kaprio, J., Koskenvuo, M., Putkonen, P. & Langinvainio, H. (1983). Genetic and environmental determination of human sleep. *Sleep*, **6**(3), 179–185.

Peyron, C., Faraco, J., Rogers, W., et al. (2000). A mutation in a case of early onset narcolepsy and a generalized absence of hypocretin peptides in human narcoleptic brains. *Nat Med*, **6**(9), 991–997.

Redline, S. & Tishler, P.V. (2000). The genetics of sleep apnea. *Sleep Med Rev*, **4**(6), 583–602.

Riha, R.L., Brander, P., Vennelle, M., et al. (2005). Tumour necrosis factor-alpha (-308) gene polymorphism in obstructive sleep apnoea-hypopnoea syndrome. *Eur Respir J*, **26**(4), 673–678.

Tafti, M. (2009). Genetic aspects of normal and disturbed sleep. *Sleep Med*, **10**(Suppl 1), S17–S21.

Tafti, M. & Franken, P. (2002). Invited review: genetic dissection of sleep. *J Appl Physiol*, **92**(3), 1339–1347.

Taheri, S. & Mignot, E. (2002). The genetics of sleep disorders. *Lancet Neurol*, **1**(4), 242–250.

Toh, K.L., Jones, C.R., He, Y., et al. (2001). An hPer2 phosphorylation site mutation in familial advanced sleep phase syndrome. *Science*, **291**(5506), 1040–1043.

Vgontzas, A.N., Bixler, E.O. & Chrousos, G.P. (2003). Metabolic disturbances in obesity versus sleep apnoea: the importance of visceral obesity and insulin resistance. *J Intern Med*, **254**(1), 32–44.

Viola, A.U., Archer, S.N., James, L.M., et al. (2007). PER3 polymorphism predicts sleep structure and waking performance. *Curr Biol*, **17**(7), 613–618.

Chapter 13

The sociology of sleep

S. Williams, R. Meadows, and S. Arber

Introduction

Sleep, until recently, has been a neglected topic or issue within sociology and the social sciences and humanities in general. At first glance this may seem unsurprising given the predominant waking assumptions, concerns, or preoccupations of these disciplines. Further reflection, however, reveals the shortcomings of any such neglect or dismissal of sleep as a topic worthy of sociological attention. Sleep is a socially, culturally, and historically variable phenomenon. How we sleep, when we sleep, where we sleep, what meaning and value we accord sleep, let alone with whom we sleep, are all important topics of sociological investigation which do not simply vary around the world, both past and present, but within different segments of society and within and between cultures. The nature, quantity, and quality of sleep, moreover, are clearly important both for the individual and society in terms of health and safety, productivity and performance, and quality of life and well-being.

In part a response to this past neglect, and in part a response to broader social trends and transformations regarding sleep, sociologists and others in the social sciences and humanities are now turning their attention to what might broadly be termed the 'sleep and society' agenda (Williams, 2005, 2008). Sleep, in this respect, is not simply a rich and fascinating sociological topic in its own right, but a valuable new window or way of approaching a range of existing sociological research agendas on issues as diverse as work, health, gender, ageing, and family life. This work in turn opens up significant new opportunities to explore the dynamic interrelations between social and biological factors regarding sleep and sleep disruption across the life course. In these and many other ways then, a sociological approach to sleep is not simply long overdue, but a timely and valuable complement to work in related fields of inquiry such as sleep epidemiology and public health which, in similar fashion, take us far beyond the sleep laboratory or sleep clinic to broader issues concerning sleep, health, and society.

It is therefore to a further consideration and elaboration of this newly emerging sleep and society agenda within sociology that we now turn in this chapter. We outline several strands of recent sociological work—starting with some preliminary points regarding the very conceptualization and measurement of 'sleep' as a methodological backdrop to the sociological themes and issues that follow.

Methodological matters: the meaning and measurement of sleep in everyday life

It is little wonder perhaps, given the complex, multifaceted nature of sleep, and its rich social, cultural, moral, metaphorical, metaphysical, even mystical heritage, that problems of meaning or conceptualization, let alone measurement, abound.

Sleep science, of course, has taught us to think of not one but two distinct types of sleep (i.e. rapid eye movement [REM] and non-rapid eye movement [NREM]) with the latter itself split or sub-divided into four further stages, with standardized terminology, techniques, and scoring systems for each sleep stage. This is the sleep, in other words, of theta waves, delta waves, sleep spindles, K-complexes, and the like, captured through elaborate monitoring and recording devices such as electroencephalogram (EEG), electromyogram (EMG), electrooculogram (EOG), in the modern day sleep laboratory. To this we may add a variety of other operationalized definitions and measures of various dimensions of sleep, sleepiness, and the like—such as watch actigraphy (a proxy measure in fact which records movement rather than sleep), the multiple sleep latency test (Carskadon et al., 1977), the Epworth Sleepiness Scale (Johns, 1991), and the Pittsburgh Sleep Quality Index (Buysse et al., 1989). We also now, of course, have a growing lexicon of sleep 'disorders', from narcolepsy to restless legs syndrome, obstructive sleep apnoea to shift-work sleep disorder (SWSD), judged and adjudicated through internationally agreed criteria (American Sleep Disorders Association, 2005).

Behind this seemingly stable or objective reality of sleep and its disorders, however, lies a rich and fascinating history of changing ideas, theories, understandings, and explanations of sleep, and techniques and technologies designed to record, measure, or treat it: a history, that is to say, of 'knowing sleep' in which sleep itself has been turned or transformed into an 'object of scientific knowledge' (Kroker, 2007). It is not simply the shifting or variable nature of 'sleep' as an object of scientific investigation or medical practice that we must attend to or bear in mind, but the multiple and diverse meanings of sleep and associated terms of reference in everyday life. Although many of the foregoing definitions and measures of sleep, for example, are reliable and valid, and while the correspondence between these objective and subjective measures is generally good, there is clearly a need for more detailed (sociological) research on the diverse or multiple meanings people bring to bear, in the context of their daily lives, regarding 'sleep', sleep 'problems', 'sleepiness', 'sleeplessness', and associated terms such as 'fatigue', 'tiredness', or 'exhaustion'. Although, 'tiredness' and 'sleepiness', for instance, are clearly separate states, they are frequently equated or conflated in everyday life (Widerberg, 2006). These meanings in turn are likely to be gendered and to differ according to other sociological or sociodemographic factors such as class, occupation, education, and age. Similarly, we need to know much more about people's own definitions and normative expectations regarding 'ideal', 'adequate', or 'enough' sleep, which themselves may be context dependent.

One may point, in this respect, to important social as well as biological dimensions of 'sleep', which cannot neatly or simply be mapped on to one another (Williams, 2007). Wiggs (2007), for example, elaborating on this latter point in relation to children's sleep, has recently suggested that 'sleepiness' might best be conceptualized in two distinct ways: first, the biological dimensions of sleepiness, which have objective implications for sleep quantity and quality in relation to biologically established sleep needs or norms; second, socially defined sleepiness, which involves deviations from socially defined/desired sleep hours or standards which themselves are shaped and influenced by a variety of social and cultural norms, values, and expectations. Both dimensions of course, as Wiggs rightly comments, are important to consider here in any full and proper assessment, particularly when deciding whether or not children or adults are getting 'enough' sleep, and what should be 'done' about it. This moreover, Wiggs reminds us, becomes doubly important in the case of proxy reporting (which frequently happens when parents report on their child's sleep 'problems'), where complainant and sufferer are not one and the same person.

These issues in turn require a sociological focus not simply on sleep, defined or measured, but the 'doing' of sleeping in everyday/night life: a shift, that is to say, from sleep itself, to all the things that surround it, including both pre- and post-sleep practices, rituals, and routines, and their relationship to everyday roles and responsibilities. It also suggests that one prime (though not sole, of course) sociological focus should be on 'normal' sleep and its 'disturbance' or 'disruption' through social roles, responsibilities, and relationships across the life course, rather than on sleep 'disorders' as such. This moreover, in contrast to much sleep research to date, includes a *dyadic* focus on sleep in relation to sleep partners, rather than a focus solely or simply on the individual. Again, to repeat, this takes us far beyond the artificial environments of the sleep laboratory or sleep clinic, to the logic and relations of sleep and sleeping in everyday/night life, thereby providing a valuable complement to work within both sleep epidemiology and public health.

This shift in focus brings with it the need for methodological innovation, which may include new tools to measure an individual's objective sleep, as well as new methods which focus on the social dimensions and variable and shifting meanings surrounding sleep. Thus, it could be suggested that to understand fully the meanings and experiences of poor sleep, epidemiologists should consider enlarging their methodological armoury to include qualitative methodologies, such as focus groups and in-depth interviews. In addition, there is value in developing new qualitative tools to study subjective experiences of sleep, for example through audio sleep diaries (Hislop et al., 2005), in which participants record their own narratives of the night soon after waking each morning.

Given the shared nature of many sleeping environments (discussed later), Venn et al. (2008) show the particular value of interviewing couples together, so that each partner can provide accounts of the other's sleep, while also interviewing each partner separately about his/her own and the partner's sleep. These dual couple and separate individual interviews also provide insights into how sleeping practices and disturbances relate to power and inequalities within the couple relationship (Meadows et al., 2008b; Venn et al., 2008), for example whether certain issues are spoken of in each context and the different ways they are articulated with/without the presence of the partner. When studying sleep among couples, audio sleep diary data from both partners for the same night revealed the different ways in which the same night was experienced by each partner, such as the influence of disruptions from children or a partner snoring (Venn et al., 2008).

Since sleep represents a physiological process and to some extent is unknown and unknowable to the sleeper, inter-disciplinary research on sleep is particularly important, integrating surveys with the collection of qualitative interview data and audio sleep diaries, and with actigraphy. For example, actigraphic data can be linked to data from audio-sleep diaries to provide insights into the nature and extent of sleep disturbance for each partner during the night (Meadows et al., 2005).

At the very least then, the sociology of sleep invites or encourages a broader conceptualization and engagement with sleep or sleeping in everyday/night life, including the potential refinement of existing methods and measures or the development of new ones (Meadows et al., 2008a; Hislop et al., 2005), both quantitative and qualitative, objective and subjective, in order to better capture, clarify, or convey these complex, socially contingent, and contextually dependent matters. These are issues we shall return to, illustrate, and elaborate upon throughout the course of this chapter, starting with a consideration of the broader sociological parameters of sleep, risk, and social change.

Sleep, risk, and social change: the sleep deprivation debate

One obvious point of sociological entry concerning sleep and society pertains to questions of social change, particularly with regard to ongoing debates as to the nature and extent of sleep deprivation and its costs and consequences for society.

It is certainly possible to point towards elements of both social continuity and social change which, singly or in combination, are likely to have an adverse bearing or influence on our sleep.

This, for example, includes: (i) long-standing negative attitudes towards sleep and their associa-tion with work-time, work-culture, and work-ethics (Steger and Brunt, 2003; Brunt and Steger, 2008); (ii) the emergence of around the clock 24/7 economies or societies (Moore-Ede, 1993); (iii) the information technology revolution and the advent of the 'wired' world (Summers-Bremner, 2008); and (iv) associated processes of globalization, instaneity, and intensification (Gleick, 2000). Sleep deprivation, in this respect, is said to be a widespread and growing problem in contemporary society, the costs and consequences of which have yet to be fully counted (see also Chapters 5, 6, 15–18, and 21).

A number of sources may be pointed to in this respect, some more scientifically credible than others. The eminent American sleep scientist William Dement (Dement, 2000), for example, claims that:

◆ We are a 'sleep sick society'.
◆ People now sleep on average 1½ hours less each night than they would have a century ago.
◆ There is an 'epidemic' of sleep deprivation in our midst.
◆ Most people in advanced industrialized countries are walking around with an accumulated 'sleep deficit' of between 25 and 30 hours.

These claims in turn are echoed in official reports by bodies such as the *US National Commission on Sleep Disorders Research*, whose 'Wake Up America: A National Sleep Alert' (NCSDR, 1993) estimated that as many as 70 million Americans were suffering from sleep 'deprivation' or some form of 'sleep problem'.

Other scientists and commentators also take a strong moral line here. Coren, for example, in his tellingly entitled book *'Sleep Thieves'*, unequivocally states that sleepiness:

> … is a health hazard to individuals. It may also be a danger to the general public because of the probabil-ity that a sleepy individual might cause a catastrophic accident…Perhaps someday society will act to do something about sleepiness. It may even come to pass that someday the person who drives or goes to work sleepy will be viewed as reprehensible, dangerous, or even criminally negligent like the person who drives or goes to work while drunk. If so perhaps the rest of us can all sleep a little bit more soundly.

> (Coren, 1996)

A litany of supposedly 'sleepy' people is singled out for attention here, including: sleepy drivers, pilots, doctors, parents, children, teachers, and politicians. The invisible hand of sleep deprivation, moreover, has been linked to various large-scale accidents, catastrophes, or national disasters such as the Exxon Valdez oil spill, the Challenger Space Shuttle disaster, and the Chernobyl nuclear meltdown. Sleep-related accidents, as this suggests, are costly on many counts. Mitler et al. (2000), for example, in purely financial terms, estimate this to be in the region of $56 billion each year in the United States alone, excluding lost productivity, medical illness, or shortened life span.

Is this however, we may ask, a distinctly American problem or crisis? There is certainly plenty of campaigning or lobbying about sleep-related matters in North America, through bodies such as the National Sleep Foundation (<<http://www.sleepfoundation.org>>). North America, moreover, has been at the forefront of sleep science and sleep medicine over the past half-century or so (Kroker, 2007), with membership of the Academy of Sleep Medicine at an all time high and a burgeoning number of sleep clinics (Norbutt, 2004). Sleep deprivation nonetheless, according to a variety of studies and sources, is a widespread and growing problem in many if not all advanced industrial societies and 24-hour economies in the global interconnected, 'wired' world, age, or era. Martin (2002), for example, drawing on studies in countries as diverse as Australia, Sweden, Poland, Finland, France, and Japan, concludes 'overall' that it is safe to say at least 'one in ten adults in the general population (you, me, and the people next door) are currently affected by moderate or severe daytime sleepiness. Some scientists believe the situation is much worse, with up to one in three adults suffering from significant sleepiness'. These findings in turn are echoed and amplified in other specially commissioned surveys and public opinion polls. For example, a recent report by the British Association of Counselling and Psychotherapy (2005), entitled '*Insomniac Britain—Does Anybody Sleep Here Anymore?*' claims 'the nation is "sleep deprived"', based on findings that:

♦ People report they only get on average 6 hours 53 minutes of sleep per night.

♦ 12+ million people in Britain (27% of adult population) experience at least 3 bad nights sleep in an average week.

♦ There is a 'nighttime gender divide'—women are significantly worse sleepers than men.

'We are prosperous', the report concludes, but live in an 'anxiety society' which it claims is 'penetrating' our sleeping lives and acting as a 'barrier' to peaceful sleep for many.

Similarly, a Demos report entitled '*Dream On: Sleep in the 24/7 Society*' (Leadbeater, 2004), finds that:

♦ 39% of British adults say they 'do not get enough sleep'.

♦ Sleep deficit/deprivation is most concentrated in the 25–54 age bracket (i.e. those of working age who are likely to have family responsibilities); amongst managers and white-collar workers (51%) and full-time workers (49%).

♦ Self-reported consequences of sleep deprivation included irritability and shouting, mistakes at work and behind the wheel, and falling asleep at work.

♦ Key disrupters identified were children (reported by 41% of parents), worry at work (15% of managers), and noise.

The recommendations of this report are also instructive, given they include a broad range of measures for taking sleep seriously at home and at work, including:

♦ Better education targeted particularly at parents and children about sleep.

♦ Greater employer responsibility for helping employees get the sleep they need, including provision of workplace naps.

♦ Better public napping facilities, particularly on motorways, etc. to help reduce sleepiness-related accidents.

♦ Greater role for government in the regulation of working hours for more groups of people (i.e. beyond pilots, lorry drivers, etc.) and the enhancement of rights to insist on family and sleep-friendly hours of work, particularly for parents of young children.

♦ Politicians, managers, and other public figures to lead by example, transforming themselves from 'poor role models' into exemplars of a new sleep-friendly ethos/ethic.

Politicians, as this suggests, are frequently criticized as 'poor role models' given a macho political culture where sleep is seen as for 'wimps' (e.g. Thatcher legacy), and sleep deprivation treated as a sign of virtue, dedication, determination, drive. An article in the UK's *Guardian* newspaper (14th October, 2008) entitled 'Sleepless in SW1', for example, in the midst of the financial crisis/credit crunch, notes that:

The financial crisis is keeping politicians (such as Alistair Darling and Gordon Brown) from their beds with rounds of all-night meetings'.

But then proceeds to ask:

Is this wise?
How much sleep deprivation can anyone take before their judgement takes a fall?

The media, in this respect, play a crucial role here as articulators and amplifiers of these issues surrounding sleep in contemporary society, including both the construction of sleep(iness) as a matter of public concern and an 'at-risk' state (Williams et al., 2008; Seale et al., 2007; Kroll-Smith, 2003).

This in turn suggests a need for caution with respect to many of these claims regarding sleep and society in both scientific and popular culture. Horne (2006), for example, highlights a number of important points to consider here in response to both current evidence and assumptions of a '(chronically) sleep-deprived society'. These include:

◆ The limits of historical comparative data and the quality as well as quantity of sleep.
◆ The problem of asking people about their sleep.
◆ The costs versus benefits, at a public health level, of encouraging people to get more sleep (instead of more exercise).
◆ Problems of anxiety inflation through sleep awareness campaigns and the like, which paradoxically may result in more rather than less insomnia/sleep problems!

With respect to the first of these issues, for example, the partial or patchy available historical data make firm claims about the quantity or quality of our sleep relative to our ancestors, at best difficult and at worst impossible in anything other than the most general terms. It may well be indeed, as Ekirch (2005) notes, that the quality of our sleep has improved over time—through adequate housing, heating, bedding, pain relief, and so on—even if, and it is still a big if, its quantity has declined. Many people today indeed, as Klug rightly notes, 'can hardly imagine the various threats our medieval ancestors were exposed to in the dormant part of their lives, given the warmth and security of modern day centrally heated bedrooms and our safely locked if not gated houses or apartments' (Klug, 2008)—see also Cox (2008) on the perils and potential of sleep in the eighteenth century.

Caution is also needed on this historical count, in relation to our so-called long work-hours culture. The picture in fact, unsurprisingly perhaps, is considerably more complex than this, depending on sector or occupation, and the time period in question. Generally, working hours have declined over time, even if work intensification has increased (Wainwright and Calnan, 2002). Measures such as the European Work Time Directive (EWTD), despite important loopholes or exemptions which the British Government seeks to maintain, are serving to exert further downward pressure on work hours, including those of junior hospital doctors (which is proving particularly controversial) (see also Chapter 18).

The problems of asking people about their sleep also return us to some of the issues raised earlier about the meaning and measurement of sleep. Self-reports of sleep deprivation, in this respect, may have a variable relationship to other more 'objective' measures of biological sleep need. Just because people say they are 'tired' or 'sleepy' or not getting 'enough' sleep, in other words, does not mean they need 'more' sleep or therefore, as a corollary, that more sleep would be a worthwhile investment of their time (compared to other possible investments). Most evidence anyway, as Horne (2006) himself stresses, seem to show that, whatever people say, they actually get between 7 and 7½ hours per night which, depending on quality, the majority of sleep experts would probably deem to be adequate for most healthy adults. The UK 2000 Time Use Survey, for example, points to a fairly constant 8 hours per night for adults until people get into their 60s, when it begins to rise to an average of 9 hours (with women, on the whole, appearing to sleep longer than men, particularly in the 30–60 age range). This survey is, however, far from unproblematic in terms of sleep, recording as it does 'sleep' from duration of 'time in bed', which includes 'trying to sleep' and 'lying awake', and therefore overestimates sleep duration (Chatzitheochari and Arber, 2009).

The final point about anxiety inflation is also a sociologically important one to stress and bear in mind, given the aforementioned proliferation of discussion and debate in professional and popular culture about sleep (or lack of it) as a matter of public concern, both for adults and children. At the very least, this suggests a need for caution here in relation to any so-called 'sleep awareness' campaigns which sleep scientists and health professionals, including public health specialists, should bear in mind or factor into the cost-benefit calculus.

What we see here then from a sociological perspective is the manner in which:

- Sleep(iness) is now being problematized if not politicized in contemporary society through discourses of risk, if not crisis or catastrophe (i.e. sleep(iness) as an 'at-risk' state).
- The construction of sleep as a significant public health and safety issue.
- The potential for further anxiety inflation which public health campaigns around sleep may fuel, however well intentioned.

We also glimpse here the manner in which sleep(iness), at one and the same time, is becoming:

- a point of articulation for a range of other social and cultural concerns and anxieties about life and living in the contemporary 'interconnected' if not 'incessant', 'wired' or 'runaway' world.

In these and other ways then, sleep is intimately bound up with issues of risk, health, and social change.

Cultures of sleeping: comparative and popular perspectives

It is not just social trends and transformations regarding sleep and society that are important to consider here, but cultural variations in sleeping patterns and practices too.

Steger and Brunt (2003), for example, usefully refer here to three different types of sleeping cultures around the world, both past and present. In 'monophasic' sleeping cultures, sleep in the main is concentrated or consolidated into a single block of usually nocturnal sleep with a widespread cultural norm or ideal of around 8 hours per night. 'Biphasic' or 'siesta' sleeping cultures, in contrast, usually involve a short afternoon nap or snooze coupled with a longer sleep at nighttime. In 'polyphasic' sleeping cultures, napping may occur at any time, as and when the social situation allows or permits, albeit with an 'anchor sleep' still at night. A high level of tolerance therefore, compared to mono or biphasic sleeping cultures, is evident in polyphasic sleeping cultures regarding the possibility or permissibility of daytime napping.

The monophasic sleeping pattern is commonly found or practiced in Northern Europe and North America. Historically speaking, as Ekirch's (2005) careful analysis of sleep in pre-industrial times suggests, it is a rather recent arrival—not only was public, undisciplined, daytime napping common, but nighttime slumber itself was segmented into a so-called 'first' and 'second' (or 'morning') sleep, with a period for quiet contemplation or other nocturnal activity (prayer, divination, or other [il]licit activity under the cover of night) interspersed in between. Even today, many Westerners take daytime naps. Shift-work too is now common, with nighttime sleep frequently sacrificed in the service of one's occupation. The need to protect nighttime sleep as the normative reference point or cultural ideal, remains 'quite strong' in monophasic sleeping cultures—a process which itself is intimately bound up with the privatization or sequestration of sleep in the bedroom behind the scenes of social or public life, with the transition to and from the sleep role (Schwartz, 1970) to the waking role 'comparably long and elaborate' (Steger and Brunt, 2003).

Siesta cultures, in contrast, are characteristic of Spain and other societies with Spanish speaking cultural influences, as well as Italy and other Mediterranean cultures. Climatic influence may seem the obvious factor here for the adoption of this sleeping pattern, yet as Steger and Brunt

(2003) rightly note, the siesta is 'neither restricted to countries near the equator, as the example of China shows, nor is it habit found everywhere in Southern regions—neighbouring Portugal, for example, hardly adheres to a socially set afternoon nap, whereas Greece does'. In siesta cultures, on the whole, there is a far greater tolerance of late night activities, given the siesta provides an important resource to draw upon, or 'buffer zone', for such late night pursuits. The siesta none-theless, these authors note, is now increasingly at risk in the global era, given the move towards the 'international clock' which is no respecter of local customs, timetables, or traditions.

Polyphasic sleeping cultures are perhaps the most geographically dispersed around the world today, and can be found not simply in 'every continent' but 'under different climatic and socio-economic conditions' (Steger and Brunt, 2003). The emphasis here is on highly *flexible* or poly-morphic sleeping patterns that adapt to or fit around other social roles, activities, duties, and obligations. With regard to China and Japan, for example, Steger and Brunt suggest at least two different kinds of sleep can be distinguished: the first involving the separation of sleeper from waking activities; the second involving a form of quasi-sleep known as *inemuri*, in which the sleeper remains present in a social situation which is meant for something other than sleep, but where this form of sleep or napping is socially tolerated if not sanctioned as long as the sleeper is prepared to relinquish his/her sleep as and when his/her full attention is required (see also Steger, 2003a, b). In India too, Brunt (2008) observes, people 'fall in and out of sleep just like they fall in and out of conversation'. Despite more or less generally accepted 'sleeping times', 'nobody seems to claim that sleeping is something one should only do during certain periods', or we might add in certain places. Sleeping in India, in this respect, has a 'public or semi-public character' and in contrast to the Western norms or ideals, it seems 'perfectly natural to sleep in public—with either intimates or complete strangers around'. Even in these countries where public sleeping is toler-ated, there are many social situations and occasions, as Steger and Brunt (2003) note, in which napping is not allowed or sanctioned.

Sleeping then, to repeat, may well be a universal need or imperative, but when we sleep, let alone where and with whom we sleep, are all socially, culturally, and historically variable matters. Sleeping cultures themselves, as the foregoing discussion suggests, are complex if not contradic-tory, with important variations towards sleep and sleeping within as well as between cultures and societies over time. Although napping, for example, is becoming increasingly popular in a number of countries around the world today—as an efficient, flexible if not 'smart' way to organize our sleep given the rapid pace of modern life in general, and the demands and dictates of the modern day economy or workplace in particular—it remains a highly variable practice which, as Baxter and Kroll-Smith (2005) rightly note, depends on factors such as economic sector, stage of eco-nomic development, and the sociocultural context of change. A reversal of the traditional for-tunes of napping may well be occurring between Asia and the West. Instructive comparisons, for instance, may be drawn between pressures on the midday nap in rapidly modernizing countries such as China, and the growing appreciation if not art or practice of napping in the West—a trend that is not simply evident in safety-critical occupations and various types of shift-work, but in a wide range of other occupations and working environments where mental rather than manual labour is prized.

Advertising agencies, computer software companies, and corporate law firms, for example, are now beginning to introduce official napping practices and facilities into the workplace (i.e. nap-ping as an acceptable part of work culture) in recognition of the fact that a nap may boost the creativity, productivity, and performance of its employees. These trends in turn are both fuelled and reflected through a range of self-help or self-improvement materials in popular culture, including books such as *The Art of Napping* (Anthony, 1997) or *The Art of Napping at Work* (Anthony and Anthony, 2001), and the provision of sleeping pods or facilities through dedicated companies such as *MetroNaps*. A growing number of companies, moreover, now provide health and well-being packages or programmes to their employees, which frequently include aspects of good 'sleep hygiene', if not the merits of napping.

Viewed in this light then, the changing fate and fortunes of (workplace) napping provide an instructive lens through which to view both sleeping cultures in general and contemporary aspects of work time, work culture, and work ethics in particular, both locally and globally. Various future scenarios regarding sleeping cultures, as Brunt and Steger (2008) suggest, are possible given globalizing pressures and processes. One possibility, for example, might be the continuing decline or disappearance of the siesta from countries such as Spain and the rest of the Mediterranean, and the drift towards monophasic sleeping cultures in other napping cultures such as China, Japan, and India. Alternatively, the campaign or culture of napping (or 'power-napping' as it is now commonly known in the West) might become so successful, that 'all societies will change into napping cultures', a process these authors speculate which may itself be aided and abetted by scientific and medical assumptions which point to the merits of napping.

It is not simply a case of when we sleep, or even where we sleep, but of how we sleep and with whom we sleep. Children and adults, for example, often have their own special bedtime rituals or routines, or what Ben-Ari (2008) terms 'key cultural scenarios', which help ready or prepare them for sleep, with similar more or less elaborate routines or rituals following sleep in order to facilitate the passage or transition back into waking roles. The very word 'bedtime' however is somewhat problematic or misleading here, given that in some countries or cultures people sleep in beds while in others people sleep on some kind of mattress on the floor, or even, in the case of napping cultures such as India, in rickshaws, handcarts, trucks, benches, or on medium height walls (Brunt, 2008)! Patterns of co-sleeping are also socially and culturally variable. In India for example, as Brunt (2008) observes, co-sleeping is perfectly normal, including public napping in groups. In countries such as the United States, in contrast, children are taught from a relatively early age to sleep on their own (Ben-Ari, 2008); a pattern which is only broken in adulthood with respect to one's intimate partner.

Popular culture is another important reference point here in relation to sleep and sleeping, including the role of the mass media and the proliferation of self-help books and Internet websites of a 'how to...' kind regarding sleep matters (Brown, 2004). Kroll-Smith (2003), for example, has documented the role of the mass media and Internet in the social construction of 'excessive daytime sleepiness' as a significant public health problem. Williams et al. (2008) and Seale et al. (2007) have also, through a series of publications, demonstrated the role of the media, particularly the print news media, in the social construction and social mediation of a range of sleep-related problems and issues in modern society. The media, in this respect, appear to play a variety of roles in the articulation and amplification of cultural concerns and anxieties about sleep, depending on both the media and topic in question, including discourses and debates which reflect both the increasing 'medicalization' of sleep problems (i.e. the cultural framing of sleep problems as medical matters), and broader cultural trends or tendencies towards the 'healthicization' of sleep (i.e. the construction of sleep as a key part of healthy, happy, productive lives and lifestyles)—see also Woloshin and Schwartz (2006) on media constructions of restless legs syndrome and Weisgerber (2004) on the role of Internet websites for sleep paralysis sufferers.

Media portrayals and constructions of sleep-related pharmaceuticals, such as the wakefulness promoting agent Modafinil, have also been examined in recent sociological research, particularly in relation to media concerns about the blurring of the boundaries between treatment and enhancement, which these drugs threaten or promise in a 24/7 competitive society where staying awake is culturally prized and vigilance is valorized (Williams et al., 2008). Media constructions of pharmaceuticals in this respect, as previous studies have shown, are deeply ambivalent, if not contradictory, often moving from idealization to stigmatization, if not demonization, over time through recourse to 'oppositional extremes' (Seale, 2004).

The media therefore, as this suggests, are important to consider in relation to sleep and public health, given the critical role they play in the articulation and amplification of a broad range of advice as well as anxieties about sleep and society in popular culture. Questions of audience reception amongst diverse publics, however, remain to be addressed in much of this research, and as such merit further study in future sociological work of this kind.

Sleep across the life course

Another important strand of sociological work has begun to examine sleep across the life course. At least two rationales underpin a life course approach to sleep. First, as a sizeable body of scientific literature and physiological evidence demonstrates, sleep duration, patterns, and stages vary across the life course, and generally deteriorate as one ages. Second, a life course perspective on sleep brings into sharp focus sociological issues of power, status, and control across the life course, from childhood, through youth and working life, and into later life (Arber et al., 2007a; Williams, 2005). In addition, it emphasizes how sleep is embedded in the social context of everyday life, although until recently little research had examined sleep within family contexts, or had recognized how gender and the life course are inextricably linked (Arber et al., 2003). Throughout this section, we consider the gendered aspects of sleep and sleeping, and show how a close analysis of sleep illuminates gender roles and gender inequalities within families.

One key challenge or opportunity for sociologists of sleep, in addition to a sole or primary focus on the social dimensions of sleep, is to explore the dynamic interplay between the social and biological or neurobiological aspects of sleep across the life course and how this interlinks with gender. It is to sociological research on these fronts, therefore, that we now turn, starting with children, young people, and sleep.

Children, young people, and sleep

Sleep, as we know, consumes a large proportion of children's time, particularly the very early years of a child's life. It is nonetheless, romanticized constructions of bedtime for children in the Euro-American middle classes notwithstanding (Ben-Ari, 2008), often an area or issue of considerable contest or conflict, if not anxiety, in childhood, for both parents and children alike (Furedi, 2002). Children, for example, who do not obtain sufficient nighttime sleep, are now increasingly constructed as a social, health, or educational 'problem'. At the same time, children's bedrooms have become a site of increasing activity, with televisions, computer games, mobile phones, and other forms of communication transforming them into networked zones of social connectivity (Van den Bulck, 2004; Venn and Arber, 2008), thereby posing risks of nighttime sleep disruption which itself often remains hidden from parents' gaze.

The very notion of whether children are getting 'enough' sleep, as Wiggs (2007) notes, is itself complex if not controversial, particularly as noted earlier when 'socially defined sleeplessness' is considered alongside 'biologically defined sleeplessness'. This in turn becomes all the more complex when complainant, in this case parent, and sufferer, in this case children, are not one and the same person, thereby bringing into play the role of parental perceptions and parental or family sleeping patterns in the very definition of children's own sleep problems.

Other recent sociological research, partly in recognition of these limits, has taken a more child-centred focus regarding children's own accounts, perspectives, and experiences of their sleep and the construction of their 'nighttime worlds' (Williams et al., 2007; Moran-Ellis and Venn, 2007; Venn and Arber, 2008). This research has highlighted a number of important issues, including the embedding of children's sleep in complex and changing family forms (e.g. more complex family structures of step-siblings and other household members, teenagers and young people living at home for longer periods, etc.), the influence of other family members (particularly siblings) on children's sleep, and the 'mobile' nature of children's own sleeping arrangements in relation to multiple family and friendship networks. Discussions in families surrounding when and where young people should sleep are influenced 'firstly, by changes that have been taking place in the United Kingdom to family composition, and secondly, through the negotiation for increased autonomy by young people as they make the transition into adulthood and beyond' (Venn and Arber, 2008). The increasing autonomy or negotiability of bedtimes can result in a delay in sleep time, as young people frequently choose to do other things in their bedroom than sleep. Escalating demands regarding these young peoples' daytime activities (school, jobs, etc.), at one and the same time, mean that they are awakening sooner than most would have liked. What we see here then are the complexities of familial negotiations of sleep within complex household structures.

Another particularly revealing finding, given the weight of expert opinion, concerns the role of technology which, for some of the children in Williams et al.'s (2007) study at least, was thought to *facilitate* rather than delay or disrupt their sleep—a finding which echoes Kaji et al.'s (2007) research in Japan on the role of mobile phones and other 'knickknacks' as items seen to assist rather than interrupt sleep through the reassurance and security they provide. Issues of privacy, self-determination, and control over the material space of sleep also appear to be crucial factors here for children, as Moran-Ellis and Venn (2007) show, particularly with respect to intergenerational and sibling relationships, and in terms of children's ability to construct their own-night worlds as distinct from those of adults—see also Williams et al. (2007) on children's battles for bedroom space and privacy, and various incursions or infringements of these rights. According to Venn and Arber's (2008) research with young people—'The combination of interacting with social networks, usually via mobile phones, worries, and their frequently phase-delayed sleep cycle, left many of the young adult children talking of being "totally exhausted", "very, very tired", and even "depressed"'.

The sleep of parents

The sleep of children and young people is intimately tied to the quality of their parents' sleep, gender inequalities, and ideologies of 'parenting'. It is well known, at least in Western societies, that infants and small children disturb parents' sleep. Research with heterosexual couples illustrates the lack of explicit negotiation between partners about who provides care for children at night (Venn et al., 2008). It is almost tacitly assumed that women should get up in the night to deal with, for example, nappy changing or settling anxious children. Even when women return to employment or full-time education, they continue to undertake most of the child-care at night, significantly disturbing their own sleep. These nighttime roles are not restricted to the direct provision of care, such as attending to the physical needs of children, but also relate to women's engagement in the emotional labour of worrying about and anticipating the nighttime needs of their family members.

Less widely reported is how the complexity of everyday household living arrangements impact on all family members' sleep. Although parents of young children have access to plenty of advice about how to get children to sleep, how to keep them asleep, and how to manage on very little sleep, parents of teenagers and young adult children are left largely bereft of such resources. Many parents in Venn and Arber's (2008) study were surprised by the way in which their older, seemingly more autonomous or independent children, 'continued to keep them awake, and in some instances interrupted their sleep even more than when they were young'. Worries about their teenage children's whereabouts, and their safety, were particularly important sources of parental sleep disturbance in this respect, with fathers in particular voicing these concerns (Venn et al., 2008). Late night noise and door slamming also contributed to parental sleep disturbance, as well as occasional late night phone calls from young people in need of help.

Cultural differences also influence to what extent children disturb parents' sleep. For example, in Mediterranean cultures, adult children tend to leave their family of origin at an older age, prolonging co-habitation with their parents. The percentage of young people (age 20–29) living in the parental home is 75% in Italy and Spain, compared to 31% in the United Kingdom and The Netherlands (Becker et al., 2004). In Italy, this relates to both economic difficulties facing young people and strong cultural pressure for adult children to remain living with their parents until marriage. Bianchera and Arber's (2007) research shows that for Italian women, no matter their age, as long as a child lives under the same roof, worries about adult children out at night disturbed their sleep. These midlife women recounted diverse techniques to minimize anxiety and check if adult children were home, which included checking if the car was in the garage, checking the child's bed, calling them on their mobile phone, and waiting up until they came home. Current trends in the United Kingdom for young adults to remain living in the parental home for longer, due to economic pressures, may have the unanticipated consequence of leading to greater disruption of their parent's sleep.

Gender, couples, and co-sleeping

Today, most adults do not sleep alone (Martin, 2002; Hislop, 2007). Yet, for the majority of its history, sleep research has paid little attention to marriage/co-habitation and the co-sleeping of partners, and almost 'everything that has been published in the social and behavioural sciences and in medicine about adult sleep has looked at adult sleep as an individual phenomenon' (Rosenblatt, 2006). However, some research suggests that co-sleeping negatively impacts on sleep duration and sleep quality. Nearly 40 years ago, Monroe (1969) found that lone sleeping significantly increased the amount of stage 4 sleep and reduced the number of awakenings by 60%. More recently, Meadows et al. (2009) quantified the dyadic interdependence of couples sharing a bed by analyzing actigraphically recorded variables collected over a 1-week period. Amongst other things, results suggested that about one-third of nocturnal awakenings are similar for bed partners.

It has largely been left to sociological work to explore issues of co-sleeping further. Discussing 'sleep timing' Crossley (2004) suggests that 'in situations of co-presence the parties to that situation need to secure cooperation from one another for their own sleep ritual, whether this means common bedtimes and sleep conditions or different but complementary patterns, with each party respecting the needs of the other'. Crossley's choice of terminology is not meant to imply the absence of power, status, or social control. For example, it may well be that it is left to the female partner to alter her bedtime towards the male partner's preferred bedtime (Vaughan et al., 2006).

Once in bed, sleep can be disturbed by a multitude of bedfellows' behaviours (Strawbridge et al., 2004). Hislop (2007), for example, uses qualitative data collected with 40 couples to show how a range of aspects of the sleeping environment have to be explicitly, or more often implicitly, negotiated between partners, from the amount of light in the room to appropriate 'bedtimes'. This can lead to the double bed becoming a site of potential sleep disruption through partner snoring, hogging the bed covers, going to the toilet, having the TV/radio on, etc. (see also Meadows, 2005).

Parties to co-presence can also be disturbed by their own response to bedfellows' behaviours. Although, the sleep of many couples is disturbed by nighttime behaviours of their partner, it is seen as a 'last resort' for a partner to re-locate to sleep in another room (or on the sofa) on either a temporary or permanent basis, even when partners recognize that sleeping alone may lead to better quality sleep (Hislop and Arber, 2003a). The norm that partners 'should' share a double bed are inherently tied to intimacy and the 'culture of togetherness' in contemporary western societies (Hislop, 2007). Further to this, Venn (2007) argues that the strategies women develop to cope with their partners' snoring can actually prolong their own sleep disturbance. These strategies, which are in line with normative expectations of femininity and of women being adaptive and passive, include prodding (but not waking their partner), passivity, and (occasionally) re-location.

It would, however, be wrong to suggest that all bedfellow impacts are perceived as negative. A small scale study by Cartwright (2008) found that continuous positive airway pressure (CPAP) compliance in married men is (positively) related to the frequency with which his partner co-sleeps with him (although, no comment is made about whether the wife's sleep was adversely affected by her husband's CPAP use). Further to this, Pankhurst and Horne (1994) found that people often seem unaware of the impact bed partners can have on their sleep and report sleeping better when their partner is there.

Gender, paid employment, and sleep

We will not discuss the extensive research on shift-work here, but note that the relationship between 'normal' paid employment and sleep is complex. On the one hand, reports stress the negative impact that 'long work hours' presently have on sleep quality and quantity. On the other hand, there is a need for caution with respect to many of these types of arguments, as noted earlier. Historical data suggest that working hours have actually declined over time.

Recent empirical research has further highlighted these complexities. Chatzitheochari and Arber (2009) analyzed UK Time Use Survey data on 2,882 workers aged 20–60 years, finding an inverse relationship between length of working hours and short sleep duration (under 6.5 hours), which was stronger for men than women. Social class was a significant predictor of short sleep for men, with those at either end of the class spectrum more likely to report short sleep. The results suggest a gender difference with working men more likely than women to obtain under 6.5 hours of sleep on a typical weekday, although the few women who worked very long hours (over 10 hours) were also likely to have short sleep duration. However, it is important to consider how *both* work and family responsibilities may impinge on women's sleep *quality* (Venn et al., 2008) as well as sleep *duration*, and to note that time-use data tend to overestimate sleep duration.

Recent research also suggests that employment impacts upon the meanings we attribute to sleep and highlights the 'powerful internalizing role of labour' in experiences of sleep (Henry et al., 2008). Put slightly differently, 'paid work' may be bound up with subjective understandings and attitudes towards sleep—regardless of whether or not it is objectively affecting sleep. Meadows et al. (2008b), for example, illustrate how men link 'sleep need' with the ability to 'function' (especially in terms of paid labour). The same men also identified paid work as one of the key causes of their poor sleep (both in terms of work constraints and work stresses). Research has also shown that patient explanatory models of insomnia revolve around 'work'. In Henry et al.'s (2008) small-scale study of 24 patients (19 female and 5 male) who were receiving treatment for insomnia, paid work was offered as the primary causal agent in the development of their insomnia, the primary reason for needing good sleep, the reason for seeking medical help, and the reason why individuals complied with medical regimens. Perhaps most surprisingly, at least for these authors, 'even retired informants couched their illness experience in terms of work' (Henry et al., 2008).

Gender, ageing, and sleep

Throughout adulthood and later life, sleep continues to be marked by changes, transitions, and negotiations. Drawing on qualitative data from women aged 40 to their 80s, Hislop and Arber (2006) summarize many of these transitions and negotiations and propose a framework of four temporal dynamics that impact on sleep in later life:

1. *Biological or physiological ageing*: Physiological changes with age include increasing frailty, reduction in strength, impairment, increasing levels of chronic illness and for women, the menopause.
2. *Institutional structures*, such as engagement in paid work or education, vary by age and gender, but their form and impact differ over time and between societies.
3. *Relational structures*, which are associated with an individual's roles and relationships with partners, children, parents, and friends. These not only differ by gender but often change with age and life course stage, for example, children leaving home or frail parents requiring care.
4. *Biographical transitions*, which are associated with life events and other transitions, such as marriage, parenthood, retirement, divorce, and widowhood, all of which may impact on sleep.

Biological or physiological age-dependent transformations in sleep have been well documented (Bliwise, 2005) and are known to include shifts in sleep architecture as well as increased susceptibility to certain sleep disorders. As we age the amount of time spent in deep, slow wave sleep diminishes, along with a decrease in REM (dreaming) sleep, and the time spent in lighter, stage 1 and stage 2 sleep increases. Therefore, older people often find it takes longer to get to sleep, have more fragmented sleep, and wake up earlier (Bliwise, 2005). In addition, a major physiological reason for poorer sleep quality with increasing age is because chronic ill-health, disability, and impairment cause pain and discomfort at night, resulting in sleep complaints and difficulties (Davidson et al., 2002; Stewart et al., 2006; Vitiello et al., 2002).

Ageing is also associated with increased daytime sleep via napping or dozing. It remains unclear whether the change in nighttime sleep experienced by older people leads to a propensity for daytime napping (Münch et al., 2005), or has no effect on whether older people sleep during the day or not (Klerman and Dijk, 2008). Increased napping/dozing in later life may result from a combination of factors, some being physiological changes, others related to release from institutional structures (of work), and lack of stimulating activities or boredom.

Regarding 'institutional structures', retired people no longer have the constraints of institutionalized time; they no longer 'need' to be woken by the alarm clock to get to work and therefore have to determine their own sleeping times and routines. Biographical transitions, such as widowhood or divorce, mean a person no longer experiences the potential disruptions of sleeping with a partner. However, their sleep may be disturbed through missing the intimacy and sense of security of co-sleeping, with sleeping *alone* in the 'double bed' making more poignant what they have lost. They may also experience worries and anxieties from the experience of divorce/widowhood and having to 'cope alone'.

The four temporal dynamics in Hislop and Arber's schema mentioned above primarily relate to impacts on sleep duration and sleep quality. Returning to our earlier debates, we could extend this framework to incorporate two other 'domains'. The first concerns 'discourses' and the politics of scientific truth claims. As Martin (1987) suggests, discussing science generally, 'it is no accident that "natural" facts about women, in the form of claims about biology, are often used to justify social stratification based on gender'. The second concerns subjective meanings. Each of the four temporal dynamics could be extended to examine how they intersect with individuals' understandings and meanings. As Bliwise (2000) suggests, 'whether an aged person views 75% sleep efficiency as insomnia or merely accepts this as a normal part of ageing may depend largely on the individual's perspective on growing old and what that means to him or her' (see also Davis et al., 2007).

This may, in turn, help shed light on controversies regarding the nature of gender differences in sleep quality in later life. Physiological changes in sleep with ageing are often said to differ by biological 'sex'. Meta-analysis of polysomnographic data collected in sleep laboratories (an abnormal sleeping context), for example, suggests that older women sleep better than men and that, from a sleep physiological perspective, it is the quality of sleep in men that deteriorates most with ageing (Bliwise, 2000; Dijk, 2005; Redline et al., 2004). However, a representative survey of 1,158 people aged 65 years and over, conducted as part of the SomnIA (Sleep In Ageing) project, found higher rates of poor sleep among women than men using the PSQI: 58% of older women compared to 44% of men had a PSQI score of >5 signifying clinically poor sleep (SomnIA, 2009). Analysis of in-depth interviews (in the SomnIA project) is exploring the ways that subjective views of sleep among older people are related to their PSQI scores and how these differ by gender.

Caring for (older) relatives and sleep

Among older and disabled people, not only is their own sleep likely to be disrupted by ill-health, but also the sleep of their family members and caregivers. Caregiving for partners and older relatives can have a profound impact on the carers' sleep. Care at night may include helping an older person to use the toilet, cleaning an older person (and/or changing their bed) following incontinence, turning or repositioning, and medication administration. The care recipients' nighttime activities or behaviours, such as wandering or shouting at night, may also disturb the carers' sleep. Such nighttime disturbances may also engender stress and anxiety in the caregiver, further compromising their sleep quality.

Extensive research has shown that women are more likely than men to be caregivers (Arber and Ginn, 1991; Wolff and Kasper, 2006; Sims-Gould et al., 2008). Therefore nighttime care provision, which involves practical tending, emotional labour, and surveillance/monitoring at night, is more likely to affect women's sleep quality, continuity, and duration.

The relationship between 'caring' and sleep can be influenced by the nature and context of the caregiving role, including 'cultural' setting. In their study of sleep disruption among women over age 40 in Italy, Bianchera and Arber (2007) illustrate how, compared to the United Kingdom, 'care provided in Italy is more intense, first because of Italy's family oriented culture, and second because of gaps in the Italian welfare system, resulting in minimal state support for care delivery and an informal familiarized care model'. Thus, Italian women's sleep is particularly adversely affected by intensive care provision often over lengthy periods.

Bianchera and Arber (2007, 2008) describe how caregivers' sleep can be disrupted by having to deal with the nighttime physical needs of the care receiver, and the worries and anxieties connected to the role of carer. They also suggest that these negative impacts on sleep can continue long after the caregiving role has ended. This is partly because women get into the 'habit' of light sleep, listening out, and experiencing sudden awakenings, and because women continued to be 'haunted by distressing images of caring, especially during terminal phases, when their relative was undignified and vulnerable' (Bianchera and Arber, 2007). See also, albeit in a different context, the long-lasting impacts of domestic violence on family members' sleep, even when the perpetrator has long since left the family home or the family has relocated (Lowe et al., 2007).

Sleep in institutional contexts

Most sleep takes place in the privacy of an individual's home. However, some people sleep in institutional settings, whether hospitals, care homes or prisons. Here, their sleep is to a considerable extent under the control of others rather than themselves. Goffman (1961) suggested that in 'normal' adult life an individual 'sleeps, works, and plays' in different places, each with different sets of other social actors (Williams, 2005). In 'total institutions', these activities all tend to occur in the same setting, operating according to timetables laid down by the institution, rather than under the personal control of the individual.

Research has shown that nursing home residents have poor sleep quality (Ancoli-Israel et al., 1989; Fetviet and Bjorvatn, 2002). Care home residents frequently do not have control over the time they go to bed or are woken up in the mornings. The routines of the care home and timing of staff shifts take precedence in determining residents' sleep timing, especially for residents who are more physically disabled, for example, requiring a hoist to get them into and out of bed. Resident surveillance through routine checks, together with changing incontinence pads, and associated changes in lighting levels and noise of doors opening, often seriously disturb residents' sleep. In care homes, there is a tension between staff concerns for 'risk' and the routine surveillance this engenders, which conflicts with residents' privacy, autonomy, and control at night (Martin and Bartlett, 2007).

Thus in later life, having to be 'cared for', whether in one's own home or in a residential setting, can impact on sleep quality and duration. This is not just because of associations with poor health, but also because sleep is controlled by the routines and priorities of others. Since women are more likely than men to have disabilities that require care in later life, are more likely to be caregivers, and are more likely to be resident in care homes (Arber and Ginn, 1991), they are particularly vulnerable to sleep disruption and lack of control over their own sleep in the latter phases of their life.

Summary—gender, sleep, and the life course

This section has shown that sleep is influenced by numerous social factors across the life course, as well as by transitions, such as marriage/co-habitation, parenthood, caregiving, and widowhood. Sleep always takes place in a social context, whether a family or institutional context, and it is essential to consider how that context, and others in that context, impact on the quality of a person's sleep. This section has also discussed the importance of considering how gender impacts on sleep, and the nature of power in negotiations about sleep.

More work is required here, however. Much of the work on marriage and couples, for example, has focused solely on heterosexual couples. Without more complete comparisons, it remains difficult to separate 'gender' effects from more general 'co-sleeping' effects.

Sleep and worry

A theme running throughout the discussion above relates to how sleep is often linked to 'worry'. Sleep research and epidemiology has long been alert to the impact that worries can have on sleep. For example, our analysis of the UK *Psychiatric Morbidity Survey* shows that, until 65–69 years of age, 'worry/thinking' is the largest, single, self-reported cause of sleep loss (see Fig. 13.1), after which it is surpassed by 'illness/discomfort', which increases markedly with age as a cause of sleep loss.

However, we need to be mindful that worry/thinking can cover a range of differing factors. In a sociologically informed survey of 1,445 women over age 40, Arber et al. (2007b) examined the self-reported impact that seven different types of worry had on sleep (concerns about the future, family concerns, feelings of loneliness, money concerns, relationship concerns, safety concerns, and work concerns). The authors found that it was family concerns which had the largest impact on women's self-reported sleep quality.

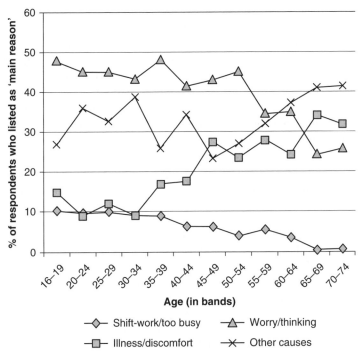

Fig. 13.1 Self-reported causes of poor sleep (by age band).
Authors' analysis: The question analyzed asked respondents to identify the main cause of their poor sleep. The question was asked only of those people who said that they 'had problems with sleeping in past month' and 'at least one night of sleep problems in the past week' and 'knows why they were having sleep problems'. 'Other causes' includes the following self-reported causes of poor sleep—noise, needing to go to the toilet, having to do something (e.g. look after baby), tired, medication, and other.
Source: UK *Psychiatric Morbidity Survey* (2000) (*n* = 2,400).

Further to this, worry as a cause of sleep disturbance may be experienced differentially by men and women. First, in relation to prevalence—our analysis of the UK *Psychiatric Morbidity Survey* (2000) shows how, despite worry/thinking being a dominant cause of poor sleep for both men and women, the figures for women are higher at all ages except for age 16–19. Second, in relation to type of worry, men may, for example, worry more about financial matters, while women may worry more about family concerns and caring for aged parents.

Worries are therefore an important source of sleep disturbance and are implicated in the gender difference in self-reported sleep problems (Arber et al., 2009). Women's sleep is particularly likely to be disturbed by worries associated with their role as mothers or wives, and their concern for the well-being of family members (Hislop and Arber, 2003a,b; Arber et al., 2007b). Previous sleep research has tended to view 'worries' as a mark of anxiety or psychological problems, but it may be more appropriate to see worries as embedded within gender roles and responsibilities, as well as influenced directly by the socioeconomic circumstances of an individual's everyday life.

Socioeconomic status (SES) and sleep

Socioeconomic status (SES) has relevance for individual's sleep throughout their life course, as well as influencing the nature and prevalence of worries, which as noted above are key sources of sleep disturbance. It has long been held that SES and health are strongly correlated. As Young (2004) suggests, the best known feature of the SES-health association is the fact that it takes the shape of a 'gradient'. In other words, 'it is not a problem of a threshold effect that separates the very poor [for example] from the rest of the distribution' (Young, 2004), rather there is a stepwise relationship of higher levels of health with, for example, each year of schooling or income increment. Other features of the SES-health association include social differentials in mortality rates for most diseases, 'life course effects' (education continues to predict self-reported health for older people), and 'impervious effects' (education and income continue to be predictors despite the inclusion of a wide range of possible determinants) (Young, 2004).

It has recently been acknowledged that SES affects sleep duration, sleep quality, and acceptance of sleep-related treatments. Research has, for example, illustrated how lower educational qualifications, unemployment, and low income are all independently associated with poorer quality sleep (Hartz et al., 2007; Arber et al., 2009). Research has also shown that low SES patients are less receptive to CPAP treatment (Simon-Tuval et al., 2009).

The linear associations between reported sleep problems and educational qualifications and household income are illustrated in Table 13.1 (from Arber et al., 2009, based on analysis of the UK *Psychiatric Morbidity Survey*, 2000). A quarter of women with no qualifications report sleep problems on 4 or more nights a week compared with only 15% of women with a degree (Table 13.1a). At each educational level, more women report sleep problems than men. Following

Table 13.1 Reported sleep problems on four or more nights per week by (a) highest educational qualifications and (b) household income (age 16–74)

	% reporting sleep problems on four or more nights per week		Odds Ratio (OR) of reporting sleep problems on four or more nights per week	
	Men	**Women**	**Age and sex adjusted[a]**	**Fully adjusted[b]**
(a) Educational qualifications				
No qualifications	18.7	25.1	1.97**	1.31*
Lower qualifications	15.2	17.9	1.45**	1.31*
Professional/A levels	10.7	17.2	1.21	1.17
Degree	9.4	14.7	1.00	1.00
(b) Household income per week[c]				
Under £150	24.9	25.7	2.94**	1.12
£150 < £300	16.7	19.8	1.91**	0.95
£300 < £500	11.2	18.2	1.49*	1.09
£500 < £750	10.0	16.8	1.31*	1.19
≥£750	9.2	11.9	1.00	1.00
All	14.2	19.7		
N =	3851	4727	8240	8240

[a]Adjusted for sex and age (in 10-year age groups).

[b]Adjusted for sex, age (in 10-year age groups), marital status, number of children, other socioeconomic variables (educational qualifications, household income, housing tenure, employment status), smoking, worries, self-assessed health, number of chronic illnesses, health worries, and depression.

[c]Household income per week is the sum of personal gross income from all sources for each household member, equivalized by household composition using the McClements Scale.

*$P < .05$, **$P < .01$ (difference from reference category).

Source: From Arber et al. (2009), analysis of the UK *Psychiatric Morbidity Survey* (2000).

adjustment for age and gender, the odds ratio (OR) of sleep problems for those with no qualifications is twice as high as for those with a degree. An OR of 1.31 remains for those with no qualifications following adjustment with a full range of potential mediators (marital status, children, other socioeconomic variables, smoking, worries, physical and psychological health variables). Table 13.1b shows a strong linear relationship between household income (equivalized for household composition) and self-reported sleep problems, but here the income-sleep relationship is fully mediated by other intervening variables.

Sociological work has sought to *explore* the SES-sleep relationship. For example, Arber et al. (2009) examined whether SES relationships with sleep quality are confounded by poor health among those with lower SES. They found that the association between sleep problems and both household income and housing tenure is fully mediated by differences in other SES characteristics, smoking, worries, health, and depression. However, the unemployed, economically inactive, and those with low educational qualifications report significantly greater sleep problems even after adjusting for the full range of other potential mediators.

There is a strong gender difference in self-reported sleep problems, which Arber et al. (2009) found was halved after adjustment for socioeconomic characteristics (education, income, employment status, and housing), indicating that a major reason for women's greater reported sleep problems related to their more disadvantaged socioeconomic circumstances. These findings support Sekine et al.'s (2006) Japanese research and cast doubt on the sole importance of a physiological basis for the gender difference in reported sleep quality, while supporting our earlier discussion which emphasizes the differential social roles and socioeconomic characteristics of men and women.

Hitherto there has been little attempt to *understand* the SES-sleep relationship. Biomedical explanations of the SES-health relationship tend to suggest that education, income, etc. operate through proximate determinants (Young, 2004), arguing that an organism is endowed with defences, but that these resistances can be enhanced by social determinants. In contrast, sociological explanations of the SES-health association tend to discuss 'structural' models, for example, Young (2004) proposes that greater 'years of schooling' result in superior 'problem-solving' capacity, which in turn moderates behaviours, resulting in improved health.

Applying sociological thinking specifically to the SES-sleep association, Arber et al. (2009) propose several types of mechanisms which may underlie associations between socioeconomic variables and reported sleep problems:

i. *Structural disadvantage.* Living in disadvantaged material circumstances has direct adverse effects on sleep quality—in crowded households, family members may disturb each other's sleep; smaller, poorer quality housing leads to greater likelihood of nighttime noise disturbance from neighbours; disadvantaged neighbourhoods have greater problems of nighttime noise, crime, anti-social behaviour, safety, and security.

ii. *Psychological distress associated with structural disadvantage.* Low SES—for example, unemployment, poor housing, disadvantaged neighbourhoods, poverty—are all likely to increase worries, anxieties, and psychological distress, which in turn impact on sleep quality.

iii. *Education and knowledge of sleep promoting strategies.* More education may be associated with greater knowledge about sleep hygiene practices and awareness of strategies to improve sleep.

iv. *Lifestyle—individual behaviours.* Low SES is linked to lifestyle behaviours (smoking, alcohol consumption, poor diet, less exercise), which may in turn adversely affect sleep quality. However, Lallukka et al. (2010) and Arber et al. (2009) found no evidence that lifestyle behaviours mediated the association between SES and sleep complaints.

Given the significance for public health of the relationship between low SES and ill-health/mortality, and increasing evidence of the link between sleep and health/well-being, we suggest that further research is needed to assess to what extent disrupted sleep (or sleep duration) may be one potential mechanism through which social class is causally related to health inequalities.

Conclusion

A sociological approach to sleep, as this chapter clearly attests, sheds valuable new light on how sleep and society are related, with important implications for current and future research, policy and practice in epidemiology, and public health. A number of conclusions may be drawn here in this respect.

First, sleep as we have seen occurs in a social context, whether public or private, and is socially, culturally, and historically variable. To the extent, moreover, that sleeping together is the norm, in adult life at least if not childhood, this suggests the need for a dyadic rather than monadic focus on couples' sleep and relations between sleeping partners, particularly with respect to sleep loss and sleep disruption. To the extent, furthermore, that subjective perceptions and definitions of sleep need and sleep loss are related to socially variable norms and values, then relations between the sociological and biological dimensions of sleep need and sleep loss are likely to be multiple, complex, and variable.

A second conclusion therefore concerns the need for both qualitative and quantitative methodologies in order to capture these complexities and access these issues in the context of people's everyday/night lives outside the sleep laboratory or the sleep clinic. This, as we have seen, includes the use of qualitative interviews and audio-sleep diaries, as well as other more standardized measures, such as the PSQI and watch actigraphy.

Third, at the empirical level, recent sociological research has clearly shown that sleep is influenced by numerous social factors across the life course, as well as by transitions, such as marriage/co-habitation, parenthood, caregiving, and widowhood. This, moreover, includes the importance of considering how gender impacts on sleep, and the nature of power in negotiations about sleep. Sociological work is also now occurring on the SES-sleep association, including several proposed mechanisms which may underlie associations between socioeconomic variables and reported sleep problems, namely: (i) structural disadvantage; (ii) psychological distress associated with structural disadvantage; (iii) education and knowledge of sleep promoting strategies; and (iv) lifestyle—individual behaviours.

This in turn suggests two further conclusions regarding current and future public health research, policy, and practice. First, while caution is undoubtedly needed, as we have suggested, regarding general claims (amplified by the media) that society is 'chronically sleep deprived', or that sleep deprivation has reached 'epidemic' proportions today, and while public awareness campaigns or sleep alerts may themselves fuel or inflate public anxieties about sleep loss, poor sleep (particularly prolonged sleep loss) clearly has important implications for both individuals and society in terms of health, well-being, safety, productivity, and performance. Sleep, therefore, is a critical issue for public health and public policy, which demands far greater attention than it has hitherto received. Second, given the significance for public health of the low SES-morbidity/mortality relationship, and growing evidence of the link between sleep and health/well-being, further research is clearly needed to assess whether disrupted sleep (or sleep duration) may be one potential mechanism through which social class is causally related to health inequalities.

Sleep then, to conclude, is an important yet all too often neglected dimension of sociological study. Sociology, in this respect, in conjunction with public health, has an important role to play in putting sleep on the public and policy agenda. To the extent that sleep constitutes a crucial yet hidden dimension of social and health inequalities, then this redoubles the need to take sleep seriously as a matter of public concern.

Summary box

♦ Sleep occurs in a *social context* and is socially, culturally, and historically variable.

♦ Researching sleep in the context of people's everyday lives requires the use of *qualitative* as well as *quantitative* methodologies, including interviews, focus groups, and sleep diaries as well as other more standardized or objective measures such as watch actigraphy. A *relational* or *dyadic* focus on *couples' sleep* is also called for given that sleeping together is the norm in adult life.

♦ Sleep is influenced by numerous social factors across the *life course*, as well as by *transitions*, such as marriage/co-habitation, parenthood, caregiving, and widowhood. This includes the importance of how *gender* and *socioeconomic inequalities* impact on sleep, and the nature of *power in negotiations* about sleep.

♦ Relations between the sociological and (neuro)biological dimensions of sleep are complex and variable and, as such, sleep research needs to be based on well-thought through methodologies. The diverse or multiple meanings people bring to bear regarding sleep, suggests that epidemiological research, especially which uses survey methods, should prioritize the use of multiple indicators for the same construct.

♦ Although caution is needed (on conceptual, methodological, and empirical grounds) regarding claims that society is chronically sleep deprived, and while public awareness/sleep alertness campaigns may fuel sleep anxieties, sleep (loss) is a *critical public health and safety issue* which demands far greater attention in terms of policy and practice.

References

American Sleep Disorders Association (2005). *International Classification of Sleep Disorders: Diagnostic Classification Steering Committee*. Wetscheter, IL: American Academy of Sleep Medicine.

Ancoli-Israel, S., Parker, L., Sinaee, R., Fell, R.L. & Kripke, D.F. (1989). Sleep fragmentation in patients from a nursing home. *J Gerontol*, 44, M18–M21.

Anthony, W.A. (1997). *The Art of the Napping*. New York, NY: Larson Publications.

Anthony, C. & Anthony W.C. (2001). *The Art of Napping at Work*. London: Souvenir Press.

Arber, S. & Ginn, J. (1991). *Gender and Later Life*. London: Sage.

Arber, S., Davidson, K. & Ginn, J. (2003). Changing approaches to gender and later life. In: Arber, S., Davidson, K. & Ginn, J. (eds.), *Gender and Ageing: Changing Roles and Relationships*. Maidenhead: Open University Press, pp. 1–14.

Arber, S., Hislop, J. & Williams, S. (2007a). Editor's introduction: gender, sleep and the life course. *Soc Res Online*, 12(5). Available at: http://www.socresonline.org.uk/12/5/19.html (accessed 28 September, 2009).

Arber, S., Hislop, J., Bote, M. & Meadows, R. (2007b). Gender roles and women's sleep in mid and later life: a quantitative approach. *Soc Res Online*, 12(5). Available at: http://www.socresonline.org.uk/12/5/3.html. (accessed 28 September 2009)

Arber, S., Bote, M. & Meadows, R. (2009). Gender and social-economic patterning of self-reported sleep problems in Britain. *Soc Sci Med*, 68, 281–289.

Baxter, V. & Kroll-Smith, S. (2005). Napping at work: shifting boundaries between public and private time. *Curr Sociol*, 53(1), 33–55.

Becker S., Bentolila, S., Fernandes, A. & Ichino, A. (2004). Job insecurity and children emancipation: the Italian puzzle. CESinfo working paper no. 1144, category 4: Labour Markets.

Ben-Ari, E. (2008). It's bedtime in the world's urban middle classes, around the world. In: Brunt, L. & Steger, B. (eds.), *Worlds of Sleep*. Berlin: Frank & Timme, pp. 175–192.

Bianchera, E. & Arber, S. (2007). Caring and sleep disruption among women in Italy. *Soc Res Online*, **12**(5). Available at: http://www.socresonline.org.uk/12/5/4.html. (accessed 28 September 2009)

Bianchera, E. & Arber, S. (2008). Women's sleep in Italy: the influence of caregiving roles. In: Brunt, L. & Steger, B. (eds.), *Worlds of Sleep*. Berlin: Frank & Timme, pp. 131–151.

Bliwise, D.L. (2000). Normal aging. In: Kryger, M.H., Roth, T. & Dement, W.C. (eds.), *Principles and Practice of Sleep Medicine*. Third edition. Philadelphia, PA: Elsevier Saunders.

Bliwise, D.L. (2005). Normal aging. In: Kryger, M.H., Roth, T. & Dement, W.C. (eds.), *Principles and Practice of Sleep Medicine*. Fourth edition. Philadelphia, PA: Elsevier Saunders, pp. 24–38.

British Association of Counselling and Psychotherapy (2005). *Insomniac Britain*. Available at: http://www. bacp.co.uk/media/index.php?newsId=300 (accessed March 12, 2009).

Brown, M. (2004). Taking care of business: self-help and sleep medicine in American corporate culture. *J Med Humanit*, **25**(3), 173–187.

Brunt, L. (2008). Sote hug log: in and out of sleep in India. In: Brunt, L. & Steger, B. (eds.), *Worlds of Sleep*. Berlin: Frank & Timee, pp. 153–174.

Brunt, L. & Steger, B. (2008). Introduction. In: Brunt, L. & Steger, B. (eds.), *Worlds of Sleep*. Berlin: Frank & Timee, pp. 9–30.

Buysse, D.J., Reynolds, C.F., Monk, T.H., Buman, S.R. & Kupfer, D.J. (1989). Pittsburgh Sleep Quality Index: a new instrument for psychiatric practice and research. *Psychiatry Res*, **28**,193–213.

Carskadon, M.A. & Dement, W.C. (1977). Sleep tendency: an objective measure of sleep loss. *Sleep Res*, **6**, 200.

Cartwright, R. (2008). Sleeping together: a pilot study of the effects of shared sleeping on adherence to CPAP treatment in obstructive sleep apnea. *J Clin Sleep Med*, **4**, 123–127.

Chatzitheochari, S. & Arber, S. (2009). Lack of sleep, work and the long hours culture: evidence from the UK Time Use Survey. *Work Employ Soc*, **23**, 30–48.

Coren, S. (1996). *Sleep Thieves*. New York, NY: The Free Press.

Cox, R.S. (2008). The suburbs of eternity: on visionaries and miraculous sleepers. In: Brunt, L. & Steger, B. (eds.), *Worlds of Sleep*. Berlin: Frank & Timee, pp. 53–74.

Crossley, N. (2004). *Sleep, Reflexive Embodiment and Social Networks*. Paper presented at the first ESRC 'Sleep and Society' seminar, 3 December, University of Warwick.

Davidson, J.R., MacLean, A.W., Brundage, M.D. & Schulze, K. (2002). Sleep disturbance in cancer patients. *Soc Sci Med*, **54**, 1309–1321.

Davis, B., Moore, B. & Bruck, D. (2007). The meanings of sleep: stories from older women in care. *Soc Res Online*, **12**(5). Available at: http://www.socresonline.org.uk/12/5/7.html. (accessed 28 September 2009)

Dement, W.C. (with Vaughan, C.) (2000). *The Promise of Sleep*. London: Macmillan.

Dijk, D.J. (2005). Sleep of ageing women and men: back to basics. *Sleep*, **29**,12–13.

Ekirch, R. (2005). *A Day's Close; Night in Times Past*. New York, NY: W.W. Norton.

Fetviet, A. & Bjorvatn, B. (2002). Sleep disturbance among nursing home residents. *Int J Geriatr Psychiatry*, **17**, 604–609.

Furedi, F. (2002). *Paranoid Parenting: Why Ignoring the Experts May Be Best for Your Child*. Chicago, IL: Chicago Review Press, Inc.

Gleick, J. (2000). *Faster: The Acceleration of Just About Everything*. London: Abacus.

Goffman, E. (1961). *Asylums: Essays on the Social Situation of Mental Patients and Other Inmates*. Harmondsworth: Penguin.

Hartz, A.J., Daly, J.M., Kohatsu, N.D., Stromquist, A.M., Jogerst, G.J. & Kukoyi, O.A. (2007). Risk factors for insomnia in a rural population. *Ann Epidemiol*, **17**, 940–947.

Henry, D., McClellen, D., Rosenthal, L., Dedrick, D. & Gosdin, M. (2008). Is sleep really for sissies? Understanding the role of work in insomnia in the US. *Soc Sci Med*, **66**, 715–726.

Hislop, J. (2007). A bed of roses or a bed of thorns? Negotiating the couple relationship through sleep. *Soc Res Online*, **12**(5). Available at: http://www.socresonline.org.uk/12/5/2.html. (accessed 28 September 2009)

Hislop, J. & Arber, S. (2003a). Sleepers Wake! The gendered nature of sleep disruption among mid-life women. *Sociology*, **37**, 695–711.

Hislop, J. & Arber, S. (2003b). Understanding women's sleep management: beyond medicalization-healthicization? *Sociol Health Illn*, **26**, 815–837.

Hislop, J. & Arber, S. (2006). Sleep, gender and aging. In: Calsanti, T.M. & Slevin, K.L. (eds.), *Age Matters: Realigning Feminist Thinking*. New York, NY: Routledge, pp. 225–246.

Hislop, J., Arber, S., Meadows, R., & Venn, S. (2005). Narratives of the night: the use of audio diaries in sleep research. *Soc Res Online*, **10**, 4.

Horne, J. (2006). *Sleepfaring*. Oxford: Oxford University Press.

Johns, M.W. (1991). A new method for measuring daytime sleepiness: the Epworth sleepiness scale. *Sleep*, **14**, 540–545.

Kaji, M., Shigeta, M. & Takada, Y. (2007). Knickknacks for sleeping (nemuri-komono) in contemporary Japan. Paper presented at workshop at University of Vienna, June 2007. *New Directions in the Social and Cultural Study of Sleep*. Vienna: Austria.

Klerman, E.B. & Dijk, D.-J. (2008). Age-related reduction in the maximal capacity for sleep—implications for insomnia. *Curr Biol*, **18**, 1118–1123.

Klug, G. (2008). Dangerous doze: sleep and vulnerability in medieval German literature. In: Brunt, L. & Steger, B. (eds.), *Worlds of Sleep*. Berlin: Frank & Timee, pp. 31–52.

Kroll-Smith, S. (2003). Popular media and 'excessive daytime sleepiness': a study of rhetorical authority in medical sociology. *Soc Health Illn*, **25**(6), 625–643.

Kroker, K. (2007). *The Sleep of Others*. Toronto: University of Toronto Press.

Lallukka, T., Rahkonen, O., Lahelma, E. & Arber, S. (2010). Sleep complaints in middle-aged women and men: the contribution of working conditions and work-family conflicts. *J Sleep Res*, **19**, (online).

Leadbeater, C. (2004). *Dream On—Sleep in the 24/7 Society*. London: Demos.

Lowe, P., Humphreys, C. & Williams, S.J. (2007). Night terrors: women's experiences of (not) sleeping where there is domestic violence. *Violence Against Women*, **13**(6), 549–561.

Martin, E. (1987). *The Woman in the Body*. Milton Keynes: Open University Press.

Martin, P. (2002). *Counting Sheep: The Science and Pleasures of Sleep and Dreams*. London: HarperCollins.

Martin, W. & Bartlett, H. (2007). The social significance of sleep for older people with dementia in the context of care. *Soc Res Online*, **12**(5). Available at: http://www.socresonline.org.uk/12/5/11.html. (accessed 28 September 2009)

Meadows, R. (2005). The 'negotiated night': an embodied conceptual framework for the sociological study of sleep. *Sociol Rev*, **53**, 240–254.

Meadows, R., Venn, S., Hislop, J., Stanley, N. & Arber, S. (2005). Investigating couples' sleep: an evaluation of actigraphic analysis techniques. *J Sleep Res*, **14**, 377–386.

Meadows, R., Arber, S., Venn, S. & Hislop, J. (2008a). Engaging with sleep: male definitions, understandings and attitudes. *Soc Health Illn*, **30**, 696–710.

Meadows, R., Arber, S., Venn, S. & Hislop, J. (2008b). Unruly bodies and couples' sleep. *Body Society*, **14**, 75–92.

Meadows, R., Arber, S., Venn, S., Hislop, J. & Stanley, N. (2009). Exploring the interdependence of couples' rest-wake cycles: an actigraphic study. *Chronobiol Int*, **26**, 80–92.

Mitler, M.M., Dement, W.C. & Dinges, D.F. (2000). Sleep medicine, public policy and public health. In: Kruger, M.H., Roth, T. & Dement, W.C. (eds.), *Principles and Practices of Sleep Medicine*. Third edition. Philadelphia, PA: W.B. Saunders.

Monroe, L.J. (1969). Transient changes in EEG sleep patterns of married good sleepers: the effects of altering sleeping arrangement. *Psychophysiology*, **6**, 330–337.

Moore-Ede, M. (1993). *The 24/7 Society*. London: Piatkus.

Moran-Ellis, J. & Venn, S. (2007). The sleeping lives of children and teenagers: night-worlds and arenas of action, *Soc Res Online*, **12**(5). Available at: http://www.socresonline.org.uk/12/5/9. (accessed 28 September 2009)

Münch, M., Cajochen, C. & Wirz-Justice, A. (2005). Sleep and circadian rhythms in ageing. *Zeitschrift für Gerontologie und Geriatrie*, **38**(Suppl 1), 121–123.

National Commission on Sleep Disorders Research (1993). *Wake Up America: A National Sleep Alert. V1: Executive Summary and Executive Report of the NCSDR*. Washington, DC: NCSDR.

Norbutt, M. (2004). Waking up to sleep clinics. *American Medical Association News*, 5th January. Available at: www.ama-assn.org/amednews/2004/01/05/bisa015.html. (accessed 28 September 2009)

Pankhurst, F.P. & Horne, J.A. (1994). The influence of bed partners on movement during sleep. *Sleep*, **17**, 308–315.

Redline, S., Kirchner, H.L., Quan, S.F., Gottlieb, D.J., Kapur, V. & Newman, A. (2004). The effects of age, sex, ethnicity, and sleep-disordered breathing on sleep architecture. *Arch Intern Med*, **164**, 406–418.

Rosenblatt, P.C. (2006). *Two in a Bed: The Social System of Couple Bed Sharing*. Albany, NY: State University of New York Press.

Seale, C. (2004). *Media and Health*. London: Sage.

Seale, C., Boden, S., Williams, S.J., Lowe, P. & Steinberg, D.L. (2007). Media constructions of sleep and sleep disorders: a study of UK national newspapers. *Soc Sci Med*, **65**, 418–430.

Schwartz, B. (1970). Notes on the sociology of sleep. *Sociol Q*, **11**, 485–499.

Sekine, M., Chandola, T., Martikainen, P., Marmot, M. & Kagamimori, S. (2006). Work and family characteristics as determinants of socioeconomic and gender inequalities in sleep: the Japanese Civil Servants Study. *Sleep*, **29**, 206–216.

Simon-Tuval, T., Reuveni, H., Greenberg Dotan, S., Oksenberg, A., Tal, A. & Tarasiuki, A. (2009). Low socioeconomic status is a risk factor for CPAP acceptance among adult OSAS patients requiring treatment, *Sleep*, **32**, 545–552.

Sims-Gould, J., Martin-Matthews, A. & Rosenthal, C.J. (2008). Family caregiving and helping at the intersection of gender and kinship. In: Martin-Matthews, A. & Phillips, J.E. (eds.), *Ageing and Caring at the Intersection of Work and Home Life*. New York, NY: Lawrence Erlbaum Associates, pp. 65–83.

SomnIA (2009). Poor sleep among community dwelling older people. Workpackage 2, *SomnIA Briefing Paper 2*. Centre for Research on Ageing and Gender (CRAG), University of Surrey.

Steger, B. (2003a). Negotiating sleep patterns in Japan. In: Steger, B. & Brunt, L. (eds.), *Night-time in Asia and the West: Exploring the Dark Side of Life*. London: Routledge Curzon.

Steger, B. (2003b). Getting away with sleep—social and cultural aspects of dozing in parliament. *Soc Sci Jpn J*, **6**, 181–197.

Steger, B. & Brunt, L. (2003). Introduction: into the night and the world of sleep. In: Steger, B. & Brunt, L. (eds.), *Night-time and Sleep in Asia and the West: Exploring the Dark Side of Life*. London: Routledge Curzon, pp. 1–23.

Stewart, R., Besset, A., Bebbington, R., et al. (2006). Insomnia comorbidity and impact and hypnotic use by age group in a national survey population aged 16 to 74. *Sleep*, **29**, 1391–1397.

Strawbridge, W.J., Shema, S.J. & Roberts, R.E. (2004). Impact of spouses sleep problems on partners. *Sleep*, **27**, 527–531.

Summers-Bremner, E. (2008). *Insomnia: A Cultural History*. London: Reaktion Books.

Van den Bulck, J. (2004). Television viewing, computer game playing and Internet use and self-reported time to bed and time out of bed in secondary-school children. *Sleep*, **27**, 101–104.

Vaughan, V., Meadows, R., Archer, S., Skene, S.N. & Arber, S. (2006). Diurnal preference in couples: negotiating sleep timing. *J Sleep Res*, **15**(Suppl 1), 95.

Venn, S. (2007). It's okay for a man to snore: the influence of gender on sleep disruption in couples. *Soc Res Online*, **12**(5). Retrieved December 12, 2008 from http://www.socresonline.org.uk/12/5/1.html.

Venn, S. & Arber, S. (2008). Conflicting sleep demands: parents and young people in UK households. In: Steger, B. & Brunt, L. (eds.), *Worlds of Sleep*. Berlin: Frank & Timme, pp. 105–129.

Venn, S., Arber, S., Meadows, R. & Hislop, J. (2008). The fourth shift: exploring the gendered nature of sleep disruption in couples with children. *Br J Sociol*, **59**, 79–97.

Vitiello, M.V., Moe, K.E. & Prinz, P.N. (2002). Sleep complaints cosegregate with illness in older adults. Clinical research informed by and informing epidemiological studies of sleep. *J Psychosom Res*, **53**, 555–559.

Wainwright, D. & Calnan, M. (2002). *Work Stress*. Buckingham: Open University Press.

Weisgerber, C. (2004). Turning to the internet for help on sensitive medical problems: a qualitative study of the construction of a sleep disorder through online interaction. *Inform Commun & Soc*, **7**(4), 554–574.

Widerberg, K. (2006). Embodying modern times: investigating tiredness. *Time Soc*, **15**(1), 105–120.

Wiggs, L. (2007). Are children getting enough sleep? Implications for parents. *Soc Res Online*, **12**(5). Retrieved December 9, 2008 from http://www.socresonline.org.uk/12/5/13.html.

Williams, S.J. (2005). *Sleep and Society: Sociological Ventures into the (Un)known*. Abingdon: Routledge.

Williams, S.J. (2008). The sociological aspects of sleep; progress, problems, prospects. *Sociology Compass*, **2**(2), 639–653.

Williams, S., Lowe, P. & Griffiths, F. (2007). Embodying and embedding children's sleep: some sociological comments and observations. *Soc Res Online*, **12**(5). Available at: http://www.socresonline.org.uk/12/5/6.html. (accessed 28 September 2009)

Williams, S.J., Seale, C., Boden, S., Lowe, P., & Steinberg, D.L. (2008). Medicalisation and beyond: The social construction of insomnia and snoring in the news. *Health*, **12**(2), 251–268.

Wolff, J.L. & Kasper, J.D. (2006). Caregivers of frail elderly: updating a national profile. *Gerontologist*, **46**, 344–356.

Woloshin, S. & Schwartz, L.M. (2006). Giving legs to restless legs: a case study of how the media help make people sick. *PLoS Med*, **3**(4), 170–178.

Young, F.W. (2004). Socioeconomic status and health: the problem of explanation and a sociological solution. *Soc Theory Health*, **2**, 123–141.

Chapter 14

Misdiagnosis of sleep disorders in adults and children: implications for clinical practice and epidemiology

G. Stores

Preamble: misdiagnosis is a common problem

The rate of 'non-trivial' diagnostic error in developed countries could be as high as 15% (Graber and Berner, 2008). In a 2009 Sunday Times article, headed 'One in six patients "given wrong diagnosis"', a similar figure (and possibly higher) was quoted for the United Kingdom, based on the opinion of British researchers at the Imperial Centre for Patient Safety and Service Quality (MacDonald, 2009). The most common misdiagnosed illnesses include epilepsy, ovarian cancer, meningitis, dementia, and osteoporosis.

The American Journal of Medicine statement was part of a Supplement which contained a collection of articles and commentaries concerned with the possible reasons why such errors come about, as well as strategies for overcoming the problem (Graber and Berner, 2008). If this error rate occurs in such conditions as those mentioned, about which teaching is traditionally well provided, how much more common are errors likely to be concerning sleep disorders in view of their striking neglect in medical education and training? (see also Chapter 19).

This present chapter is concerned with the risk of diagnostic error in the sleep disorders field. Few statistics are available on this point, only conjectures—but then the same largely applies in the more conventional medical specialties. As another commentator has stated, 'There is no comprehensive system for ensuring we collect information about problems with diagnosis. In any part of the UK, there is no legal requirement to report incidents that affect patients, be it misdiagnosis or any other mistake, error or omission. We want action, misdiagnosis must be tackled' (Walsh, 2009). These comments are just some of the flurry of recent concerns expressed in the United Kingdom and also in the United States (Wachter and Holmboe, 2009).

Basic issues

Before examples are given of possible misdiagnoses of sleep disorders, the following relevant general points will be discussed in this section:

- Sleep disturbance is extremely common, especially in some sections of the population.
- The importance of sleep and the various adverse effects of sleep disturbance demonstrates that sleep disorders can be at least as important for health and well-being as other types of clinical disorders.
- Sleep disorders are not of marginal relevance to clinical practice in general. In view of their high prevalence, either as the main symptom or as a complication of other illnesses, they can

be considered to be of basic importance in primary care and in hospital and community medicine.

♦ In addition to the general clinical importance of sleep disorders they have serious implications for the national economy, including the cost of providing clinical services to which diagnostic error makes a significant contribution.

♦ Generalizations about 'disturbed' sleep are rarely justified. Assessment of the risk of diagnostic error (as well as the provision of appropriate advice and treatment) have to be based on an accurate account of specific sleep disorders of which many types are now officially described.

♦ A major reason for diagnostic error is the almost universal neglect of sleep and its disorders in public health education and the teaching and training of health professionals.

♦ A further source of diagnostic error, even on the part of those familiar with adult sleep disorders, can be failure to appreciate that children's sleep disorders are different from those in adults including their manifestations. In some instances, the clinical features of the same type of disorder are very different. Examples include the increase of activity and other attention deficit hyperactivity disorder (ADHD) behaviours in sleep-deprived children in contrast to reduced activity in sleepy adults, the fact that only the minority of children with obstructive sleep apnoea (OSA) are overweight and snore loudly, and the many manifestations of childhood narcolepsy may be far removed from the classical narcolepsy syndrome in adults (Stores, 2006).

Sleep disturbance is widespread

Surveys, such as the National Sleep Foundation 'Sleep in America' polls carried out in recent years (<<www.sleepfoundation.org>>) indicate very high rates of sleep disturbance in both adults and children—an overall prevalence rate of about 30% possibly being an underestimation with much higher rates in certain subgroups.

More than 50% of elderly people complain of not sleeping well, the reasons being a combination of medical and psychological problems in later life (Phillips and Ancoli-Israel, 2001). Particularly high rates are reported in people with psychiatric conditions (Abad and Guilleminault, 2005), chronic physical illness (Chokroverty, 2000), or learning disability (Didden and Sigafoos, 2001). Reliable epidemiological information about specific sleep disorders is limited by diagnostic inaccuracy (Partinen and Hublin, 2005), perhaps (as discussed later) especially in cases of excessive sleepiness and the parasomnias. Epidemiological aspects are considered in more detail in Chapters 1, 3–5, and 8.

Sleep is important in many ways

Examination of the entries for sleep in, for example, the Oxford Dictionary of Quotations (Knowles, 2003) demonstrates the enduring fascination with sleep, sometimes concerning its importance; at other times concern (even dread) about being deprived of it. Both aspects are dramatically conveyed by Lady Macbeth following her husband's murder of the king, Duncan:

> *Methought I heard a voice cry, 'Sleep no more!*
> *Macbeth does murder sleep', the innocent sleep,*
> *Sleep that knits up the ravell'd sleave of care,*
> *The death of each day's life, sore labour's bath,*
> *Balm of hurt minds, great nature's second course,*
> *Chief nourisher in life's feast.*

W. Shakespeare, *Macbeth*, Act 2, Scene 2

A less dramatic expression of the importance of sleep, this time for children, is provided by the sixteenth century physician, Thomas Phaire, in the first textbook of paediatrics published in English (The Boke of Chyldren):

> Slepe is the nourishment & foode of a sucking child,
> and asmuch requisite as ye very teate, wherefore wha
> It is depruiued of the naturall rest, all the hole body
> falleth in distemper: cruditie and weakenes, it procedeth
> commonly by corrupcion of the mylke, or to muche
> aboundance, whiche ouerladeth the stomacke, and for
> lacke of good digestion, vapours and fumes aryse into
> the head, and infect the braine, by reason wherof the
> child can not slepe, but turneth & vexeth it self w^t crying.

Thomas Phaire, 1545

Since the relatively recent scientific approach to sleep and its disorders, mainly extending over only the last several decades (Thorpy, 2000; Shepard et al., 2005), much has been discovered about the nature of sleep and the many ways in which it can be disturbed, as well as the consequences, prevention, and treatment of such disturbance (Kryger et al., 2005; Stores, 2001a).

On the basis of such observations, the functions of sleep have become clearer, although the details and underlying mechanisms often remain a matter of conjecture. Various theories have emphasized different possibilities: physical and psychological restoration and recovery, energy conservation, memory consolidation, discharge of emotions, brain growth, and various other basic biological functions including somatic growth and repair, as well as immune systems (see also Chapters 2 and 11).

No one theory accounts for all the complexities of sleep and it seems likely that sleep serves multiple purposes with some variation according to species. Function also seems to vary with type of sleep (Siegel, 2005), non-rapid eye movement (NREM) sleep being mainly important for energy conservation and central nervous system (CNS) recuperation. The role of rapid eye movement (REM) sleep is less clearly defined although memory and learning processes seem to be implicated especially in very early development when this type of sleep is particularly prominent.

The continuing debate about the relative importance of these various functions apart, it is clear that sleep is essential not only for psychological and physical well-being but even for survival: sleep deprivation in rodents can cause death more quickly than food deprivation (Rechtschaffen, 1998). The fundamental importance of sleep is also evident from the fact that adult humans spend about a third of their lives asleep—and children, especially infants, much more than that.

The complexity of the brain processes and mechanisms adds further weight to the belief that sleep is intrinsically important in many ways. Sleep is not simply the suspension of daytime processes as once thought; onset of sleep and waking, as well as switching from NREM to REM sleep repeatedly, involves complicated biochemical processes and activation of complex pathways in various parts of the brain.

At the psychological level, as discussed next, the wide-ranging consequences of sleep loss or disruption further illustrates the importance of sleep: the adverse effects on mood, behaviour, and cognitive function can be substantial, with consequences for personal, social, occupational, educational, and family functioning. It is for these reasons that failure to recognize and treat sleep disorders (the point of emphasis in this chapter) is so important.

Sleep disturbance has many adverse consequences

Review of these effects is appropriate as a background to discussion of the consequences of mistaking sleep disorders for other conditions such that the sleep disturbance persists.

Psychological effects of sleep disturbance

Clinical and experimental evidence has consistently shown that sustained sleep disturbance in the form of loss of sleep, poor quality sleep (i.e. disruption or 'fragmentation' of sleep architecture, or inappropriate timing of the sleep period in relation to day-night rhythms) can have serious adverse psychological effects (Bonnet, 2005; Dinges et al., 2005).

Experimental studies of *total sleep loss* demonstrate a progressive deterioration in cognitive function, mood, and behaviour related to length of sleep loss. However, inter- and also intra-individual differences in susceptibility are seen, reflecting such factors as motivation, personality, and usual sleep requirements. Task characteristics (e.g. brief or prolonged and monotonous tasks), timing of the task in relation to the circadian sleep-wake rhythm, and physical environmental factors such as noise and other distracting stimuli, are also important.

For similar reasons, individual differences are observed in *partial sleep deprivation* (much closer to real-life sleep disturbance) caused by social activities, job demands, and other aspects of modern lifestyle. These studies raise the issues of how much sleep is needed for optimal daytime functioning and whether these requirements are not being met. It has been argued that there is 'national sleep debt' in the United States and other western countries, and that by sleeping longer than they do habitually, many people would increase their performance and improve their well-being during the day.

Irritability, fatigue, poor concentration, and depression are usual subjective effects of sleep disturbance. More dramatic effects are described with prolonged and severe sleep disturbance, such as disorientation, illusions, hallucinations, persecutory ideas, and inappropriate behaviour with impaired awareness ('automatic behaviour'). Psychometric studies have shown that sleep disturbance can produce a range of cognitive impairments, again depending on its duration and individual susceptibility. Sustained attention (vigilance) is particularly vulnerable and possibly abstract thinking and creativity.

These experimental findings are in keeping with the results of studies of various occupational groups including medical staff (Philibert, 2005), night shift-workers—who commonly suffer both sleep deprivation and poor quality sleep (Åkerstedt, 2003) (see also Chapters 15–18),—and drivers of various types of vehicle. In these and other groups, impaired performance or accidents are associated with sleep disturbance. Some industrial and engineering disasters have been attributed to sleep loss and impaired performance on the part of key personnel.

Neuropsychological studies of people with certain specific sleep disorders have produced additional evidence that sleep disturbance affects daytime functioning. Examples include the excessive daytime sleepiness caused by OSA in both adults and children (Engleman and Douglas, 2004; Blunden et al., 2001) and narcolepsy (Stores, 2010).

When return to normal sleep is possible, recovery from short periods of sleep disturbance occurs after much less sleep than that originally lost, for example, after one night's sleep following sleep loss over several days and nights. Repeated sleep loss results in the accumulation of the 'sleep debt' with increasingly harmful effects. Reversal of the effects of sleep disturbance is likely to be complicated, for example, by emotional consequences of the sleep disturbance.

Many of the reported observations about the psychological effects of sleep disturbance have been made on young adult subjects or patients. Other groups (deserving more intensive study) in whom similar deficits and complications have been reported include children and the elderly, as well as people with learning disability, psychiatric disorder, dementia, or other medical conditions. Sleep disturbance and its effects further complicate the lives of those with such disorders. Contrary to common supposition by both professionals and relatives, success in treating their sleep disturbance may well be possible, given an accurate diagnosis of the type of sleep disorder involved and, preferably, early intervention.

Social effects

The adverse effects of sleep disturbance just mentioned often predispose to social problems including interpersonal difficulties in people of all ages. There are many possible examples such as:

- Irritability or other changes of behaviour can impair personal relationships at home, work, or school (see also Chapter 16).
- Night shift-work (see also Chapter 16) in particular can interfere with social activities and give rise to problems within the family including marital relationships (see also Chapter 13)
- Impaired performance at work or absenteeism may put an individual's job and livelihood at risk.
- Insomnia predisposes to depression and its psychosocial consequences and can have widespread effects on quality of life (QOL) (Colten and Altevogt, 2006) (see also Chapter 8).
- Resorting to non-prescribed drugs or other substances (including alcohol) either to promote sleep or to combat excessive sleepiness is likely to cause or worsen psychosocial difficulties.
- Daytime sleepiness may undermine the educational progress of children and adolescents and limit their career opportunities (Wolfson and Carskadon, 2003).
- Family cohesion can be seriously affected by persistent sleeplessness in young children, because of parents' own sleep loss or, for example, disagreement between them about the best way of dealing with the problem. In extreme cases, parenting practices can be severely punitive (Quine, 1992).

Physical effects

Extensive review of the health consequences of sleep loss and sleep disorders demonstrates an increased risk of a wide range of medical conditions such as hypertension, diabetes, obesity, myocardial infarction, and stroke (Colten and Altevogt, 2006) (see also Chapters 3–7, 9, and 11). OSA is the main disorder implicated in this way and can also exacerbate epilepsy (Hollinger et al., 2006). However, shift-workers are now acknowledged to be also prone to various medical and psychiatric problems such as gastrointestinal complaints, cardiovascular disease, and pregnancy problems, as well as metabolic disturbances (Knutsson, 2003) (see also Chapters 6, 15, and 16). Sleep loss can also affect immune responses (Majde and Krueger, 2005) (see also Chapter 11) and physical growth which may be compromised by, for example, early onset of sleep-disordered breathing (Bonuck et al., 2006).

Sleep disorders are commonplace in clinical practice

Despite its neglect in clinical training, sleep and its disorders can reasonably be seen as fundamentally significant throughout clinical practice. The following is merely an outline of the important connections between sleep disorders and clinical practice. Extensive coverage of these aspects of sleep in a wide range of clinical conditions is provided elsewhere (Lee-Chiong, 2006 and also Chapters 3–11).

Links between sleep disorders and general medicine, neurology, and paediatrics

- Most medical disorders in adults and children are complicated by sleep disturbance.
- Some sleep disorders are essentially medical in type, for example, OSA, nocturnal epilepsy, and also some cases of REM sleep behaviour disorder (RBD) which can foretell the emergence of neurodegenerative disorders. These conditions are considered later in this chapter.

- Certain sleep disorders predispose to medical conditions.
- As just described, some general medical drugs (e.g. those used in respiratory disease, cardiac disease, hypertension, or Parkinson's disease) are reported to cause sleep loss or disruption (Welsh and Fugit, 2006; Pagel, 2006). Parasomnias may be triggered by beta-blockers and anti-parkinsonian agents (nightmares) (Schenck and Mahowald, 2000) or by treatments for neurodegenerative disease (RBD) (Schenck and Mahowald, 2002).

Sleep disorders in psychiatry

- Reference has been made to the fact that sleep disturbance commonly causes psychological problems resulting from effects on emotional state and behaviour, cognitive function and performance at work or at school, family and social life, and QOL in general. Severe, sustained sleep loss can even induce psychotic phenomena.
- Disturbed sleep (often to a serious extent) is a common feature of actual psychiatric disorder at all ages (Abad and Guilleminault, 2005; Ivanenco et al., 2006) (see also Chapter 8).
- Sleep disturbance, including circadian sleep-wake rhythm disturbance, can have a profound effect on the pattern and course of psychiatric disorders (Boivin, 2000), and insomnia or hypersomnia can be the harbinger of the onset or recurrence of depression and other psychiatric illnesses (Nutt et al., 2008).
- Unwanted effects of certain psychiatric medications include sleep disturbance which can be severe. Examples include: insomnia caused by some selective serotonin re-uptake inhibitors (SSRIs) and excessive sleepiness produced by sedating tricyclic drugs. Withdrawal from sedative-hypnotic substances can cause 'rebound insomnia'. Detailed reviews of psychotropic drugs and other medications that induce insomnia or sleepiness have been published recently (Welsh and Fugit, 2006; Pagel, 2006).
- Some psychotropic drugs may also precipitate parasomnias. Certain anti-depressants, lithium, and zolpidem, as well as other CNS-depressant medication, have been reported to precipitate sleepwalking episodes or nightmares (Schenck and Mahowald, 2000) and anti-depressants may also increase periodic limb movements in sleep, decreasing its restorative value. An acute form of RBD (see later) has been associated with intoxication with anti-depressants and withdrawal from sedative-hypnotic abuse as well as alcohol (Schenck and Mahowald, 2002).
- As discussed later, sleep disorders can be misinterpreted as psychiatric conditions.

Sleep disorders and their consequences cost the nation dearly

Of particular significance in the global economic plight at the time of writing is the estimated enormous socioeconomic cost to each nation of sleep disturbance in view of its high prevalence, often severe complications and persistence in untreated cases (Hossain and Shapiro, 2002).

Overall costing attempts to take into account direct, indirect, and related expenses of sleep disturbance. Direct expenses include those for all aspects of the provision of healthcare services for the diagnosis and treatment of sleep disorders. Indirect costs are incurred, for example, when sleep disorders result in impaired productivity and mishaps at work, vehicular accidents, or ill-health of a psychiatric or physical nature. Related costs arise from other personal (including financial) consequences to the individual of having a sleep problem. It is not surprising that the estimated total cost of all these aspects is so considerable—and yet the figures quoted may well be underestimated given the difficulties of determining the true prevalence rates of many sleep disorders.

There are many causes of sleep disturbance to consider: sleep problems and sleep disorders

There are just three basic sleep *problems* or complaints (insomnia, excessive daytime sleepiness, and disturbed behaviour or abnormal experiences associated with sleep, i.e. parasomnias). In contrast, nearly 100 possible causes of these problems (sleep *disorders*) are now described in the latest revision of the International Classification of Sleep Disorders or ICSD-2 (American Academy of Sleep Medicine, 2005a, b, c). The grouping of these sleep disorders is shown in Table 14.1.

Table 14.1 ICSD-2 groups of sleep disorders*

Insomnias

The many psychological and physical causes of difficulty getting off to sleep, not staying asleep, early morning wakening, and feeling unrefreshed by sleep are included here including stress, poor sleep habits, and various mental and medical conditions.

Sleep-related breathing disorders

This group includes the common condition of obstructive sleep apnoea in adults and in children which often causes excessive daytime sleepiness and other serious effects including changes in mood and behaviour. Central apnoea and various types of hypoventilation/hypoxaemic syndromes are also part of this group.

Hypersomnias of central origin not due to a circadian rhythm sleep disorder, sleep-related breathing disorder, or other cause of disturbed nocturnal sleep.

Included here are narcolepsy and the causes of intermittent or recurrent hypersomnia such as the Kleine-Levin syndrome.

Circadian rhythm sleep disorders

These disorders are characterized by a mistiming (and often disruption) of the sleep period, resulting in insomnia and/or hypersomnia: a prominent example is the DSPS common in adolescence. The ASPS can be seen in the elderly in whom the sleep period begins in the evening with waking early when sleep requirements have been met. Irregular sleep-wake rhythms may be the result of an ill-organized way of life and substance abuse. Jet lag and night shift-work disorder are further examples of sleep problems caused by disturbance of the biological clock controlling the sleep-wake cycle.

Parasomnias

These are abnormal behaviours or experiences during or otherwise closely related to sleep. Many can be categorized according to the stage of sleep with which they are usually associated, for example, NREM sleep (sleepwalking) and REM sleep (nightmares, RBD). Other parasomnias of particular psychiatric interest include sleep-related dissociative disorders and sleep-related eating disorders.

Sleep-related movement disorders

These include the restless legs syndrome and periodic limb movement disorder.

Isolated symptoms, apparently normal variants and unresolved issues

Other sleep disorders

The classificatory scheme also includes an appendix on sleep disorders associated with conditions classifiable elsewhere such as sleep-related epilepsy, headaches, gastroesophageal reflux. A further appendix is concerned with other psychiatric and behavioural disorders frequently encountered in the differential diagnosis of sleep disorders. This appendix covers mood disorders, anxiety disorders, somatoform disorders, schizophrenia, and other psychotic disorders, personality disorders, and disorders of a psychiatric or behavioural type first diagnosed in infancy, childhood, or adolescence.

*See text for fuller accounts of disorders mentioned in the table.

To be meaningful, discussion of sleep disturbance, including the misinterpretation theme of this chapter, has to be mainly in terms of sleep disorders rather than sleep problems, not least of all because appropriate advice and treatment depends on accurate diagnosis of the cause or type of condition underlying the sleep problem.

Sleep and its disorders are neglected in health education and training

Despite the compelling clinical and socioeconomic reasons for viewing sleep and its disorders as a priority subject and the repeated calls for it to be taken more seriously (Dement and Mitler, 1993), it features relatively little in health education for both the general public and professionals as emphasized in two comprehensive reviews which have called for the correction of this serious shortcoming: Wake Up America: A National Sleep Alert (National Commission on Sleep Disorders Research, 1993, 1994) and Sleep Disorders and Deprivation: An Unmet Public Health Problem (Colten and Altevogt, 2006) (see also Chapter 19). Both have argued fervently for better teaching and training, as well as increased research funding, in the sleep disorders field as means of improving standards of patient care. Although the situation improved somewhat between these two reports, and continues to improve to some extent, progress remains very slow internationally and many inadequacies remain in the recognition of the importance of sleep disorders and the provision of clinical services.

Lack of public awareness

A fundamental limitation to the improvement of standards is the general public's very limited knowledge about sleep, the ways in which it can be disturbed and the consequences of this, as well as the fact that sleep problems can often be solved or, indeed, prevented. Diet has become a preoccupation in public health education but Thomas Phaire's awareness of the importance of sleep is not shared by many people for lack of even basic information on the topic.

The above 1993 report stated 'No existing program is responsible for general public awareness about the importance of sleep hygiene, the risks of inadequate rest, or the recognition of a sleep problem as a symptom of a medical disorder'. The same is true today. Prospective parents hear little or nothing about how to deal with their child's sleep, sleep does not usually feature in biology courses at school, and teenagers very rarely have advice about their sleep despite the frequency with which it is disturbed with potentially serious consequences (see later).

Professional neglect

The same report also highlighted widespread deficiencies in the training of professionals whose daily work frequently brings them in touch with individuals whose sleep is disturbed. The result is also still the same. As the report states: 'most Americans with sleep disorders have no recourse but to suffer from the disorder'. There is no reason to believe that this problem is confined to the United States.

Consistently, it has been found that the amount of time devoted to sleep and its disorders in undergraduate medical student courses in North America has been very limited (Rosen et al., 1998). A study of UK medical schools found that out of a typical 5-year undergraduate course, the median total time given to sleep and its disorders was 5 minutes, for pre-clinical teaching 15 minutes and zero for clinical teaching (Stores and Crawford, 1998) (see also Chapter 19).

With very few notable exceptions, it seems that the situation has remained the same in more recent times, nor is there reason to believe that these deficiencies are made up significantly in higher training in primary care or hospital specialties. It is no surprise, then, that history taking and even basic knowledge about sleep disorders are reported to be neglected or wanting regarding both adult and paediatric patients (Namen et al., 2001; Owens, 2001). This results in failure to even recognize patients' sleep disorders (Rosen et al., 2001) let alone diagnose or treat them appropriately (Chervin et al., 2001).

The same unfortunate story can be told for other clinical groups including nursing staff (Cohen et al., 1992) (although some health visitors have now taken the initiative and set up sleep clinics for young children and their parents), and clinical psychologists (Stores and Wiggs, 1998). Teachers can be added to the list despite the fact that they will encounter in the classroom the effects of sleep disturbance in children and adolescents.

The consequences of this continuing widespread educational shortcoming, now increasingly recognized as a public health problem but at a slow pace, include the following:

- The general public often fail to see sleep disturbance as requiring professional advice. For example, only a minority of adults with such a serious sleep disorder as OSA seek medical attention and parents often omit to see the doctor about their child's sleep problems (Blunden et al., 2004), therefore depriving them of the help that usually can be given. This is often the case with parents of children with neurodevelopmental disorders who think that their sleep problems are particularly inevitable and cannot be prevented or treated—which is not the case (Wiggs and Stores, 1996). As discussed later, parents may well interpret the consequences of partly biologically based sleep disturbance in teenagers as 'typical adolescent waywardness' (Stores, 2009a).
- Teachers and educational psychologists encounter the school problems of some children and adolescents without necessarily realizing that they are often the result (especially in adolescence) of inadequate sleep (Wolfson and Carskadon, 2003).
- Both general practitioners and specialist physicians, including psychiatrists, also might be unaware of the extent to which symptoms of sleep disorders can overlap with those of other conditions with the inevitable risk of (at least) diagnostic uncertainty.

There was no shortage of suggestions in the 1993 report for correcting these serious public education and professional training shortcomings, and the Executive Summary of the 2006 report set out clearly the requirements in research and training for remedying the situation. Hopefully, it is not over-optimistic to think that, sooner rather than later, they will be acted upon with the appropriate sense of urgency!

Children are not little adults

The progress in disseminating knowledge about sleep disorders is limited regarding adults but more so where children's sleep disorders are concerned. This is reflected in the largely adult orientation of ICSD-2, which concedes to some extent that special considerations are required in describing children. Nevertheless, children remain under-represented in sleep conference programmes and publications, sometimes with the implication that what applies to adults also applies to younger patients.

In fact, there are many differences according to age regarding sleep and its disorders, including, as mentioned previously, the manifestations of basically the same type of sleep disorder. OSA is a good example (Marcus, 2000). This can give rise to misinterpretation even by those with a sound understanding of sleep disorder manifestations in adults.

Other contrasts, depending on developmental level, include sometimes profound differences in sleep physiology, patterns of occurrence of specific sleep disorders, aetiological factors, effects on the individual child and the family, and treatment possibilities, as well as prognosis (Stores, 2009b). Awareness of all these differences has important implications for both clinical practice and epidemiological studies.

Examples of misinterpretation of sleep disorders and their psychosocial and medical consequences

The remainder of the chapter is concerned with examples across the age span of the various possible consequences of failure to recognize or to misdiagnose the nature of sleep disorders. With the exception of the few instances where these mistakes have been studied empirically (see OSA and narcolepsy later), this account is based on clinical impression and reasonable supposition.

Given the generally limited awareness of the diversity and nature of the many sleep disorders, possibly all are to some extent at risk of their manifestations and consequences being misconstrued. Necessarily, this present account has had to be selective, emphasizing a combination of those sleep disorders which are relatively common, dramatic, and/or especially prone to misinterpretation. To structure the account, rather than simply provide a list of examples, those chosen are grouped under the headings of the three basic sleep problems mentioned earlier.

Misinterpretation of sleep disorders underlying insomnia

As described earlier, persistently not being able to sleep well (including not being refreshed by sleep) is likely to cause tiredness, fatigue, irritability, poor concentration, depression, or impaired performance perhaps leading to injuries or accidents at work or while driving. Of the various possible explanations for such changes, sleep disturbance may well be overlooked with failure to appreciate that, with an improvement in sleep (which is usually possible with the correct advice), such problems will often be resolved.

The features of individual sleep disorders in this insomnia category are open to misinterpretations of a more specific nature. The following are examples of this. The first three are examples of circadian sleep-wake cycle disorders (Reid and Zee, 2005), which tend to cause both insomnia and excessive daytime sleepiness.

- The *delayed sleep phase syndrome or DSPS* is considered in the next section.
- Because of body clock changes occurring in old age, there is a tendency to fall asleep in the evening (*advanced sleep phase syndrome* or ASPS—opposite to the effect of body clock changes at puberty) (Bloom et al., 2009). The early morning waking when sleep requirements have been met should not be mistaken for the early morning waking associated with depression where the total amount of sleep is reduced.
- *Jet lag* (Arendt, 2009) is another circadian rhythm sleep-wake cycle disorder which, like DSPS, causes both insomnia and excessive daytime sleepiness. These effects are usually short-lived, but travellers who frequently cross several time zones on each flight can develop chronic sleep disturbances with serious effects on mood, performance, and physical well-being, the true cause of which may not be appreciated.
- *Bedtime problems* are very common in young children. Many are 'behavioural' in origin including parental failure to set limits to their child's delaying tactics about going to bed, or lack of an evening routine leading to their child being relaxed and ready for sleep. However, other, very different possibilities might be revealed if the situation is carefully assessed. These include the bedroom being associated with recriminations about bedtime, nighttime fears (Gordon et al., 2007), or putting the child to bed too early when the biological clock dictates that it is not yet time to sleep—the 'forbidden zone' (Lavie, 1986). Clearly, very different advice is required for each of these different explanations.

Misinterpretation of excessive daytime sleepiness

Excessive sleepiness, whatever its cause out of the many possibilities (Black et al., 2007), is often misjudged as laziness, loss of interest, daydreaming, lack of motivation, depression, intellectual failure, or other unwelcome states of mind. This applies to adults and also younger people (Fallone et al., 2002). Sometimes, in very sleepy states, periods of 'automatic' behaviour occur, that is, prolonged, complex, and often inappropriate behaviour with impaired awareness of events and, therefore, amnesia for them. Such episodes can easily be misconstrued as reprehensible or dissociative behaviour, or prolonged seizure states. The paradoxical effect in young children of sleepiness causing overactivity has sometimes led to a diagnosis of ADHD and inappropriate treatment with stimulant drugs instead of correction of the sleep disorder (Lewin and Di Pinto, 2004). As mentioned earlier, circadian sleep-wake cycle disorders can cause a combination of insomnia and excessive sleepiness both of which are common in psychiatric patients including children (Kotagal, 2009).

The following sleep disorders provide examples of the general tendency to misconstrue the cause of excessive sleepiness.

◆ The *delayed sleep phase syndrome* or *DSPS* (Crowley et al., 2007), said to be common in adolescents in particular, is a case in point. At puberty, the biological clock which controls the timing of the sleep-wake cycle undergoes a change so that the onset of nighttime sleepiness shifts to a later time ('sleep phase delay'). Also, the previous steady reduction with age of the amount of sleep needed is halted and, indeed, in some teenagers the amount of sleep required might actually increase to something in excess of 9 hours. Late-night socializing or entertainment, or regularly studying late, increases the sleep phase delay and is likely to cause much difficulty waking up in the morning for school, college, or work because of inadequate sleep.

The longer this situation goes on, the more a 'sleep debt' accumulates with excessive sleepiness and under-functioning during the day, and possibly the other consequences of disturbed sleep such as behaviour and mood problems, poor performance at school, college, or work, and even accidents.

American studies have reported that 80% of adolescents obtain less than adequate sleep (i.e. 9 hours), 25% less than 6 hours and over 25% fall asleep in class. Students with insufficient sleep generally achieve lower school grades (Wolfson and Carskadon, 2003).

The main signs of DSPS are persistent severe difficulty getting to sleep until very late, then sleeping soundly, very difficult to wake up (may resist vigorously), missing school or repeatedly late, sleepiness, under-functioning, disturbed behaviour during the day, and sleeping in very late at weekends.

DSPS should be treatable (by resetting the body clock by various means) provided the individual and the family concerned are sufficiently motivated and capable of doing what is required. Sometimes the young person has a vested interest in maintaining the abnormal sleep pattern (e.g. to avoid school) in which case treatment has to be based on a thorough understanding of the situation and help to improve the overall situation.

It is important that the DSPS condition is not misjudged by parents and others and professionals including psychiatrists and teachers, but it seems that this often happens. Possible misinterpretations of the situation are that not sleeping until late at night and reluctance to get up in the morning are just 'difficult adolescent behaviour', the more usual form of school refusal, or possibly depression or substance misuse—all of which misinterpretations are destined to make a difficult situation worse.

◆ Over 20% of employees work in shifts. Night shift-workers, in particular, suffer from inadequate and poor quality sleep because they are required to work when their body clock

indicates that they should be asleep (see also Chapters 15 and 16). Their daytime sleep is usually shorter and of poorer quality than that previously obtained at night. This *shift-work disorder* (Åkerstedt, 2003), another circadian sleep-wake cycle disorder, is associated with various
forms of physical ill-health. The psychological effects of inadequate or poor quality sleep,
compounded by the disruptive influence of shift-work on family and social life, are commonplace in shift-workers (see also Chapter 13).

These physical health issues and unfortunate psychosocial consequences can easily overshadow
and distract from the true origins of the shift-worker's primary problems and lead to referral
exclusively to medical or psychiatric services without advice about the underlying sleep disorder.

- *OSA* (Netzer et al., 2003) affects about 4% of men, at least 2% of women, and perhaps 2% of
children. It can cause excessive sleepiness, changes of personality, and adverse effects on social
life and performance at work, as well as intellectual deterioration to the extent that sometimes
dementia is suspected. Only about a tenth of adults with OSA seek medical advice, probably
because many others do not realize that their daytime problems are the result of their disrupted sleep. Those who have sought medical advice may well have been treated initially
(before their sleep disorder was recognized) for the complications of their OSA, such as hypertension or depression, rather than the OSA itself (Smith et al., 2002). Clearly, early recognition
of this treatable condition is highly desirable (see also Chapters 5 and 7).

The same is true of OSA in children, the usual cause of which at this age is enlarged tonsils and
adenoids. Learning and behaviour problems are commonly reported (Lewin and Di Pinto, 2004)
but these can improve following adenotonsillectomy which allows the child to sleep better
(Garetz, 2008). Failure to realize this link between poor sleep and psychological problems is
likely to mean that other, more usual causes are the explanation with referral to an educational
psychologist or child psychiatrist. OSA, usually of more varied origins, complicates many forms
of learning disability, notably Down syndrome (Stores, 2001b) (see also Chapter 10).

- *Narcolepsy* (Thorpy, 2001) is characterized mainly by sleep attacks, as well as more general
sleepiness. It is not the rarity once supposed—prevalence in Western societies is in the order of
0.02–0.05% which is only somewhat less than Parkinson's disease or multiple sclerosis. Cataplexy,
with recurrent loss of tone causing collapse or weakness of one part of the body or another,
usually in response to strong emotion, is usually also present. This offers even more scope for
mistakes as it can be misconstrued as syncope, epilepsy, or attention-seeking behaviour.

Other possible components of the narcolepsy syndrome (namely, hallucinations, which can
be especially vivid, and sleep paralysis, as well as associated automatic behaviour) are also
open to misinterpretation. The same is true of the secondary effects of experiencing nar-
colepsy/cataplexy symptoms such as mood disorders, nighttime fears, loss of self–esteem, and
other social difficulties or impaired performance at work or at home (Stores, 2010). All these
problems have a variety of possible causes which are more likely to be considered rather than
the sleep disorder itself.

It has been reported that, in the year prior to the diagnosis being definitively made at a sleep
disorders centre, narcolepsy had been considered in only 38% of cases (Kryger et al., 2002).
Incorrect diagnoses had included other neurological disorders, such as epilepsy, and a variety
of psychiatric problems especially neurosis and depression. Neurologists had made the correct
diagnosis in 55% of the cases they had seen, internists in 23.5%, general practitioners in
21.9%, and psychiatrists in 11%. Paediatricians had failed to recognize the condition as narcolepsy in all the children they had seen, possibly because of the special difficulties that can be
encountered in recognizing the condition at an early age (Stores, 2006), but also because it is

not usually realized that the onset of narcolepsy occurs before adulthood in at least a third of cases. Hypothyroidism and hypoglycaemia are other possible misdiagnoses of narcolepsy.

◆ The episodic, prolonged sleepiness in the *Kleine-Levin syndrome* (Arnulf et al., 2005) accompanied by often bizarre and out of character behaviour when the patient is awake, understandably causes confusion in the minds of those who are unfamiliar with the condition. Some people with this disorder have initially been thought to perhaps have encephalitis, cerebral tumour, epilepsy, drug addiction, or a psychiatric problem including conduct disorder (Pike and Stores, 1994).

Misinterpretation of the parasomnias

This category of sleep disorders deserves special attention because parasomnias are particularly at risk of diagnostic confusion (Mahowald et al., 2004). Without careful description, the many different types of parasomnias (about 30 of which are now described in ICSD-2) can easily be confused with each other or with other conditions of a very different nature.

Many parasomnias are primary sleep phenomena ('primary parasomnias'): others are manifestations of medical or psychiatric conditions ('secondary parasomnias'). The behaviour and subjective experience in some is subtle but in others dramatic.

Primary parasomnias

The following group of parasomnias occur predominantly when falling asleep or when waking up. Seemingly they are more common in the general population than might be supposed. Despite their possibly alarming and worrying nature giving rise to unnecessary concern, they are very rarely associated with medical or psychiatric disorder.

◆ *Sleep starts* (American Academy of Sleep Medicine, 2005b) usually consist of single jerks of the limbs or other parts of the body when going to sleep ('hypnic jerk') possibly accompanied by a feeling of falling, or an intense sensory experience, such as a flash of light, a loud bang, or sudden pain, also when going off to sleep ('the exploding head syndrome') (Evans and Pearce, 2001). Such experiences may mistakenly be thought to imply something neurologically abnormal such as stroke or epilepsy.

Frequent hypnic jerks have been described in brain-damaged children in whom they may well be interpreted as epileptic in nature (Fusco et al., 1999) although the two conditions may co-exist in this group of children.

◆ *Sleep-related hallucination* (Ohayon et al., 1996)—'hypnagogic' when falling asleep; 'hypnopompic' when waking up—occur in a dream-like state in which objects (including people or animals) may be seen, heard, felt, smelled, tasted, or distorted. Personal body-image distortions might also occur. These experiences are also common and can be alarming especially if combined with sleep paralysis (see below).

◆ 'Isolated' sleep paralysis (Cheyne, 2005) (i.e. other than that associated with narcolepsy when they can be particularly intense and terrifying), which occurs briefly when going to sleep or on waking up, is not uncommon but often unreported unless it is frequent. It consists of recurrent brief episodes of inability to move or speak. Eye movements are possible but there is a sensation of not being able to breathe. The episodes end spontaneously after several seconds or longer, or with external stimulation such as being touched or moved. In rare cases the condition is familial.

Although actually benign, sleep paralysis also can generate much anxiety and fear of having a stroke or other neurological problem. If sleep paralysis is combined with complex hallucinatory experiences, the experience can be so complicated and bizarre (including conversations with people or other beings, as well as feelings of threat and dread or an alien presence) that a psychotic process, especially of a schizophrenic nature, may well be mistakenly suspected (Stores, 1998).

Sleep paralysis seems to be a universal phenomenon which, especially when combined with hallucinatory experiences, in some cultures is interpreted as being caused by mystical influences such as visitation by demons, spirits, or witches.

- Parents of the many young children who bang their heads or roll about rhythmically usually in the pre-sleep period but also sometimes after waking during the night may worry that this is a sign of an emotional problem or neurological disorder, particularly epilepsy. In fact, this *rhythmic movement disorder* (Hoban, 2003) is also benign and usually remits spontaneously by the age of 3–4 years although occasionally it persists into adult life. This condition in otherwise normal children should not be confused with the often continuous rhythmic movements occurring during the day associated with severe neurodevelopmental disorders.

- So-called *'arousal disorders'* (Mahowald and Schenck, 2005), that is, confusional arousals, sleepwalking, and sleep terrors, may well be confused with other parasomnias, especially those of a dramatic nature, and mistakenly thought to be the result of an underlying psychological or medical condition which is rarely the case. They are very common in childhood persisting into adult life in the minority of cases. Onset in adolescence or adult life occurs in only a few.

'Arousal' does not mean that the person wakes up; the arousal is, in fact, a partial arousal usually from deep NREM sleep to another, lighter stage of sleep. In such arousals, various behaviours can occur which are either simple in nature (e.g. sitting up in bed and mumbling) or complicated such as rushing out of the house in a highly agitated state. Other, even more complex behaviours include aggressive acts and sleep-related eating disorders.

The person remains asleep during the episode itself, failing to recognize others present or be comforted by them, although waking sometimes occurs at the end of it, particularly in older patients.

The main predisposing factor is genetic: a first-degree family history of partial arousals has been reported in the vast majority of cases. Precipitating factors (Pressman, 2007), in constitutionally predisposed individuals, include fever, systemic illness, CNS-depressant medication or other substances (possibly including alcohol although this has been disputed recently) (Pressman et al., 2008), internal or external sleep-interrupting stimuli (such as a full bladder, sleeping in an unfamiliar environment, or being woken forcefully by a sudden noise), and other sleep disorders in which sleep is interrupted such as sleep-related breathing disorders. Psychological factors may precipitate or maintain the occurrence of the episodes and also influence their severity. Medications reported to be capable of inducing arousal disorder episodes include zolpidem, benzodiazepines, some SSRIs, and lithium.

Clinically, all three forms of arousal disorder have in common a curious combination of features suggestive of being simultaneously awake and asleep. Despite seeming to be alert (indeed, sometimes highly aroused), the patient appears confused and disoriented and relatively unresponsive to environmental events including attempts to communicate. There is little or (usually) no recall of events during each episode of disturbed behaviour.

- *Confusional arousals* occur mainly in infants and toddlers a high proportion of whom have such episodes. An episode may begin with movements and moaning and then progress to agitated and confused behaviour with crying (perhaps intense), calling out, or thrashing about. Typically, although appearing very alert, the child does not respond when spoken to; more forceful attempts to intervene may meet with resistance and increased agitation.

Parents are often very alarmed and, mistakenly thinking their child is awake and distressed, want to console him/her, and may make vigorous attempts to waken him/her, without success or only with much trying. In fact, such efforts may actually prolong the arousal and, if the child is woken to some extent, he/she is likely to be confused and frightened. The young children who have confusional arousals may well be thought by their parents to be ill in some way because of the degree of behavioural disturbance involved.

◆ *Sleepwalking* is said to occur occasionally in 20–40% of children and frequently in another 3–4%; the rate in adults is 4–10%—higher than previously thought.

The young child may crawl or walk about in his/her cot. Older children and adults may calmly walk around the bedroom or into other parts of the house such as to the toilet. The patient may appear downstairs or be found standing on the landing or elsewhere in the house, looking vague, with eyes open but with a glassy stare, at most partially responsive. Movements are often clumsy and urinating in inappropriate places or other inappropriate behaviour is common.

Some sleepwalkers are found asleep in various parts of the house or further afield. Quite complicated routes may be followed if well-known, or other complex habitual behaviour (automatism) may occur, possibly extending over long periods of time. Accidental injury in sleepwalking (e.g. from falling downstairs or through a bedroom window) is a serious risk.

Although sleepwalking may involve calm walking about in a semi-purposeful confused manner, sleepwalking may take an agitated form (similar to sleep terrors) which may be worsened by attempts to intervene and with an even greater risk of injury from crashing through windows or glass doors, for example. Some sleepwalkers do much more complex things such as making themselves drinks or meals, following complicated routes outside the house, or even driving a car. Other sleepwalkers develop an eating disorder with excessive weight gain due to the amount of food they consume while they are still asleep at night (Howell et al., 2009).

Yet others behave in an aggressive or destructive way and, at times, sexual or other serious offences have been committed during a sleepwalking or confusional arousal episode (and, indeed, in some other sleep disorders). There has been increasing interest in recent times in the notion of 'sexomnia', that is, sexual activity while still asleep, which has been entered as a defence for sexual offences (Schenck et al., 2007). Guidelines have been suggested for the recognition of sleepwalking automatisms, mainly for medico-legal purposes (Mahowald et al., 2005).

◆ *Sleep terrors* occur in about 3% of children, mainly in later childhood, and about 1% of adults. Classically, parents are woken by their child's piercing scream which marks the very sudden onset of the partial arousal. The child (or adult) appears terrified, with staring eyes, intense sweating, rapid pulse, and cries or other vocalizations suggesting intense distress. He/She may jump out of bed and rush about frantically and crying out, as if trying to escape from danger. Injury from running into furniture or jumping through windows is again a serious risk. The event usually lasts no more than a few minutes at most before typically ending abruptly with the patient then settling back to sleep. If the person wakes up at the end of the episode, he/she may describe feelings of primitive threat or danger, but not the extended narrative of a nightmare.

If it is not known that a wide variety of complicated actions are compatible with still being asleep, it is likely to be assumed that, during the partial arousal episodes, the person was awake at the time and aware of what was happening and what he/she was doing, and, therefore, responsible for what had happened. Alternatively, the episodes might be thought to be epileptic in nature, the result of some other physical or psychiatric state or, indeed, pretence.

◆ *Nightmares* (American Academy of Sleep Medicine, 2005b), an example of a REM (or 'dreaming') sleep-related parasomnia, are frightening dreams that awaken the sleeper in a highly distressed state. 'Bad dreams' are also disturbing without waking the patient. The two may coexist and typically occur in the later part of overnight sleep when REM sleep is most abundant.

A nightmare consists of a frightening or otherwise very upsetting sequence of dream events (i.e. a narrative) the distressing effect of which increases as the events unfold until the patient wakes up, very frightened, fully alert, and able to describe the dream experience. The feeling of distress persists preventing a return to sleep for some time, although reassurance and comfort can usually be provided.

The content of the nightmare varies with age. In childhood they tend to become increasingly complex, that is, monsters or other frightening creatures at an early age, progressing to dreams based on frightening TV or film content, or events at home or school. Common adult themes include being in danger, pursued, trapped, or threatened in other ways. The responsible traumatic experience (or part of it) is likely to be re-lived in the dream where nightmares follow trauma.

Possibly everyone has experienced a nightmare at least once in their life. However, 10–50% of young children are reported to have nightmares severe enough to disturb their parents, and 2–8% of the general population are said to have a current problem with nightmares.

Typically, nightmares begin between 3 and 6 years of age, peaking about 6–10, and then diminishing although some people are lifelong sufferers. Generally, such dreams occur infrequently, possibly with no apparent cause, and without any serious psychological significance. They may be spontaneous or (like arousal disorders) precipitated by illness or psychological stress of any sort.

There seems to be a genetic predisposition to nightmares, and women tend to be more affected than men. Nightmares may be associated with other sleep disorders such as OSA, sleep terrors, or narcolepsy. In addition, various medications (e.g. beta-blockers, anti-parkinsonian agents, and SSRIs) are reported to be capable of triggering nightmares and bad dreams.

The term 'nightmare' can be a source of confusion and diagnostic inaccuracy when it is used for any sort of dramatic nocturnal episode in which the patient appears to be very frightened. For example, sometimes nightmare and sleep terror are used synonymously despite the fact that they are very different parasomnias (see Table 14.2).

A distinction must be made between a child's reluctance to go to bed as part of a behavioural problem as distinct from being fearful of nighttime for whatever reason (Gordon et al., 2007) including experiencing nightmares.

Secondary parasomnias

A number of non-convulsive types of epilepsy are closely related to sleep. These, like many cases of RBD, are 'secondary parasomnias' in that they are or can be manifestations of a medical disorder. All can give rise to dramatic behaviour which is easily construed as some other type of nighttime disturbance.

- Benign partial epilepsy with centro-temporal spikes or *Rolandic epilepsy* (Panayiotopoulos, 2002) is thought to account for up to 24% of children with epilepsy. The distinctive features of the seizures are hemifacial motor or sensory abnormal movements or sensations, pharyngo-laryngeal symptoms, excess salivation, and speech impairment. These symptoms are in keeping with the centro-temporal location of the source of seizure discharge. Generalized tonic-clonic seizures may also occur.

  The seizures are brief and occur exclusively during sleep in 75% of cases, most frequently on falling asleep, and shortly before or on waking. The experiences are likely to cause much distress for both the child and his/her parents.

  The frequency of attacks is very variable. Onset is usually between 3 and 13 years, peaking at 7–10 years. Prospects for seizure remission are generally thought to be excellent in most cases. Overall intelligence is not usually impaired but some specific neuropsychological deficits

Table 14.2 Comparison of the main features of arousal disorders, nightmares, and sleep-related seizures

	Arousal disorders	Nightmares	Sleep-related seizures*
Age of onset (years)	1–8	3–6	Any age
Gender	Both	Both	Both
Family history	Common	Sometimes	Variable
Prevalence	Common	Common	Much less common
Usual stage of sleep	Deep NREM	REM	Variable
Time of the night	Usually first third of the night	Middle to last third of the night	Variable
Episodes at night	Usually one	Usually one	One to many
Episodes/month	Usually sporadic	Usually sporadic	Sporadic to many
Behaviour	Variable but usually dramatic with intense autonomic arousal (apart from calm sleepwalking); often inaccessible and cannot be comforted; may resist intervention	Little movement during dreams but distressed on awakening, accessible and welcomes, comforting; autonomic arousal usually marked	Variable, may be undirected violence or distress during or after attack in state of impaired consciousness; autonomic arousal can be considerable
Level of consciousness	Unaware during episode, confused if awakened or following episode	Asleep during episode, fully awake afterwards	Variable, may be impaired during or after attack
Memory for events	None or fragmentary	Vivid recall	Variable
Stereotyped	Somewhat	Somewhat	Often
Likelihood of injury	Moderate to high in agitated sleepwalking and sleep terrors	Low	Overall low to moderate
Prognosis	Good	Good	Good to poor

*In view of the wide range of types of epileptic seizures associated with sleep, the descriptions given are no more than generalizations with certain clear exceptions to the general rule (see text).

have sometimes been reported, for example, aspects of memory function or educational attainments.

Although the features of these Rolandic seizures are distinctive, limited familiarity with them leads to their confusion with other dramatic parasomnias such as arousal disorders or 'nightmares' in the loose meaning of the term, or with other seizure disorders of a focal or partial type which may be due to a structural brain lesion. In fact, Rolandic seizures are usually benign and remit spontaneously by about age 16 years.

- *Nocturnal frontal lobe epilepsy (NFLE)* (Provini et al., 2000), described in both adults and in children (Stores et al., 1991), is often misdiagnosed mainly because of the complicated motor manifestations (e.g. kicking, hitting, rocking, thrashing and cycling, or scissor movements of the legs) and vocalizations (from grunting, coughing, muttering, or moaning to shouting, screaming, or roaring) that characterize many attacks. They are very different from other seizure types. Such episodes are stereotyped and occur in clusters within any one night. The abrupt onset and termination, short duration of the attacks (different from seizures of temporal lobe origin) and, sometimes, preservation of consciousness can also suggest a non-epileptic basis for the attacks. Often they are misdiagnosed as nightmares, sleep terrors, or 'hysteria'.

The correct diagnosis of NFLE rests on awareness of this form of epilepsy and recognition of the unusual clinical manifestations in the attacks as described above. Electroencephalography (EEG) recordings are of limited diagnostic value because they can show no definite abnormality even during the episodes. This has sometimes confirmed the mistaken impression that the episodes are psychological in origin. Neuroimaging reveals no abnormality in most cases.

◆ In REM sleep behaviour disorder (RBD) (Schenck and Mahowald, 2002), muscle tone is pathologically retained during REM sleep, allowing dreams to be acted out (most dreaming occurs during REM sleep). Violent dreams are likely to cause injury to the patient or bed partner.

Although some cases of RBD seem to be idiopathic (i.e. a primary parasomnia), increasingly the term 'cryptogenic' is preferred because an underlying condition is identified or eventually comes to light (Thomas et al., 2007). RBD has a strong association with neurodegenerative disorders such as Lewy body disease, multiple system atrophy, Parkinson's disease, and also with narcolepsy. There is also a link with some forms of medication, including anti-depressants. Although mainly described in elderly males, it has also been reported at other ages, including children, and in women.

The condition (which is eminently treatable, mainly with clonazepam, even in the presence of neurodegenerative disease) may well be confused with other dramatic parasomnias despite their different, distinctive features. Especially if the bed partner is attacked, a psychological motive may be wrongly suspected.

◆ A combination of sleepwalking and night terrors, as well as RBD (*parasomnia overlap disorder*) has been described in some individuals (Schenck et al., 1997). This can increase the degree of diagnostic uncertainty.

A recurrent theme in the above account of the risk of misdiagnosis of the parasomnias is the likelihood of confusion between those parasomnias of a dramatic nature. There are many which fit this description. However, perhaps the main distinctions in this respect are those that can be made between the clinical characteristics of arousal disorders, nightmares, and epileptic seizures. Table 14.2 summarizes these differences which need to be appreciated in order to avoid such confusion. More general guidance for distinguishing between nocturnal epilepsy and non-epileptic episodes at night is provided elsewhere (Tinuper et al., 2007; Derry et al., 2006).

A number of other parasomnias are secondary to psychiatric disorders.

◆ *Nocturnal panic attacks* (Craske and Tsao, 2005) are an example. They are characterized by sudden awakening in a highly aroused state with dizziness, difficulty breathing, sweating, trembling, and palpitations, as well as a fear of an impending and possibly fatal heart attack or stroke. If panic attacks occur only at night, they might well be misdiagnosed as some other form of dramatic parasomnia such as sleep terror or nightmare.

◆ The prevalence of frequent *nightmares* is increased in sufferers from anxiety states including post-traumatic stress disorder (PTSD) in whom nightmares are a cardinal feature, people subject to persistent psychological stress or other psychiatric disorders, and chronic alcoholics and drug users including during their withdrawal phase.

◆ In *dissociative states* (i.e. states of apparently impaired awareness for psychological rather than physical reasons), dramatic behaviour, sometimes bizarre or violent, occurs at night but while the patient is actually awake as shown by polysomnography (PSG) (Schenck et al., 1989).

◆ Episodes while awake resembling sleepwalking, epilepsy, or narcolepsy have been reported in both adults and children (Molaie and Deutsch, 1997; Thacker et al., 1993; Hvidsten and Bates, 2008). These parasomnias can pose particularly difficult diagnostic challenges but, clearly, the correct diagnosis is essential to determine what particular type of help is required. In such cases, the possibility of *dissociation or malingering* must be considered.

Detection and assessment of sleep disorders

The risk of misdiagnosis can be lessened by being acquainted with the various sleep disorders including an awareness of their main characteristic features. A patient may have a combination of sleep disorder and other conditions of a different nature (and, indeed, more than one type of sleep disorder), especially in the elderly. Therefore, it is all the more important that each complaint and its cause, including the possibility of sleep disorder, is assessed adequately.

Sleep history

The cornerstone of assessment is a sleep history which traditionally has been neglected (Namen et al., 2001). The following outline illustrates the main clinical enquiries that should supplement usual history-taking schedules in primary care and specialist settings. A more detailed account is provided elsewhere (Malow, 2005); a modified approach is required in the case of children (Stores, 2001c).

Three basic screening questions for any patient are:

◆ Do you sleep long enough or well enough?
◆ Are you very sleepy during the day?
◆ Do you do unusual things or have strange experiences at night?

The patient's bed partner or other relative should also be questioned.

Positive answers call for a detailed sleep history, essential elements of which are:

◆ The precise nature of the sleep complaint, its onset, and development.
◆ Medical or psychological factors at the start of the sleep problem or which might be maintaining it.
◆ Patterns of occurrence of the sleep problem including provoking or ameliorating factors, and differences in sleep patterns between weekdays and weekends.
◆ The sleeping environment, regularity of sleep habits, and other aspects of 'sleep hygiene', i.e. practices that are conducive to sleep (Hauri, 1998).
◆ Effects on mood, work, social life, and other family members.
◆ Effects of past and present treatments for the sleep problem, and medications taken now or in the past for other conditions.
◆ Details of the patient's typical 24-hour sleep-wake pattern, starting with evening events leading up to bedtime, time and process of getting to sleep, events during the night, time and ease of waking up, daytime sleepiness (including naps), as well as mental state and behaviour during the day.
◆ Estimation of the duration and soundness of overnight sleep.
◆ Features of particular diagnostic importance such as a combination of obesity, loud snoring or snorting and apnoeic episodes (OSA), wide discrepancy between weekday and weekend sleep patterns (DSPS), sleep attacks and cataplexy (narcolepsy), repeated jerking at night (periodic limb movements in sleep), or violent dreams and behaviour during sleep (RBD).

Other aspects of assessment

A screening *questionnaire* for use with adults (Buysse et al., 1989) or younger patients (Owens et al., 2000) can be a useful starting point in assessment. A structured *sleep diary*, recording day and night events for, say, 1–2 weeks, might also reveal further valuable information.

Additional potentially relevant details may be contained in the patient's *medical, psychiatric, and social histories* including occupational factors and also habits (such as caffeine, alcohol, or nicotine consumption and use of illicit drugs) which might affect sleep. A family history of sleep disorders might also be revealing.

These enquiries should be accompanied by a *review of systems*, as well as physical and mental state examination. It is important to identify any neurological, general medical, or psychiatric disorder likely to affect sleep, or physical anomalies of possible importance such as those which predispose to OSA, especially obesity and nasopharyngeal abnormalities.

Clinical information from these sources may well be sufficient to at least provisionally formulate the problem correctly. In a proportion of cases, special investigations will be required such as actigraphy (monitoring of body movements to show the pattern of periods of sleep or wakefulness) or PSG if more physiological detail is required. Diagnostically difficult cases will need referral to a specialized sleep disorders service.

Improvements in public and professional knowledge about sleep and its disorders

There is much more to be said about ways of achieving this than is possible in the present chapter. The following sources can be seen as simply starting points. More complete coverage of educational aspects is provided in Chapter 19.

Regarding *public education*, the websites of the American Academy of Sleep Medicine (AASM) (<<www.sleepeducation.com>>) and the National Sleep Foundation (<<www.sleepfoundation.org>>) provide valuable information for the general public about a variety of basic aspects of sleep and its disorders across the age range from infants through older children and adolescents to adults into old age.

Most books published for the general public have been about young children but recently others have covered a wider childhood age range, or adults in general in a form which is also suitable as a primer for others, including professionals with limited knowledge of the sleep disorders field (Stores, 2009c, d). Such reading material can be valuable but there remains the need for 'live' contact between professionals well versed in sleep disorders and the public in the form of talks and seminars for prospective parents, school children, and the various adult groups.

As mentioned earlier, websites such as the AASM reflect the thought that has been given (mainly in the United States) to *professional education* mainly for physicians at undergraduate and postgraduate levels, and also for others who need to know about sleep disorders. Various means of achieving this have been formulated including sources of information and model curricula (Sateia and Avidan, 2002), and ways in which the success of such teaching and training can be assessed have been devised (Zozula et al., 2001). Accreditation in sleep disorders is well-established in America and moves in that direction are now being made in Europe. Despite these efforts, there is still a long way to go.

Summary box

♦ Disturbed sleep is a common problem of relevance to primary care and medical specialties alike.

♦ It is probable that the clinical manifestations of the many types of sleep disorders in adults and children are often not recognized for what they really are and, being misconstrued, the patient receives inappropriate advice or treatment—or no help at all!

♦ The main reason for this is that the general public and professionals do not have an adequate appreciation of the importance of sleep and its disorders because the topic is neglected in health education and professional training.

♦ There is no lack of knowledge about the importance of sleep, the psychological, social, and physical consequences of sleep disturbance, the many manifestations of sleep disorders, and preventive and treatment possibilities—the problem is that this knowledge is poorly disseminated.

♦ The main clinical 'take home message' from this chapter is that, whatever the nature of a person's problem (be it psychological or medical, and whether it be a child or an adult), sleep disturbance must be included in the list of possible explanations. Needless to say, this principle also has important implications for epidemiological studies of sleep and its disorders.

References

Abad, V.C. & Guilleminault, C. (2005). Sleep and psychiatry. *Dialogues Clin Neurosci*, 7, 291–303.

Åkerstedt, T. (2003). Shift work and disturbed sleep/wakefulness. *Occup Med*, 53, 89–94.

American Academy of Sleep Medicine (2005a). *The International Classification of Sleep Disorders: Diagnostic and Coding Manual*. Second edition. Westchester, IL: American Academy of Sleep Medicine.

American Academy of Sleep Medicine (2005b). Sleep starts. In: *The International Classification of Sleep Disorders: Diagnostic and Coding Manual*. Second edition. Westchester, IL: American Academy of Sleep Medicine, pp. 208–210.

American Academy of Sleep Medicine. (2005c). Nightmare disorder. In: *The International Classification of Sleep Disorders: Diagnostic and Coding Manual*. Second edition. Westchester, IL: American Academy of Sleep Medicine, pp. 155–158.

Arendt, J. (2009). Managing jet lag: some of the problems and possible new solutions. *Sleep Med*, 13, 249–256.

Arnulf, I., Zeitzer, J.M., File, J., et al. (2005). Kleine-Levin syndrome: a systematic review of 186 cases in the literature. *Brain*, 128, 2763–2776.

Black, J., Duntley, S.P., Bogan, R.K., et al. (2007). Recent advances in the treatment and management of excessive daytime sleepiness. *CNS Spectr*, 12(Suppl 2), 1–16.

Bloom, H.G., Ahmed, I., Alessi, C.A., et al. (2009). Evidence-based recommendations for the assessment and management of sleep disorders in older persons. *J Am Geriatr Soc*, 57, 761–789.

Blunden, S., Lushington, K. & Kennedy, D. (2001). Cognitive and behavioural performance in children with sleep-related obstructive breathing disorders. *Sleep Med Rev*, 5, 447–461.

Blunden, S., Lushington, K., Lorenzen, B., et al. (2004). Are sleep problems under-recognised in general practice? *Arch Dis Child*, 89, 708–712.

Boivin, D.B. (2000). Influence of sleep-wake and circadian rhythm disturbances in psychiatric disorders. *J Psychiatry Neurosci*, 25, 446–458.

Bonnet, H. (2005). Acute sleep deprivation. In: Kryger, M.H., Roth, T. & Dement, W.C. (eds.), *Principles and Practice of Sleep Medicine*. Fourth edition. Hoboken, NJ: Elsevier Saunders, pp. 51–66.

Bonuck, K, Parikh, S. & Bassila, M. (2006). Growth failure and sleep disordered breathing: a review of the literature. *Int J Pediatr Otorhinolaryngol*, 70, 769–778.

Buysse, D.J., Reynolds, C.F., Monk, T.H., et al. (1989). The Pittsburgh Sleep Quality Index: a new instrument for psychiatric practice and research. *Psychiatry Res*, **28**, 193–213.

Chervin, R.D., Archbold, K.H., Panahi, P., et al. (2001). Sleep problems seldom addressed at two pediatric clinics. *Pediatrics*, **107**, 1375–1380.

Cheyne, J.A. (2005). Sleep paralysis episode frequency and number, types, and structure of associated hallucinations. *J Sleep Res*, **14**, 319–324.

Chokroverty, S. (2000). Medical sleep-wake disorders. In: Gelder, M.G., Lopez-Ibor, J.J., Jr. & Andreasen, N. (eds.), *New Oxford Textbook of Psychiatry*. Oxford: Oxford University Press, pp. 1026–1031.

Cohen, F.L., Merritt, S.L., Nehring, W.M., et al. (1992). Curricular sleep content in graduate and undergraduate nursing programs. *Sleep Res*, **21**, 187.

Colten, H.R. & Altevogt, B.M. (eds.) (2006). Chapter 3: extent and health consequences of chronic sleep loss and sleep disorders and Chapter 4: functional and economic impact of sleep loss and sleep-related disorders. *Sleep Disorders and Sleep Deprivation: An Unmet Public Health Problem*. Washington, DC: National Academies Press, pp. 67–209. Available at: http://www.nap.edu/catalog/11617.html. (accessed 27 April 2010)

Craske, M.G. & Tsao, J.C. (2005). Assessment and treatment of nocturnal panic attacks. *Sleep Med Rev*, **9**, 173–184.

Crowley, S.J., Acebo, C. & Carskadon, M.A. (2007). Sleep, circadian rhythms, and delayed sleep phase in adolescence. *Sleep Med*, **8**, 602–612.

Dement, W.C. & Mitler, M.M. (1993). It's time to wake up to the importance of sleep disorders. *J Am Med Assoc*, **269**, 1548–1550.

Derry, C.P., Davey, M. & Johns, M. (2006). Distinguishing sleep disorders from seizures: diagnosing bumps in the night. *Arch Neurol*, **63**, 705–709.

Didden, R. & Sigafoos, J. (2001). A review of the nature and treatment of sleep disorders in individuals with developmental disabilities. *Res Dev Disabil*, **22**, 255–1031.

Dinges, D.F., Rogers, N.L. & Baynard, M.D. (2005). Chronic sleep deprivation. In: Kryger, M.H., Roth, T. & Dement, W.C. (eds.), *Principles and Practice of Sleep Medicine*. Fourth edition. Hoboken, NJ: Elsevier Saunders, pp. 67–76.

Engleman, H.M. & Douglas, N.J. (2004). Sleepiness, cognitive function, and quality of life in obstructive sleep apnoea/hypopnoea syndrome. *Thorax*, **59**, 612–622.

Evans, R.W. & Pearce, J.M. (2001). Exploding head syndrome. *Headache*, **41**, 602–603.

Fallone, G., Owens, J.A. & Deane, J. (2002). Sleepiness in children and adolescents: clinical implications. *Sleep Med Rev*, **6**, 287–306.

Fusco, L., Pachatz, C., Cusmai, R. & Vigevano, F. (1999). Repetitive sleep starts in neurologically impaired children: an unusual non-epileptic manifestation in otherwise epileptic subjects. *Epileptic Disord*, **1**, 63–67.

Garetz, S.L. (2008). Behavior, cognition, and quality of life after adenotonsillectomy for pediatric sleep-disordered breathing: summary of the literature. *Otolaryngol Head Neck Surg*, **138**(Suppl 1), S19–S26.

Gordon, J., King, N., Gullone, E., et al. (2007). Nighttime fears of children and adolescents: frequency, content, severity, harm expectations, disclosure, and coping behaviours. *Behav Res Ther*, **45**, 2464–2472.

Graber, M.A. & Berner, E.S. (2008). Diagnostic error: is overconfidence the problem? *Am J Med*, **121**(Suppl 5), S2–S23.

Hauri, P.J. (1998). Insomnia. *Clin Chest Med*, **19**, 157–168.

Hoban, T.F. (2003). Rhythmic movement disorder in children. *CNS Spectr*, **8**, 135–138.

Hollinger, P., Khatami, R., Gugger, M., et al. (2006). Epilepsy and obstructive sleep apnoea. *Eur Neurol*, **55**, 74–79.

Hossain, J.L. & Shapiro, C.M. (2002). The prevalence, cost implications, and management of sleep disorders: an overview. *Sleep Breath*, **6**, 85–101.

Howell, M.J., Schenk, C.H. & Crow, S.J. (2009). A review of nighttime eating disorders. *Sleep Med Rev*, **13**, 23–34.

Hvidsten, S. & Bates, G. (2008). Pseudonarcolepsy in an 11-year old boy. *Clin Child Psychol Psychiatry*, 13, 585–591.

Ivanenco, A., Crabtree, V.M., Obrien, L.M., et al. (2006). Sleep complaints and psychiatric symptoms in children evaluated at a pediatric mental health clinic. *J Clin Sleep Med*, 15, 42–48.

Knowles, E. (2003). *The Concise Oxford Dictionary of Quotations*. Revised Fourth edition. Oxford: Oxford University Press.

Knutsson, A. (2003). Health disorders of shift workers. *Occup Med*, 53, 103–108.

Kotagal, S. (2009). Hypersomnia in children: interface with psychiatric disorders. *Child Adolesc Psychiatr Clin N Am*, 18, 967–977.

Kryger, M.H., Walld, R. & Manfreda, J. (2002). Diagnoses received by narcolepsy patients in the year prior to diagnosis by a sleep specialist. *Sleep*, 25, 36–41.

Kryger, M.H., Roth, T. & Dement, W.C. (eds.) (2005). *Principles and Practice of Sleep Medicine*, Fourth edition. Philadelphia, PA: Elsevier Saunders.

Lavie, P. (1986). Ultra short sleep-waking schedule. III. 'Gates' and 'forbidden zones' for sleep. *Electroencephalogr Clin Neurophysiol*, 63, 414–425.

Lee-Chiong, T. (2006). *Sleep. A Comprehensive Handbook*. Hoboken, NJ: Wiley-Liss.

Lewin, D.S. & Di Pinto, M.S. (2004). Sleep disorders and ADHD: shared and common stereotypes. Editorial. *Sleep*, 27, 188–189.

MacDonald, S. (2009). One in six patients 'given wrong diagnosis'. *Sunday Times,* 20th September.

Mahowald, M.W. & Schenck, C.K. (2005). Non-rapid eye movement sleep parasomnias. *Neurol Clin*, 23, 1077–1106.

Mahowald, M.W., Bornemann, M.C. & Schenck, C.H. (2004). Parasomnias. *Semin Neurol*, 24, 283–292.

Mahowald, M.W., Schenck, C.H. & Cramer Bornemann, M.A. (2005). Sleep-related violence. *Curr Neurol Neurosci Rep*, 5, 153–158.

Majde, J.A. & Krueger, J.M. (2005). Links between the innate immune system and sleep. *J Allergy Clin Immunol*, 116, 1188–1198.

Malow, B.A. (2005). Approach to the patient with disordered sleep. In: Kryger, M.H., Roth, T. & Dement, W.C. (eds.), *Principles and Practice of Sleep Medicine*. Fourth edition. Philadelphia, PA: Elsevier Saunders, pp. 589–593.

Marcus, C.L. (2000). Obstructive sleep apnea syndrome: differences between children and adults. *Sleep*, 23(Suppl 4), 140–141.

Molaie, M. & Deutsch, G.K. (1997). Psychogenic events presenting as parasomnia. *Sleep*, 20, 402–405.

Namen, A.M., Landry, S.H., Case, D., et al. (2001). Sleep histories are seldom documented on a general medical service. *South Med J*, 94, 874–879.

National Commission on Sleep Disorders Research (1993 and 1994). *Wake Up America: A National Sleep Alert*, Vols. 1 and 2. Washington, DC: National Commission on Sleep Disorders Research, United States Department of Health and Human Services.

Netzer, N.C., Hoegel, J.J., Loube, D., et al. (2003). Prevalence of symptoms and risk of sleep apnoea in primary care. *Chest*, 124, 1406–1414.

Nutt, D., Wilson, S. & Paterson, L. (2008). Sleep disorders as core symptoms of depression. *Dialogues Clin Neurosci*, 10, 329–336.

Ohayon, M.M., Priest, R.G., Caulet, M., et al. (1996). Hypnagogic and hypnopompic hallucinations: pathological phenomena? *Br J Psychiatry*, 169, 459–467.

Owens, J.A. (2001). The practice of pediatric sleep medicine: results of a community survey. *Pediatrics*, 108, E51.

Owens, J.A., Spirito, A. & McQuinn, M. (2000). The Children's Sleep Habits Questionnaire (CSHQ): psychometric properties of a survey instrument for school-aged children. *Sleep*, 23, 1043–1051.

Pagel, J.F. (2006). Medications that induce sleepiness. In: Lee-Chiong, T. (ed.), *Sleep: A Comprehensive Handbook*. Hoboken, NJ: Wiley-Liss, pp. 175–182.

Panayiotopoulos, C.P. (2002). Benign childhood epilepsy with centrotemporal spikes. In: Panayiotopoulos, C.P. (ed.), *A Clinical Guide to Epileptic Syndromes and their Treatment*. Chipping Norton: Bladon Medical Publishing, pp. 90–95.

Partinen, M. & Hublin, C. (2005). Epidemiology of sleep disorders. In: Kryger, M.H., Roth, T. & Dement, W.C. (eds.), *Principles and Practice of Sleep Medicine*. Fourth edition. Philadelphia, PA: Elsevier Saunders, pp. 626–647.

Phaire, T. (1545). *The Boke of Chyldren*. Translated by A.V. Neale & H.R.E.Wallis. Edinburgh: Livingstone, 1955.

Philibert, I. (2005). Sleep loss and performance in residents and nonphysicians: a meta-analytic examination. *Sleep*, **28**, 1392–1402.

Phillips, B. & Ancoli-Israel, S. (2001). Sleep disorders in the elderly. *Sleep Med*, **2**, 99–114.

Pike, M. & Stores, G. (1994). Kleine-Levin syndrome: a case of diagnostic confusion. *Arch Dis Child*, **71**, 355–357.

Pressman, M.R. (2007). Factors that predispose, prime and precipitate NREM parasomnias in adults: clinical and forensic implications. *Sleep Med Rev*, **11**, 5–30.

Pressman, M.R., Mahowald, M.W. & Schenck, C.H. (2008). No scientific evidence that alcohol causes sleepwalking. *J Sleep Res*, **17**, 473–474.

Provini, F., Plazzi, G., Montagna, P., et al. (2000). The wide clinical spectrum of nocturnal frontal lobe epilepsy. *Sleep Med Rev*, **4**, 375–386.

Quine, L. (1992). Severity of sleep problems with severe learning difficulties: description and correlates. *J Community Appl Soc Psychol*, **2**, 247–268.

Rechtschaffen, A. (1998). Current perspectives on the function of sleep. *Perspect Biol Med*, **41**, 359–390.

Reid, K.J. & Zee, P.C. (2005). Circadian disorders of the sleep wake cycle. In: Kryger, M.H., Roth, T. & Dement, W.C. (eds.), *Principles and Practice of Sleep Medicine*. Fourth edition. Philadelphia, PA: Elsevier Saunders, pp. 691–701.

Rosen, R., Mahowald, M., Chesson, A., et al. (1998). The Taskforce 2000 survey on medical education in sleep and its disorders. *Sleep*, **21**, 235–238.

Rosen, R.C., Zozula, R., Jahn, E.G., et al. (2001). Low rates of recognition of sleep disorders in primary care: comparison of a community-based versus clinical academic setting. *Sleep Med*, **2**, 47–55.

Sateia, M.J. & Avidan, A.Y. (2002). Tools for sleep medicine education: the MEDSleep site. *Sleep Med*, **3**, 379–381.

Schenck, C.H. & Mahowald, M.W. (2000). Parasomnias: managing bizarre sleep-related behaviour disorders. *Postgrad Med*, **107**, 145–156.

Schenck, C.H. & Mahowald, M.W. (2002). REM sleep behavior disorder: clinical, developmental, and neuroscience perspectives 16 years after its formal identification. *Sleep*, **25**, 120–138.

Schenck, C.H., Milner, D.M., Hurwitz, T.D., et al. (1989). Dissociative disorders presenting as somnambulism: polysomnographic, video, and clinical documentation (8 cases). *Dissociation*, **4**, 194–204.

Schenck, C.H., Boyd, J.L. & Mahowald, M.W. (1997). A parasomnia overlap disorder involving sleepwalking, sleep terrors, and REM sleep behavior disorder in 33 polysomnographically confirmed cases. *Sleep*, **20**, 927–981.

Schenck, C.H., Arnulf, I. & Mahowald, M.W. (2007). Sleep and sex: what can go wrong? A review of the literature on sleep related disorders and abnormal sexual behaviors and experiences. *Sleep*, **30**, 683–702.

Shepard, J.W., Buysse, D.J., Chesson, A.L., et al. (2005). History of the development of sleep medicine in the United States. *Clin Sleep Med*, **1**, 61–82.

Siegel, J.M. (2005). Clues to the functions of mammalian sleep. *Nat Insight*, **437**, 1264–1271.

Smith, R., Ronald, J., Delaive, K., et al. (2002). What are obstructive sleep apnea patients being treated for prior to this diagnosis? *Chest*, **121**, 164–172.

Stores, G. (1998). Sleep paralysis and hallucinosis. *Behav Neurol*, **11**, 109–112.

Stores, G. (2001a). *A Clinical Guide to Sleep Disorders in Children and Adolescents*. Cambridge: Cambridge University Press.

Stores, G. (2001b). *Sleep-wake function in children with neurodevelopmental and psychiatric disorders. Semin Pediatr Neurol*, 4, 188–197.

Stores, G. (2001c). Assessment of sleep disorders. In: Stores, G. (ed.), *A Clinical Guide to Sleep Disorders in Children and Adolescents*. Cambridge: Cambridge University Press, pp. 42–52.

Stores, G. (2006). The protean manifestations of childhood narcolepsy and their misinterpretation. *Dev Med Child Neurol*, 48, 307–310.

Stores, G. (2009a). Sleep disorders in general and in adolescence. *J Fam Health*, 19, 51–53.

Stores, G. (2009b). Sleep disorders in children and adolescents. In: Gelder, M.G., Andreasen, N.C. & Lopez-Ibor, J.J., Jr. (eds.), *New Oxford Textbook of Psychiatry*. Second edition, Vol. 2. Oxford: Oxford University Press, pp. 1693–1702.

Stores, G. (2009c). *Sleep Problems in Children and Adolescents: The Facts*. Oxford: Oxford University Press.

Stores, G. (2009d). *Insomnia and Other Adult Sleep Problems: The Facts*. Oxford: Oxford University Press.

Stores, G. (2010). Psychosocial impact of narcolepsy in children and adolescents. In: Goswami, M., Pandi-Perumal, S.R. & Thorpy, M.J. (eds.), *Narcolepsy: A Clinical Guide*. New York: Humana Press, pp. 181–187.

Stores, G. & Crawford, C. (1998). Medical student education in sleep and its disorders. *J R Coll Physicians Lond*, 32, 149–153.

Stores, R. & Wiggs, L. (1998). Sleep education in clinical psychology courses in the UK. *Clin Psychol Forum*, 119, 14–18.

Stores, G., Zaiwalla, Z. & Bergel, N. (1991). Frontal lobe complex partial seizures in children: a form of epilepsy at particular risk of misdiagnosis. *Dev Med Child Neurol*, 33, 998–1009.

Thacker, K., Devinsky, O., Perrine, K., et al. (1993). Nonepileptic seizures during apparent sleep. *Ann Neurol*, 33, 414–418.

Thomas, A., Bonnani, L. & Onofri, M. (2007). Symptomatic REM sleep behaviour disorder. *Neurol Sci*, 28(Suppl 1), S21–S36.

Thorpy, M.J. (2000). Historical perspective on sleep and man. In: Culebras, A. (ed.), *Sleep Disorders and Neurological Disease*. New York, NY: Marcel Dekker, pp. 1–36.

Thorpy, M. (2001). Current concepts in the etiology, diagnosis and treatment of narcolepsy. *Sleep Med*, 2, 5–17.

Tinuper, P., Provini, F. & Bisulli, F., et al. (2007). Movement disorders in sleep: guidelines for differentiating epileptic from non-epileptic motor phenomena arising from sleep. *Sleep Med Rev*, 11, 255–267.

Wachter, R.M. & Holmboe, E.S. (2009). Diagnostic errors and patient safety. *J Am Med Assoc*, 302, 258.

Walsh, P. (2009). Quoted by S. MacDonald. *Sunday Times*, 20th September.

Welsh, C.H. & Fugit, R.V. (2006). Medications that can cause insomnia. In: Lee-Chiong, T. (ed.), *Sleep: A Comprehensive Handbook*. Hoboken, NJ: Wiley-Liss, pp. 103–109.

Wiggs, L. & Stores, G. (1996). Sleep problems in children with severe intellectual disabilities: what help is being provided? *J Appl Res Intellect Disabil*, 9, 160–165.

Wolfson, A.R. & Carskadon, M.A. (2003). Understanding adolescent sleep patterns and school performance: a critical appraisal. *Sleep Med Rev*, 7, 491–506.

Zozula, R., Bodow, M., Yatcilla, D., et al. (2001). Development of a brief, self-administered instrument for assessing sleep knowledge in medical education: 'The ASKME Survey'. *Sleep*, 24, 227–233.

Chapter 15

Sleep and shift-work

J. Axelsson, G. Kecklund, and M. Sallinen

Introduction

Increasing demands for emergency and health services, energy supply, economic returns, and flexibility to travel and carry out activities such as eating out, have resulted in a rapid development of the so-called 24-hour society, which is particularly present in the industrialized world. A 'shift-worker' is, broadly speaking, someone who works beyond the conventional 8–9 hours work day, often into the night or with very early starting times. Shift-work includes permanently displaced work hours (e.g. night work), rotating shift-work (typically alternation in 8 hours or 12 hours shifts across the 24-hour cycle) and other types of unscheduled working hours (Åkerstedt et al., 1984). About 30% of the working force in the European countries have atypical schedules (weekend work and irregular schedules) and 14% have long shifts (at least 10 hours) on a regular basis (Boisard et al., 2002; Stevens et al., 2004). A number of studies, some based on stratified samples, report that about 15–30% of the workers can be classified as shift-workers (Drake et al., 2004; Karlsson et al., 2001; Bureau, 2005); a number that comes down slightly if only including workers having night shifts on a regular basis. In a Finnish study of randomly selected healthy young adults, 25% of women and 22% of men were shift-workers (Puttonen et al., 2009).

Shift-work is particularly common in transportation and in emergency/health services, and includes many security sensitive professions such as nurses, physicians, police officers, fire fighters, pilots, and power plants operators (Barger et al., 2009). Many of these workers have been 'forced' to be shift-workers as there are few opportunities to get a day job in these professions without extensive experience. Indeed, up to 80% of the shift-workers would have preferred to work days and only one in five choose shift-work for personal preference (Bureau, 2005).

Sleep patterns and disturbances in shift-work

Shift-worker's sleep, as any other person's sleep, is determined by a number of factors relating to his or her ability to sleep, need for sleep, opportunities to sleep, and motivation to sleep (Fig. 15.1).

The mechanisms underlying the regulation of the sleep-wake rhythm will be discussed in detail later. For the shift-worker, the 'opportunity for sleep' is strongly limited compared to day workers, since the timing of shifts requires at intervals the shift-worker to sleep during the normal waking period and to work during the normal sleeping period of the human body (Fig. 15.1).

Sleep-wake pattern in connection with various shifts

Shift-worker's sleep is most affected in connection with the morning and night shifts, as these shifts overlap with the normal human sleep period. *Prior to the early morning shift* (start time at 6:00 or earlier), the main pattern is the curtailment of sleep by, on average, 2 hours, even if the

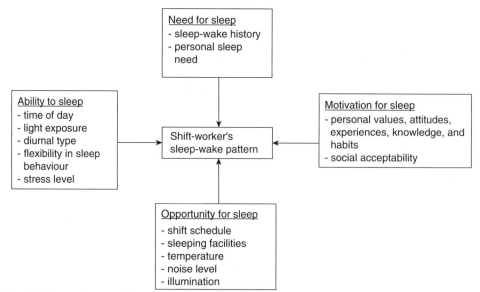

Fig. 15.1 Determinants of the sleep-wake pattern in shift work.

amount of an actual curtailment depends largely on the start time of the shift. Advancing the start time by an hour leads to a shortening of nocturnal sleep by about 45 minutes (Ingre et al., 2008; Sallinen et al., 2003). Also, postponing the start time to later than 6:00 leads to an extension of sleep (Ingre et al., 2008; Rosa et al., 1996).

Due to the short sleep prior to the early morning shift, it is quite common for the shift-worker to experience difficulties in awakening and non-refreshing sleep even if electroencephalography-based indicators usually show no impairments in sleep quality within the sleep period (Åkerstedt et al., 1991; Kecklund et al., 1997). Afternoon napping is a relatively common way to compensate for inadequate nocturnal sleep: about one-fourth of the shift-workers take a nap in the afternoon after the early morning shift (Åkerstedt et al., 1991). The prevalence of napping can, however, be much higher, up to 70–90%, if the morning shift is followed by, for example, a night shift that starts on the same day (Sallinen et al., 2003; Garbarion et al., 2002).

Prior to the first night shift, about 50% of the shift-workers take an afternoon or evening nap (Åkerstedt and Torsvall, 1985; Rosa, 1993). Consequently, the other half of the shift-workers have stayed awake for 24 hours or even more without any sleep before going to bed after the first night shift. A rule of thumb seems to be that the later the start time of the night shift, the more likely is napping prior to the shift (Sallinen et al., 2003).

Daytime sleep between two successive night shifts is usually 4–5 hours in duration and usually starts an hour after the end of the shift (Åkerstedt et al., 1991; Knauth and Rutenfranz, 1981; Tilley et al., 1982). This amount of sleep can be considered to be far too little, in particular since the shift-worker is under sleep loss already before going to bed after the night shift. Compared to nocturnal sleep, day sleep contains less stage 2 and rapid eye movement (REM) sleep, while the amount of slow wave sleep (SWS) remains relatively unchanged (Åkerstedt et al., 1991). Afternoon napping between two successive night shifts is less common than napping prior to the first night shift: it occurs in about one-fourth of the cases (Åkerstedt et al., 1991; Rosa, 1993) (Fig. 15.2).

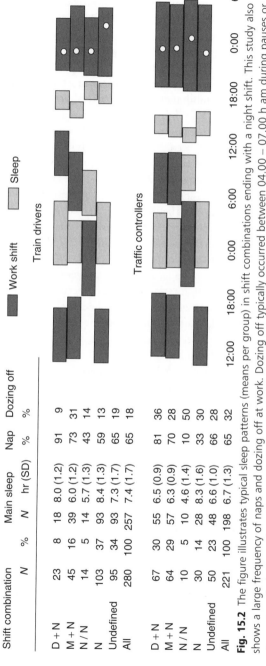

Shift combination	N	%	Main sleep N	hr (SD)	Nap %	Dozing off %
D + N	23	8	18	8.0 (1.2)	91	9
M + N	45	16	39	6.0 (1.2)	73	31
N / N	14	5	14	5.7 (1.3)	43	14
N	103	37	93	8.4 (1.3)	59	13
Undefined	95	34	93	7.3 (1.7)	65	19
All	280	100	257	7.4 (1.7)	65	18
D + N	67	30	55	6.5 (0.9)	81	36
M + N	64	29	57	6.3 (0.9)	70	28
N / N	10	5	10	4.6 (1.4)	10	50
N	30	14	28	8.3 (1.6)	33	30
Undefined	50	23	48	6.6 (1.0)	66	28
All	221	100	198	6.7 (1.3)	65	32

Fig. 15.2 The figure illustrates typical sleep patterns (means per group) in shift combinations ending with a night shift. This study also shows a large frequency of naps and dozing off at work. Dozing off typically occurred between 04.00 – 07.00 h am during pauses or stops at stations (Reproduced from Sallinen et al., 2003, with permission).

Sleep-wake pattern in connection with various shift combinations and cycles

It is not only the start and end times of a single shift that affect sleep, but also the combinations and cycles certain shifts construct. An example of this is given in Fig. 15.2 that shows the average sleep-wake rhythm of train drivers and railway traffic controllers in various shift combinations (Sallinen et al., 2003). Different shift systems can be divided into the following categories: regular three-shift-work, irregular three-shift-work (usually schedules are done in periods of a couple of weeks), regular two-shift-work, and permanent night work. In addition, there is a variety of alternatives to organize work hours within each of these categories.

A short rest period between two successive shifts is one of the most common characteristics of shift combinations that jeopardises the fulfilment of shift-workers' sleep need (Axelsson et al., 2004; Roach et al., 2003; Sallinen et al., 2003). The relationship between the duration of a break and the amount of sleep gained during the break is dependent on the timing of the break. The study of Roach et al. (2003) on train drivers showed that a mean of 8 hours of sleep or more was obtained during a 12-hour break that began between 20:00 and 22:00, during a 16-hour break that began between 18:00 and 22:00, and during almost all 24-hour break irrespective of their start time. In all, a 12-hour break seems to be often too short to allow even a minimum of 6 hours of sleep between two shifts: only a 12-hour break that starts between 20:00 and 0:00 is likely to lead to the fulfilment of this minimum criterion of sleep duration. In shift-work, evening shift-morning shift combinations, including only an 8- to 10-hour break, are quite widespread and the amount of sleep obtained between these shifts is usually less than 6 hours (Axelsson et al., 2004; Sallinen et al., 2003).

A number of consecutive shifts that overlap with the standard nocturnal sleep period often cause an accumulation of sleep loss. In case of, for example, five consecutive night shifts, the amount of sleep loss can be around 2.5 hours per 24-hour day, which makes a total of 10 hours at the beginning of the last night shift. A similar pattern can be found in association with several consecutive early morning shifts. The severity of sleep loss is, of course, dependent on the individual's capacity and possibilities to phase shift his or her circadian rhythms. For example, an individual with a good capacity to phase delay while working a spell of consecutive night shifts is in a more favourable position to sleep between the shifts than his or her counterpart with a limited capacity. In addition, exceptional circumstances, such as working on an oil rig, may facilitate sleeping during daytime due to low social demands during daytime and good possibilities to avoid exposure to morning light.

Two of the most studied shift cycle characteristics with respect to sleep are *the direction and speed of shift rotation.* Systematic reviews by Driscoll et al. (2007) and Bambra et al. (2008) concluded that a change from backward-rotating shifts to forward-rotating shifts results in improvements in sleep. These improvements are seen in sleep quality and possibly in sleep length on night shift days, in particular. It may also be that fast shift rotations are preferable to slow rotations. The best solution is probably achieved when these two characteristics of shift schedule—fast and forward shift rotation—are both present. In a study by Härmä et al. (2006), this kind of intervention was performed with relatively encouraging results: the replacement of a slowly backward-rotating shift system (E [evening shift] E E E F [free day] M [morning shift] M M M F N [night shift] N N N) with a rapidly forward-rotating system (e.g. M M E E N N F F F F) improved sleep quality, whereas the amount of sleep remained quite the same.

Another typical change in shifts is *to replace 8-hour shifts with 12-hour shifts.* Results from the effects of this change are somewhat mixed and the present conclusion is that no dramatic changes occur in sleep following this shift rescheduling, given that the amount of weekly work hours remains the same in the shift change (Smith et al., 1998). A reason for this result may be that a change from 8-hour shifts to 12-hour shifts also makes the shift schedule more regular, prevents the occurrence of quick changeovers and double shifts, and provides workers with a sufficient recovery period between two consecutive shift cycles.

Permanent night work is a remedy to cover all 24 hours of the day without shift rotations from day to night. Results from the effects of permanent night work on sleep suggest that permanent night workers sleep somewhat more than the rotating shift-workers in association with night shifts, but if one takes the whole shift cycle into account no such difference can be observed (Folkard, 2008). It is also important to notice that the permanent night workers are a highly selected group of people, which makes it difficult to compare their results with the results of rotating shift-workers.

Shift-workers who have the same shift schedule can have very different sleep-wake rhythms. For example, a study by Daurat and Foret (2004) showed that nurses who worked 12-hour day and night shifts had two main sleep-wake rhythms in association with the night shift. A half of the nurses took a nap during the night shift and averaged 3 hours of sleep between two successive shifts, while the other half did not take a nap during the night shift but slept twice as long as the night-nappers after the night shift. Similarly, Darwent et al. (2008) found some differences in the train drivers' sleep strategies during an extended freight-haul operation.

In real life, there are often several options for a sleep strategy in various shift system and it may be difficult to recommend one strategy over some others (Åkerstedt, 1998a). The most important principles are to gain sleep as much as possible prior to the early morning and night shifts and also sleep for 1–2 hours close to the beginning of the night shift. Some of the recommended sleep strategies are discussed later in Chapter 16.

During the first days off after a shift spell, the nocturnal sleep period is usually 0.5–1 hours longer than habitually (Axelsson et al., 2004; Härmä et al., 2006). However, in extreme circumstances the sleep-wake rhythm on the recovery days may be different to this pattern. For example, after working 14 consecutive night shifts on an oil rig, shift-workers' nocturnal sleep at home can be quite short for a couple of days (around 6 hours) and prolong just after that as their wake-up time gradually delays (Bjorvatn et al., 1998). Also, sleep quality can be reduced for several days in this case. In practice, the number of days needed for the complete recovery from a shift spell depends on a variety of individual and shift system related factors (see Chapter 16).

Individual differences in sleep disturbances in shift-work

Sleep disturbances experienced by the average shift-worker are far less severe than those reported by the average insomniac, non-shift-working patient (Åkerstedt et al., 2008). Compared to day workers, the prevalence rate of insomnia symptoms (difficulties in initiating and maintaining sleep and advanced awakenings) is around 10% higher for shift-workers (Drake et al., 2004; Garbarino et al., 2002). However, when looking at these results, one should bear in mind that the above-mentioned results are based on questions about sleep disturbances in general, while sleep disturbances occur mostly in connection with the night and early morning shifts. In practice, the experiences of 'too little sleep', premature awakening, and non-refreshing sleep are very common in association with the night and early morning shift.

When assessing sleep disturbances in shift-work it is important to be aware of the individual differences in adaptation to shift-work. For example, in some shift-workers, sleep-wake disturbances are so severe that they can be diagnosed with shift-work disorder (SWD), while some others may work on shifts for decades without notable problems. There are a number of individual factors that, to some extent, explain why some individuals cope with shift-work better than some others (Härmä, 1995). Sleep is one of those factors. In particular, tolerance to sleep loss, sleep need, sleep flexibility (the ability to sleep at irregular times and in unusual places), and preference for the start and end times of daily sleep have been proposed to influence shift-workers' tolerance to their working hours (Costa et al., 1989; Folkard and Monk, 1979; Smith et al., 2002; Van Dongen, 2006), even if prospective studies on the predictive power of these factors for shift-workers' health and well-being are largely missing. In practice, self-selection into shift-work and 'the healthy worker effect' make it difficult to estimate exactly the role of the individual factors in adaptation to shift-work.

Shift-work-related sleep disturbances usually ease or disappear after exiting shift-work. In fact, sleep quality improves more in workers with night work than in their counterparts without night work after retirement (Vahtera et al., 2009).

Sleepiness

Subjective sleepiness

Reduced alertness and impaired performance is one of the major consequences of insufficient sleep and it is therefore not surprising that shift-work is associated with excessive sleepiness (Son et al., 2008; Ursin et al., 2009; Åkerstedt, 1995). Sleepiness has been widely studied in shift-work research, however most of the studies are questionnaire-based and the designs are cross-sectional. Åhsberg et al. (2000) compared three different subjective instruments of fatigue and sleepiness and found a high degree of correspondence; thus, irrespective of the subjective instrument, sleepiness peaked at night, was lowest during the evening shift, and moderately increased during the morning shift. Some studies have addressed the question of unintentional falling asleep at work, which is an obvious sign of severe sleepiness, and found that shift-workers who work at night have a higher risk (Åkerstedt et al., 2002a; Coleman and Dement, 1986; Prokop and Prokop, 1955; Ursin et al., 2009). The study by Åkerstedt et al. (2002b) showed a moderate increased odds ratio (OR: 1.6; 95% confidence interval [CI]: 1.14–2.23) for shift-workers who had night work, whereas the OR (1.05) for those who have shift-work, which did not include night shifts, was non-significant. Interestingly, shift-work was not a risk factor for unintentional falling asleep episodes during leisure time (Åkerstedt et al., 2002b), which possibly could be related to the high frequency of intentional napping among shift-workers (Åkerstedt and Torsvall, 1985) (see also Fig. 15.3). Figure 15.3 illustrates the development of rated sleepiness in a rotating shift schedule across both work and recovery days.

Physiological sleepiness

Relatively few field studies have monitored physiological sleepiness in real-life shift-work. In a pioneering study on train drivers, Torsvall and Åkerstedt (1987) showed a clear increase in physiological sleepiness during the night shift as demonstrated by increased alpha and theta power density and higher occurrence of slow eye movements. The covariation between subjective ratings of sleepiness and physiological signs of sleepiness was high. A study on truck drivers from the same group showed similar results (Kecklund and Åkerstedt, 1993). In another study by Torsvall et al. (1989), it was found that 20% of the shift-workers (working as control room operators) dozed off (mean sleep time was 43 minutes) during the night. Interestingly, those that dozed off at work tended to report that the work shift included more passive supervision, which suggests that work conditions may play an important role on whether unintentional sleep events will occur. Most falling asleep incidents started around 3:00 (±30 minutes). The peak in physiological sleepiness during late night and early morning hours was also observed in a power plant simulator study by Gillberg et al. (2003) on real shift-workers. Mitler et al. (1997) made a large-scale study on truck drivers where they compared four different shift systems of which one only included

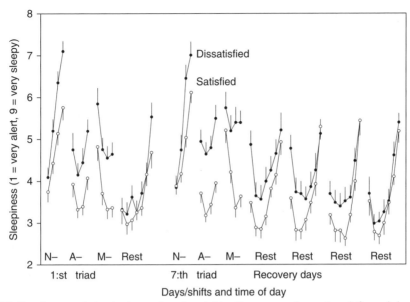

Fig. 15.3 Sleepiness and standard error bars for night, afternoon and morning shifts and days off during the first and seventh triads of shifts for both tolerant (satisfied) and intolerant shift workers (dissatisfied with their shift system). The first four days of recovery are also presented. Satisfied (open circles) and dissatisfied (closed circles) shift workers. (Reproduced from Axelsson et al., 2004, with kind permission from Springer Science+Business Media).

daytime work. During daytime, the prevalence of video-recorded sleepiness events was low (1.5% of the entire recording time), whereas the highest prevalence of sleepiness events (11.6%) occurred for the permanent night group. Eighty-five percent of the sleepiness events occurred during evening and nighttime. The individual differences were also noteworthy and only a small group (10% of the participants) of the drivers accounted for 54% of the sleepiness events. More recently, Lockley et al. (2004) carried out an intervention study in which interns working more than 80 hours (involving 24-hour shifts) during the traditional schedule reduced their maximum shift length to 16 hours and the weekly working hours to 65 hours. Physiological sleepiness, which they called attentional failures, during on-call nights was reduced by approximately 50% (from 5.5 failures per intern overnight to 2.6 failures per intern overnight) after the intervention.

Early morning and sleepiness

Early morning work is also associated with increased sleepiness, although studies using physiological sleepiness recordings are rare. Härmä et al. (2002) examined self-rated sleepiness (Karolinska Sleepiness Scale [KSS] ratings) and found that severe sleepiness (KSS ratings ≥ 7) peaked at nighttime and was much lower in the afternoon, whereas morning shifts were in-between. In another paper from the same study, Sallinen et al. (2005) found that early start time of the morning shift increased sleepiness. The latter finding was also demonstrated in a study by Ingre et al. (2004) in which the train drivers were experimentally scheduled to the same trip but with three different start times of the shift. This means that work characteristics were very similar between the experimental conditions. A large majority (82%) of the drivers in the earliest shift (start time at 5:49) rated severe sleepiness (KSS ratings ≥ 7) at least once during the work shift. However, severe sleepiness was also relatively common towards the end of the late day shift (start time at 9:49) that finished around 22:00.

Shift system and sleepiness

The characteristics of the shift system are an important determinant for sleepiness. Thus, some intervention studies show decreased levels of sleepiness when the shift schedule has changed from a slowly, backward-rotating system to a rapidly, forward-rotating system (Härmä et al., 2006; Viitasalo et al., 2008). It has also been argued that permanent night worker are less sleepy compared to rotating three-shift-workers (Wilkinson, 1992), because such a shift system facilitates circadian adaptation to night work. However, Folkard (1992) has argued against this conclusion and in a recent paper he showed that very few (<5%) of the permanent night workers demonstrated complete circadian adaptation to working at night. In fact, most of the night workers did not seem to adjust their circadian rhythm to the permanent night shift system. Some recent studies show that short (<11 hours) break time between the shifts increases sleepiness (Axelsson et al., 2004; Lowden et al., 1998; Sallinen et al., 2003). As mentioned earlier, early start time of the morning shift also increases sleepiness (Ingre et al., 2004; Sallinen et al., 2003) although an advanced changeover time between the night and the morning shift may result in a slight reduction of sleepiness during the night (Rosa et al., 1996). There are also many studies that have evaluated a change from 8-hour shifts to 12-hour shifts (Smith et al., 1998). The results are, however, quite inconsistent and some studies show increased sleepiness (Rosa, 1995), whereas others show no change or that sleepiness decreases (Lowden et al., 1998; Peacock et al., 1983; Tucker et al., 1996). Some recent studies on train drivers, who have highly irregular shift systems, have identified length of the shift as a significant determinant of sleepiness (Sallinen et al., 2003). Kecklund and Åkerstedt (1993) also found that the length of night shift was the strongest predictor of both physiological sleepiness (alpha power density) and subjective sleepiness (KSS ratings) in a field study of long-distance truck drivers.

It has been argued, based on laboratory studies on cumulative sleep restriction, that sleepiness may accumulate across shifts (Axelsson et al., 2008). However, there are surprisingly few studies showing such a pattern. Paley and Tepas (1994) show an increase in subjective sleepiness across a 2-week period of night work and afternoon work but not when they worked day shifts. In contrast to their finding, a recent paper by Son et al. (2008) observed that the peak in (subjective) severe sleepiness occurred on the first night shift and then slightly decreased across the 5–7 consecutive days with night work. The pattern for the day shift was quite similar, although a peak was observed during the 7th day shift in a small sub-sample. Also studies on oil rig workers have shown that sleepiness decreased across a sequence of 14 consecutive night shifts (Bjorvatn et al., 1998) or in a shift system based on 7 night shifts followed by 7 consecutive day shifts (Bjorvatn et al., 2006).

Operational performance and safety

There are very few studies on real work performance in shift-work (Folkard and Tucker, 2003). Bjerner et al. (1955) found a peak in reading errors during the night shift for operators at a gas plant. The previously mentioned study by Torsvall and Åkerstedt (1987) observed errors such as signals passed at danger that coincided with the physiological sleepiness events during nighttime. Similar results were demonstrated in other studies on train drivers (Hildebrandt et al., 1974; Kogi and Ohta, 1975). An intervention study related to reduced weekly working hours for interns (with on-call work at night) also decreased the number of serious medical errors by approximately 30% in intensive care units (Landrigan et al., 2004) (Chapter 17). However, there are also studies that do not show any significant increase in errors during the night shift (Gillberg et al., 2003; Monk and Embrey, 1981). It has been suggested that the lack of effect on real work performance during the night shift may be related to lower work demands and less risk of mistakes (Gillberg et al., 2003). In many occupations it is difficult to obtain good measures of real work performance and they have therefore used short performance tests as a proxy for work performance. The most used tests are psychomotor vigilance test (PVT)-related tests such as simple reaction time tasks. The results are somewhat inconsistent between studies but in general lapses (extended reaction times) peak towards the end of the night shift, although the increase sometimes fails to reach significance (Axelsson et al., 1998, 2004; Bjorvatn et al., 2006; Bonnefond et al., 2006; Gillberg et al., 2003; Härmä et al., 2006; Rosa and Bonnet, 1993; Tilley et al., 1982).

Injuries and accidents

Since shift-work is clearly associated with severe sleepiness, it is not surprising that night work increases the risk of accidents and injuries (Åkerstedt et al., 2002a; Dembe et al., 2006; Hamelin, 1987; Smith et al., 1994) (Chapter 16). Folkard et al. (2005) estimated, based on a review of several studies, that the risk of an accident is 30% higher during the night shift and 18% higher during the evening shift (the morning shift was the reference). The increased risk associated with the evening shift is somewhat surprising since sleepiness normally is rather low at this shift. However, the epidemiological study by Dembe et al. (2006) also observed a robust increase risk of injuries during the evening shift (hazard ratio [HR]: 1.43). Thus, it is possible that the safety risk during the evening shifts is related to other factors than sleepiness, for example, specific work tasks, staffing levels, or length of work shift. Some of the major industrial disasters, such as Chernobyl, Three Mile Island, the Exxon Valdez, and Bhopal, have identified difficult shift systems (in particular related to the night shift) as important contributing factors, which suggest anecdotal evidence of a relationship between shift-work and accidents (Mitler et al., 1988).

Some papers have related the accident risk to specific shift system characteristics such as length of shift, type of shift system, and whether several consecutive night shifts increase the risk (Folkard et al., 2005; Folkard and Tucker, 2003). Several studies show that long working hours, both long work days (e.g. due to having 12-hour shifts) and long working week (>60 hours) increases the risk of accidents (Dembe et al., 2005, 2009; Folkard and Tucker, 2003; Hänecke et al., 1998). Folkard and Tucker (2003) observed a trend indicating that the accident risk increases across successive shifts, particularly during the night. Thus, they estimate that the accident risk is 36% higher on the fourth night shift compared to the first night shift. Dembe et al. (2006, 2009) compare the accident risk for different shift systems but did not find any clear pattern. Thus, it is so far not possible to conclude whether permanent night work has a higher accident risk than rotating shift systems. Moreover, it is not possible to draw any conclusions of whether rapidly rotating shift systems are superior to slowly backward-rotating shift systems, despite the fact that several studies show that the latter shift system often is associated with improved sleep and less sleepiness (Driscoll et al., 2007).

Night work is also associated with increased accident risks outside work. Stutts et al. (2003) showed that shift-work was a risk factor for sleepiness-related car crashes in general. Barger et al. (2005) and Gold et al. (1992) found increased risk of reporting a motor vehicle crash (or a near miss incident) when they returned home from a long work shift or night shift. Simulator studies of shift-workers driving home after the night shift supported the findings by Barger et al. and Gold et al. (Åkerstedt et al., 2005; De Valck et al., 2007). Thus, lane crossings and lane variability, subjective sleepiness, and blink duration (as a marker of physiological sleepiness) increased after the night shift compared to driving after a normal night sleep, or compared to simulator driving after a morning shift or an afternoon shift.

Shift-work disorder

Shift-work disorder is a circadian rhythm sleep disorder caused by the clash between the working schedule and the endogenous sleep-wake cycle of the worker. The main symptoms are excessive sleepiness during work, or on the commute to/from work, or insomnia during daytime sleep. The diagnosis of SWD, defined by the International Classification of Sleep Disorders (ICSD-2) (American Academy of Sleep Medicine, 2005) is based on four criteria: (1) complaint of insomnia or excessive sleepiness temporally associated with a recurring work schedule that overlaps the usual time for sleep, (2) symptoms must be associated with the shift-work schedule over the course of at least 1 month, (3) circadian and sleep time misalignment as demonstrated by sleep log or actigraphic monitoring for ≥7 days, and (4) sleep disturbance is not explainable by another sleep disorder, a medical or neurological disorder, mental disorder, medication use or substance use disorder. The criteria do not include degree or severity of the problems.

Although there are many studies on sleep-wakefulness and shift-work, only a few have made an attempt to estimate the prevalence of SWD (Schwartz and Roth, 2006). Furthermore, the limited number of studies on shift-work and SWD show rather inconsistent results. On the one hand, one could argue that the majority of the shift-workers suffer from the symptoms of SWD as many as three-fourths of the shift-workers have impaired wakefulness and/or insufficient sleep during night work or early morning work (Åkerstedt, 1998b). On the other hand, some recent epidemiological studies show that the difference in sleep-wake complaints between shift-workers and daytime workers maybe relatively small. In a national representative sample of 3,400 Swedish workers, Åkerstedt et al. (2008) found that shift-workers did not report as many sleep problems as expected. In fact, the difference to day workers was only marginal and shift-workers only reported slightly more problems with insufficient sleep and nodding off at work. Similar results have also been obtained in other studies (Tepas and Mahan, 1989). The Swedish study also included clinically diagnosed insomniacs as a reference group and found that a very small proportion of night workers had a prevalence of sleep disturbances similar to those seen in insomniacs. The authors suggest that many shift-workers may perceive their sleep disturbances and wakefulness problems as a part of their job, which may lead to under-reporting of sleep-wake complaints.

In a representative community-based sample of 2,570 adults, Drake et al. (2004) estimated that about 10% of the shift-workers suffer from SWD. Even though they found that 32% of night workers and 26% of the rotating shift-workers fulfilled the criteria of SWD, so did 18% of the day workers. This study did not specifically ask whether the workers had insomnia or excessive sleepiness associated to their work schedule, and assuming that 18% of the shift-working population also suffer from insomnia, as found in the day working group, the 'over risk' was around 10% in the shift-working group. Both the study by Drake et al. and the study by Åkerstedt et al. show that it is difficult to accurately estimate the prevalence of SWD if one is not specifically asking for problems related to the working hours.

In a recent publication of 104 oil rig workers, Waage et al. (2009) reported that 23% fulfilled the criteria of SWD using questions based on the ICSD-2 criteria, namely: (1) Do you experience either difficulties sleeping or excessive sleepiness? (yes or no), (2) Is the sleep or sleepiness problem related to the work schedule that makes you work when you normally would sleep? (yes or no), (3) Have you had this sleep or sleepiness problem related to the work schedule for at least 1 month? (yes or no). Subjects were classified as having SWD when they responded 'yes' to all three questions. The resulting prevalence of 23% is considerably higher than the studies not specifically asking about work-related problems of sleep and wakefulness. This suggests that studies not specifically asking for work-related problems probably underestimate the amount suffering from SWD.

The 'healthy worker' effect is probably one reason for the rather low prevalence of SWD reported in many studies. A healthy worker effect would result in fewer insomniacs amongst shift- than day workers as those developing insomnia-related problems are likely to drop out. Indeed, Waage et al. argue that the number suffering from SWD is probably higher than 23% in other shift-working populations since oil rig workers go through health and drug screenings every second year, hence limiting the workers with insomnia-related problems or other clinical diseases.

Taken together, it is difficult to estimate the prevalence of SWD. One problem is probably due to the shift-workers' own subjective definition of an insomnia problem. Although it is clear that the majority of the shift-workers have severely shortened day sleep—surpassing the effects seen in most insomniacs by far—many may not see this as a problem related to quality of life or their well-being. It is likely that the workers see their disturbed sleep and wakefulness as a natural part of their working life. As such, this does not mean that they are not suffering from SWD, it merely says that they have accepted the sleep disturbances and sleepiness associated with certain shifts. Thus, SWD is probably more common than previously reported. There is also a lack of knowledge on the causes of SWD. For example, do the shift system and the workload play a role? Early morning work is often associated with severe reduction of sleep, poor sleep quality, and high levels of sleepiness (Härmä et al., 2002; Ingre et al., 2004, 2008; Åkerstedt, 1991). Hence, SWD may not necessarily be associated with only night work but can probably also appear during other shifts, in particular when the work schedule interferes with the endogenous circadian sleep-wake cycle or when the break time between shifts is restricted (Roach et al., 2003). See Fig. 15.4 for illustration of individuals experiencing severe sleepiness in a forward-rotating shift system with limited recovery time between shifts.

The clinical relevance of SWD is, today, mainly related to safety issues; severe impairments of wakefulness are related to worse performance and accidents. The effects of SWD on clinical health are less explored. It has been observed that workers with SWD also report more mental and physical health complaints (Drake et al., 2004; Waage et al., 2009). However, these data are limited to cross-sectional self-reports and there are no data on more objectively measured health outcomes or in prospective studies on the long-term health consequences of SWD.

Thus, longitudinal studies are clearly needed in which individuals are followed when they enter shift-work, and compared with a well-matched control group including only daytime workers.

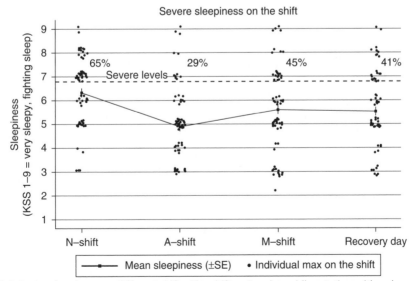

Fig. 15.4 Severe sleepiness on different shifts. The shift system is rapidly rotating with only 8–9 hours off between shifts. The percentage shows how many workers that have experienced severe sleepiness (ratings of 7 or above on the Karolinska Sleepiness scale = KSS) on the shift (or between 10.00 h and 22.00 h on the day off).

Table 15.1 Shift-work and health risks compared to day work

	Relative risk	Evidence*
Transient insomnia and short sleep	12	+++
Fatigue and accidents	1–2	+++
Cardiovascular disease	0.9–2.3	++
Coronary risk factors	about 2	++
Metabolic syndrome	1.6–1.7	++
Obesity	1–2	++
Peptic ulcer	About 2	++
General poor health	2–3.2	++
Prostate cancer	1.1–3.0	++
Breast cancer	1.0–1.8	++
Other cancer forms	?	+
Type 2 diabetes	About 2	+
Rheumatoid arthritis	1.3	+
Long-term sleep disorders	2.8	+
Preterm birth	1–2	++
Low birth weight	1.0–1.6	+
Miscarriage	1.4	+
Mortality	1.2–2.6	++
Depression	?	(+)
Cerebral infarction	?	(+)

*+++ = strong evidence, ++ = moderate evidence, + = weak evidence, (+) = no evidence.

Long-term health consequences of shift-work

On top of the immediate effects on sleep and wakefulness, shift-work has also been shown to cause general poor health (Ingre and Åkerstedt, 2004; van Amelsvoort et al., 2004) as well as a wide range of short- and long-term health problems. The most prominent ones are disturbed sleep (which can become chronic), cardiovascular and gastrointestinal diseases (such as gastric and duodenal ulcers), and metabolic disturbances (such as obesity and metabolic syndrome) (see Table 15.1). The recent classification of shift-work by the World Health Organization (WHO) as being probably carcinogenic has rendered further interest in the health aspects of shift-work (Straif et al., 2007). Other health-related problems with weaker links are birth-related problems (such as preterm birth and low birth weight) (Knutsson, 2003) and possibly diabetes (Mikuni et al., 1983) and all-over mortality (Knutsson et al., 2004).

Sleep

Several researchers have proposed that the acute sleep disturbances seen in shift-workers would increase the risk for developing chronic sleep disturbances. A twin study of elderly (+65 years) monozygotic twins, discordant on the exposure to night work, confirms a rather potent risk (relative risk [RR]: 2.8) for chronic sleep disturbances in the twin who had worked shifts (Ingre and

Åkerstedt, 2004). A comparison of 13 nurses who had worked night for at least 10 years had less SWS when compared to a group of 15 nurses with day work (Dumont et al., 1997). The few studies on this issue indicate a risk for shift-workers to develop chronic sleep disturbances.

Cardiovascular disease

A number of studies have analyzed how shift-work affects cardiovascular disease. Although several negative findings have been reported (Boggild et al., 1999; McNamee et al., 1996; Hermansson et al., 2007), many studies have shown an increase of approximately 40% (Tenkanen et al., 1997; Kawachi et al., 1995; Boggild and Knutsson, 1999). Several studies show that the risk increases with exposure, but the effect seems to vary largely from no effect (McNamee et al., 1996) to a significant increase starting from 6 years (Kawachi et al., 1995), 11–15 years (Knutsson et al., 1986), or even 30 years (Karlsson et al., 2005). There are less data on female than male shift-workers, but a Danish study using a random sample from the general population showed a similar increase of both men and women (about 30%) (Tuchsen et al., 2006), exactly repeating the risks that was found in Swedish case control study (Knutsson et al., 1999). In a study of 79,000 female American nurses, the risk of shift-work for cardiovascular disease was significant already after 6 years of shift-work, the RR then being 1.5 (Kawachi et al., 1995). In a recent prospective randomized cross-over trial, it was shown that physicians having 'on–call' night shifts had a higher rate of ventricular premature beats and a greater diastolic blood pressure, all pointing to an increased risk profile for cardiovascular disease (Rauchenzauner et al., 2009). It has also been shown that shift-work is particularly harmful for workers with high systolic blood pressure, which suggests that hypertension might be a mechanism by which shift-work increases the risk of cardiovascular disease (Virkkunen et al., 2007). Evidence from a population-based study of 1,543 young adults (25–39 years) suggests that male (but not female) shift-workers already have observable subclinical atherosclerosis before the age of 40 (Puttonen et al., 2009). This included higher thickness of the common carotid artery intima-media and an OR of 2.2 for carotid plaque.

It should be noted, however, that a recent review of the epidemiological evidence concludes that the causal evidence are limited and that more studies are needed (Frost et al., 2009). The main reason being that many of the studies suffer from limitations, particularly about information about exposure to night/shift-work and the use of confounders. There is an ongoing debate whether some lifestyle-related risk behaviours are confounders (non-shift-related risk factors) or mediators (risk factors caused by shift-work) amongst shift-workers. For example, smoking has been shown to be both a confounder as well as mediator between shift-work and cardiovascular disease. Although shift-workers are more prone to start smoking (van Amelsvoort et al., 2006), it has also been shown that smoking is more common in shift-workers even prior to starting working shifts (Nabe-Nielsen et al., 2008). Other probable mediators include metabolic disturbances.

Endocrine and metabolic disturbances

Both experimental and epidemiological studies have shown that shift-work leads to an alteration of wide number of endocrine and metabolic hormones. A rather consistent finding is that shift-workers often have higher levels of triglycerides, cholesterol, and worse blood lipids than day workers (Biggi et al., 2008; Karlsson et al., 2001, 2003; Puttonen et al., 2009; Nakamura et al., 1997). An early study of 33 railway workers showed that serum levels of glucose, cholesterol, uric acids, and total lipoproteins increase during night work (Theorell and Åkerstedt, 1976), effects that seem transient as the levels returned to baseline when the workers went back to day work.

Melatonin is lower in shift-workers during night shifts as well as during days off, 24-hour urine samples were taken during the second night shift and second day off (Hansen et al., 2006).

The adaptation of the circadian system to night work seems incomplete, as measured with melatonin. The melatonin rhythm has not adapted even amongst permanent night workers measured directly after the last night shift of a working week (Sack et al., 1992; Weibel et al., 1997), and with a large variation in the adaptation between individuals (Weibel et al., 1997). Oil rig workers seem to adapt better to a work week with night shifts, probably because of better control of light conditions, but the re-adaptation back to day work was very problematic amongst the majority (Gibbs et al., 2007). Three major patterns were seen during re-adaptation to day work, one-third phase-advanced, one-third phase-delayed further, and one-third showed little changes of their phase.

It has recently been shown that shift-workers younger than 50 have worse markers of insulin resistance than day workers (Nagaya et al., 2002). Endocrine and metabolic disease are about twice as common in shift-workers than day workers, as for example seen in Australian oil refinery workers, 3.5% versus 1.5% (Koller et al., 1978). Only a few studies exist on shift-work and diabetes, but there is some support for a slight increased prevalence of diabetes amongst shift-working female nurses (Kawachi et al., 1995), and Japanese male factory workers, the latter having a RR of about 2.3 (Mikuni et al., 1983). A Swedish cohort study of 2,354 shift-workers and 3,088 day workers showed an increased risk of mortality with diabetes as the underlying cause amongst shift-workers (Karlsson et al., 2005). The risk increased with exposure in this study having an extremely long follow-up period of up to 65 years. It has also been suggested that selection processes may reduce the chances of finding effects of shift-work on diabetes. Kivimäki and colleagues (2006) have shown that it was twice as common for shift-workers with prevalent diabetes or risk factors for diabetes to leave the organization within 2–4 years compared to those without diabetes or related risk factors. Several studies have showed that shift-work is related to weight gain, increased body mass index (BMI), or worse hip-waist ratio (Di Lorenzo et al., 2003; Nakamura et al., 1997; Niedhammer et al., 1996; Suwazono et al., 2008), and BMI has been shown to increase with exposure (van Amelsvoort et al., 1999). However, many studies have failed to find significant relationships between shift-work and weight changes, and the overall evidence must be seen as weak (Boggild and Knutsson, 1999). On the whole, there is rather clear evidence that shift-work-related behaviours cause endocrine and metabolic disturbances with limited adaptation of the circadian system and large problems of readapting after a period of night work.

Gastrointestinal disorders

Gastrointestinal disorders are more common in shift-workers than day workers (Scott and LaDou, 1994; Knutsson, 2003), but also in other non-day working groups (Tuchsen et al., 1994). Peptic ulcer has been a traditionally well-known problem amongst many shift-workers (Harrington, 1978) and especially in occupations related to shift-work such as taxi and truck drivers, railway employees, and factory workers. In a study of 11,567 Japanese workers, it was shown that the prevalence of peptic ulcers (diagnosed with X-ray) was doubled in shift-workers compared to day workers, the prevalence being 3.75% amongst shift-workers, 2.14% for former shift workers, and 1.72% amongst day workers (Segawa et al., 1987). On the other hand, a study of 1,754 aged Italian hospital workers showed a decreased risk of self-reported gastrointestinal disorder (Conway et al., 2008). Other common complaints amongst shift-workers are constipation and diarrhoea, which seem transiently related to the night shifts (Knutsson, 2003), indicating that the main problems are related to night work and probably night eating.

Cancer

Both female and male night shift-workers seem to have an increased risk of developing a number of different malignancies including breast (Hansen, 2001; Davis et al., 2001; Schernhammer et al.,

2001, 2006), colon, (Schernhammer et al., 2003) prostate (Kubo et al., 2006), and endometrial cancer (Viswanathan et al., 2007). It seems that the relative risk (RR) for cancer varies between 1.3 and 1.8, and that exposure needs to be around 20–30 years before significant effects are found (Hansen, 2001; Davis et al., 2001; Schernhammer et al., 2001, 2006), and with an increased risk with the frequency of night shifts (Davis et al., 2001). This work has lead to that the International Agency for Research on Cancer (IARC), a part of the World Health Organization, recently declared shift-work as probably carcinogenic to humans (group 2a classification) (Straif et al., 2007). However, a few studies have failed to find a significant relationship between shift-work and breast cancer (O'Leary et al., 2006; Schwartzbaum et al., 2007); and a recent review concluded that there is only support for a moderate link between shift-work and breast cancer, and then mainly for long-term exposure of 20–30 years (Kolstad, 2008). Interestingly, one study found that women who frequently turned on lights at home during sleep had an increased risk of breast cancer (O'Leary et al., 2006).

Data on a link between shift-work and prostate cancer have shown strong effects, RRs of 2.3 and 3.0 amongst fixed night workers and shift-workers, respectively (Kubo et al., 2006), marginal increases, (RR: 1.2) (Conlon et al., 2007), or no increase (RR: 1.19) (Schwartzbaum et al., 2007). Shift-work also show a marginal link to all over cancer, but not to colon cancer (Kolstad, 2008). The high prevalence of many cancer forms warrants further studies on the relationships and underlying mechanisms. There is particular need for studies with good control of exposure to shift-work and in more occupational groups than in previous studies (Kolstad, 2008).

Infections and sick leave

There is limited support for a link between shift-work and infections, although a slight increase for common infections has been shown (Mohren et al., 2002). A vulnerability to infections amongst shift-workers fits with recent data showing that shorter (<7 hours) or more disturbed sleep (reports collected for 14 days) increases the risk between 294% and 550%, respectively, for developing the common cold after being exposed to nasal drops with rhinovirus (Cohen et al., 2009). An increased sensitivity to infections might explain why some studies have reported more frequent sick leave amongst shift-workers than day workers. In interviews of 817 psychiatric staff, it was shown that 52% of the shift-workers had sick leave in the previous 12 months while this number was 38% in the day workers (Ohayon et al., 2002). A link between shift-work or exposure to shift-work and sick leave was not confirmed in a study of industry workers in Norway (Kleiven et al., 1998). A Danish study has shown that shift-work moderately increases the risk of disability pension in women (Tuchsen et al., 2008). A recent study has shown shift-work to increase the risk of female shift-workers to develop rheumatoid arthritis (a chronic inflammatory disease; RR: 1.33), but not in men (Puttonen et al., 2010b). The study was based on 229 new cases of rheumatoid arthritis (but only few men) in a sample of 70,376 government employees. This suggests that shift-work-related behaviours are related to the development of chronic inflammations.

Only a few studies are concerned with how shift-work affects the immune functions. Based on experimental studies, disturbed sleep has many potent effects on the immune system (Bryant et al., 2004), but epidemiological studies have shown rather inconsistent and moderate effects of disturbed sleep on inflammatory markers such as interleukin-6 and C-reactive protein. For example, in an analysis of 4,600 individuals from the Whitehall II Study, sleep had no effect on these inflammatory markers in men, but both increased in women sleeping extremely short (5 hours or less) (Miller et al., 2009) (Chapter 11). Studies on shift-workers are considerably smaller (lacking power) and suffer from methodological problems. A recent study of 208 Japanese male workers showed that white blood cell count was higher in shift-workers than day workers (Nishitani and

Sakakibara, 2007), which was suggested to relate to disturbed sleep but no other sleep parameters. Despite having control over the time of day for the samplings, it was not possible to exclude any circadian effects on their findings. To summarize, shift-workers may be more vulnerable to infections, as well as having increased risk of developing more chronic inflammatory disease.

Birth-related problems

Several studies have shown that shift-work is linked to low birth weight (−79 g) (Axelsson et al., 1989; MacDonald et al., 1988; Xu et al., 1994), preterm birth (about a doubled risk) (MacDonald et al., 1988; Xu et al., 1994), spontaneous abortion (MacDonald et al., 1988), miscarriage (RR = 1.44 and 3.2, respectively) (Axelsson et al., 1984; Mamelle et al., 1984), and irregular menstruation (Uehata and Sasakawa, 1982). These studies have included 60 occupational groups in Canada (MacDonald et al., 1988), textile workers in China (Xu et al., 1994), birth givers at two hospitals in France (Mamelle et al., 1984), and hospital staff and laboratory workers in Sweden (Axelsson et al., 1984, 1989). In a study of American nurses, shift-work was not related to menstrual irregularities on the whole, but nurses who had noticed menstrual irregularities also reported shorter and more disturbed sleep (Labyak et al., 2002). A recent population-based study in almost 40,000 Danish women only found marginal effects of shift-work on birth weight, a slight increased excess of small gestational-age babies (OR: 1.1) (Zhu et al., 2004). This study also found that fixed night workers prolonged the duration of pregnancy (OR: 1.3), and that this effect was mediated by industrial work. A recent review concluded that the larger studies have found smaller effects, and their pooled effects for the best quality studies were 1.26 for preterm delivery and non-significant for low birth weight (Bonzini et al., 2007). The authors also propose that it would be prudent to advice against long working hours, prolonged standing, and heavy physical work, particularly late in pregnancy.

Mortality

In a classical study by Taylor and Pocock (1972), the authors could not find a significant effect of shift-work on mortality, but a re-analysis of the same data set found ex-shift-workers to have increased risk of mortality, RR 1.2 (Knutsson et al., 2004), a risk that increased to 1.5 in the age group of 47–54 years. In a recent study of 22,411 Swedish individuals, it was shown that female shift-working white collar workers had an increased mortally risk of 2.61, while an increase was not seen amongst female blue collar workers or any of the male groups (Åkerstedt et al., 2004). Although total mortality has not been shown to be related to all-over mortality in all studies (Karlsson et al., 2005), the fact that shift-work is related to disease with severe outcomes suggests that shift-work is related to overall mortality, particularly as short/disturb sleep is related to increased mortality (Hublin et al., 2007). A more recent study failed to find any effects of shift-work on mortality (or chronic disease) for shift-works being part of a larger medical program specifically targeting to help shift-workers (Oberlinner et al., 2009).

Mechanisms: why the problems occur

The mechanisms by which disturbed sleep and circadian disruption affect sleep, sleepiness, and health are more thoroughly reviewed elsewhere in the book (Chapters 2–10), but a short summary is included below. The main reason for reduced alertness during the night and short day sleep is the misalignment between the circadian system, working hours, and sleep (Åkerstedt, 1998b). Long waking hours, often more than 20 hours, is an extra burden particularly affecting alertness and performance during the first night shift. Day sleep after night work are about 2–3 hours shorter due to the interference of the circadian system, hence resulting in an increased sleep pressure affecting the oncoming waking period.

The mechanisms by which shift-work causes health problems are less explored, but probably include circadian disruption, insufficient sleep, behavioural disturbances, and disturbed socio-temporal patterns (Knutsson, 2003). A central problem with circadian misalignment (Hampton et al., 1996), insufficient sleep (Spiegel et al., 1999), and irregular eating habits—all common amongst shift-workers, is that they all lead to metabolic disturbances. For example, both glucose and lipid metabolism have time of day-dependent variations with reduced metabolism at night, which can contribute to higher levels of serum triglycerides, cholesterol, and impaired glucose metabolism frequently seen in shift-workers. The negative consequences of eating during the night have been suggested before (Lennernäs et al., 1994), then as it is related to worse blood lipids, but has rendered new interest since eating has been shown to be a strong zeitgeber for circadian clocks in the periphery (Schibler et al., 2003), although very few data exist in humans (Cermakian and Boivin, 2009). Whether eating during the night is related to a desynchronization between central and peripheral clocks remains to be studied. With respect to cardiovascular disease, already young male shift-workers under the age of 40 have accelerated processes of atherosclerosis (Puttonen et al., 2009) suggesting that the effects of shift-work are rather imminent. It has been proposed that shift-work affects myocardial metabolism by disrupting molecular and genetic regulation (Martino and Sole, 2009). In a recent review it was suggested that poor recovery and shift-work related behaviours such as smoking and weight gain are key mechanisms in the development of cardiovascular disease amongst shift workers (Puttonen et al., 2010). The increased risk of cancer has been suggested to be related to light exposure and/or reduced levels of melatonin (Kolstad, 2008). Other mechanisms may be related to those of shifting sleep to the daytime, which results in a desynchronization of sleep-related hormones (such as growth hormone, prolactin, and testosterone), hormones largely regulated by the circadian system (such as cortisol and melatonin), and hormones regulated by both sleep and the circadian system (such as thyrotropin). It has for example, been shown that intolerant shift-workers have lower testosterone levels than their tolerant colleagues (Axelsson et al., 2003). Taken together, the understanding of the involved mechanisms will improve as we obtain a better understanding of the mechanisms by which disturbed sleep and circadian desynchronization affects long-term health. There is a need for prospective studies with a focus on mechanisms and long-term clinical outcomes to understand why some individuals are more vulnerable to shift-work than others.

Potential interventions to improve alertness, sleep, and health in shift-workers

Several strategies, such as napping, caffeine, modafinil, and bright-light exposure, have been proposed as effective countermeasures against sleepiness and performance decrements, either directly via alertness-enhancing effects or indirectly via adaptation to night work or improved sleep. Although most knowledge is based on laboratory findings in non-shift-working populations, few studies have actually been carried out on how effectively these countermeasures are in real-life situations. Many interventions can be made on the organizational level, such as improved working schedules, bright light exposure, and also on the individual levels, such as sleep strategies (mainly napping), pharmacological therapies, and an improved lifestyle.

Organizational interventions

Organizational interventions can include a variety of improvements of the work situation/environment such as better shift schedules, artificial light at work/home, sleep facilities, back-up for persons taking a nap, less noise, and prevention programs for improving lifestyle factors such as smoking, training, and alcohol habits. Several reviews (Knauth and Hornberger, 2003) have discussed different aspects of shift systems such as: order of rotation (forward rotating vs. backward rotating), speed of rotation (fast vs. slowly rotating shifts), shift length (8-hour shifts vs. 12-hour shifts), number of consecutive night shifts, timing of shifts (6:00 or 7:00 in the morning), and time off between shifts (16 hours, 12 hours, or even as little as 8 hours off between shifts). Although a number of studies have compared different aspects, few studies have used well-controlled investigations on most of the shift characteristics above. There is today rather little evidence that order of rotation and number of consecutive shifts have any major impact on alertness and health. A very important aspect is 'time off between shifts', where only 8 or 9 hours off between shifts has strong negative effects on sleep duration and subjective sleepiness (Axelsson et al., 1998; Loweden et al., 1998) and accidents (Garbarino et al., 2002). With respect to length of shifts, there is compelling evidence that it is efficient to reduce extremely long working hours. There is recent evidence that limiting the medical interns maximal working hours from 30 to 16 has very positive effects on sleep duration (Lockley et al., 2004) and medical errors (Landrigan et al., 2004) (Chapters 17 and 18). A wider approach can also be very effective. Böggild and Jeppesen (2001) found improved lipoproteins 6 months after introducing more ergonomic shifts in four hospital wards. The ergonomic principles included: (1) a maximum of three to four consecutive night shifts followed by an extra day off for full recovery, (2) more regular and predictable schedules, (3) reducing from three shifts to two shifts (workers could chose to work either day and night or evening and night), and (4) minimizing weekend work. In a recent review of neurobehavioral and physiological aspects of shift-work systems, it was concluded that the rotation of the shift system should be forward rotating rather than backward rotating, hence avoiding the short recovery periods of 8–9 hours off between shifts, and that there was a lack of neurobehavioral evidence for most other aspects of shift-work (Driscoll et al., 2007).

Bright light exposure and/or melatonin to improve adaptation to night work

Melatonin, bright light, and avoidance of daylight can been used to treat circadian sleep rhythm disorders, including SWD (recently reviewed by Bjorvatn and Pallesen, 2009), but also to improve adaptation to longer periods with night shifts (reviewed by Boivin and James, 2005). The reason for improving adaptation to night work is that very few (less than 3%) seem to adapt completely to night work (Folkard, 2008), and that a longer period of night work results in a circadian misalignment between activity, sleep, and the circadian system, and an accumulation of sleep debt (Burgess et al., 2002). The exception seem to be oil rig workers, a group who are seldom exposed to day light in the morning after the night shift, who adapt to night work rather fast even in the absence of bright light treatment or melatonin (Bjorvatn et al., 1998, 2006). Indeed, bright light or melatonin have only modest positive effects on sleep and sleepiness in oil rig workers (Bjorvatn et al., 2007), hence not confirming the rather strong effects seen in the laboratory, or, alternatively, that oil rig workers are in no need for help in adapting to night work. On the other hand, oil rig workers have large problems to adapt back to day life after a period of night work (Bjorvatn et al., 1998; Gibbs et al., 2002). Similar problems to adapt back to day life have been reported in workers who have adapted to night work with help of bright light (Budnick et al., 1995). Workers who have adapted to night work should be offered help to re-adapt efficiently after a period with night work, particularly if they have adapted to night work with help of bright light or melatonin in the first place. Although few studies exist, bright light on days off can speed up re-adaptation in workers who have adjusted to night work (Bjorvatn et al., 1999). Another approach may be to use bright light to only partially adapt to night work so that the circadian low occurs after the night shift and the travel home from work (Smith et al., 2009). Although bright light and melatonin are well-tolerated in the short term, there is lack of more long-term effects and possible drug interactions (Bjorvatn and Pallesen, 2009). Perhaps the most important aspect that has not yet been answered is whether regular adaptation and re-adaptation to night work has any long-term health consequences.

Napping

The most natural countermeasure to fight sleepiness is obviously sleep (i.e. naps), that can be taken before or during the night shift (Ficca et al., 2009). It is not surprising that up to 65% of the shift-workers take a nap before the first night shift, and around 30% before subsequent night shifts. A number of laboratory studies with shift-workers and nap studies in operational settings have shown that long naps before the night shift or short naps, around 30 minutes, during the night shift can improve nighttime alertness and performance, effects that often last for the commute home as well (Schweitzer et al., 2006; Sallinen et al., 1998). Napping seems to be particularly valuable in extended work shifts and in shift combinations when a night shift is preceded by a morning shift the same day (Ficca et al., 2009). Up to 92% of the workers takes a nap in the latter shift combination, which also lowers accident risk (Garbarino et al., 2002).

Napping is not always feasible in operational settings, and a major drawback may be sleep inertia that may last for a considerable time upon awakening. On the other hand, it is possible to limit sleep inertia by using rather short naps (20–30 minutes) and place them before or during the first half of the night shift. Laboratory findings have also shown that caffeine can reduce inertia from later naps, but this needs to be confirmed in operational settings. Another suggested drawback of napping is poorer daytime sleep after the night shift. On the other hand, the total sleep is not disturbed if including the nap itself, and studies with shorter naps (30 minutes) have not found any negative effects on subsequent sleep (Sallinen et al., 1998; Purnell et al., 2002). In fact, a slight negative effect on subsequent sleep should also be seen as positive as it suggests that the workers have been more alert on the commute home. Still, napping can be difficult to manage in the workplace because of cultural and practical reasons (e.g. noise and lack of back-up personnel), and many individuals can be considered as no nappers. Taken together, napping is a cheap and efficient method to improve sleepiness and performance, and most likely with very few side effects except for inertia.

Pharmacological therapies

Caffeine is the most widely used drug in the world and particularly common amongst shift-workers. Caffeine, which is an adenosine receptor antagonist, has strong alerting properties, both objectively and subjectively, that may last for many hours (Landolt et al., 2004; Schweitzer et al., 2006). To improve nighttime alertness and performance, the caffeine dose should occur between 22:30 and 1:20 with a dosage of 250–400 mg (Walsh et al., 1995). This protocol will have alerting properties for the entire shift and on the commute home, but will have limited effects on subsequent day sleep. Although most studies have been carried out in the lab, a recent study confirms the positive effects of caffeine in operational settings (Schweitzer et al., 2006). One should preferably avoid caffeine later during the night shift as this can disturb the subsequent sleep period, and day sleep periods seem more vulnerable for caffeine than normal night sleep (Carrier et al., 2007). Taken together, caffeine is a cheap, effective, readily available drug that is also highly accepted amongst workers, and can as such serve as useful method to improve alertness amongst the majority of shift-workers. However, further studies need to evaluate how habitual caffeine intake before the night shift affects caffeine intake meant to improve night shift alertness, as well as possible long-term effects.

Other pharmacological stimulants include *amphetamines*, *modafinil*, and *armodafinil*. Although amphetamines and metamphetamines can enhance alertness and performance, they have also been related to disturbed sleep, hypersomnia, adverse cardiovascular effects and development of tolerance (Schwartz and Roth, 2006), and are hence not optimal for regular use in shift-workers. A few recent placebo-controlled studies of shift-workers with SWD have shown that modafinil and armodafinil can improve alertness and performance during nighttime and on the commute home without compromising sleep (Czeisler et al., 2005, 2009). These studies have been carried out in the field and also included follow-up periods of 3 months without any obvious health consequences, perhaps with the exclusion of headaches. It should be noted that modafinil is not advised for individuals with cardiovascular disease and those taking oral contraceptives (Schwartz and Roth, 2006).

Hypnotics have also been used to improve sleep in shift-workers, with the idea that improved sleep will result in less sleepiness (recently reviewed by Schwartz and Roth, 2006). However, the effects are somewhat mixed and the use is limited as they may cause unwanted rebound insomnia and the risk of adverse withdrawal effects.

Improving lifestyle

Based on the facts that many risk factors potentiate each other and that many shift-workers have a rather unhealthy lifestyle, preventive programs are generally considered important for shift-workers (Boggild and Knutsson, 1999). Lack of exercise, poor eating habits, smoking, and high alcohol consumption are risk factors that may potentiate the risk of shift-work, for example for cardiovascular disease. The advice is that lifestyle improvements are more effective for shift-workers than for day workers.

Combination of countermeasures/interventions

In real-life situations, workers are free to combine several countermeasures to improve their on-shift alertness. However, few studies have investigated the combined effects of more than one countermeasure in a systematic manner. In a recent study by Schweitzer et al. (2006), it was shown that an individualized nap and caffeine intervention can be successfully introduced. Workers at different work sites were instructed to take a 1- to 2-hour nap at home before the first two night shifts and combine this with a 300 mg of caffeine at the beginning of the shift. The effects included less sleepiness and better performance at the end of the shift. Although this study could not confirm that the combination of napping and caffeine is superior to the use of either a nap or caffeine, several laboratory studies indicate that this is the case (Schweitzer et al., 2006; Reyner and Horne, 1997). The previously discussed intervention studies in medical interns (Landrigan et al., 2004; Lockley et al., 2004) did not only include a limitation of working hours, from 30 to 16 hours, but also information of napping strategies. These studies indicate that napping can boost the positive effects of other countermeasures/interventions suggesting that napping strategies should be a natural part of all fatigue management strategies. Nevertheless, further studies are required if we are to understand the combinatory effects of different countermeasures to maximize alertness at crucial time points.

Individual differences

A critical question is to evaluate possible long-term health consequences of different countermeasures. For example, it is possible that a countermeasure can improve alertness and safety acutely, but also increase the risk of long-term health problems. The preferred countermeasure should be evaluated from several perspective including mood, performance, safety, as well as long-term health. There is today poor knowledge of how individual characteristics affect the outcomes of interventions, and more studies are needed if we are to understand which interventions are most beneficial, and for whom.

Taken together, employers should focus on providing a shift system that allows recovery on a regular basis and only support circadian adaptation to longer periods with night work. The workplace should preferably allow for naps in a noise-free environment and good back-up systems, particularly if errors are related to safety risks. The shift-workers themselves should try to minimize their sleep debt before work, that is, taking rather long naps before the night shift. In workers with most severe sleepiness, that is, individuals suffering from SWD, there is support for a positive effect of modafinil and armodafinil, but caffeine is probably an equal alternative for many workers (Wesensten et al., 2005).

Summary box

- About 15–30% of the working population work shift-work.
- Night work and early morning work decreases sleep with 2–4 hours and increases work-related sleepiness.
- Sleepiness in connection with the night shift increases the risk for errors and accidents, and may have a negative impact on work productivity.
- Shift-workers suffering from excessive sleepiness during work or insomnia during daytime sleep can be classified as having shift-work disorder, if not suffering from any other disturbance or disorder that can explain their symptoms. The criteria do not include degree or severity of the problems.
- The prevalence of shift-work disorder is largely unknown, but earlier estimations of 10–23% are probably underestimating the numbers suffering from work-related insomnia and excessive sleepiness.
- Shift-work has been related to increased risk for long-term health consequences such as cardiovascular disease, endocrine and metabolic disturbances, gastrointestinal disorder, breast cancer, and prostate cancer.
- The main reason for reduced alertness during the night and short day sleep is the misalignment between the circadian system, working hours, and sleep.
- The mechanisms by which shift-work causes health problems are less explored, but probably include circadian disruption, insufficient sleep, behavioural disturbances (including eating habits), and disturbed sociotemporal patterns.
- There is still a poor knowledge of why some individuals are more vulnerable to shift-work than others.
- Employers should focus on providing a shift system that allows recovery on a regular basis and only support circadian adaptation to longer periods of night work.
- A shift system that minimizes circadian disruption and offers sufficient sleep opportunities is associated with lower levels of disturbed sleep and higher alertness. Thus, the design of a sleep-friendly shift system should be rapidly, forward-rotating, avoid long (>12 hours) work shifts and long weekly working hours (>48 hours), and have at least 12 hours of rest time between shifts.
- Several strategies, such as napping, caffeine, modafinil, and bright-light exposure, have been proposed as effective countermeasures against sleepiness and performance decrements, either directly via alertness-enhancing effects or indirectly via adaptation to night work or improved sleep.
- The workplace should preferably allow for naps in a noise-free environment and good back-up systems, particularly if errors are related to safety risks. The shift-workers themselves

Summary box *(continued)*

should try to minimize their sleep debt before work, that is, taking rather long naps before the night shift.

◆ Promising data suggest that combining caffeine and napping can effectively counteract sleepiness during work and the commute to and from work. However, further studies are required if we are to understand the combinatory effects of different countermeasures to maximize alertness at crucial time points.

References

Åhsberg, E., Kecklund, G., Åkerstedt, T. & Gamberale, F. (2000). Shiftwork and different dimensions of fatigue. *Int J Ind Ergon*, **26**, 457–465.

Åkerstedt, T. (1995). Work hours, sleepiness and the underlying mechanisms. *J Sleep Res*, **4**(suppl. 2), 15–22.

Åkerstedt, T. (1998a). Is there an optimal sleep-wake pattern in shift work? *Scand J Work Environ Health*, **24**(Suppl 3), 18–27.

Åkerstedt, T. (1998b). Sleepiness. *Sleep Med Rev*, **2**, 1–2.

Åkerstedt, T. (1991). Sleepiness at work: effects of irregular work hours. In: Monk, T. (ed.), *Sleep, Sleepiness and Perfomance*. New York, NY: Wiley.

Åkerstedt, T. & Torsvall, L. (1985). Napping in shift work. *Sleep*, **8**, 105–109.

Åkerstedt, T., Knutsson, A., Alfredsson, L. & Theorell, T. (1984). Shift work and cardiovascular disease. *Scand J Work Environ Health*, **10**, 408–414.

Åkerstedt, T., Kecklund, G. & Knutsson, A. (1991). Spectral analysis of sleep electroencephalography in rotating three-shift work. *Scand J Work Environ Health*, **17**, 330–336.

Åkerstedt, T., Fredlund, P., Gillberg, M. & Jansson, B. (2002a). A prospective study of fatal occupational accidents—relationship to sleeping difficulties and occupational factors. *J Sleep Res*, **11**, 69–71.

Åkerstedt, T., Knutsson, A., Westerholm, P., Theorell, T., Alfredsson, L. & Kecklund, G. (2002b). Work organisation and unintentional sleep: results from the WOLF study. *Occup Environ Med*, **59**, 595–600.

Åkerstedt, T., Kecklund, G. & Johansson, S.E. (2004). Shift work and mortality. *Chronobiol Int*, **21**, 1055–1061.

Åkerstedt, T., Peters, B., Anund, A. & Kecklund, G. (2005). Impaired alertness and performance while driving home from the night shift—a driving simulator study. *J Sleep Res*, **14**, 17–20.

Åkerstedt, T., Ingre, M., Broman, J.E. & Kecklund, G. (2008). Disturbed sleep in shift workers, day workers, and insomniacs. *Chronobiol Int*, **25**, 333–348.

American Academy of Sleep Medicine (2005). *The International Classification of Sleep Disorders: Diagnostic and Coding Manual*. Second edition, Westchester, IL: American Academy of Sleep Medicine.

Axelsson, G., Lutz, C. & Rylander, R. (1984). Exposure to solvents and outcome of pregnancy in university laboratory employees. *Br J Ind Med*, **41**, 305–312.

Axelsson, G., Rylander, R. & Molin, I. (1989). Outcome of pregnancy in relation to irregular and inconvenient work schedules. *Br J Ind Med*, **46**, 393–398.

Axelsson, J., Kecklund, G., Åkerstedt, T. & Lowden, A. (1998). Effects of alternating 8-and 12 hour shifts on sleep, sleepiness, physical effort and performance. *Scand J Work Environ Health*, **24**(Suppl 3), 62–68.

Axelsson, J., Åkerstedt, T., Kecklund, G., Lindqvist, A. & Attefors, R. (2003). Hormonal changes in satisfied and dissatisfied shift workers across a shift cycle. *J Appl Physiol*, **95**, 2099–2105.

Axelsson, J., Åkerstedt, T., Kecklund, G. & Lowden, A. (2004). Tolerance to shift work-how does it relate to sleep and wakefulness? *Int Arch Occup Environ Health*, **77**, 121–129.

Axelsson, J., Kecklund, G., Åkerstedt, T., Donofrio, P., Lekander, M. & Ingre, M. (2008). Sleepiness and performance in response to repeated sleep restriction and subsequent recovery during semi-laboratory conditions. *Chronobiol Int*, **25**, 297–308.

Bambra, C.L., Whitehead, M.M., Sowden, A.J., Akers, J. & Petticrew, M.P. (2008). Shifting schedules: the health effects of reorganizing shift work. *Am J Prev Med*, **34**, 427–434.

Barger, L.K., Cade, B.E., Ayas, N.T., et al. (2005). Extended work shifts and the risk of motor vehicle crashes among interns. *N Engl J Med*, **352**, 125–134.

Barger, L.K., Lockley, S.W., Rajaratnam, S.M. & Landrigan, C.P. (2009). Neurobehavioral, health, and safety consequences associated with shift work in safety-sensitive professions. *Curr Neurol Neurosci Rep*, **9**, 155–164.

Biggi, N., Consonni, D., Galluzzo, V., Sogliani, M. & Costa, G. (2008). Metabolic syndrome in permanent night workers. *Chronobiol Int*, **25**, 443–454.

Bjerner, B., Holm, Å. & Swensson, Å. (1955). Diurnal variation of mental perfomance. A study of three-shift workers. *Br J Ind Med*, **12**, 103–110.

Bjorvatn, B. & Pallesen, S. (2009). A practical approach to circadian rhythm sleep disorders. *Sleep Med Rev*, **13**, 47–60.

Bjorvatn, B., Kecklund, G. & Åkerstedt, T. (1998). Rapid adaptation to night work at an oil platform, but slow readaptation after returning home. *J Occup Environ Med*, **40**, 601–608.

Bjorvatn, B., Kecklund, G. & Åkerstedt, T. (1999). Bright light treatment used for adaptation to night work and re-adaptation back to day life. A field study at an oil platform in the North Sea. *J Sleep Res*, **8**, 105–112.

Bjorvatn, B., Stangenes, K., Oyane, N., et al. (2006). Subjective and objective measures of adaptation and readaptation to night work on an oil rig in the North Sea. *Sleep*, **29**, 821–829.

Bjorvatn, B., Stangenes, K., Oyane, N., et al. (2007). Randomized placebo-controlled field study of the effects of bright light and melatonin in adaptation to night work. *Scand J Work Environ Health*, **33**, 204–214.

Boggild, H., & Jeppesen, H.J. (2001). Intervention in shift scheduling and changes in biomarkers of heart disease in hospital wards. *Scand J Work Environ Health*, **27**(2), 87–96.

Boggild, H. & Knutsson, A. (1999). Shift work, risk factors and cardiovascular disease. *Scand J Work Environ Health*, **25**, 85–99.

Boggild, H., Suadicani, P., Hein, H.O. & Gyntelberg, F. (1999). Shift work, social class, and ischaemic heart disease in middle aged and elderly men; a 22 year follow up in the Copenhagen Male Study. *Occup Environ Med*, **56**, 640–645.

Boisard, P., Cartron, D., Gollac, M. & Valeyre, A. (2002). *Time and Work: Duration of Work*. Dublin: European Foundation for the Improvement of Living and Working Conditions.

Boivin, D.B. & James, F.O. (2005). Light treatment and circadian adaptation to shift work. *Ind Health*, **43**, 34–48.

Bonnefond, A., Härmä, M., Hakola, T., Sallinen, M., Kandolin, I. & Virkkala, J. (2006). Interaction of age with shift-related sleep-wakefulness, sleepiness, performance, and social life. *Exp Aging Res*, **32**, 185–208.

Bonzini, M., Coggon, D. & Palmer, K.T. (2007). Risk of prematurity, low birthweight and pre-eclampsia in relation to working hours and physical activities: a systematic review. *Occup Environ Med*, **64**, 228–243.

Bryant, P.A., Trinder, J. & Curtis, N. (2004). Sick and tired: Does sleep have a vital role in the immune system? *Nat Rev Immunol*, **4**, 457–467.

Budnick, L.D., Lerman, S.E. & Nicolich, M.J. (1995). An evaluation of scheduled bright light and darkness on rotating shiftworkers: trial and limitations. *Am J Ind Med*, **27**, 771–782.

Bureau of Labour Statistics Workers on Flexible and Shift Schedules in May 2004 (2005). Available at: http://www.bls. gov/news.release/pdf/flex.pdf (accessed November 22, 2009).

Burgess, H.J., Sharkey, K.M. & Eastman, C.I. (2002). Bright light, dark and melatonin can promote circadian adaptation in night shift workers. *Sleep Med Rev*, **6**, 407–420.

Carrier, J., Fernandez-Bolanos, M., Robillard, R., et al. (2007). Effects of caffeine are more marked on daytime recovery sleep than on nocturnal sleep. *Neuropsychopharmacology*, **32**, 964–972.

Cermakian, N. & Boivin, D.B. (2009). The regulation of central and peripheral circadian clocks in humans. *Obes Rev*, **10**(Suppl 2), 25–36.

Cohen, S., Doyle, W.J., Alper, C.M., Janicki-Deverts, D. & Turner, R.B. (2009). Sleep habits and susceptibility to the common cold. *Arch Intern Med*, **169**, 62–67.

Coleman, R.M. & Dement, W.C. (1986). Falling asleep at work: a problem for continous operations. *J Sleep Res*, **15**, 265.

Conlon, M., Lightfoot, N. & Kreiger, N. (2007). Rotating shift work and risk of prostate cancer. *Epidemiology*, **18**, 182–183.

Conway, P.M., Campanini, P., Sartori, S., Dotti, R. & Costa, G. (2008). Main and interactive effects of shiftwork, age and work stress on health in an Italian sample of healthcare workers. *Appl Ergon*, **39**, 630–639.

Costa, G., Lievore, F., Casaletti, G., Gaffuri, E. & Folkard, S. (1989). Circadian characteristics influencing interindividual differences in tolerance and adjustment to shiftwork. *Ergonomics*, **32**, 373–385.

Czeisler, C.A., Walsh, J.K., Roth, T., et al. (2005). Modafinil for excessive sleepiness associated with shift-work sleep disorder. *N Engl J Med*, **353**, 476–486.

Czeisler, C.A., Walsh, J.K., Wesnes, K.A., Arora, S. & Roth, T. (2009). Armodafinil for treatment of excessive sleepiness associated with shift work disorder: a randomized controlled study. *Mayo Clin Proc*, **84**, 958–972.

Darwent, D., Lamond, N. & Dawson, D. (2008). The sleep and performance of train drivers during an extended freight-haul operation. *Appl Ergon*, **39**, 614–622.

Daurat, A. & Foret, J. (2004). Sleep strategies of 12-hour shift nurses with emphasis on night sleep episodes. *Scand J Work Environ Health*, **30**, 299–305.

Davis, S., Mirick, D.K. & Stevens, R.G. (2001). Night shift work, light at night, and risk of breast cancer. *J Natl Cancer Inst*, **93**, 1557–1562.

De Valck, E., Quanten, S., Berckmans, D. & Cluydts, R. (2007). Simulator driving performance, subjective sleepiness and salivary cortisol in a fast-forward versus a slow-backward rotating shift system. *Scand J Work Environ Health*, **33**, 51–57.

Dembe, A.E., Erickson, J.B., Delbos, R.G. & Banks, S.M. (2005). The impact of overtime and long work hours on occupational injuries and illnesses: new evidence from the United States. *Occup Environ Med*, **62**, 588–597.

Dembe, A., Erickson, J., Delbos, R. & Banks, S. (2006). Nonstandard shift schedules and the risk of job-related injuries. *Scand J Work Environ Health*, **32**, 232–240.

Dembe, A., Delbos, R. & Erickson, J. (2009). Estimates of injury risks for health care personnel working night shifts and long hours. *Qual Saf Health Care*, **18**, 336–340.

Di Lorenzo, L., De Pergola, G., Zocchetti, C., et al. (2003). Effect of shift work on body mass index: results of a study performed in 319 glucose-tolerant men working in a Southern Italian industry. *Int J Obes Relat Metab Disord*, **27**, 1353–1358.

Drake, C.L., Roehrs, T., Richardson, G., Walsh, J. & Roth, T. (2004). Shift work sleep disorder: Prevalence and consequences beyond that of symptomatic day workers. *Sleep*, **27**, 1453–1462.

Driscoll, T., Grunstein, R.R. & Rogers, N.l. (2007). A systematic review of the neurobehavioural and physiological effects of shiftwork systems. *Sleep Med Rev*, **11**, 179–194.

Dumont, M., Montplaisir, J. & Infante-Rivard, C. (1997). Sleep quality of former night-shift workers. *Int J Occup Environ Health*, **3**, S10–S14.

Ficca, G., Axelsson, J., Mollicone, D.J., Muto, V. & Vitiello, M.V. (2009). Naps, cognition and performance. *Sleep Med Rev*.

Folkard, S. (1992). Is there a 'best compromise' shift system? *Ergonomics*, **35**, 1453–1463.

Folkard, S. (2008). Do permanent night workers show circadian adjustment? A review based on the endogenous melatonin rhythm. *Chronobiol Int*, **25**, 215–224.

Folkard, S. & Monk, T. (1979). Toward a predictive test of adjustment to shiftwork. *Ergonomics*, **22**, 79–91.

Folkard, S. & Tucker, P. (2003). Shift work, safety and productivity. *Occup Environ Med*, **53**, 95–101.

Folkard, S., Lombardi, D.A. & Tucker, P.T. (2005). Shiftwork: safety, sleepiness and sleep. *Ind Health*, **43**, 20–23.

Frost, P., Kolstad, H.A. & Bonde, J.P. (2009). Shift work and the risk of ischemic heart disease—a systematic review of the epidemiologic evidence. *Scand J Work Environ Health*, **35**, 163–179.

Garbarino, S., De Carli, F., Nobili, L., et al. (2002). Sleepiness and sleep disorders in shift workers: a study on a group of Italian police officers. *Sleep*, **25**, 648–653.

Gibbs, M., Hampton, S., Morgan, L. & Arendt, J. (2002). Adaptation of the circadian rhythm of 6-sulphatoxymelatonin to a shift schedule of seven nights followed by seven days in offshore oil installation workers. *Neurosci Lett*, **325**, 91–94.

Gibbs, M., Hampton, S., Morgan, L. & Arendt, J. (2007). Predicting circadian response to abrupt phase shift: 6-sulphatoxymelatonin rhythms in rotating shift workers offshore. *J Biol Rhythms*, **22**, 368–370.

Gillberg, M., Kecklund, G., Göransson, B. & Åkerstedt, T. (2003). Operator performance and signs of sleepiness during day and night work in a simulated thermal power plant. *Int J Ind Ergon*, **31**, 101–109.

Gold, D.R., Rogacz, S., Bock, N., et al. (1992). Rotating shift work, sleep, and accidents related to sleepiness in hospital nurses. *Am J Public Health*, **82**, 1011–1014.

Hamelin, P. (1987). Lorry driver's time habits in work and their involvement in traffic accidents. *Ergonomics*, **30**, 1323–1333.

Hampton, S.M., Morgan, L.M., Lawrence, N., et al. (1996). Postprandial hormone and metabolic responses in simulated shift work. *J Endocrinol*, **151**, 259–267.

Hansen, J. (2001). Increased breast cancer risk among women who work predominantly at night. *Epidemiology*, **12**, 74–77.

Hansen, M.A., Garde, H.A. & Hansen, J. (2006). Diurnal urinary 6-sulfatoxymelatonin levels among healthy Danish nurses during work and leisure time. *Chronobiol Int*, **23**, 1203–1215.

Harrington, J. (1978). *Shift Work and Health*. London: Her Majesty's Stationery Office.

Hermansson, J., Gillander Gadin, K., Karlsson, B., Lindahl, B., Stegmayr, B. & Knutsson, A. (2007). Ischemic stroke and shift work. *Scand J Work Environ Health*, **33**, 435–439.

Hildebrandt, G., Rohmert, W. & Rutenfranz, J. (1974). 12 and 24 hour rhythms in error frequency of locomotive drivers and the influence of tiredness. *Int J Chronobiol*, **2**, 175–180.

Hublin, C., Partinen, M., Koskenvuo, M. & Kaprio, J. (2007). Sleep and mortality: a population-based 22-year follow-up study. *Sleep*, **30**, 1245–1253.

Hänecke, K., Tiedemann, S., Nachreiner, F. & Grzech-Sukalo, H. (1998). Accident risk as a function of hour at work and time of day as determined from accident data and exposure models for the German working population. *Scand J Work Environ Health*, **24**(Suppl 3), 43–48.

Härmä, M. (1995). Sleepiness in shiftwork: individual differences. *J Sleep Res*, **4**, 57–61.

Härmä, M., Sallinen, M., Ranta, R., Mutanen, P. & Müller, K. (2002). The effect of an irregular shift system on sleepiness at work in train drivers and railway traffic controllers. *J Sleep Res*, **11**, 141–151.

Härmä, M., Hakola, T., Kandolin, I., Sallinen, M., Virkkala, J. & Bonnefond, A. (2006). A controlled intervention study of the effects of a very rapidly forward rotating shift system on sleep-wakefulness and well-being among young and elderly shift workers. *Int J Psychophysiol*, **59**, 70–79.

Ingre, M. & Åkerstedt, T. (2004). Effect of accumulated night work during the working lifetime, on subjective health and sleep in monozygotic twins. *J Sleep Res*, **13**, 45–48.

Ingre, M., Kecklund, G., Åkerstedt, T. & Kecklund, L. (2004). Variation in sleepiness during early morning shifts: a mixed model approach to an experimental field study of train drivers. *Chronobiol Int*, **21**, 973–990.

Ingre, M., Kecklund, G., Åkerstedt, T., Söderström, M. & Kecklund, L. (2008). Sleep length as a function of morning shift-start time in irregular shift schedules for train drivers: self-rated health and individual differences. *Chronobiol Int*, **25**, 349–358.

Karlsson, B., Knutsson, A. & Lindahl, B. (2001). Is there an association between shift work and having a metabolic syndrome? Results from a population based study of 27,485 people. *Occup Environ Med*, **58**, 747–752.

Karlsson, B.H., Knutsson, A.K., Lindahl, B.O. & Alfredsson, L.S. (2003). Metabolic disturbances in male workers with rotating three-shift work. Results of the WOLF study. *Int Arch Occup Environ Health*, **76**, 424–430.

Karlsson, B., Alfredsson, L., Knutsson, A., Andersson, E. & Toren, K. (2005). Total mortality and cause-specific mortality of Swedish shift- and dayworkers in the pulp and paper industry in 1952-2001. *Scand J Work Environ Health*, **31**, 30–35.

Kawachi, I., Colditz, G.A., Stampfer, M.J., et al. (1995). Prospective study of shift work and risk of coronary heart disease in women. *Circulation*, **92**, 3178–3182.

Kecklund, G. & Åkerstedt, T. (1993). Sleepiness in long distance truck driving: an ambulatory EEG study of night driving. *Ergonomics*, 36, 1007–1017.

Kecklund, G., Åkerstedt, T. & Lowden, A. (1997). Morning work: effects of early rising on sleep and alertness. *Sleep*, **20**, 215–223.

Kivimäki, M., Virtanen, M., Elovainio, M., Vaananen, A., Keltikangas-Jarvinen, L., & Vahtera, J. (2006). Prevalent cardiovascular disease, risk factors and selection out of shift work. *Scand J Work Environ Health*, **32**(3), 204–208.

Kleiven, M., Boggild, H. & Jeppesen, H.J. (1998). Shift work and sick leave. *Scand J Work Environ Health*, **24**(Suppl 3), 128–133.

Knauth, P. & Rutenfranz, J. (1981). Duration of sleep and related to the type of shift work. In: Reinberg, A., Vieux, N. & Andlauer, P. (eds.), *Advances in the Biosciences, Vol. 30. Night and Shiftwork Biological and Social Aspects*. Oxford: Pergamon Press.

Knauth, P. & Hornberger, S. (2003). Preventive and compensatory measures for shift workers. *Occup Med (Lond)*, **53**, 109–116.

Knutsson, A. (2003). Health disorders of shift workers. *Occup Med*, **53**, 103–108.

Knutsson, A., Åkerstedt, T., Jonsson, B.G. & Orth-Gomér, K. (1986). Increased risk of ischemic heart disease in shift workers. *Lancet*, **12**(2), 89–92.

Knutsson, A., Hallquist, J., Reuterwall, C., Theorell, T. & Åkerstedt, T. (1999). Shiftwork and myocardial infarction: a case-control study. *Occup Environ Med*, **56**, 46–50.

Knutsson, A., Hammar, N. & Karlsson, B. (2004). Shift workers' mortality scrutinized. *Chronobiol Int*, **21**, 1049–1053.

Kogi, K. & Ohta, T. (1975). Incidence of near accidental drowsing in locomotive driving during a period of rotation. *J Hum Ergol*, **4**, 65–76.

Koller, M., Kundi, M. & Cervinka, R. (1978). Field studies of shift work at an Austrian oil refinery. I: Health and psychosocial wellbeing of workers who drop out of shiftwork. *Ergonomics*, **21**, 835–847.

Kolstad, H.A. (2008). Nightshift work and risk of breast cancer and other cancers—a critical review of the epidemiologic evidence. *Scand J Work Environ Health*, **34**, 5–22.

Kubo, T., Ozasa, K., Mikami, K., et al. (2006). Prospective cohort study of the risk of prostate cancer among rotating-shift workers: findings from the Japan collaborative cohort study. *Am J Epidemiol*, **164**, 549–555.

Labyak, S., Lava, S., Turek, F. & Zee, P. (2002). Effects of shiftwork on sleep and menstrual function in nurses. *Health Care Women Int*, **23**, 703–714.

Landolt, H.P., Retey, J.V., Tonz, K., et al. (2004). Caffeine attenuates waking and sleep electroencephalographic markers of sleep homeostasis in humans. *Neuropsychopharmacology*, **29**, 1933–1939.

Landrigan, C.P., Rothschild, J.M., Cronin, J.W., et al. (2004). Effect of reducing interns' work hours on serious medical errors in intensive care units. *N Engl J Med*, **351**, 1838–1848.

Lennernäs, M., Åkerstedt, T. & Hambraeus, L. (1994). Nocturnal eating and serum cholesterol of three-shift workers. *Scand J Work Environ Health*, **20**, 401–406.

Lockley, S.W., Cronin, J.W., Evans, E.E., et al. (2004). Effect of reducing interns' weekly work hours on sleep and attentional failures. *N Engl J Med*, **351**, 1829–1837.

Lowden, A., Kecklund, G., Axelsson, J. & Åkerstedt, T. (1998). Change from an 8-hour shift to a 12-hour shift, attitudes, sleep, sleepiness and performance. *Scand J Work Environ Health*, **24**(Suppl 3), 69–75.

Macdonald, A., Mcdonald, J., Armstrong, B., Cherry, N., Nolin, A. & Robert, D. (1988). Prematurity and work in pregnancy. *Br J Ind Med*, **45**, 56–62.

Mamelle, N., Laumon, B. & Lazar, P. (1984). Prematurity and occupational activity during pregnancy. *Am J Epidemiol*, **119**, 309–322.

Martino, T.A. & Sole, M.J. (2009). Molecular time: an often overlooked dimension to cardiovascular disease. *Circ Res*, **105**, 1047–1061.

McNamee, R., Binks, K., Jones, S., Faulkner, D., Slovak, A. & Cherry, N.M. (1996). Shiftwork and mortality from ischaemic heart disease. *Occup Environ Med*, **53**, 367–373.

Mikuni, E., Ohoshi, T., Hayashi, K. & Miyamura, K. (1983). Glucose intolerance in an employed population. *Tohoku J Exp Med*, **141**(Suppl), 251–256.

Miller, M.A., Kandala, N.B., Kivimaki, M., et al. (2009). Gender differences in the cross-sectional relationships between sleep duration and markers of inflammation: Whitehall II study. *Sleep*, **32**, 857–864.

Mitler, M.M., Carskadon, M.A., Czeisler, C.A., Dement, W.C., Dinges, D.F. & Graeber, R.C. (1988). Catastrophes, sleep and public policy: concensus report. *Sleep*, **11**, 100–109.

Mitler, M.M., Miller, J.C., Lipsitz, J.J., Walsh, J.K. & Wylie, C.D. (1997). The sleep of long-haul truck drivers. *N Engl J Med*, **337**, 755–761.

Mohren, D.C., Jansen, N.W., Kant, I.J., Galama, J., Van Den Brandt, P.A. & Swaen, G.M. (2002). Prevalence of common infections among employees in different work schedules. *J Occup Environ Med*, **44**, 1003–1011.

Monk, T.H. & Embrey, D.E. (1981). A field study of circadian rhythms in actual and interpolated task performance. In: Reinberg, A., Vieux, N. & Andlauer, P. (eds.), *Night and Shift Work: Biological and Social Aspects*. Oxford: Pergamon Press.

Nabe-Nielsen, K., Garde, A.H., Tuchsen, F., Hogh, A. & Diderichsen, F. (2008). Cardiovascular risk factors and primary selection into shift work. *Scand J Work Environ Health*, **34**, 206–212.

Nagaya, T., Yoshida, H., Takahashi, H. & Kawai, M. (2002). Markers of insulin resistance in day and shift workers aged 30-59 years. *Int Arch Occup Environ Health*, **75**, 562–568.

Nakamura, K., Shimai, S., Kikuchi, S., et al. (1997). Shift work and risk factors for coronary heart disease in Japanese blue-collar workers: serum lipids and anthropometric characteristics. *Occup Med (Lond)*, **47**, 142–146.

Niedhammer, I., Lert, F. & Marne, M.J. (1996). Prevalence of overweight and weight gain in relation to night work in a nurses' cohort. *Int J Obes Relat Metab Disord*, **20**, 625–633.

Nishitani, N. & Sakakibara, H. (2007). Subjective poor sleep and white blood cell count in male Japanese workers. *Ind Health*, **45**, 296–300.

O'Leary, E.S., Schoenfeld, E.R., Stevens, R.G., et al. (2006). Shift work, light at night, and breast cancer on Long Island, New York. *Am J Epidemiol*, **164**, 358–366.

Oberlinner, C., Ott, M.G., Nasterlack, M., et al. (2009). Medical program for shift workers—impacts on chronic disease and mortality outcomes. *Scand J Work Environ Health*, **35**, 309–318.

Ohayon, M.M., Lemoine, P., Arnaud-Briant, V. & Dreyfus, M. (2002). Prevalence and consequences of sleep disorders in a shift worker population. *J Psychosom Res*, **53**, 577–583.

Paley, M.J. & Tepas, D.I. (1994). Fatigue and the shiftworker: firefighters working on a rotating shift schedule. *Hum Factors*, **36**, 269–284.

Peacock, B., Glube, R., Miller, M. & Clune, P. (1983). Police officers' responses to 8 and 12 hour shift schedules. *Ergonomics*, **325**, 479–493.

Prokop, O. & Prokop, L. (1955). Ermüdung und Einschlafen am Steuer. *Zentralblatt für Verkehrsmedizin, Verkehrspsychologie und angrenzende Gebiete*, **1**, 19–30.

Purnell, M.T., Feyer, A.-M. & Herbison, G.P. (2002). The impact of a nap opportunity during the night shift on the performance and alertness of 12-h shift workers. *J Sleep Res*, **11**, 219–227.

Puttonen, S., Kivimäki, M., Elovainio, M., et al. (2009). Shift work in young adults and carotid artery intima-media thickness: The Cardiovascular Risk in Young Finns study. *Atherosclerosis*, **205**, 608–613.

Puttonen, S., Harma, M., & Hublin, C. (2010). Shift work and cardiovascular disease - pathways from circadian stress to morbidity. *Scand J Work Environ Health*, **36**(2), 96–108. Epub 20 Jan 2010.

Puttonen, S., Oksanena, T., Vahteraa, J., et al. (2010b). Is shift work a risk factor for rheumatoid arthritis? The Finnish Public Sector Study. *Ann Rheum Dis*, **69**(4), 779–780.

Rauchenzauner, M., Ernst, F., Hintringer, F., et al. (2009). Arrhythmias and increased neuro-endocrine stress response during physicians' night shifts: a randomized cross-over trial. *Eur Heart J*, **30**, 2606–2613.

Reyner, L.A. & Horne, J.A. (1997). Suppression of sleepiness in drivers: combination of caffeine with a short nap. *Psychophysiology*, **34**, 721–725.

Roach, G.D., Reid, K.J. & Dawson, D. (2003). The amount of sleep obtained by locomotive engineers: effect of break duration and time of break onset. *Occup Environ Med*, **60**(12), e17.

Rosa, R.R. (1993). Napping at home and alertness on the job in rotating shift workers. *Sleep*, **16**, 727–735.

Rosa, R.R. (1995). Extended work shifts and excessive fatigue. *J Sleep Res*, **4**(suppl 2), 51–56.

Rosa, R.R. & Bonnet, M.H. (1993). Performance and alertness on 8h and 12h rotating shifts at a natural gas utility. *Ergonomics*, **36**, 1177–1193.

Rosa, R.R., Härmä, M., Pulli, K., Mulder, M. & Nasman, O. (1996). Rescheduling a three shift system at a steel rolling mill: effects of a one hour delay of shift starting times on sleep and alertness in younger and older workers. *Occup Environ Med*, **53**, 677–685.

Sack, R.L., Blood, M.L. & Lewy, A.J. (1992). Melatonin rhythms in night shift workers. *Sleep*, **15**, 434–441.

Sallinen, M., Härmä, M., Åkerstedt, T., Rosa, R. & Lillqvist, O. (1998). Promoting alertness with a short nap during a night shift. *J Sleep Res*, **7**, 240–247.

Sallinen, M., Härmä, M., Mutanen, P., Ranta, R., Virkkala, J. & Muller, K. (2003). Sleep-wake rhythm in an irregular shift system. *J Sleep Res*, **12**, 103–112.

Sallinen, M., Härmä, M., Mutanen, P., Ranta, R., Virkkala, J. & Müller, K. (2005). Sleepiness in various shift combinations of irregular shift systems. *Ind Health*, **43**, 114–122.

Schernhammer, E.S., Laden, F., Speizer, F.E., et al. (2001). Rotating night shifts and risk of breast cancer in women participating in the nurses' health study. *J Natl Cancer Inst*, **93**, 1563–1568.

Schernhammer, E.S., Laden, F., Speizer, F.E., et al. (2003). Night-shift work and risk of colorectal cancer in the nurses' health study. *J Natl Cancer Inst*, **95**, 825–828.

Schernhammer, E.S., Kroenke, C.H., Laden, F. & Hankinson, S.E. (2006). Night work and risk of breast cancer. *Epidemiology*, **17**, 108–111.

Schibler, U., Ripperger, J. & Brown, S.A. (2003). Peripheral circadian oscillators in mammals: time and food. *J Biol Rhythms*, **18**, 250–260.

Schwartz, J.R. & Roth, T. (2006). Shift work sleep disorder: burden of illness and approaches to management. *Drugs*, **66**, 2357–2370.

Schwartzbaum, J., Ahlbom, A. & Feychting, M. (2007). Cohort study of cancer risk among male and female shift workers. *Scand J Work Environ Health*, **33**, 336–343.

Schweitzer, P.K., Randazzo, A.C., Stone, K., Erman, M. & Walsh, J.K. (2006). Laboratory and field studies of naps and caffeine as practical countermeasures for sleep-wake problems associated with night work. *Sleep*, **29**, 39–50.

Scott, A.J. & Ladou, J. (1994). Health and safety in shift workers. In: Zenz, C., Dickerson, O.B. & Horvath, E.P. (eds.), *Occupational Medicine*. St. Louis, MO: Mosby.

Segawa, K., Nakazawa, S., Tsukamoto, Y., et al. (1987). Peptic ulcer is prevalent among shift workers. *Dig Dis Sci*, **32**, 449–453.

Smith, L., Folkard, S. & Poole, C.J.M. (1994). Increased injuries on night shift. *Lancet*, **344**, 1137–1139.

Smith, L., Folkard, S., Tucker, P. & Macdonald, I. (1998). Work shift duration: a review comparing eight hour and 12 hour shift systems. *Occup Environ Med*, 55, 217–229.

Smith, C., Folkard, S., Schmieder, R.A., et al. (2002). Investigation of morning-evening orientation in six countries using the preferences scale. *Pers Individ Dif*, 32, 949–968.

Smith, M.R., Fogg, L.F. & Eastman, C.I. (2009). A compromise circadian phase position for permanent night work improves mood, fatigue, and performance. *Sleep*, 32, 1481–1489.

Son, M., Kong, J.O., Koh, S.B., Kim, J. & Härmä, M. (2008). Effects of long working hours and the night shift on severe sleepiness among workers with 12-hour shift systems for 5 to 7 consecutive days in the automobile factories of Korea. *J Sleep Res*, 17(4), 385–394.

Spiegel, K., Leproult, R. & Van Cauter, E. (1999). Impact of sleep debt on metabolic and endocrine function. *Lancet*, 354, 1435–1439.

Stevens, J., Brown, J. & Lee, C. (2004). The Second Work-Life Balance study: results from the Employees' Survey. London: MORI Social Research Institute.

Straif, K., Baan, R., Grosse, Y., et al. (2007). Carcinogenicity of shift-work, painting, and fire-fighting. *Lancet Oncol*, 8, 1065–1066.

Stutts, J.C., Wilkins, J.W., Scott Osberg, J. & Vaughn, B.V. (2003). Driver risk factors for sleep-related crashes. *Accid Anal Prev*, 35, 321–331.

Suwazono, Y., Dochi, M., Sakata, K., et al. (2008). A longitudinal study on the effect of shift work on weight gain in male Japanese workers. *Obesity (Silver Spring)*, 16, 1887–1893.

Taylor, P.J. & Pocock, S.J. (1972). Mortality of shift and day workers 1956–68. *Br J Ind Med*, 29, 201–207.

Tenkanen, L., Sjoblom, T., Kalimo, R., Alikoski, T. & Härmä, M. (1997). Shift work, occupation and coronary heart disease over 6 years of follow-up in the Helsinki Heart Study. *Scand J Work Environ Health*, 23, 257–265.

Tepas, D.I. & Mahan, R.P. (1989). The many meanings of sleep. *Work Stress*, 3, 93–102.

Theorell, T. & Åkerstedt, T. (1976). Day and night work: changes in cholesterol, uric acid, glucose and potassium in serum and in circadian patterns of urinary catecholamine excretion. A longitudinal cross-over study of railway workers. *Acta Med Scand*, 200, 47–53.

Tilley, A.J., Wilkinson, R.T., Warren, P.S., Watson, B. & Drud, M. (1982). The sleep and performance of shift workers. *Hum Factors*, 24, 629–641.

Torsvall, L. & Åkerstedt, T. (1987). Sleepiness on the job: continuously measured EEG changes in train drivers. *Electroencephalogr Clin Neurophysiol*, 66, 502–511.

Torsvall, L., Åkerstedt, T., Gillander, K. & Knutsson, A. (1989). Sleep on the night shift: 24-hour EEG monitoring of spontaneous sleep/wake behavior. *Psychophysiology*, 26, 352–358.

Tuchsen, F., Jeppesen, H.J. & Bach, E. (1994). Employment status, non-daytime work and gastric ulcer in men. *Int J Epidemiol*, 23, 365–370.

Tuchsen, F., Hannerz, H. & Burr, H. (2006). A 12 year prospective study of circulatory disease among Danish shift workers. *Occup Environ Med*, 63, 451–455.

Tuchsen, F., Christensen, K.B., Lund, T. & Feveile, H. (2008). A 15-year prospective study of shift work and disability pension. *Occup Environ Med*, 65, 283–285.

Tucker, P., Barton, J. & Folkard, S. (1996). Comparison of eight and 12 hour shifts: impacts on health, wellbeing, and alertness during the shift. *Occup Environ Med*, 53, 767–772.

Uehata, T. & Sasakawa, N. (1982). The fatigue and maternity disturbances of night workwomen. *J Hum Ergol (Tokyo)*, 11(Suppl), 465–474.

Ursin, R., Baste, V. & Moen, B. (2009). Sleep duration and sleep-related problems in different occupations in the Hordaland health study. *Scand J Work Environ Health*, 35, 193–202.

Vahtera, J., Westerlund, H., Hall, M., et al. (2009). Effect of retirement on sleep disturbances: the GAZEL prospective cohort study. *Sleep*, 32, 1459–1466.

van Amelsvoort, L.G., Schouten, E.G. & Kok, F.J. (1999). Duration of shiftwork related to body mass index and waist to hip ratio. *Int J Obes Relat Metab Disord*, 23, 973–978.

van Amelsvoort, L.G., Jansen, N.W., Swaen, G.M., Van Den Brandt, P.A. & Kant, I. (2004). Direction of shift rotation among three-shift workers in relation to psychological health and work-family conflict. *Scand J Work Environ Health*, **30**, 149–156.

van Amelsvoort, L.G., Jansen, N.W. & Kant, I. (2006). Smoking among shift workers: More than a confounding factor. *Chronobiol Int*, **23**, 1105–1113.

Van Dongen, H.P. (2006). Shift work and inter-individual differences in sleep and sleepiness. *Chronobiol Int*, **23**, 1139–1147.

Viitasalo, K., Kuosma, E., Laitinen, J. & Härmä, M. (2008). Effects of shift rotation and the flexibility of a shift system on daytime alertness and cardiovascular risk factors. *Scand J Work Environ Health*, **34**, 198–205.

Virkkunen, H., Härmä, M., Kauppinen, T. & Tenkanen, L. (2007). Shift work, occupational noise and physical workload with ensuing development of blood pressure and their joint effect on the risk of coronary heart disease. *Scand J Work Environ Health*, **33**, 425–434.

Viswanathan, A.N., Hankinson, S.E. & Schernhammer, E.S. (2007). Night shift work and the risk of endometrial cancer. *Cancer Res*, **67**, 10618–10622.

Waage, S., Moen, B.E., Pallesen, S., et al. (2009). Shift work disorder among oil rig workers in the North Sea. *Sleep*, **32**, 558–565.

Walsh, J.K., Muehlbach, M.J. & Schweitzer, P.K. (1995). Hypnotics and caffeine as countermeasures for shiftwork-related sleepiness and sleep disturbance. *J Sleep Res*, **4**, 80–83.

Weibel, L., Spiegel, K., Gronfier, C., Follenius, M. & Brandenberger, G. (1997). Twenty-four-hour melatonin and core body temperature rhythms: their adaptation in night workers. *Am J Physiol*, **272**, R948–R954.

Wesensten, N.J., Killgore, W.D. & Balkin, T.J. (2005). Performance and alertness effects of caffeine, dextroamphetamine, and modafinil during sleep deprivation. *J Sleep Res*, **14**, 255–266.

Wilkinson, R.T. (1992). How fast should the night shift rotate? *Ergonomics*, **35**, 1425–1446.

Xu, X., Ding, M., Li, B. & Christiani, D.C. (1994). Association of rotating shiftwork with preterm births and low birth weight among never smoking women textile workers in China. *Occup Environ Med*, **51**, 470–474.

Zhu, J.L., Hjollund, N.H. & Olsen, J. (2004). Shift work, duration of pregnancy, and birth weight: the National Birth Cohort in Denmark. *Am J Obstet Gynecol*, **191**, 285–291.

Chapter 16

Sleepiness, alertness, and performance

T. Åkerstedt

Introduction

Sleep attracts considerable public attention and is a focus of much medical intervention. However, the traditional reason for the interest in sleep is its ability to suppress sleepiness (or its related performance impairment). Despite this, we know relatively less about sleepiness than we know about sleep. Sleepiness, or its relative, 'fatigue', is also the main reason for seeking primary health care (Wessely et al., 1997).

There are many definitions of sleepiness, but a reasonable one is 'the tendency to fall asleep' (Carskadon and Dement, 1982). This has subjective (the feeling), physiological (the speed of switching to physiological patterns of sleep), and behavioural (absences, gaps in performance, slowness) manifestations, and these may differ. Thus, the manifestations of sleepiness need to be kept apart in discussions of prevalence, causes, countermeasures, etc. A related concept is *excessive daytime sleepiness* (EDS), which essentially means 'being sleepy when one is not expected to be sleepy' (Arand et al., 2005). For individuals active during non-day hours the term *excessive sleepiness* (ED) may be more suitable.

One probably cannot discuss the concept of sleepiness without mentioning the concept of 'fatigue'. It seems to refer to a situation in which energy loss exceeds energy availability (Piper, 1986). The distinction between sleepiness, tiredness, and fatigue is often blurred and there is no consensual definition. Fatigue seems to be a broader concept, referring to a situation in which demands for activity exceed the present resources. It is debated whether tiredness, fatigue, and sleepiness are different dimensions on the same continuum (Dement, 2003) or if they are qualitatively distinguished from each other (Horne, 2003). Here, however, the focus is on sleepiness.

The present review is focused on sleepiness at a population level, that is, prevalence and prediction of sleepiness using epidemiological approaches. However, field experiments and naturalistic studies with relevance to population issues will also be discussed. With respect to performance/safety there are very little data available on direct relations with sleepiness. Rather, most information is inferential in its character, that is, sleepiness is inferred from contexts of disturbed sleep or sleep loss. Another observation is that, at population level, the most readily available material involves simple self-ratings of habitual/retrospective sleepiness. However, data on repeated instantaneous self-ratings and to some extent data obtained with electrophysiological techniques are also available.

Concerning the causes of sleepiness, the field is dominated by settings in which the sleep-wake pattern is altered, as occurs, for example in shift-work or in voluntary sleep restriction, or in outright sleep pathology (sleep apnoea, insomnia, narcolepsy). Other possible causes of sleepiness are rarely studied but there is scant evidence relating sleepiness to demographics, work environment factors, or to diseases in general. A particular field, in which sleepiness research has seen an impressive increase in the number of papers, is driving safety—a number of studies have looked at measurement techniques and risk factors (usually sleep pathology, altered sleep-wake patterns, and drugs). Other chapters in the present volume will contain somewhat overlapping material, such as those on shift-work, respiratory diseases, sleep deprivation, and measurement of sleepiness.

Background

Measurement

The measurement of sleepiness has been called the holy grail of sleep medicine (Bliwise, 2001). The reason is that it may be the main or most obvious consequence of sleep quality or sleep duration. Many other approaches have also been tried.

Habitual subjective sleepiness is usually measured via some type of combination of questions, such as the popular Epworth Sleepiness Scale (ESS) (Johns, 1991). This scale contains 10 descriptions of situations and the respondent is asked to rate the likelihood of him/her falling asleep in that situation (e.g. during a boring lecture, at the red light while driving a car, etc.). Values above 10 are considered excessive/pathological. The ESS does not, however, seem to be strongly linked to subjective sleep quality or to polysomnography (PSG) (Sangal et al., 1999; Buysse et al., 2008). Frequently, questionnaire studies have simply asked questions on how frequently sleepiness occurs or how frequently the respondent 'nods off' or has 'involuntary sleep'. These questions are usually not part of validated scales.

With respect to *momentary* sleepiness measured repeatedly across time, a classical way has been to use visual analogue scales (Monk, 1989), or Likert type scales, like the Stanford Sleepiness Scale (SSS) (Hoddes, 1973) or the Karolinska Sleepiness Scale (KSS) (Åkerstedt, 1990). The first consists of a 100 mm line with anchors like 'very sleepy' and 'very alert'. The numerical value is the number of millimeters measured from one end of the scale to a mark placed by the respondent that corresponds to his/her perceived level of sleepiness. The KSS varies from 'very alert' to 'very sleepy, fighting sleep, an effort to remain awake' in 9 steps. The SSS varies from 'very alert' to 'completely exhausted, cannot function efficiently' in 7 steps.

The *physiological* way of measuring sleepiness is the time taken to fall asleep while lying down (while electroencephalogram [EEG], electrooculogram [EOG], and electromyogram [EMG] is recorded) (Carskadon and Dement, 1902). This constitutes the so-called multiple sleep latency test (MSLT). It is usually run for 20 minutes or until the first epoch of sleep occurs (while lying down). Normal latency in the day time is around 15 minutes, while a shorter period than 5 minutes suggests too low a level of alertness (Carskadon et al., 1986). An alternative is the maintenance of wakefulness test (MWT) (Mitler et al., 1982), which involves an instruction to try to stay awake while sitting in a chair. The duration is twice that of the MSLT. Although useful in the laboratory, it is often not feasible to use the MSLT (or MWT) in real field studies for practical reasons.

In another modification, one measures intrusions of EEG and EOG while the subject keeps his/her eyes open and while performing a task (Åkerstedt and Gillberg, 1990), the Karolinska drowsiness test (KDT). Other developments include various ways of quantifying sleep intrusions during normal work situations. These methods usually involve subjecting EEG recordings to spectral analysis, using the 4–8 Hz and 8–12 Hz frequency bands as indicators of sleepiness. This has been used to quantify physiological sleepiness in truck drivers (Kecklund and Åkerstedt, 1993) and train drivers (Torsvall and Åkerstedt, 1987) during night work, as well as in subjects in driving simulators after sleep loss (O'Hanlon and Kelly, 1974; Horne and Reyner, 1996; Lal and Graig, 2002; Otmani et al., 2005).

Blink duration is another interesting indicator of sleepiness. It increases with sleep loss in field studies of driving (Mitler et al., 1997; Klauer et al., 2006) and in driving simulators (Wierwille and Ellsworth, 1994; Åkerstedt et al., 2005; Anund et al., 2008; Caffier et al., 2003; Schleicher et al., 2008). The latter showed strong effects on the delay of lid opening and lid closure speed. Saccades were not as responsive, although Russo et al. (2005) and Rowland et al. (2005) have found effects. Blink rate has shown both an effect (Summala et al., 1999) and a lack of effect of sleep loss (Torsvall and Åkerstedt, 1988). On the whole, measures related to blink duration seem most responsive to sleepiness.

Performance tests are often used to assess fatigue, they do not in fact measure fatigue as such, but rather its consequences. Still they are very important in sleepiness research. On the whole, tests which require constant attention are externally paced and boring and they seem to be most sensitive to manipulations of sleep (Balkin et al., 2004), so-called vigilance tasks, reaction time tasks, tracking tasks, etc. In real life, such tasks correspond to driving a vehicle, monitoring screens for deviations in signals (healthcare, security situations), but many other tasks are conceivable. Probably, the most used laboratory test of sleepiness is simple serial reaction time, in one version labelled as 'the Psychomotor Vigilance Task' (PVT) (Dinges, 1992).

Sleepiness regulation

Sleepiness is mainly determined by circadian phase, time awake, and amount of sleep. The amount of prior sleep is directly related to subjective, physiological, and behavioural sleepiness (Wilkinson et al., 1966; Härmä et al., 1998a; Jewett et al., 1999). However, 1 hour of reduction (from 8 hours of sleep) has hardly any discernible effects, while 2 hours of reduction may be noticed and 3 hours of loss will have clear effect. Thus, the recuperative value falls with each hour of sleep. With respect to accumulation of partial sleep loss, it appears that effects become noticeable when total sleep time falls below 7 hours (Van Dongen et al., 2003). Fragmentation of sleep, that is, frequent awakenings, leads to effects similar to those of sleep reduction (Bonnet and Arand, 2003). However, the rate of awakenings needs to exceed 5/hour in order to cause significant effects on sleepiness.

The number of hours spent awake will have similar effects on the different types of sleepiness (Fröberg, 1977; Dijk and Czeisler, 1995). The pattern is one of a large decrease of alertness the first hour after rising, followed by a gradual flattening out after 24 hours. Both these studies also demonstrated the pronounced circadian modulation of sleepiness, with increased levels during the daytime and decreased levels during nighttime. The combination of such effects has been brought together in mathematical models that predict sleepiness after manipulations of one or more of the primary components (Åkerstedt et al., 2004; Folkard and Åkerstedt, 1991). Possibly, also the amount of sleep stages 3 + 4 are important for alertness since enhancement of such sleep has been shown to increase MSLT values (i.e. increased sleepiness) (Walsh et al., 2008).

Time on task is another important factor, but which has not been extensively investigated. Classical studies of performance show the so-called 'vigilance decrement', that is a gradual impairment of performance with time on task (Mackworth, 1950). It is present in all types of performance, for example, reaction time (Kribbs and Dinges, 1994) or driving a simulator (Horne and Reyner, 1996). Real driving has been studied only once and it was demonstrated that during night driving unintended line crossing occurred with increasing time of driving (8 hours, 4 hours, and 2 hours) (Sagaspe et al., 2008). Subjective ratings or EEG/EOG variables are less common, but EEG or EOG indicators of sleepiness show a rather steep increase with time on task in the typical boring vigilance test situation (Horne and Reyner, 1996; Åkerstedt et al., 2005).

Finally, several other aspects of the situation will affect alertness. Thus, lighting and temperature, position (standing, lying), and level of activity are important contributors (Johns, 2002).

Physiological structures

The brain changes behind sleepiness are not well investigated. Earlier positron emission tomography (PET) studies showed that sleep deprivation led to reduced metabolism in frontal, thalamic, and parietal areas under memory performance tests (Thomas et al., 2000). This seemed to constitute an attractive explanation behind subjective sleepiness and behavioural impairment. Studies using functional magnetic resonance imaging (fMRI) techniques have modified this notion and it appears that sleep loss may cause increased activity in the structures involved in a particular task, but with increased recruitment of other cortical areas, presumably to support the loss of efficiency in the designated cells, involving frontal, parietal, and other areas (Olbrich et al., 2009; Vandewalle et al., 2009). In the latter study, a Per3 polymorphism showed that the recruitment was broader and performance was not maintained, whereas individuals without this polymorphism showed a more moderate increase in recruitment and an ability to maintain performance (on a 3-back memory load). It is not clear if the fMRI changes described is exactly the same as sleepiness, but it seems likely. Slater (2008) proposed that one purpose of sleep would be to reduce 'drowsiness', that is, to return from the recruitment of large brain areas for a task to activity in the main designated structures for that activity.

Prevalence of sleepiness

There are a number of survey studies on sleepiness, but conclusions on prevalence are quite difficult to draw. The reason is that there is no agreement on the definition of sleepiness. There are essentially two types of studies of sleepiness. One is concerned with excessive amounts of sleep and the other with the tendency to fall asleep during times when sleep is not intended (Ohayon, 2008). There are a few studies of the former type and the prevalence seems to be around 4% (Ohayon, 2008). This type of hypersomnia is not, however, the focus of the present report.

The most common approach to excessive sleepiness has been to ask respondents to indicate the *frequency* of sleepiness symptoms. The questions have been of the type 'sleepiness independent of mealtimes (8.7%)' and 'a strong need to sleep during the day (21.5%). In other studies, prevalences have been 16.7% for 'moderate sleepiness' and 5.7% in a male sample (Gislason et al., 1988). Similar wordings have yielded 15.2% and 5.5%, respectively (Ohayon et al., 1997) and 7.7% and 11.8% in a third study (Nugent et al., 2001). Or 8.7% and 3.8% in a fourth study (Ohayon et al., 2002).

Using frequency of EDS, 'very often sleepy during the daytime' was found in 5.3% (Liljenberg et al., 1988), 'sleepiness often' occurred in 26.1% (Zielinski et al., 1999), and being 'excessively sleepy often or always' occurred in 15% of the sample (Liu et al., 2000). Daytime sleepiness occurring at least 3 days per week was found in 20.6% (5% daily or almost daily) occurrence of daytime sleepiness in the Finnish twin cohort (Hublin et al., 1996). Tendency to fall asleep easily during the daytime and almost anywhere was 4% at least 3 days per week (Ohayon et al., 2002). Periods of sudden and irresistible sleep during the daytime occurred at least 3 days per week in 3.8% in the same study.

A more palpable indicator of sleepiness may be *falling asleep* at work. Åkerstedt et al. (2002a, b) showed that the percentage of subjects falling asleep unintentionally during work several times per month or more was 7% versus 93% never or seldom doing so. 'Falling asleep during the day occurs in 12%', 'falling asleep when you must not sleep occurs in 2.5% (Kaneita et al., 2005)', 'unintentionally falling asleep during leisure time often' occurs in 23%, whereas 77% never or seldom do so. In the 2002 Sleep in America Poll, it was determined that 16% of adults experience sleepiness severe enough to interfere with their work several times per week (NSF, 2002). The same survey also showed that 51% of drivers admitted to driving while drowsy, 17% admitted to dozing off while driving, and 1% admitted to having had a crash due to dozing off or fatigue.

The ESS is particularly interesting because of its widespread use. In a Polish study the mean ESS score was 8.5, EDS in passive situations was 22.3% and in active situations 0.7% (Zielinski et al., 1999). The latter attests to the importance of the context. A Japanese study found that 8.9% had abnormal ESS scores (Takegami et al., 2005). In a Norwegian representative sample, ESS had a mean of 6.9 and 17.7% had more than 10 (Pallesen et al., 2007). Gander et al. (2005) found in a large (10,000) sample a mean of ESS 6.0 and prevalence of 13.9% of scores above ESS 10 in non-Maoris, and 7.5 and 23.9, respectively, in Maoris.

The prevalence data are obviously heavily dependent on the particular definition of sleepiness, but it seems that EDS occurring at least 3 days per week has been reported in 4–20% of the population, while severe EDS is reported in about 5%.

Predictors of sleepiness

The main causes of sleepiness were discussed above, but it is an interesting question how sleepiness manifests itself in different demographic and occupational groups as well as in individuals with different lifestyles. It is difficult to summarize this knowledge systematically and in this context the results will be organized according to study.

Pilcher et al. (2000b) found that that sleep duration did not correlate well with measures of sleepiness, but that subjective sleep quality did. Kim and Young (2005) looked at dimensions of sleepiness and correlates in the general population in 2,913 individuals to general sleepiness (feeling sleepy, not rested, need for coffee) and sleepiness behaviours—active (dozing off while talking) or passive (dozing off when listening to a lecture). The predictors of general sleepiness were: female gender, younger age, higher body mass index (BMI), and lower education. Active sleep propensity was related to male gender, older age, higher BMI. Passive sleep propensity was related to male gender, older age, higher BMI, lower education. With regard to MSLT, general sleepiness was not related (!) while both active and passive sleep propensity was negatively related. Note that women complained of general sleepiness (including not feeling rested) but did not show increased sleep propensity. More general sleepiness was found in the young but a higher sleep propensity was found in older individuals.

Theorell-Haglöw et al. (2006) studied daytime sleepiness in women (5,508 women) and found that 16.1% showed excessive sleepiness and 13.3% physical fatigue. EDS decreased with increasing age and increased with anxiety, depression, insomnia, somatic disease, snoring, being overweight, being on sick leave, being a student, being unmarried (similar for fatigue). EDS was also related to reduced work performance (Johns and Hocking, 1997) and general health (Asplund and Aberg, 1998). Smoking, habitual alcohol consumption, physical activity, number of children (unexpectedly), having a job, early retirement were not related to sleepiness.

In a Norwegian representative sample (Pallesen et al., 2007), logistic regression showed that predictors of EDS were: being male, living in southern Norway, working nights, being young, having symptoms of cataplexy, restless legs, PLMS (periodic limb movements of sleep) in sleep, breathing pauses, depression. All except restless legs remained significant in multiple logistic regression. BMI, socioeconomic group, insomnia were not significant. Using the same Norwegian database, Ursin et al. (2009) showed that craft workers, plant operators, and drivers had an increased risk of daytime sleepiness (odds ratio [OR]: 1.5, 1.8, and 1.8, respectively) and of falling asleep at work (OR: 1.6, 2.1, and 2.0, respectively). The analyses were adjusted for shift-work and number of work hours. It is not clear why the particular occupational groups would be more susceptible to sleepiness, but both operators and drivers have vigilance type sedentary tasks. Shift-workers had an increased risk of falling asleep at work and insomnia.

Gander et al. (2005), using ESS >10 as a criterion, found that the best predictors (mutually adjusted for) in a large New Zealand national sample were snoring, sleep apnoeas, not getting enough sleep, not waking up refreshed, being Maori, being above 59 years, sleeping <6.5 hours, being a non-drinker, and being male. Smoking was not a significant predictor. The inclusion of the three sleep sufficiency variables probably caused some confounding, however. Bartlett et al. (2008), using ESS >10 as criterion, found in a representative Australian sample the best predictors to be voluntarily short sleep duration, symptoms of insomnia, and depression.

Åkerstedt et al. (2002b) studied the predictors of involuntary sleep at work and found that the risk of falling asleep at work was related to disturbed sleep, having shift-work, being young, being male, being a non-smoker. Work demands, decision latitude at work, physical load, sedentary work, solitary work, having extra work, and having overtime work were not related to falling asleep at work. With respect to falling asleep during leisure time, disturbed sleep, snoring, high work demands, being a smoker, not exercising, and higher age (>45 years) were the risk indicators. In a study of 16,583 individuals in Pennsylvania (Bixler et al., 2005), ranking predictors of EDS resulted in: depression, BMI, (low) age, habitual sleep duration, diabetes, smoking, and sleep apnoea.

Hublin et al. (1996) studied a large representative of Finnish sample (11,354) and found that the predictors of feeling sleepy almost every day were insomnia most days of the week, major depression (both with ORs > 10), hypnotic use, tranquillizer use (both with ORs > 5), apnoeas >3 nights weekly, snoring >3 nights weekly. Kaneita et al. (2005) studied a sample of 28,714 Japanese and found the best predictors to be snoring, rated insufficient sleep, stress, unpleasant sensations in the legs, short sleep duration, being male, being young (i.e. a curvilinear relation). Hasler et al. (2005) demonstrated in a longitudinal study that new cases of EDS were related to prior insomnia, as well as anxiety. Cross–sectionally, very high relations were seen between EDS and sleep disturbances and many health variables.

Psychosocial workload increases sleepiness in workers (Takahashi et al., 2006). A similar finding was made in a study of a week with high stress, compared to a week with low stress (Dahlgren et al., 2005). A sedentary lifestyle seems to be related to sleepiness in shift and day workers (Härmä et al., 1998b).

Pack et al. (2006) studied risk factors for EDS in the elderly (65+) and found pain (OR: 5.9), wheezing chest, sleep quality, number of medications, being male and (apnoea-hypopnoea index [AHI] > 20 events per hour). High consumption of alcohol reduced the risk. Restless legs or periodic leg movements did not predict EDS.

Shift-work is a major cause of sleepiness since night shifts place work at the circadian trough, extends the time awake, and frequently is preceded by a reduced prior sleep (Pilcher et al., 2000a). The latter occurs because the circadian rise in metabolism during the daytime curtails day sleep (Czeisler et al., 1980; Åkerstedt and Gillberg, 1981). The overwhelming majority of shift-workers experience sleepiness in connection with night shift-work, whereas day work is associated with no, or marginal, sleepiness (Thiis-Evensen, 1957; Andersen, 1970; Verhaegen et al., 1986; Paley and Tepas, 1994).

In many studies, a majority of shift-workers admit to having experienced involuntary sleep on the night shift, whereas this is rare on day-oriented shifts (Prokop and Prokop, 1955; Coleman and Dement, 1986). Between 10% and 20% report falling asleep during night work. The ESS has not been used very frequently in relation to shift-work, but one recent study showed values of 9.2 in night workers, 8.6 in rotating shift-workers, and 8.0 in day workers (Drake et al., 2004). The differences are small, however. In a national representative sample in Sweden, shift-workers and day workers were compared using a sleep questionnaire. Very few differences from day workers were seen except for a small excess of 'involuntary sleep at work' and of 'insufficient amounts of sleep' (Åkerstedt et al., 2008a).

Another major cause of sleepiness is sleep disorders. This is, however, not the focus of this chapter (see Chapters 3–5, 7–9 for more details).

The predictors of sleepiness vary between studies but, apart from actual sleep disorders, short sleep (or reports of insufficient sleep), awakenings, snoring, night shifts, also seem important. Gender and age seem to yield inconclusive results.

Field studies of momentary subjective sleepiness

The instantaneous (here and now) sleepiness adds information beyond that of questionnaires on habitual sleepiness. This is important for describing the pattern of sleepiness across the day and for describing effects of factors that cause acute sleepiness, for example, acute sleep loss, or monotony, drugs, etc. We here draw on some of our own studies, where we use the same rating scale. The KSS (Åkerstedt and Gillberg, 1990), that was mentioned initially.

The most obvious observation in this type of study is the high level of sleepiness in the morning, low levels during the afternoon (4–4.5 units), and return to relatively high levels of sleepiness in the evening. Figure 16.1 describes this pattern in a group of healthy normals and a group high on burnout (Söderström et al., 2004). Note the similarity of burnout subjects and controls during the working week and the large difference during the weekend. The control groups show values below 3 (alert) during much of the day, whereas the burnout group remains at working week levels. The reason for the latter is not clear but there is a substantial increase in sleep duration and a delay of the time of rising, which may be the likely causes.

Figure 16.2 shows the effect of night shifts on subjective sleepiness (KSS) (Lowden et al., 1998). The maximum, towards the end of the night shifts, is well above level 7, at which sleep intrusions into the EEG usually occur and performance starts to be impaired (Åkerstedt and Gillberg, 1990). During the days off there is a gradual return to low levels of sleepiness.

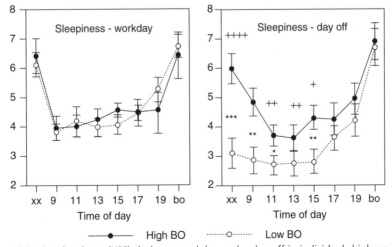

Fig. 16.1 Subjective sleepiness (KSS) during a workday and a day off in individuals high on burnout (but still working) and controls.

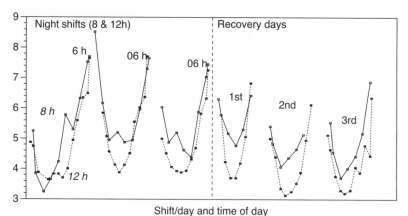

Fig. 16.2 Subjective sleepiness (KSS) during 3 days with traditional night shifts (22:00–6:00 hours) and 3 days off. The leftmost curve starts with rising around 7:00 hours and continues during the day and continues through the night shift. The second curve starts upon rising from day sleep around 13:00 hours.
Source: Adapted from Åkerstedt, T. & Gillberg, M. (1990). Subjective and objective sleepiness in the active individual. *Int J Neurosci*, **52**, 29–37.

Early morning work has a similar effect (reaching values between 5 and 6 units) (Ingre et al., 2008). The latter actually was a field experiment in which train drivers had their start times experimentally scheduled. Interestingly, these levels are similar to those seen in individuals on sick leave with burnout (Ekstedt et al., 2006), and in individuals after 5 days of sleep restricted to 4 hours per night (Axelsson et al., 2008). The values were around 5–6 units during daytime and around 8 towards bedtime. Total sleep deprivation leads to higher levels of sleepiness.

The sleepiness pattern during the shift-work situation above did not show any adjustment. This is a common observation and occurs because the exposure to daylight after the night shift prevents circadian adjustment. However, when day light is excluded as it may be on North Sea oil production platforms, pronounced gradual adjustment takes place (Bjorvatn et al., 1998).

Interestingly, overtime may exacerbate the effects of night work on sleepiness. In a field study of shift-workers, Son et al. (2008) showed strong effects of night shifts and overtime work on high levels of subjective sleepiness (KSS > 7). A similar finding was made by Dahlgren et al. (2006) during a week of experimental overtime work. Also monotonous work increases sleepiness (Sallinen et al., 2004).

Physiological sleepiness

Studies of multiple sleep latency test

The major measure of physiological sleepiness, the MSLT was developed for clinical applications and that is where it has been used almost exclusively. As discussed previously, MSLT values below 5 minutes are considered pathological and are often included in the diagnoses of narcolepsy, sleep apnoea, idiopathic hypersomnia, and related states, while insomnia is associated with increased MSLTs (Littner et al., 2005; Arand et al., 2005). The latter was a 'pseudo' metareview of MSLT and MWT work. It concluded that these tests, while sensitive to sleep loss and many other factors, 'do not discriminate well' between individuals with sleep disorders and the normal population. An illustration of the complexity may be found in a study of insomniacs (Edinger et al., 2008) in which it was found longer MSLTs, but higher daytime subjective sleepiness than in healthy controls. Also performance was impaired. Objective PSG measures from the preceding night predicted performance, particularly the amount of wake after sleep onset.

The Arand et al. (2005) review also established that in connection with manipulations of sleep and other parameters, MSLT increases with stress/anxiety, continuous positive airways pressure (CPAP) treatment for sleep apnoea, and with increases in sleep duration (6 hours vs. 7.5 hours resulted in MSLTs of 9.8 minutes vs. 11.2 minutes) and absence of sleep fragmentation. Most hypnotic and sedative drugs reduce MSLT. MSLT also increases with age, but does not differ with respect to gender. One of the largest single studies on non-clinical groups was carried out in 100 normals tested with a 30-minute variety of the MSLT (5 times per day) (Geisler et al., 2006). The results showed no gender difference but higher latencies in young (11.7 minutes) and older adults (12.7 minutes) and short latencies in intermediate age groups (8.3 minutes), using the 20-minute criterion. Occupational status, marital status, and education did not show any differences. No correlations were seen with the ESS, which could depend on exclusion of subjects with excessive sleepiness. The results still mean that ESS-MSLT measures do not measure the same thing in normals.

Among other factors than sleep problems, Kronholm et al. (1995) studied MSLT in a community study and found the best predictors (multiple regression) of short latencies to be low psychological distress, BMI, thyroid-stimulating hormone (TSH), high age (and daytime tiredness). Gender, reported sleep duration, heart rate, health index, breathing disturbances index were not related to the MSLT.

Very few studies of MSLT and shift-work have been carried out, but Surani et al. (2008) found that post-night-shift nurses had MSLT values around 4.7 minutes, compared to day working nurses with 10.9 minutes. Also the ESS score was higher (8.7 vs. 3.9). Torsvall et al. (1989) found similar, short, MSLT values for night sleep after a night shift. Czeisler et al. (2005) found that shift-workers with shift-work disorder (see section 'Shift-work (sleep) disorder') had a mean MSLT during the night shift of 2 minutes, which is very short. However, the measures were not made in the workplace but in a lab environment away from work.

Continuous electroencephalogram measurement

Monotonous work causes sleepiness in terms of EEG/EOG changes, as well as in subjective ratings (Sallinen et al., 2004). The effect was similar to that of a 50% sleep reduction. Changing the shift schedule from 3 days on each of the three shifts to 1 day with a fast forward rotation M-E-N caused a reduction of sleepiness during work hours (Viitasalo et al., 2008). Presumably, the reason is that the new schedule gives a possibility for speedy recovery immediately after the morning and night shifts.

With regard to other indicators of physiological sleepiness in shift-workers, several studies indicate clear effects in ambulatory recording of EEG/EOG. In process operators we found not only sleepiness-related increases in alpha and theta activity, but also full-fledged sleep during the night shift (but not during other shifts) (Torsvall et al., 1989). Such incidents of proper sleep occurred in approximately one-fourth of the subjects. Usually, they occurred during the second half of the night shift and never in connection with any other shift. Importantly, sleep on the job was not condoned by the company, nor was there any official awareness that sleep would or could occur during work hours. Interestingly, the subjects were unaware of having slept, but were aware of sleepiness (see also Chapters 15 and 18).

Furthermore, hospital interns on call showed 'attentional failures' (defined as sleep intrusions in the EEG) particularly during early morning work (Landrigan et al., 2004). This was reduced when continuous on-call duty across days was broken up to permit relatively normal amounts of sleep each day (see also Chapter 17). Increased alpha and theta activity during night driving has also been demonstrated in truck drivers during highway driving (Kecklund and Åkerstedt, 1993; Mitler et al., 1997), as well as driving a truck simulator (Gillberg et al., 1996), or in train drivers (Torsvall and Åkerstedt, 1987) or in airline pilots (Rosekind et al., 1995). It has also been demonstrated in power station operators during a night shift (Gillberg et al., 2003), or in shift-workers 'driving a simulator' home after a normal night shift (Åkerstedt et al., 2005). All studies also showed large increases in subjective sleepiness and the driving simulator studies showed impaired performance in the form of increased variation in lateral position (see also Chapter 15).

The cause of sleepiness in shift-work

Sleepiness in field studies of shift-work—whether physiological or subjective—seems pronounced. However, the exact cause is not clear (see also Chapter 15). Reduced sleep is one possibility, but meta-analyses of the average amount of sleep in connection with night and morning shifts indicate a duration of 6 hours (Pilcher et al., 2000a) and so do PSG studies, but this amount should not cause much of an impairment of alertness, at least not after one or two night shifts (Van Dongen et al., 2003; Belenky et al., 2003). A stronger cause may be work at the circadian low, which has pronounced effect, as well as an extended time awake (Dijk and Czeisler, 1995). The latter should be powerful in relation to the first night shift, the end of which is often preceded by 22 hours of time awake.

Shift-work (sleep) disorder

As noted above, the effects of shift-work are relatively pronounced, for example a reduction by 1.5–2 hours on the night shift and considerable sleepiness (reaching 2–3 minutes of MSLT or subjective sleepiness around 7 on the 1–9 level on the KSS) (see also Chapter 15). Clearly, however, some individuals are more afflicted than others. Thus, there is a diagnostic category called 'shift-work sleep disorder' (SWSD), defined by the Diagnostic and Statistical Manual of Mental Disorders (DSM IV) (APA, 2000) as 'report of difficulty falling asleep, staying asleep, or non-restorative sleep for at least 1 month'; and it must be associated with 'a work period that occurs during the habitual sleep phase'. The International Classification of Sleep Disorders (ICSD) (AASM, 2001) basis the diagnosis of shift-work disorder (SWD—'sleep' has been dropped) on four criteria: (1) complaint of insomnia or excessive sleepiness temporally associated with a recurring work schedule that overlaps the usual time for sleep, (2) symptoms must be associated with the shift-work schedule over the course of at least 1 month, (3) circadian and sleep-time misalignment as demonstrated by sleep log or actigraphical monitoring for 7 days or more, and finally (4) sleep disturbance is not explainable by another sleep disorder, a medical or neurological disorder, mental disorder, medication use or substance use disorder. An important point is that the change from SWSD to SWD has changed the focus somewhat from 'sleep' to insufficient restitution from sleep. This means to a large effect that fatigue and sleepiness have come into focus.

The prevalence of SWD is not clear since there is a lack of operational definition of the criteria (Sack et al., 2007). However, one estimate arrives at 10%, using the ICSD-1 criteria (sleep difficulties or sleepiness sometimes or often at a severity level of 6 on a 1–10 scale) (Drake et al., 2004). In another study, a figure of 8% was found when using 'a very negative or rather negative attitude to the present work hours' as a criterion (Axelsson et al., 2004). Czeisler et al. (2005) did not estimate the prevalence but used ICSD-1 criteria as well as MSLT values of <6 minutes during the night, as well as a sleep efficiency of <87.5% during day sleep (8 hours time in bed) after a night shift. The resulting group showed a mean MSLT during the night shift of 2 minutes, a sleepiness rating of 7 on the KSS (Åkerstedt and Gillberg, 1990) and sleep duration of 6 hours. MSLT and sleepiness ratings are clearly at levels indicating excessive sleepiness, whereas the sleep duration seems very similar to most other studies. Waage et al. (2009) made an estimate of 23.3% in a sample of shift-workers on North Sea oil platforms. Although these studies give some information on individuals who may suffer from SWD, they do not seem to have ruled out underlying primary insomnia (seen during non-shift-work periods) and there still has been no attempt to set clear operational and quantitative criteria.

Countermeasures

Another question concerns the countermeasures of night shift fatigue/sleepiness. Napping is one possibility (Schweitzer et al., 2006; Garbarino et al., 2004; Purnell et al., 2002). The effects are usually pronounced. Recent work on alertness-enhancing drugs, like modafinil, is another possibility (Czeisler et al., 2005), even if it seems unlikely that it would be acceptable to treat healthy individuals with potent pharmacological agents. The case is probably the same with the 'chronobiotic' melatonin (Skene, 2003; Smith et al., 2005). Light treatment is a third possibility, but very few field studies have been carried out (Lowden et al., 2004).

The relation between subjective ratings and physiology or performance

The relation between subjective sleepiness and performance or physiology is important since subjective ratings of sleepiness might be a convenient way of investigating sleep-related risks of accidents or impaired performance. Indeed, most studies show a rather strong correlation between subjective ratings and physiological changes and performance. Thus, the average longitudinal correlation between subjective sleepiness and EEG alpha activity has been shown to be high during truck (Gillberg et al., 1996) and train driving (Torsvall and Åkerstedt, 1987) and in a number of laboratory situations (Marzano et al., 2007; Kaida et al., 2008; Carskadon and Dement, 1979; Torsvall and Åkerstedt, 1987) or with performance measures of sleepiness (Cajochen et al., 1999; Ingre et al., 2006a).

However, it has been suggested that the relation may be rather moderate (Dorrian et al., 2000; Rogers and Dinges, 2003; Dinges, 1989). One reason for low correlations may be the effect of context (Dinges, 1989), although this has not been studied systematically. There are observations on monotony, for example, showing that driving a car simulator is associated with increased subjective sleepiness over time (Reyner and Horne, 1997). Physical activity, such as walking, will increase alertness (Eriksen et al., 2005) and will reduce the correlation with performance (Matsumoto et al., 2002). Sitting, lying, resisting, or inviting sleep will have strong effects on the MSLT. Thus, the value will be 10.5 minutes (regular MSLT) after instructions to lie and to try to fall asleep, 17 minutes after instructions to sit and to fall asleep, 21 minutes after instructions to lie down but to stay awake, and 29 minutes after the instruction to sit and try to stay awake (MWT). Social interaction and other factors are likely to have similar effects (Kaida et al., 2007; Åkerstedt et al., 2008b). Recently, Yang et al. (2004) demonstrated that introducing a minute of quiet sitting with closed eyes before rating sleepiness would improve correlations with subsequent performance results.

Another finding that may affect intercorrelations is the shape of the relation. An interesting finding is that the relation between perceived sleepiness and physiological or variables is curvilinear. Thus, using the KSS in a laboratory situation there was no relation to EEG alpha or theta power density or prevalence of slow eye movements on lower levels of the KSS (1–6). However, at level 7 alpha and theta activity started to increase, as did the amount of slow eye movements (Åkerstedt and Gillberg, 1990). At level 9 the EEG/EOG recording was dominated by such changes. A very similar such pattern was seen between KSS and long eye closure durations, lateral variability, and line crossings in a driving simulator (Ingre et al., 2006b). Similar findings have been presented by Ingre et al. (2006b) against long eye blink durations. The results suggest that subjective sleepiness may not be properly perceived until sleep intrusions occur in the waking brain and that high ratings may be indicators of such changes. The results also suggest that unless high levels of sleepiness are reached, the correlations between perception of sleepiness and physiology/behaviour will be quite poor.

Another observation on subjective, physiological, and behavioural sleepiness is the interindividual consistency, that is, the extent to which individuals tend to respond consistently to sleep loss across measurements/time. Van Dongen et al. (2003) noted clear individual differences in the ability to perform during partial sleep loss during 2 weeks. A similar observation was made in a driving simulator study (Ingre et al., 2006b). Individuals differed with respect the level of subjective sleepiness that was associated with driving incidents, lane drifting, and eye closure durations. Interestingly, both studies showed a very high interindividual consistency in ratings of subjective sleepiness. A peculiar point with the study by Van Dongen et al. (2003) is that the difference in performance as a result of sleep loss differs with the type of test; the group that is resilient with respect to, for example, a reaction time test may not be most resilient using a different type of test.

The results above suggest that the situation in which sleepiness ratings are given will affect the results. Logically, a 10-minute performance test under strict environmental control while exerting a burden of monotony on the individual should bring out levels of sleepiness that may have little in common with a 10-second rating under relatively uncontrolled conditions without any particular extra load.

Sleepiness and risk

Sleepiness measures and risk

Few studies have directly tried to link measures of sleepiness risk or other outcomes. However, Melamed and Oksenberg (2002) studied non-shift-workers and found that EDS (ESS > 10) predicted occupational accidents (OR: 2.23) after controlling for type of factory, heaviness of work, age, tenure, etc. A lecture and assessment of sleep problems reduced the risk in subsequent years.

Most of the studies on risk have been carried out in relation to driving. In a rather unique case-control study, Connor et al. (2002) interviewed individuals who had been involved in a car accident and found that retrospective sleepiness ratings from before a crash showed high OR for higher sleepiness (OR: 8.2) compared to drivers who had been interviewed without having been involved in a crash. Also night driving and short prior sleep increased the accident risk. Crummy et al. (2008) carried out a somewhat similar study. They interviewed 112 injured drivers and found that 50% had at least one sleep-related risk factor; 20% had two or more. Being a shift-worker, driving at night, and reporting high sleepiness (KSS > 5) were related to sleep-related accidents.

Using another approach, field studies have been carried out with long-term video recording of the driver and the traffic situation, fatigue/sleepiness (estimated through video scoring). The results suggest that inattention and frequently sleepiness are the most prevalent causes of near accidents (Hanowski et al., 2003; Klauer et al., 2006). Philip et al. (2005) equipped cars with lane trackers and conducted driving experiments on French motorways. A reduction to 2 hours of sleep caused a considerable increase in 'illegitimate' line crossings and in subjective sleepiness, presumably related to accident risk.

The link between sleepiness and risk/performance has also been studied extensively in simulator studies and both subjective sleepiness as well as increased alpha or theta activity or long eye blink durations are associated with unintentional line crossings (Reyner and Horne, 1998; Ingre et al., 2006a). As discussed above the relation is almost exponential, that is, incidents/accidents seem to occur only at the highest level of sleepiness, that of 'fighting sleep'. In a systematic driving simulator study of sleepiness and 'hitting' a rumble strip, it was found a clear relation between 'hits' and subjective sleepiness, lateral variability of the vehicle, and EEG/EOG indications of sleepiness (Anund et al., 2008). The hits occurred on the average at 8.1 units of the KSS.

Among nurses maintaining a diary for sleep, sleepiness, and errors, it was found that days with 'struggle to stay awake' (which may be seen as an indicator of sleepiness) coincided with days with errors at work (Dorrian et al., 2008). A finding of a different character than accident risk is that EDS appears to be a stable predictor of later cognitive impairment or diagnosis with dementia in older age groups (Foley et al., 2001; Ohayon and Vecchierini, 2002).

Risk and sleepiness inferred from disturbed sleep

Most knowledge of sleepiness and risk derive from studies which infer sleepiness from altered sleep-wake patterns. Thus, in the two studies that seem to have been the first to study disturbed sleep and safety, Lavie (1981) and Lavie et al. (1982) showed that EDS and frequent awakenings showed several times the risk of non-complainers with respect to having several occupational accidents. The type of accident was not specified but driving accidents do not seem to have been included. Sleep apnoea seems to be behind the effects but there seems to be an increased risk for complaints of 'mid-sleep awakenings' although this was not specifically tested. Although interesting, these data did not control for BMI or work characteristics.

A cross-sectional study 3,514 Japanese workers responded to questions on sleep and on being involved in an accident during the previous year (yes/no) (Nakata et al., 2005). Controlling for a large number of confounders (alcohol, stress, depression, and others), it was found that 'sleeping poorly at night', 'insufficient sleep', 'insomnia symptoms', and 'over 30 minutes to fall asleep' predicted accidents. Sleep duration <6 hours and 'difficulty breathing' did not. The risk ratios were moderate 1.4–1.5. The effects were pronounced in men and non-significant in women. Possibly, the retrospective character of the study may have been a problem. On the other hand, Doi et al. (2003) in a cross-sectional study of 5,090 Japanese white collar workers failed to find a significant relation between 'disturbed sleep' and accidents, but the accident prevalence was low.

In a case-control study of 2,610 French railway workers, 'sleep disorders' (short sleep, not sleeping well, hypnotics) predicted 'occupational injury' with an OR of 1.29 (95% confidence interval [CI]: 1.07–1.56) controlling for age, BMI, experience, smoking (Chau et al., 2004a, b). Stress, shift-work, and physical workload seem not to have been controlled for. Interestingly, detailed analysis showed an over-risk particularly for 'physical exertion and pain due to movement' and not for tool handling, collisions/falling objects. Train drivers made up a minor portion of the group. Similar results were obtained for construction workers. The occupations with high predictive values for sleep disorder were plumbers, electricians, and civil servants. In a prospective epidemiological study, Åkerstedt et al. (2002a) related fatal occupational accidents to a number of predictors measured previously. Both disturbed sleep and shift-work had significant ORs (age, gender, socioeconomic group, stress, and physical work situation were controlled for). However, the fatal accidents did not differentiate between transport and other accidents.

Risk and sleepiness inferred from work/rest scheduling

One of the most convincing field studies of work hours and safety thus far may be that of Landrigan et al. (2004) (see also Chapter 18). They studied interns on call and showed that reduction of total work hours from 80 to 60 hours per week, together with maximal shift duration of 16 hours (instead of 24–36 hours), there was found a 50% reduction in serious errors. Also sleepiness was reduced and the number of 'attention failures' (similar to 'microsleep') as indicated by EEG/EOG was greatly reduced during night work (Lockley et al., 2004). The hours of sleep per day (across a week) increased from 6.6 to 7.4 hours. It was concluded that the protection of sleep and the reduction of total hours was responsible for the effects. Interestingly, the number of hours worked per week correlated $r = 0.57$ with mean sleep duration per week; 55 hours per week seemed to be compatible with 56 hours of sleep per week (mean of 8 hours per day). At 70 hours of work per week mean sleep duration was 7 hours per day. Other research has demonstrated that fatigue/ sleepiness starts to accumulate below that level (Van Dongen et al., 2003).

Most other approaches have used accident statistics linked to information on work schedules (see also Chapter 15). Road transport is the area where the link between safety and night work sleepiness is most pronounced. Thus, Harris (1977) and Hamelin (1987) and others (Langlois et al., 1985; Horne and Reyner, 1995b) convincingly demonstrated that single vehicle accidents have, by far, the greatest probability of occurring at night (early morning). Interestingly, the accident risk is increased in the early morning for all types of accidents, except for those due to overtaking (Åkerstedt et al., 2001). The risk at that time is increased 5.5 times for all types of accidents and by 10 times for accidents leading to death. Young age increase risk several times and male gender doubles the risk (Åkerstedt and Kecklund, 2001).

Furthermore, the (US) National Transportation Safety Board (NTSB) found that 30–40% of all US truck accidents are fatigue related (and grossly underestimated in conventional reports). The latter investigation was extended to search for the immediate causes of fatigue-induced accidents (NTSB, 1995). It was found that the most important factor was the amount of sleep obtained during the proceeding 24 hours and split-sleep patterns, whereas the length of time driven seemed to play a minor role. The NTSB also found that the Exxon Valdez accident in 1989 was due to fatigue, caused by reduced sleep and extended work hours (NTSB, 1990). The extent of fatal, fatigue-related accidents is considered to lie around 30% (NTSB, 1999). This is compared with approximately the same level of incidence in the air-traffic sector, while equivalent accidents at sea are estimated at slightly below 20%.

It is also believed that the (nighttime) nuclear plant meltdown at Chernobyl was due to human error related to work scheduling (Mitler et al., 1988). Similar observations have been made for the Three Mile Island reactor accident and the near miss incidents at the David Beese reactor in Ohio and at the Rancho Seco reactor in California. These are all anecdotal, however, and very little other data seem available. However, the most carefully executed study, from car manufacturing, seems to indicate a moderate increase (30–50%) in accident risk on the night shift (Smith et al., 1994). As mentioned previously, Åkerstedt et al. (2002a) showed that fatal occupational accidents were higher in shift-workers in a prospective study of shift-workers (controlling for physical workload, stress, and other factors). Several studies have tried to evaluate the costs to society of alertness-related accidents and loss of performance (which does not necessarily reflect only the costs of shift-work). One estimate exceeds $40 billion per year in the United States (Léger, 1994).

With respect to errors or impaired performance, a classic study is that of Bjerner et al. (1955) who showed that errors in meter readings over a period of 20 years in a gas works had a pronounced peak on the night shift. There was also a secondary peak during the afternoon. Similarly, Brown (1949) demonstrated that telephone operators connected calls considerably slower at night. Wojtczak-Jaroszowa and Pawlowska-Skyga (1967) found that the speed of spinning threads in a textile mill went down during the night. From conventional industrial operations less data are available (Wojtczak-Jaroszowa and Jarosz, 1987; Ong et al., 1987) but indicate that overall accidents tend to occur, not surprisingly, when activity is at its peak. But these values do not take account of exposure. Most other studies show a night shift dominance (Andlauer, 1960; Quaas and Tunsch, 1972; Smith, 1979), but not all. Dorrian et al. (2007) were able to demonstrate that the fatigue of train drivers on a particular work schedule was related to the fuel costs because of uneconomical ways of using speed and braking.

The performance decrement during simulated night work has been compared to the effects of blood alcohol levels of 0.08% (Dawson and Reid, 1997). The test was a traditional laboratory psychomotor test and it is not clear how it should be generalized to more complex work situations. It still serves as a reference in many discussions of the dangers of fatigue.

Folkard and Åkerstedt (2004) have developed a model for identifying the risk factors in shift-work scheduling using published data. The results show that, apart from the night shift, accident risk rises with the number of consecutive shifts (particularly night shifts), the duration of the shift, and the absence of breaks. Sleep loss may play a role for the effect of number of successive shifts since one may assume that each night shift contributes to an accumulation of sleep loss (Lowden et al., 2004). However, the duration of the shift and the effect of time between breaks are more likely to be fatigue effects. But this is of course speculation.

Inferred sleepiness among sleep disorder patients

The most well-established link is that between accidents and sleep apnoea (see other chapters) (Rodenstein, 2008). Several reasons can explain this high prevalence. First, in the general population the prevalence of obstructive sleep apnoea syndrome is between 2% and 4% (Young et al., 1993). In the late 80s, Findley et al. (1988) published a study on a very small population of apnoeic non-professional drivers compared to controls (29 apnoeics vs. 35 controls). A higher risk of traffic accidents was found among patients suffering from sleep-related breathing disorders compared to the controls.

In the early 90s, Haraldsson et al. (1990) published a more sophisticated study showing that untreated apnoeics had a higher single-car accident rate than controls. A questionnaire was given to 140 patients with and 142 controls without symptoms associated with the obstructive sleep apnoea syndrome (OSAS). Seventy-three of the patients had a complete triad of OSAS-associated symptoms. The ratio of drivers being involved in one or more combined-car accidents was similar for patients and control drivers, but for single-car accidents the ratio was about seven times higher for patients with a complete triad of symptoms of OSAS compared to controls ($P < 0.001$). When corrected for mileage driven, the total number of single-car accidents was almost 12 times higher among patients with sleep spells while driving, compared to controls ($P < 0.001$).

Terán-Santos et al. (1999) confirmed this finding with another case-control study on non-professional drivers. The case patients were 102 drivers who received emergency treatment at hospitals after highway traffic accidents. The controls were 152 patients randomly selected from primary care centres and matched with case patients for age and sex. As compared to those without OSAS, patients with an AHI of 10 events per hour or higher had an OR of 6.3 (95% CI: 2.4–16.2) for having a traffic accident. This relation remained significant after adjustment for potential confounders, such as alcohol consumption, visual-refraction disorders, BMI, years of driving, age, history of traffic accidents, use of medications causing drowsiness, and sleep schedule. Interestingly, chronic daytime somnolence as measured by the ESS did not show a significant relationship with the risk of traffic accidents.

Stoohs et al. (1994) performed an integrated analysis of recordings of sleep-related breathing disorders, and self-reported automotive and company-recorded automotive accidents in 90 commercial long-haul truck drivers. Truck drivers with sleep-disordered breathing had a two-fold higher accident rate per mile than drivers without sleep-disordered breathing. Accident frequency was not dependent on the severity of the sleep-related breathing disorder. If the severity of breathing disorder (AHI) or chronic daytime somnolence (ESS) is poorly related to the risk of accidents, sleepiness at the wheel seems to be the key symptom to look for in at-risk patients.

George (2001) studied the impact of CPAP treatment on traffic accidents and showed that after treatment the risk of apnoeic drivers was not different from normal subjects. Ulfberg et al. (2000) selected 704 consecutive patients suffering from sleep-related breathing disorder and compared them with 580 controls. The dependent variable was occupational accidents requiring ≥1 day of absence from work during the previous 10 years. Driving accidents were excluded, as were accidents due to external causes such as explosions or 'flying objects'. The age-adjusted OR was 6.3 (95% CI: 1.6–25.6) for sleep apnoea in males and 1.5 (95% CI: 0.9–2.6) in women. For snoring, the OR reached 3.3 (95% CI: 0.98–11.0) in males and 1.8 (95% CI: 1.1–2.9) in women. Work task and work hours were not controlled for, however.

Very few studies have investigated the risk of non-respiratory sleep disorders. In the mid-sixties, narcolepsy started to become a possible risk factor for traffic accidents (Bartels, 1965; Grubb, 1969). Aldrich (1989) in a clinical study confirmed that narcoleptic patients were more frequently involved in car accidents. Unfortunately, no study investigated the impact of pharmacological treatment on narcoleptic accident risk.

Léger et al. (2002) studied 11,372 individuals in a cross-sectional study with questionnaires and found an almost eightfold higher risk for industrial accidents in DSM-IV-diagnosed 'severe insomniacs'. Driving accidents did not differ, however. No controls for confounding appear to have been applied. Drake et al. (2005) found that insomnia (determined via questionnaire) was related to different types of accidents. However, since insomnia patients are not sleepy in terms of MSLT, it is questionable if it represents a case for the link between sleepiness and risk.

Some important sidelines

The strength of sleepiness

The literature clearly shows strong links between sleepiness and involuntary sleep and accidents. However, sleepiness does not seem to be taken seriously and there may be a notion that sleepiness is easily handled by pulling oneself together. Since accidents occur because of sleepiness and since there seems to be a clear awareness of one's sleepy state (Connor et al., 2002; Horne and Baulk, 2004; Ingre et al., 2006b), strong, overpowering sleepiness might be the explanation unless sleepy individuals do not realize that their state is dangerous. Both explanations could contribute and we know too little about sleepiness, awareness, and risk perception in real on the road driving.

However, one glimpse of the imperative nature of sleepiness comes from a driving simulator study of the effects of rumble strips after a night of reduced sleep (Anund et al., 2008). It was found that hitting a rumble strip was associated with strong pre-hit increases in eye closure durations, lateral variability of the vehicle, and high sleepiness levels (KSS = 8.1 on the 9-step scale). Thus, sleepiness was undoubtedly present. The hit immediately reduced the former two to intermediate levels of sleepiness and the vehicle was brought back to the proper lane by the driver. The increased alertness was reversed in 2–4 minutes and a new hit occurred some minutes later. The most interesting aspect is that hits were repeated seven more times on the average. Apparently, the alerting effects of a hit were extremely temporary and irresistible sleepiness returned very rapidly, despite major efforts to remain awake.

Prevalence of sleep deprivation

Inferring sleepiness from shift-work and other contexts needs some substantiation of the prevalence of insufficient sleep. Certainly, night and morning shifts involve sleep durations of 5–6 hours (Pilcher et al., 2000a); since this figure is an average, about half sleep less. Epidemiological studies of sleep duration also indicate that short sleep (≤6 hours) is quite common in the general population (Kripke, 2004; Kripke et al., 2002; Stamatakis et al., 2007; Ursin et al., 2009).

Driving may constitute a special case of sleep reduction without night work being involved. Philip et al. (1996) stopped drivers and asked about sleep duration and found that 50% of drivers had a reduced sleep duration during the last 24 hours when questioned at a rest stop in the morning. Ten percent had had no sleep at all. In a follow-up, a new set of drivers was stopped at a tollbooth and questioned and essentially the same figures were obtained again; 12.5% had a reduction of 3 hours and 2.7% had a reduction of 5 hours. Being young, commuting to work, driving a long distance, and starting the trip at night were risk factors. This agrees with the study of the NTSB (1995), showing that the mean sleep duration of drivers on American highways was below 6 hours.

The need for sleep is frequently debated, but two experimental studies suggest that with 7 hours of sleep per day there is no accumulation of fatigue. At 6 hours, no effects are seen in the first 2 days, but a slow build up is seen across days. This suggests that sleep below 7 hours may be dangerous, at least if maintained across several days. However, experiments with sleep saturation give a somewhat different result. Barbato et al. (1994) had subjects spend 14 hours in a dark room for a number of days and found that sleep duration amounted to 8.3 hours after the first days of extended sleep, probably caused by a sleep deficit from before entering the laboratory. Thus, more sleep can be taken for long periods of time but it is not clear if it is useful. More importantly, the results suggest the maximum 'sleep performance' for the average sleeper under optimal conditions. It does not, however, necessarily indicate how much sleep is needed, only how much sleep that is possible under optimal conditions. It also suggests that there is a clear saturation level for sleep homeostasis.

In a similar approach with a focus on the 'sleep performance' in relation to age, Klerman and Dijk (2008) had young (20–25 years) and old (65+ years) in a similar experiment to that of Wehr. They found that young subjects gradually adopted an 8.7-hour sleep duration versus the 6.9 hours of the older subjects. Performance remained intact. The implications are that young adults can sleep much more than older adults, or perhaps, need much more sleep to maintain an acceptable level of functioning.

Another interesting contribution to the discussion of the need for sleep in relation to sleepiness is that Horne et al. (2008) have shown that an extension of night sleep by an hour has very little effect on MSLT or reaction time, whereas a 20-minute afternoon nap or caffeine have clear effects. The implication is that extended sleep from normal levels is not cost-effective. Youngstedt and Kripke (2004) have even suggested that the population sleeps too much since long sleep seems to have a stronger relation to mortality than short sleep.

It has for a long time been a consensus on the notion that one cannot 'bank' sleep, that is, prepare for sleep loss by increasing prior sleep duration. However, Rupp et al. (2009) showed that giving subjects extra sleep before a sleep deprivation experiment led to lower levels of sleepiness and performance impairment. This suggests that 'banking' extra sleep is possible and useful.

Modeling sleepiness

Mathematical models for alertness or performance prediction have been developed mainly as tools for evaluating work or sleep-wake schedules that deviate from traditional daytime orientation. The first (two-process) model mainly addressed the question of sleep regulation and by inference, the need for sleep or fatigue/sleepiness (Borbély, 1982). Its main components were one factor representing homeostatic effects of time awake and amount of prior sleep and a circadian component representing the effect of the biological clock on metabolism and performance. The homeostatic factors are usually seen as having an exponential relation to sleepiness (e.g. a steep initial fall of alertness after awakening, with a gradual flattening out towards an asymptote of very low alertness after 24 hours of time awake). The circadian component is usually represented as a sinusoid function with a 24-hour period. For a review of present models, see Mallis et al. (2004).

The first model to focus explicitly on sleepiness was inspired by the Borbély model and also included sleep inertia and was called the Three Process Model of Alertness (TPM) (Folkard and Åkerstedt, 1987), and subsequently expanded to include sleep prediction and validated against EEG parameters and laboratory performance tests (Åkerstedt et al., 2004). Several other models predict sleepiness or fatigue and most include laboratory performance validations (Hursh et al., 2004; Roach et al., 2004; Belyavin and Spencer, 2004) and the predictive accuracy is rather similar (Van Dongen, 2004).

Obviously, the prediction of sleepiness and laboratory performance measures imply the ability to predict also accident risk. To the best of our knowledge, however, no validation against safety seems to have been carried out for any of the sleepiness prediction models. This is clearly needed. It would seem that the most suitable setting for this type of validation would be driving since the link between road accident risk and sleepiness is pronounced (Horne and Reyner, 1995a; Stutts et al., 1999; Connor et al., 2002). In particular, reduced prior sleep duration or driving close to the circadian nadir is associated with increased risk. Thus, for example, Connor et al. (2002) showed that driving between 2:00 a.m. and 5:00 a.m. carried an increased risk of OR 5.6 (95% CI: 1.4–22.7), while sleep <5 hours during the last 24 hours carried a risk of OR 2.7 (95% CI: 1.4–5.4). Logically, models that predict sleepiness and laboratory performance using precise information of time of day, time elapsed since prior sleep, and exact duration of prior sleep should be able to predict accident risk quite sensitively.

Conclusion

Sleepiness has a considerable prevalence in the population, is very sensitive to manipulations of the sleep-wake pattern, as well as to various types of sleep disturbances, and to exposure to monotony. At high levels, its effects are powerful and make it responsible for many types of accidents and performance impairment. In spite of this it is remarkably disregarded in society. There is clearly a great need for information as well as a need for reliable and simple ways of measuring sleepiness.

Summary box

- Sleepiness is subjective, physiological, and behavioural. This may lead to a certain amount of confusion in discussions of prevalence, mechanism, and societal implications.
- The prevalence of sleepiness (self-reported) may vary between 4% and 20% in population studies, depending on definition. It is usually caused by shortened sleep, fragmented sleep, long time awake, or activity during the 'circadian low' (late night), but also monotony, a warm environment, physical activity, or alcohol and other drugs may contribute.
- In society, the risk groups or risk situations are workers on schedules with night shifts, individuals who extend their active time late into the night, and individuals with other factors that restrict their sleep. However, insomniacs do not belong to this category, probably because the high physiological arousal that causes insomnia also interferes with the ability to fall asleep. The strength of sleepiness may be overpowering and although sleepiness is generally clearly perceived, the afflicted person may not be able to judge the actual risk of falling asleep. These factors contribute to the considerable impact of sleepiness on accidents.
- Recent developments include technological devices to monitor sleepiness and alertness. Thus far, however, their validity has not been well documented.

References

AASM (2001). International classification of sleep disorders—diagnostic and coding manual. *American academy of Sleep Medicine.*

Åkerstedt, T. & Gillberg, M. (1981). The circadian variation of experimentally displaced sleep. *Sleep*, **4**, 159–169.

Åkerstedt, T. & Gillberg, M. (1990). Subjective and objective sleepiness in the active individual. *Int J Neurosci*, **52**, 29–37.

Åkerstedt, T. & Kecklund, G. (2001). Age, gender and early morning highway accidents. *J Sleep Res*, **10**, 105–110.

Åkerstedt, T., Kecklund, G. & Hörte, L.-G. (2001). Night driving, season, and the risk of highway accidents. *Sleep*, **24**, 401–406.

Åkerstedt, T., Fredlund, P., Gillberg, M. & Jansson, B. (2002a). A prospective study of fatal occupational accidents—relationship to sleeping difficulties and occupational factors. *J Sleep Res*, **11**, 69–71.

Åkerstedt, T., Knutsson, A., Westerholm, P., Theorell, T., Alfredsson, L. & Kecklund, G. (2002b). Work organization and unintentional sleep: results from the WOLF study. *Occup Environ Med*, **59**, 595–600.

Åkerstedt, T., Folkard, S. & Portin, C. (2004). Predictions from the three-process model of alertness. *Aviat Space Environ Med*, **75**, A75–A83.

Åkerstedt, T., Peters, T., Anund, A. & Kecklund, G. (2005). Impaired alertness and performance while driving home from the night shift—a driving simulator study. *J Sleep Res*, **14**, 17–20.

Åkerstedt, T., Ingre, M., Broman, J.E. & Kecklund, G. (2008a). Disturbed sleep in shift workers, day workers, and insomniacs. *Chronobiol Int*, **25**, 333–348.

Åkerstedt, T., Kecklund, G. & Axelsson, J. (2008b). Effects of context on sleepiness self-ratings during repeated partial sleep deprivation. *Chronobiol Int*, **25**, 271–278.

Aldrich, M.S. (1989). Automobile accidents in patients with sleep disorders. *Sleep*, **12**, 487–494.

Andersen, J.E. (1970). *Three-shift wprk.* Copenhagen: Socialforskni ngsinstitutet

Andlauer, P. (1960). *The Effect of Shift Working on the Workers' Health. European Productivity Agency*, TU Information Bulletin, 29.

Anund, A., Kecklund, G., Vadeby, A., Hjalmdahl, M. & Åkerstedt, T. (2008). The alerting effect of hitting a rumble strip—a simulator study with sleepy drivers. *Accid Anal Prev*, **40**, 1970–1976.

APA (2000). *Diagnostic and Statistical Manual of Mental Disorders.* Fourth edition. Washington, DC: American Psychiatric Association.

Arand, D., Bonnet, M., Hurwitz, T., Mitler, M., Rosa, R. & Sangal, R.B. (2005). The clinical use of the MSLT and MWT. *Sleep*, **28**, 123–144.

Asplund, R. & Aberg, H. (1998). Daytime sleepiness in 40-64 year-old women in relation to somatic health and medical treatment. *Scand J Prim Health Care*, **16**, 112–116.

Axelsson, J., Åkerstedt, T., Kecklund, G. & Lowden, A. (2004). Tolerance to shift work—how does it relate to sleep and wakefulness? *Int Arch Occup Environ Health*, **77**, 121–129.

Axelsson, J., Kecklund, G., Åkerstedt, T., Donofrio, P., Lekander, M. & Ingre, M. (2008). Sleepiness and performance in response to repeated sleep restriction and subsequent recovery during semi-laboratory conditions. *Chronobiol Int*, **25**, 297–308.

Balkin, T.J., Bliese, P.D., Belenky, G., et al. (2004). Comparative utility of instruments for monitoring sleepiness-related performance decrements in the operational environment. *J Sleep Res*, **13**, 219–227.

Barbato, G., Barker, C., Bender, C., Giesen, H.A. & Wehr, T.A. (1994). Extended sleep in humans in 14-hour nights (LD 10:14): relationship between REM density and spontaneous awakening. *Electroencephalogr Clin Neurophysiol*, **90**, 291–197.

Bartels, E.C. & Kusakcioglu, O. (1965). Narcolepsy: a possible cause of automobile accidents. *Lahey Clin Found Bull*, **14**, 21–26.

Bartlett, D.J., Marshall, N.S., Williams, A. & Grunstein, R.R. (2008). Sleep health New South Wales: chronic sleep restriction and daytime sleepiness. *Intern Med J*, **38**, 24–31.

Belenky, G., Wesensten, N.J., Thorne, D.R., et al. (2003). Patterns of performance degradation and restoration during sleep restriction and subsequent recovery: a sleep dose-response study. *J Sleep Res*, **12**, 1–12.

Belyavin, A.J. & Spencer, M.B. (2004). Modeling performance and alertness: the QinetiQ approach. *Aviat Space Environ Med*, **75**, A93–A103; discussion 104–106.

Bixler, E.O., Vgontzas, A.N., Lin, H.M., Calhoun, S.L., Vela-Bueno, A. & Kales, A. (2005). Excessive daytime sleepiness in a general population sample: the role of sleep apnea, age, obesity, diabetes, and depression. *J Clin Endocrinol Metab*, **90**, 4510–4515.

Bjerner, B., Holm, Å. & Swensson, Å. (1955). Diurnal variation of mental perfomance. A study of three-shift workers. *Br J Ind Med*, **12**, 103–110.

Bjorvatn, B., Kecklund, G. & Åkerstedt, T. (1998). Rapid adaptation to night work at an oil platform, but slow readaptation following return home. *J Occup Environ Med*, **40**, 601–608.

Bliwise, D.L. (2001). Is the measurement of sleepiness the holy grail for sleep medicine? *Am J Respir Crit Care Med*, **163**, 1517–1519.

Bonnet, M.H. & Arand, D.L. (2003). Clinical effects of sleep fragmentation versus sleep deprivation. *Sleep Med Rev*, **7**, 297–310.

Borbély, A.A. (1982). A two-process model of sleep regulation. *Hum Neurobiol*, **1**, 195–204.

Brown, R.C. (1949). The day and night performance of teleprinter switchboard operators. *J Occup Psychol*, **23**, 121–126.

Buysse, D.J., Hall, M.L., Strollo, P.J., et al. (2008). Relationships between the Pittsburgh Sleep Quality Index (PSQI), Epworth Sleepiness Scale (ESS), and clinical/polysomnographic measures in a community sample. *J Clin Sleep Med*, **4**, 563–571.

Caffier, P.P., Erdmann, U. & Ullsperger, P. (2003). Experimental evaluation of eye-blink parameters as a drowsiness measure. *Eur J Appl Physiol*, **89**, 319–325.

Cajochen, C., Khalsa, S.B.S., Wyatt, J.K., Czeisler, C.A. & Dijk, D.-J. (1999). EEG and ocular correlates of circadian melatonin phase and human performance decrements during sleep loss. *Am J Physiol*, **277**, R640–R649.

Carskadon, M.A. & Dement, W.C. (1979). Effects of total sleep loss on sleep tendency. *Perceptual and Motor Skills*, **48**, 495–506.

Carskadon, M.A. & Dement, W.C. (1982). The multiple sleep latency test: What does it measure? *Sleep*, **5**, 67–72.

Carskadon, M.A., Dement, W.C., Mitler, M.M., Roth, T., Westbrook, P.R. & Keenan, S. (1986). Guidelines for the multiple sleep latency test (MSLT): a standard measure of sleepiness. *Sleep*, **9**, 519–524.

Chau, N., Mur, J.-M., Benamghar, L., et al. (2004a). Relationships between certain individual characteristics and occupational injuries for various jobs in the construction industry: a case-control study. *Am J Ind Med*, **45**, 84–92.

Chau, N., Mur, J.-M., Touron, C., Benamghar, L. & Dehaene, D. (2004b). Correlates of occupational injuries for various jobs in railway workers: a case-control study. *J Occup Health*, **46**, 272–280.

Coleman, R.M. & Dement, W.C. (1986). Falling asleep at work: a problem for continuous operations. *Sleep Res*, **15**, 265.

Connor, J., Norton, R., Ameratunga, S., et al. (2002). Driver sleepiness and risk of serious injury to car occupants: population based case control study. *Br Med J*, **324**, 1125.

Crummy, F., Cameron, P.A., Swann, P., Kossmann, T. & Naughton, M.T. (2008). Prevalence of sleepiness in surviving drivers of motor vehicle collisions. *Intern Med J*, **38**, 769–775.

Czeisler, C.A., Weitzman, E.D., Moore-Ede, M.C., Zimmerman, J.C. & Knauer, R.S. (1980). Human sleep: its duration and organization depend on its circadian phase. *Science*, **210**, 1264–1267.

Czeisler, C.A., Walsh, J.K., Roth, T., et al. (2005). Modafinil for excessive sleepiness associated with shift-work sleep disorder. *N Engl J Med*, **353**, 476–486.

Dahlgren, A., Kecklund, G. & Åkerstedt, T. (2005). Different levels of work-related stress and the effects on sleep, fatigue and cortisol. *Scand J Work Environ Health*, **31**, 277–285.

Dahlgren, A., Kecklund, G. & Åkerstedt, T. (2006). Overtime work and its effects on sleep, sleepiness, cortisol and blood pressure in an experimental field study. *Scand J Work Environ Health*, **32**, 318–327.

Dawson, D. & Reid, K. (1997). Fatigue, alcohol and perfomance impairment. *Nature*, 388, 235.

Dement, W.C. (2003). More on feeling tired: "Response" to Jim Horne. *Sleep*, 26, 764.

Dement, W.C., Hall, J. & Walsh, J.K. (2003). Tiredness versus sleepiness: semantics or a target for public education? *Sleep*, 26, 485–486.

Dijk, D.-J. & Czeisler, C.A. (1995). Contribution of the circadian pacemaker and the sleep homeostat to sleep propensity, sleep structure, electroencephalographic slow waves, and sleep spindle activity in humans. *J Neurosci*, 15, 3526–3538.

Dinges, D.F. (1989). The nature of sleepiness: causes, contexts, and consequences. In: Stunkard, A. & Baum, A. (eds.), *Perspectives in Behavioral Medicine: Eating, Sleeping, and Sex*. Hillsdale, NJ: Lawrence Erlbaum.

Dinges, D.F. (1992). Probing the limits of functional capability: the effects of sleep loss on short-duration tasks. In: Broughton, R.J. & Ogilvie, R.D. (eds.), *Sleep Related Disorders and Internal Diseases*. Boston, MA: Birkhäuser.

Doi, Y., Minowa, M. & Tango, T. (2003). Impact and correlates of poor sleep quality in Japanese white-collar employees. *Sleep*, 26, 467–471.

Dorrian, J., Lamond, N. & Dawson, D. (2000). The ability to self-monitor performance when fatigued. *J Sleep Res*, 9, 137–144.

Dorrian, J., Hussey, F. & Dawson, D. (2007). Train driving efficiency and safety: examining the cost of fatigue. *J Sleep Res*, 16, 1–11.

Dorrian, J., Tolley, C., Lamond, N., et al. (2008). Sleep and errors in a group of Australian hospital nurses at work and during the commute. *Appl Ergon*, 39, 605–613.

Drake, C.L., Roehrs, T., Richardson, G., Walsh, J.K. & Roth, T. (2004). Shift work sleep disorder: prevalence and consequences beyond that of symptomatic day workers. *Sleep*, 27, 1453–1462.

Drake, C.L., Roehrs, T., Richardson, G., Walsh, J.K. & Roth, T. (2005). Shift work sleep disorder: prevalence and consequences beyond that of symptomatic day workers. *Sleep*, 27, 1453–1462.

Edinger, J.D., Means, M.K., Carney, C.E. & Krystal, A.D. (2008). Psychomotor performance deficits and their relation to prior nights' sleep among individuals with primary insomnia. *Sleep*, 31, 599–607.

Ekstedt, M., Söderström, M., Åkerstedt, T., Nilsson, J., Sondergaard, H.-P. & Perski, A. (2006). Disturbed sleep and fatigue in occupational burnout. *Scand J Work Environ Health*, 32, 121–131.

Eriksen, C.A., Åkerstedt, T., Kecklund, G. & Åkerstedt, A. (2005). Comment on short-term variation in subjective sleepiness. *Percept Mot Skills*, 101, 943–948.

Findley, L.J., Unverzagt, M.E. & Suratt, P.M. (1988). Automobile accidents involving patients with obstructive sleep apnea. *Am Rev Respir Dis*, 138, 337–340.

Foley, D., Monjan, A., Masaki, K., Ross, W., Havlik, R., White, L. & Launer, L. (2001). Daytime sleepiness is associated with 3-year incident dementia and cognitive decline in older Japanese-American men. *J Am Geriatr Soc*, 49, 1628–1632.

Folkard, S. & Åkerstedt, T. (1987). Towards a model for the prediction of alertness and/or fatigue on different sleep/wake schedules. In: Oginski, A., Pokorski, J. & Rutenfranz, J. (eds.), *Contemporary Advances in Shift work Research*. Krakow: Medical Academy.

Folkard, S. & Åkerstedt, T. (1991). A three process model of the regulation of alertness and sleepiness. In: Ogilvie, R. & Broughton, R. (eds.), *Sleep, Arousal and Performance: Problems and Promises*. Boston, MA: Birkhäuser.

Folkard, S. & Åkerstedt, T. (2004). Trends in the risk of accidents and injuries and their implications for models of fatigue and performance. *Aviat Space Environ Med*, 75, A161–A167.

Fröberg, J.E. (1977). Twenty-four hour patterns in human performance, subjective and physiological variables and differences between morning and evening active subjects. *Biol Psychol*, 5, 119–134.

Gander, P.H., Marshall, N.S., Harris, R. & Reid, P. (2005). The Epworth sleepiness scale: influence of age, ethnicity, and socioeconomic deprivation. Epworth sleepiness scores of adults in New Zealand. *Sleep*, 28, 249–253.

Garbarino, S., Mascialino, B., Penco, M.S., et al. (2004). Professional shift-work drivers who adopt prophylactic naps can reduce the risk of car accidents during night work. *Sleep*, 27, 1295–1302.

Geisler, P., Tracik, F., Cronlein, T., et al. (2006). The influence of age and sex on sleep latency in the MSLT-30—a normative study. *Sleep*, **29**, 687–692.

George, C.F. (2001). Reduction in motor vehicle collisions following treatment of sleep apnoea with nasal CPAP. *Thorax*, **56**, 508–512.

Gillberg, M., Kecklund, G. & Åkerstedt, T. (1996). Sleepiness and performance of professional drivers in a truck simulator—comparisons between day and night driving. *J Sleep Res*, **5**, 12–15.

Gillberg, M., Kecklund, G., Göransson, B. & Åkerstedt, T. (2003). Operator performance and signs of sleepiness during day and night work in a simulated thermal power plant. *Int J Ind Ergon*, **31**, 101–109.

Gislason, T., Almqvist, M., Eriksson, G., Taube, A. & Boman, G. (1988). Prevalence of sleep apnea syndrome among Swedish men—an epidemiological study. *J Clin Epidemiol*, **41**, 571–576.

Grubb, T.C. (1969). Narcolepsy and highway accidents. *J Am Med Assoc*, **209**, 1720.

Grunstein, R.R. & Banerjee, D. (2007). The case of 'Judge Nodd' and other sleeping judges—media, society, and judicial sleepiness. *Sleep*, **30**, 625–632.

Hamelin, P. (1987). Lorry driver's time habits in work and their involvement in traffic accidents. *Ergonomics*, **30**, 1323–1333.

Hanowski, R.J., Wierwille, W.W. & Dingus, T.A. (2003). An on-road study to investigate fatigue in local/short haul trucking. *Accid Anal Prev*, **35**, 153–160.

Haraldsson, P.O., Carenfelt, C., Laurell, H. & Törnros, J. (1990). Driving vigilance simulator test . *Acta Otolaryngol*, **110**, 136–140.

Harris, W. (1977). Fatigue, circadian rhythm and truck accidents. In: Mackie, R.R. (ed.), *Vigilance*. New York, NY: Plenum Press.

Hasler, G., Buysse, D.J., Gamma, A., et al. (2005). Excessive daytime sleepiness in young adults: a 20-year prospective community study. *J Clin Psychiatry*, **66**, 521–529.

Hoddes, E., Zarcone, V., Smythe, H., Phillips, R. & Dement, W. (1973). Quantification of sleepiness: a new approach. *Psychophysiology*, **10**, 431–436.

Horne, J.A. & Reyner, L.A. (1995a). Driver sleepiness. *J Sleep Res*, **4**(Suppl 2), 23–29.

Horne, J.A. & Reyner, L.A. (1995b). Sleep related vehicle accidents. *Br Med J*, **310**, 565–567.

Horne, J.A. & Reyner, L.A. (1996). Counteracting driver sleepiness: effects of napping, caffeine and placebo. *Psychophysiology*, **33**, 306–309.

Horne, J. (2003). The semantics of sleepiness. *Sleep*, **26**, 763; author reply 764.

Horne, J., Anderson, C. & Platten, C. (2008). Sleep extension versus nap or coffee, within the context of 'sleep debt'. *J Sleep Res*, **17**, 432–436.

Hublin, C., Kaprio, J., Partinen, M., Heikkila, K. & Koskenvuo, M. (1996). Daytime sleepiness in an adult, Finnish population. *J Intern Med*, **239**, 417–423.

Hursh, S.R., Redmond, D.P., Johnson, M.L., et al. (2004). Fatigue models for applied research in warfighting. *Aviat Space Environ Med*, **75**, A44–A53; discussion A54–A60.

Härmä, M., Suvanto, S., Popkin, S., Pulli, K., Mulder, M. & Hirvonen, K. (1998a). A dose-response study of total sleep time and the ability to maintain wakefulness. *J Sleep Res*, **7**, 167–174.

Härmä, M., Tenkanen, L., Sjöblom, T., Alikoski, T. & Heinsalmi, P. (1998b). Combined effects of shift work and life-style on the prevalence of insomnia, sleep deprivation and daytime sleepiness. *Scand J Work Environ Health*, **24**, 300–307.

Ingre, M., Åkerstedt, T., Peters, B., Anund, A., Kecklund, G. & Pickles, A. (2006a). Subjective sleepiness and accident risk avoiding the ecological fallacy. *J Sleep Res*, **15**, 142–148.

Ingre, M., Åkerstedt, T., Peters, B., Anund, A. & Kecklund, G. (2006b). Subjective sleepiness, simulated driving performance and blink duration: examining individual differences. *J Sleep Res*, **15**, 47–53.

Ingre, M., Kecklund, G., Åkerstedt, T., Soderstrom, M. & Kecklund, L. (2008). Sleep length as a function of morning shift-start time in irregular shift schedules for train drivers: self-rated health and individual differences. *Chronobiol Int*, **25**, 349–358.

Jewett, M.E., Dijk, D.-J., Kronauer, R.E. & Dinges, D.F. (1999). Dose-response relationship between sleep duration and human psychomotor vigilance and subjective alertness. *Sleep*, **22**, 171–179.

Johns, M.W. (1991). A new method for measuring daytime sleepiness: the Epworth sleepiness scale. *Sleep*, **14**, 540–545.

Johns, M.W. (2002). Sleep propensity varies with behaviour and the situation in which it is measured: the concept of somnificity. *J Sleep Res*, **11**, 61–67.

Johns, M. & Hocking, B. (1997). Daytime sleepiness and sleep habits of Australian workers. *Sleep*, **20**, 844–849.

Kaida, K., Åkerstedt, T., Kecklund, G., Nilsson, J.P. & Axelsson, J. (2007). The effects of asking for verbal ratings of sleepiness on sleepiness and its masking effects on performance. *Clin Neurophysiol*, **118**, 1324–1331.

Kaida, K., Åkerstedt, T., Takahashi, M., et al. (2008). Performance prediction by sleepiness-related subjective symptoms during 26-hour sleep deprivation. *Sleep Biol Rhythms*, **6**, 234–241.

Kaneita, Y., Ohida, T., Uchiyama, M., et al. (2005). Excessive daytime sleepiness among the Japanese general population. *J Epidemiol*, **15**, 1–8.

Kecklund, G. & Åkerstedt, T. (1993). Sleepiness in long distance truck driving: an ambulatory EEG study of night driving. *Ergonomics*, **36**, 1007–1017.

Kim, H. & Young, T. (2005). Subjective daytime sleepiness: dimensions and correlates in the general population. *Sleep*, **28**, 625–634.

Klauer, S.G., Dingus, T.A., Neale, V.L., Sudweeks, J.D. & Ramsey, D.J. (2006). *The Impact of Driver Inattention on Near-crash/Cash-risk: An Analysis Using the 100-Car Naturalistic Driving Study Data.* Blacksburg, VA: Virginia Tech Transportation Institute.

Klerman, E.B. & Dijk, D.J. (2008). Age-related reduction in the maximal capacity for sleep—implications for insomnia. *Curr Biol*, **18**, 1118–1123.

Kribbs, N.B. & Dinges, D.F. (1994). Vigilance decrement and sleepiness. In: Harsch, J.R. (ed.), *Sleep Onset. Normal and Abnormal Processes.* Washington, DC: American Psychological Association.

Kripke, D.F. (2004). Do we sleep too much? *Sleep*, **27**, 13–14.

Kripke, D.F., Garfinkel, L., Wingard, D.L., Klauber, M.R. & Marler, M.R. (2002). Mortality associated with sleep duration and insomnia. *Arch Gen Psychiatry*, **59**, 131–136.

Kronholm, E., Hyyppä, M.T., Alanen, E., Halonen, J.-P. & Partinen, M. (1995). What does the multiple sleep latency test measure in a community sample? *Sleep*, **18**, 827–835.

Lal, S.K.L. & Graig, A. (2002). Driver fatigue: electroencephalography and psychological assessment. *Psychophysiology*, **39**, 313–321.

Landrigan, C.P., Rothschild, J.M., Cronin, J.W., et al. (2004). Effect of reducing interns' work hours on serious medical errors in intensive care units. *N Engl J Med*, **351**, 1838–1848.

Langlois, P.H., Smolensky, M.H., Hsi, B.P. & Weir, F.W. (1985). Temporal patterns of reported single-vehicle car and truck accidents in Texas, USA during 1980–1983. *Chronobiol Int*, **2**, 131–146.

Lavie, P. (1981). Sleep habits and sleep disturbances in industry workers in Israel: main findings and some characteristics of workers complaining of excessive daytime sleepiness. *Sleep*, **4**, 147–158.

Lavie, P. (1983) Incidence of sleep apnea in a presumably healthy working population: a significant relationship with excessive daytime sleepiness. *Sleep*, **6**, 312–318.

Lavie, P., Kremerman, S. & Wiel, M. (1982). Sleep disorders and safety at work in industry workers. *Accid Anal Prev*, **14**, 311–314.

Léger, D. (1994). The cost of sleep-related accidents: a report for the National Commission on Sleep Disorders Research. *Sleep*, **17**, 84–93.

Léger, D., Guilleminault, C., Bader, G., Lévy, E. & Paillard, M. (2002). Medical and socio-professional impact of insomnia. *Sleep*, **25**, 621–625.

Liljenberg, B., Almqvist, M., Hetta, J., Roos, B. & Ågren, H. (1988). The prevalence of insomnia: the importance of operationally defined criteria. *Ann Clin Res*, **20**, 393–398.

Littner, M.R., Kushida, C., Wise, M., et al. (2005). Practice parameters for clinical use of the multiple sleep latency test and the maintenance of wakefulness test. *Sleep*, **28**, 113–121.

Liu, X., Uchiyama, M., Kim, K., et al. (2000). Sleep loss and daytime sleepiness in the general adult population of Japan. *Psychiatry Res*, **93**, 1–11.

Lockley, S.W., Cronin, J.W., Evans, E.E., et al. (2004). Effect of reducing interns' weekly work hours on sleep and attentional failures. *N Engl J Med*, **351**, 1829–1837.

Lowden, A., Kecklund, G., Axelsson, J. & Åkerstedt, T. (1998). Change from an 8-hour shift to a 12-hour shift, attitudes, sleep, sleepiness and performance. *Scand J Work Environ Health*, **24**(Suppl 3), 69–75.

Lowden, A., Åkerstedt, T. & Wibom, R. (2004). Suppression of sleepiness and melatonin by bright light exposure during breaks in night work. *J Sleep Res*, **13**, 37–43.

Mackworth, N.H. (1950). Researches on the measurement of human performance. *Medical Research Council Special Report*. London: His Majesty's Stationery Office.

Mallis, M.M., Mejdal, S., Nguyen, T.T. & Dinges, D.F. (2004). Summary of the key features of seven biomathematical models of human fatigue and performance. *Aviat Space Environ Med*, **75**, A4–A14.

Marzano, C., Fratello, F., Moroni, F., et al. (2007). Slow eye movements and subjective estimates of sleepiness predict EEG power changes during sleep deprivation. *Sleep*, **30**, 610–616.

Matsumoto, Y., Mishima, K., Satoh, K., Shimizu, T. & Hishikawa, Y. (2002). Physical activity increases the dissociation between subjective sleepiness and objective performance levels during extended wakefulness in human. *Neurosci Lett*, **326**, 133–136.

Melamed, S. & Oksenberg, A. (2002). Excessive daytime sleepiness and risk of occupational injuries in non-shift daytime workers. *Sleep*, **25**, 315–322.

Mitler, M., Gujavarty, K. & Broman, C. (1982). Maintenance of Wakefulness Test: a polysomnographic technique for evaluating treatment efficacy in patients with excessive somnolence. *Electroencephalogr Clin Neurophysiol*, **1982**, 658–661.

Mitler, M.M., Carskadon, M.A., Czeisler, C.A., Dement, W.C., Dinges, D.F. & Graeber, R.C. (1988). Catastrophes, sleep and public policy: consensus report. *Sleep*, **11**, 100–109.

Mitler, M.M., Miller, J.C., Lipsitz, J.J., Walsh, J.K. & Wylie, C.D. (1997). The sleep of long-haul truck drivers. *N Engl J Med*, **337**, 755–761.

Monk, T.H. (1989). A visual analogue scale technique to measure global vigor and affect. *Psychiatry Res*, **27**, 89–99.

Nakata, A., Ikeda, T., Takahashi, M., et al. (2005). Sleep-related risk of occupational injuries in Japanese small and medium-scale enterprises. *Ind Health*, **43**, 89–97.

NSF (2002). Sleep in America Poll. National Sleep Foundation.

NTSB (1990). Grounding of the US tank ship Exxon Valdez on Bligh Reef, Prince William Sound near Valdez, Alaska, March 24, 1989. *National Transportation Safety Board. Maritime Accident Report*, NTSB/MAR-90/04.

NTSB (1995). Factors that affect fatigue in heavy truck accidents. *National Transportation Safety Board. Safety Study*, NTSB/SS-95/01.

NTSB (1999). *Evaluation of U.S. Department of Transportation: Efforts in the 1990s to Address Operation Fatigue*. Washington, DC: National Transportation Safety Board.

Nugent, A.M., Gleadhill, I., McCrum, E., Patterson, C.C., Evans, A. & MacMahon, J. (2001). Sleep complaints and risk factors for excessive daytime sleepiness in adult males in Northern Ireland. *J Sleep Res*, **10**, 69–74.

O'Hanlon, J. & Kelly, G. (1974). A psycho-physiological evaluation of devices for preventing lane drift and run-off-road accidents. *Technical Report 1736-F*, Goleta, CA: Human Factors Research Inc, Santa Barbara Research Park.

Ohayon, M.M. (2008). From wakefulness to excessive sleepiness: what we know and still need to know. *Sleep Med Rev*, **12**, 129–141.

Ohayon, M.M. & Vecchierini, M.F. (2002). Daytime sleepiness and cognitive impairment in the elderly population. *Arch Intern Med*, **162**, 201–208.

Ohayon, M.M., Caulet, M., Philip, P., Guilleminault, C. & Priest, R.G. (1997). How sleep and mental disorders are related to complaints of daytime sleepiness. *Arch Intern Med*, **157**, 2645–2652.

Ohayon, M.M., Priest, R.G., Zulley, J., Smirne, S. & Paiva, T. (2002). Prevalence of narcolepsy symptomatology and diagnosis in the European general population. *Neurology*, **58**, 1826–1833.

Olbrich, S., Mulert, C., Karch, S., et al. (2009). EEG-vigilance and BOLD effect during simultaneous EEG/fMRI measurement. *Neuroimage*, **45**, 319–332.

Ong, C.N., Phoon, W.O., Iskandar, N. & Chia, K.S. (1987). Shift work and work injuries in an iron and steel mill. *Appl Ergon*, **18**, 51–56.

Otmani, S., Roge, J. & Muzet, A. (2005). Sleepiness in professional drivers: effect of age and time of day. *Accid Anal Prev*, **37**, 930–937.

Pack, A.I., Dinges, D.F., Gehrman, P.R., Staley, B., Pack, F.M. & Maislin, G. (2006). Risk factors for excessive sleepiness in older adults. *Ann Neurol*, **59**, 893–904.

Paley, M.J. & Tepas, D.I. (1994). Fatigue and the shiftworker: firefighters working on a rotating shift schedule. *Hum Factors*, **36**, 269–284.

Pallesen, S., Nordhus, I.H., Omvik, S., Sivertsen, B., Tell, G.S. & Bjorvatn, B. (2007). Prevalence and risk factors of subjective sleepiness in the general adult population. *Sleep*, **30**, 619–624.

Philip, P., Ghorayeb, I., Stoohs, R., Menny, J.C., Dabadie, P., Bioulac, B. & Guilleminault, C. (1996). Determinants of sleepiness in automobile drivers. *J Psychosom Res*, **41**, 279–288.

Philip, P., Taillard, J., Gilleminault, C., Quera Salva, M.A., Bioulac, B. & Ohayon, M. (1999). Long distance driving and self-induced sleep deprivation among automobile drivers. *Sleep*, **22**, 475–480.

Philip, P., Sagaspe, P., Moore, N., et al. (2005). Fatigue, sleep restriction and driving performance. *Accid Anal Prev*, **37**, 473–478.

Pilcher, J.J., Lambert, B.J. & Huffcutt, A.I. (2000a). Differential effects of permanent and rotating shifts on self-report sleep length: a meta-analytic review. *Sleep*, **23**, 155–163.

Pilcher, J.J., Schoeling, S.E. & Prosansky, C.M. (2000b). Self-report sleep habits as predictors of subjective sleepiness. *Behav Med*, **25**, 161–168.

Piper, B.F. (1986). Fatigue. In: Carrieri, V., Lindsay, A. & West, C. (eds.) *Pathophysiological phenomena in nursing: Human responses to illness*. Philadelphia: W. B. Sanders & Co.

Prokop, O. & Prokop, L. (1955). Ermüdung und Einschlafen am Steuer. *Zentralbl Verkehrsmed Verkehrspsychol Luft Raumfahrtmed*, **1**, 19–30.

Purnell, M.T., Feyer, A.-M. & Herbison, G.P. (2002). The impact of a nap opportunity during the night shift on the performance and alertness of 12-h shift workers. *J Sleep Res*, **11**, 219–227.

Quaas, M. & Tunsch, R. (1972). Problems of disablement and accident frequency in shift and night work. *Studia Laboris et Salutis*, **4**, 52–65.

Reyner, L.A. & Horne, J.A. (1997). Suppression of sleepiness in drivers: combination of caffeine with a short nap. *Psychophysiology*, **34**, 721–725.

Reyner, L.A. & Horne, J.A. (1998). Falling asleep whilst driving: are drivers aware of prior sleepiness? *Int J Legal Med*, **111**, 120–123.

Roach, G.D., Fletcher, A. & Dawson, D. (2004). A model to predict work-related fatigue based on hours of work. *Aviat Space Environ Med*, **75**, A61–A69; discussion A70–A74.

Rodenstein, D. (2008). Driving in Europe: the need of a common policy for drivers with obstructive sleep apnoea syndrome. *J Sleep Res*, **17**, 281–284.

Rogers, N.L. & Dinges, D.F. (2003). Subjective surrogates of performance during night work. *Sleep*, **26**, 790–791.

Rosekind, M.R., Graeber, R.C., Dinges, D.F., Connel, L.J., Rountree, M.S. & Gillen, K. (1995). *Crew Factors in Flight Operations IX: Effects of Planned Cockpit Rest on Crew Performance and Alertness in Long-haul Operations*. Moffett Field, CA: NASA Technical Memorandum.

Rowland, L.M., Thomas, M.L., Thorne, D.R., et al. (2005). Oculomotor responses during partial and total sleep deprivation. *Aviat Space Environ Med*, **76**, C104–C113.

Rupp, T.L., Wesensten, N.J., Bliese, P.D. & Balkin, T.J. (2009). Banking sleep: realization of benefits during subsequent sleep restriction and recovery. *Sleep*, **32**, 311–321.

Russo, M.B., Stetz, M.C. & Thomas, M.L. (2005). Monitoring and predicting cognitive state and performance via physiological correlates of neuronal signals. *Aviat Space Environ Med*, **76**, C59–C63.

Sack, R.L., Auckley, D., Auger, R.R., et al. (2007). Circadian rhythm sleep disorders: part I, basic principles, shift work and jet lag disorders. An American Academy of Sleep Medicine review. *Sleep*, **30**, 1460–1483.

Sagaspe, P., Taillard, J., Åkerstedt, T., et al. (2008). Extended driving impairs nocturnal driving performances. *PLoS One*, **3**, e3493.

Sallinen, M., Harma, M., Akila, R., et al. (2004). The effects of sleep debt and monotonous work on sleepiness and performance during a 12–h dayshift. *J Sleep Res*, **13**, 285–294.

Sangal, R.B., Mitler, M.M. & Sangal, J.M. (1999). Subjective sleepiness ratings (Epworth sleepiness scale) do not reflect the same parameter of sleepiness as objective sleepiness (maintenance of wakefulness test) in patients with narcolepsy. *Clin Neurophysiol*, **110**, 2131–2135.

Schweitzer, P.K., Randazzo, A.C., Stone, K., Erman, M. & Walsh, J.K. (2006). Laboratory and field studies of naps and caffeine as practical countermeasures for sleep-wake problems associated with night work. *Sleep*, **29**, 39–50.

Skene, D.J. (2003). Optimization of light and melatonin to phase-shift human circadian rhythms. *J Neuroendocrinol*, **15**, 438–441.

Slater, J.D. (2008). A definition of drowsiness: one purpose for sleep? *Med Hypotheses*, **71**, 641–644.

Smith, L., Folkard, S. & Poole, C.J.M. (1994). Increased injuries on night shift. *Lancet*, **344**, 1137–1139.

Smith, M.R., Lee, C., Crowley, S.J., Fogg, L.F. & Eastman, C.I. (2005). Morning melatonin has limited benefit as a soporific for daytime sleep after night work. *Chronobiol Int*, **22**, 873–888.

Smith, P. (1979). A study of weekly and rapidly rotating shift workers. *Int Arch Occup Environ Health*, **43**, 211–220.

Son, M., Kong, J.O., Koh, S.B., Kim, J. & Harma, M. (2008). Effects of long working hours and the night shift on severe sleepiness among workers with 12-hour shift systems for 5 to 7 consecutive days in the automobile factories of Korea. *J Sleep Res*, **17**, 385–394.

Stamatakis, K.A., Kaplan, G.A. & Roberts, R.E. (2007). Short sleep duration across income, education, and race/ethnic groups: population prevalence and growing disparities during 34 years of follow-up. *Ann Epidemiol*, **17**, 948–955.

Stoohs, R.A., Guilleminault, C., Itoi, A. & Dement, W.C. (1994). Traffic accidents in commercial long-haul truck drivers: the influence of sleep-disordered breathing and obesity. *Sleep*, **17**, 619–623.

Stutts, J.C., Wilkins, J.W. & Vaughn, B.V. (1999). Why Do People Have Drowsy Driving Crashes? Input from Drivers Who Just Did. Washington, DC: AAA Foundation for Traffic Safety.

Summala, H., Häkkänen, H., Mikkola, T. & Sinkkonen, J. (1999). Task effects on fatigue symptoms in overnight driving. *Ergonomics*, **42**, 798–806.

Surani, S., Subramanian, S., Babbar, H., Murphy, J. & Aguillar, R. (2008). Sleepiness in critical care nurses: results of a pilot study. *J Hosp Med*, **3**, 200–205.

Söderström, M., Ekstedt, M., Åkerstedt, T., Nilsson, J. & Axelsson, J. (2004). Sleep and sleepiness in young individuals with high burnout scores. *Sleep*, **17**, 1369–1377.

TakahashI, M., Nakata, A., Haratani, T. Otsuka, Y., Kaida, K. & Fukasawa, K. (2006). Psychosocial work characteristics predicting daytime sleepiness in day and shift workers. *Chronobiol Int*, **23**, 1409–1422.

Takegami, M., Sokejima, S., Yamazak, S., Nakayama, T. & Fukuhaa, S. (2005). An estimation of the prevalence of excessive daytime sleepiness based on age and sex distribution of Epworth sleepiness scale scores: a population based survey. *Nippon Koshu Eisei Zasshi*, **52**, 137–145.

Terán-Santos, J., Jiménez-Gómez, A. & Cordero-Guevara, J. (1999). The association between sleep apnea and the risk of traffic accidents. *N Engl J Med*, **240**, 847–851.

Theorell-Haglow, J., Lindberg, E. & Janson, C. (2006). What are the important risk factors for daytime sleepiness and fatigue in women? *Sleep*, **29**, 751–757.

Thiis-Evensen, E. (1957). Shift work and health. Proceedings of the XII International Congress of Occupational Health (Helsinki). Helsinki.

Thomas, M., Sing, H., Belenky, G., et al. (2000). Neural basis of alertness and cognitive performance impairments during sleepiness. I. Effects of 24 h of sleep deprivation on waking human regional brain activity. *J Sleep Res*, **9**, 335–352.

Thorpy, M.J. (2005). Which clinical conditions are responsible for impaired alertness? *Sleep Med*, 6(Suppl 1), S13–S20.

Torsvall, L. & Åkerstedt, T. (1987). Sleepiness on the job: continuously measured EEG changes in train drivers. *Electroencephalogr Clin Neurophysiol*, 66, 502–511.

Torsvall, L. & Åkerstedt, T. (1988). Extreme sleepiness: quantification of EOG and spectral EEG parameters. *Int J Neurosci*, 38, 435–441.

Torsvall, L., Åkerstedt, T., Gillander, K. & Knutsson, A. (1989). Sleep on the night shift: 24-hour EEG monitoring of spontaneous sleep/wake behavior. *Psychophysiology*, 26, 352–358.

Ulfberg, J., Carter, N. & Edling, C. (2000). Sleep-disordered breathing and occupational accidents. *Scand J Work Environ Health*, 26, 237–242.

Ursin, R., Baste, V. & Moen, B.E. (2009). Sleep duration and sleep-related problems in different occupations in the Hordaland Health Study. *Scand J Work Environ Health*, 35, 193–202.

Van Dongen, H.P. (2004). Comparison of mathematical model predictions to experimental data of fatigue and performance. *Aviat Space Environ Med*, 75, A15–A36.

Van Dongen, H.P., Maislin, G., Mullington, J.M. & Dinges, D.F. (2003). The cumulative cost of additional wakefulness: dose-response effects on neurobehavioral functions and sleep physiology from chronic sleep restriction and total sleep deprivation. *Sleep*, 26, 117–126.

Vandewalle, G., Archer, S.N., Wuillaume, C., et al. (2009). Functional magnetic resonance imaging-assessed brain responses during an executive task depend on interaction of sleep homeostasis, circadian phase, and PER3 genotype. *J Neurosci*, 29, 7948–7956.

Verhaegen, P., Dirkx, J. & Maasen, A. (1986). The evolution of shift workers' sleep four years and twelve years after starting shift work. In: Oginski, A., Pokorski, J. & Rutenfranz, J. (eds.) *Shiftwork research '87. Contemporary advances in shiftwork research*. Krakow: Medical Academy.

Viitasalo, K., Kuosma, E., Laitinen, J. & Harma, M. (2008). Effects of shift rotation and the flexibility of a shift system on daytime alertness and cardiovascular risk factors. *Scand J Work Environ Health*, 34, 198–205.

Waage, S., Moen, B.E., Pallesen, S., et al. (2009). Shift work disorder among oil rig workers in the North Sea. *Sleep*, 32, 558–565.

Walsh, J.K., Snyder, E., Hall, J., et al. (2008). Slow wave sleep enhancement with gaboxadol reduces daytime sleepiness during sleep restriction. *Sleep*, 31, 659–672.

Wessely, S., Chalder, T., Hirsch, S., Wallace, P. & Wright, D. (1997). The prevalence and morbidity of chronic fatigue and chronic fatigue syndrome: a prospective primary care study. *Am J Public Health*, 87, 1449–1455.

Wierwille, W.W. & Ellsworth, L.A. (1994). Evaluation of driver drowsiness by trained raters. *Accident Analysis & Prevention*, 26, 571–581.

Wilkinson, R.T., Edwards, R.S. & Haines, E. (1966). Performance following a night of reduced sleep. *Psychon Sci*, 5, 471–472.

Wojtczak-Jaroszowa, J. & Jarosz, D. (1987). Time-related distribution of occupational accidents. *J Safety Res*, 18, 33–41.

Wojtczak-Jaroszowa, J. & Pawlowska-Skyga, K. (1967). Night and shift work: circadian variations in work. *Med Pr*, 18, 1–10.

Yang, C.-M., Lin, F.-W. & Spielman, A.J. (2004). A standard procedure enhances the correlation between subjective and objective measures of sleepiness. *Sleep*, 27, 329–332.

Young, T., Palta, M., Dempsey, J., Skatrud, J., Weber, S. & Badr, S. (1993). The occurrence of sleep-disordered breathing among middle-aged adults. *N Engl J Med*, 328, 1230–1235.

Youngstedt, S.D. & Kripke, D.F. (2004). Long sleep and mortality: rationale for sleep restriction. *Sleep Med Rev*, 8, 159–174.

Zielinski, J., Zgierska, A., Polakowska, M., et al. (1999). Snoring and excessive daytime somnolence among Polish middle-aged adults. *Eur Respir J*, 14, 946–950.

Chapter 17

Effect of lack of sleep on medical errors

C.P. Landrigan

Introduction: the silent epidemic

On July 17, 1996, shortly after taking off from JFK international airport in New York, TWA flight 800—a Boeing 747 en route to Paris—exploded in mid-air off the coast of the United States. All 230 people on board were killed (Wikipedia, 2009). The crash was instantly international news and the subject of major investigations by the US National Transportation Safety Board and the Federal Bureau of Investigation. The President and First Lady of the United States went in person to Long Island to comfort the victims' families and meet with investigators (Bowser, 1996). Fifteen new regulations intended to prevent future accidents due to fuel tank explosions, the putative cause of the crash, were introduced.

Although a horrific tragedy, the magnitude of the TWA flight 800 disaster pales in comparison to even the most cautious estimates of the annual number of deaths due to medical errors. Although the precise numbers of deaths and injuries due to medical errors are uncertain, the best data available suggest that between 44,000 and 98,000 Americans are killed each year due to medical error (Institute of Medicine, 1999), making it the sixth to ninth leading cause of mortality in that country—more than the number due to motor vehicle crashes, AIDS, breast cancer, homicides, or suicides (Kochanek et al., 2004).

Medical errors are likewise extremely common in the United Kingdom, occurring in more than 10% of admissions, up to half of which may be preventable (Vincent et al., 2001). Lucian Leape, one of the pioneers of the patient safety movement, notes that this is equivalent to three 747 crashes every 2 days (Leape, 1994). Yet remarkably, while the occasional error involving a celebrity (such as the 1,000-fold overdose of heparin administered to Dennis Quaid's newborn twins) (CBS News, 2009) makes the news, most go entirely unnoticed by the public. Deaths and injuries due to medical error have not garnered anywhere near the public outcry of even a single 747 crash.

A major reason for this silence is the invisibility of the patient safety epidemic. Although deaths due to medical errors are extremely common when viewed at a worldwide level, they occur quietly, one at a time, scattered among the thousands of hospitals in the United Kingdom, the United States, and throughout the world. There is no explosion, no wreckage. Especially egregious events occasionally make the local evening news, but the vast majority do not. The caregivers and family members left behind are usually the only ones who know of the error, and often even they are not entirely aware of what transpired. It is easy to dismiss a death or injury in a very sick patient as inevitable, or to write off an error as an aberration; after all, most hospitalized patients do just fine. There is always an easy explanation for any error, a reason why this case was different. Sometimes, a doctor or a nurse is blamed, but care goes on much the same as before the event occurred. Until recently, few hospitals responded to serious errors by taking hard looks at their systems of care delivery.

Because of the invisibility of medical error, change has been slow. Unlike aviation, nuclear power, and the automobile industries, which have been focused on designing systems to optimize safety for decades, concerns about the safety of the healthcare system have only recently come to the fore, and efforts to design safer systems are in their infancy. In 1999, the US Institute of Medicine (IOM) began to galvanize concerns about patient safety worldwide with the publication of its report, *To Err is Human*. This report systematically gathered together data on the frequency of medical errors, and concluded that these events were neither rare, nor the product of a few bad providers. Rather, it asserted that most errors in medicine are due to faulty systems of care. This notion challenged an implicit assumption in healthcare that errors are the by-product of insufficient training or attention to detail, and did not happen to good doctors. The traditional wisdom was that doctors who are smart, well-trained, work hard, and put their patients' needs ahead of their own do not make errors. After all, training to be a physician is highly competitive, extremely rigorous, and requires considerable self-sacrifice—individuals who make it through medical school, and then devote themselves to working day and night for a 3- to 10-year residency in the field of their choosing should emerge well enough trained, skilled enough, and devoted enough to provide safe patient care. Unfortunately, it is not this simple.

Human fallibility and system complexity

As *To Err is Human*, along with decades of research by cognitive psychologists, human factors engineers—experts in the study of the interface between individuals and the complex environments in which they work—and safety experts demonstrates, sufficient knowledge and attention to detail do not guarantee safe care. Human fallibility as well as the complexity of our care systems can induce errors even among the most highly qualified and devoted of providers.

Individual errors by physicians and nurses do not occur in a void. Rather, they are typically the product of inherent human cognitive limits, compounded by an individual's environment and working conditions, factors beyond the immediate control of providers. Cognitive psychologists have long recognized that human cognitive processes have inherent vulnerabilities (Rasmussen and Jensen, 1974; Reason, 1990). Errors in probabilistic thinking, lapses in short-term memory, slips in the execution of routine, over-learned tasks, and misapplication of rules are common human experiences that unfortunately occur routinely even among highly trained professionals. For example, after having admitted a patient with respiratory distress who unexpectedly turned out to have congestive heart failure, a healthcare provider is likely to jump prematurely to the conclusion that the next patient who comes in with respiratory distress has congestive heart failure, rather than considering all possibilities on a differential diagnosis and appropriately weighting their likelihood based on the epidemiology of illness in the community where he/she practices, the history of illness, and findings on examination. This particular logical fallibility is called the 'availability heuristic'. Moreover, having jumped to a possible diagnosis, he/she is likely to downplay data that refute his/her thinking, fully accepting only those data that support his/her initial impression, a problem known as 'confirmation bias'. The likelihood of falling for these and other logical traps is increased if one is distracted, overworked, or sleep deprived (Leape, 1994; Rasmussen and Jensen, 1974; Reason, 1990).

In addition, system complexity increases the risk of error. With multiple steps in a routine process, there is an opportunity, however small, for an error to occur at any step in this process. In the typical medication delivery system, there are 20 or more steps from the writing of a medication to its successful delivery to a patient (e.g. physician writes order, clerk transcribes it, order faxed to pharmacist, pharmacist receives order, pharmacist enters order into patient's drug list in pharmacy, pharmacist checks allergies, pharmacist checks for drug interactions, etc.). With 20 steps, and a 99% chance of each step being performed without error, the chance that a medication order makes it all the way through the system with no error occurring is only 82% ($0.99^{20} = 0.82$). Because each step in the process described is driven by human actions, error can be introduced by any individual involved along the way. An error made at an early step could be caught at a later step (and indeed most are), but a few will make it all the way through the system to cause harm to a patient.

James Reason, a pioneer in the field of human factors engineering, conceptualizes this process of failures occurring in a complex system in his 'Swiss Cheese Model' (Fig. 17.1), which suggests that in complex systems, multiple defenses (a series of barriers, represented by slices of cheese) must be penetrated (the holes in the cheese) in order for an error to cause harm (Reason, 1990, 2000).

If, for example, a junior doctor inadvertently writes the wrong route on a medication order (e.g. intravenous instead of oral), it is not the case that such an error immediately results in harm. In order for harm to occur, many secondary errors must occur: the error must (at a minimum) be missed by the clerk who transcribes the order; the pharmacist who fills the order; the pharmacy technician who sends the medication back up to the hospital floor from which it was ordered; and the nurse who receives the medication from pharmacy and administers it. Each of the individuals downstream of the initial error is part of a 'safety net'; these safety nets are imperfect, however, and from time to time they will all fail and harm may result.

Sleep deprivation and healthcare provider performance

As alluded to above, sleep deprivation increases the risk of slips, lapses, and mistakes in judgment. Healthcare providers make thousands of small decisions per day, some requiring careful judgment, and many others simply involving the accurate completion of routine tasks. Both the routine and the complex, however, are subject to the adverse effects of sleep deprivation. Even minor misjudgments or calculation errors can be consequential in tenuous hospitalized patients. In healthcare, where junior doctors, senior doctors, and nurses routinely work long shifts and long workweeks, circadian misalignment, sleep deprivation, and sleep inertia can significantly affect systemic safety.

Human alertness and performance

The daily performance of healthcare providers, like all other humans, is driven in large measure by two neurobiological systems: the sleep homeostat and the circadian system. The homeostatic system normally mediates time awake and asleep, and has a direct effect on performance of a range of

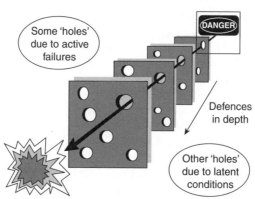

Fig. 17.1 Reason's Swiss cheese model.
Source: Reproduced from Reason, J. (2000). *Managing the Risks of Organizational Accidents*. Burlington, VT: Ashgate Publishing Company, with permission.

cognitive and motor tasks. The circadian system superimposes a near-24-hour cycle of perform-ance on top of the effects due to the sleep homeostat, with the minimum performance normally occurring a few hours prior to waking. Under regular sleep-wake conditions, the homeostatic and circadian systems work together to maintain a high level of performance throughout the waking day. Under the types of rotating and shifting sleep-wake schedules worked by healthcare providers, it has been shown that the systems can interact in a manner that causes performance deficits greater than would be observed during the standard waking day. Chronic sleep loss and sleep inertia, described below, can lead to further performance decrements. The combined effect of acute sleep deprivation and circadian forces, particularly when compounded by chronic sleep loss or sleep inertia, can lead to a critical level of drowsiness on the job that can lead both to decreased vigilance and performance, and an increased risk of fall-asleep incidents, errors, and accidents.

Circadian misalignment

Human circadian rhythms are driven by an endogenous circadian pacemaker, located in the suprachiasmatic nucleus of the hypothalamus (Klein et al., 1991) (see also Chapter 2). This light-sensitive pacemaker drives near-24-h rhythms of core body temperature, hormones such as cor-tisol and melatonin, and neurobehavioural functioning. The largest neurobehavioural performance decrements are seen near the minimum of the endogenous core body temperature rhythm, which occurs approximately 1–3 hours before habitual wake time in most individuals (Carskadon et al., 1999; Czeisler et al., 1994; Dijk et al., 1992, 1997; Jewett, 1997; Johnson et al., 1992). In addition, the ability to sleep and the timing and internal organization of sleep vary with circadian phase (Czeisler, 1978; Czeisler et al., 1980; Dijk and Czeisler, 1995; Strogatz et al., 1986, 1987). Thus, not only does circadian misalignment cause decrements in neurobehavioural performance when one is awake, it also induces impairment in sleep quality, continuity, and duration during sleep. This effect is seen commonly among healthcare providers and others who work shifts at night, who find themselves unable to sleep during daytime hours (Åkerstedt et al., 1983; Colquhoun et al., 1975; Friedman et al., 1971; Vidacek et al., 1986) (see also Chapters 15 and 16). Since alertness and performance depend heavily on sleep quality and duration (Åkerstedt et al., 1979; Aschoff et al., 1972; Dement, 1972; Wilkinson, 1969), misalignment causes neurobehavioural function to decline indirectly by way of its effects on sleep as well as directly.

Sleep homeostatis

Independent of the circadian system, acute sleep deprivation causes decrements in human alert-ness and performance (Åkerstedt et al., 1979; Angus et al., 1985; Babkoff et al., 1991; Carskadon and Dement, 1992; Dinges, 1989; Fröberg et al., 1975; Johnson, 1982; Koslowsky and Babkoff, 1992; Lorenzo et al., 1995; Pilcher and Huffcutt, 1996; Wilkinson, 1972) (see also Chapter 16). Every hour that one is awake, the drive to sleep increases, which results in deteriorating perform-ance. Compared with the first hour of driving, there is more than a 15-fold increase in the risk of a fatigue-related fatal crash after 13 hours of driving (Department of Transportation, 2000). In addi-tion, chronic sleep restriction also affects performance (Blagrove et al., 1995; Brunner et al., 1990, 1993; Carskadon and Dement, 1981; Carskadon and Roth, 1991; Gillberg and Åkerstedt, 1994; Lafrance et al., 1998). Loss of even 2 hours of sleep per night for five to seven consecutive nights causes neurobehavioural performance to degrade to a level similar to that seen after 24 hours of continuous sleep deprivation; after 2 weeks at 4 hours of sleep restriction, lapses of attention are comparable to those observed after 48 hours of total sleep deprivation (Dinges et al., 1999).

Sleep inertia

In addition to these two major drivers of performance, alertness, vigilance, and judgment can be impeded by sleep inertia (Dinges, 1993), a phenomenon of degraded performance and cognition immediately following awakening (Dinges, 1990), even in subjects who are not sleep deprived and are waking at their normal circadian phase (Achermann et al., 1995; Folkard and Åkerstedt, 1992; Jewett and Kronauer, 1999). The effect is especially strong in the first few minutes after awakening, exceeding the effects of even 24 hours without sleep (Wertz et al., 2006). In hospitals, sleep inertia may be extremely important, as providers given the opportunity to sleep overnight may be awoken and required to perform critical tasks immediately, including the performance of procedures and prescription or administration of potentially hazardous medications.

Sleep deprivation, circadian misalignment, performance, and healthcare safety

Sleep deprivation has been systematically documented to impair cognition, vigilance, mood, and reaction time in healthcare providers as well as in others. Consequently, reducing the work hours of physicians and nurses, who have historically experienced intense sleep deprivation due to their protracted work hours, is an important means of improving performance and thereby reducing the burden of harm due to medical errors.

Junior medical doctors—simulation and laboratory studies

A large number of studies have now documented the adverse effects of sleep deprivation on physicians-in-training. Measures employed in these studies have included tests of manual dexterity, memory, and reaction time. Although a few have not demonstrated decrements in performance due to sleep deprivation (Bartle et al., 1988; Deaconson et al., 1988; Reznick and Folse, 1987), the large majority have demonstrated performance worsening across a range of tasks (Beatty et al., 1977; Hart et al., 1987; Hawkins et al., 1985; Klose et al., 1985; Lewittes and Marshall, 1989; Narang and Laycock, 1986; Orton and Gruzelier, 1989). In one of the first studies of resident-physician sleep deprivation, Friedman et al. (1971, 1973) had interns read electrocardiograms when rested and when sleep deprived. Sleep-deprived interns made nearly twice the number of errors in detecting cardiac arrhythmias, a finding that subsequent studies have replicated (Deary and Tait, 1987; Lingenfelser et al., 1994). Other early studies found that the quality of the physical examination and documentation decreased with increasing time at work (Bertram, 1988). More recently, Arnedt et al. (2005) demonstrated that residents working longer than 24-hour shifts every four to five nights had a similar degree of impairment when completing neurobehavioural and driving tests as those with a blood alcohol level of 0.04–0.05%, even though these residents were not completely deprived of sleep, obtaining an average of 3 hours sleep while working intermittent overnight shifts. Compiling the results of these and many other studies of physicians' and non-physicians' performance—60 studies in total—Philibert (2005) found that residents' mean performance on clinical tasks dropped nearly two standard deviations after 24 hours of sleep deprivation, to the 7th percentile of their rested performance level, a drop of the same magnitude as a 30-point drop in IQ (Landrigan, 2005).

Junior surgeons—simulation and laboratory studies

Surgical residents are likewise susceptible to the adverse effects of sleep deprivation. More than 3 decades ago, Goldman et al. (1972) conducted video recordings of surgical procedures, and found that most surgeons who received less than 2 hours of sleep the night before surgery performed at an inferior level to those who were better rested. Simulated laparoscopic surgery studies conducted more recently also demonstrate that sleep deprivation degrades performance. Taffinder et al. (1998) found that residents awake all night made more errors and were less efficient than those who had had a full night's sleep. Grantcharov et al. (2001) found that surgical residents performing simulated laparoscopic surgery after a night without sleep made more frank errors, and performed inefficiently, a finding replicated by Eastridge et al. (2003).

Field studies: measuring the effects of junior doctor sleep deprivation in clinical settings

In a randomized controlled trial, the Harvard Work Hours, Health, and Safety Group found that first-year medical residents (interns) working traditional 30-hour shifts had twice as many electroencephalographically documented attentional failures at night, made 36% more serious medical errors, and five times as many serious diagnostic errors as those limited to 16 scheduled hours of consecutive work (Landrigan et al., 2004; Lockley et al., 2004) (Fig. 17.2).

In a nationwide cohort study, our group also found that interns working >24 hours had more than twice the odds of crashing their cars when driving home after work (Barger et al., 2005), and a 61% increased odds of suffering a percutaneous injury at work (Ayas et al., 2006). According to interns' own reports, those working more than five 24-hour shifts per month were seven times as likely to make a harmful fatigue-related medical error, and four times as likely to make a fatigue-related error that led to a patient's death (Barger et al., 2006). Extrapolating from these data (which included 1,417 person-years of data) to the full national US cohort of 100,000 physicians-in-training, there are apparently thousands of fatal, preventable fatigue-related medical errors made by residents each year.

Nurses

Sleep deprivation and circadian misalignment also impairs nurses. Gold et al. (1992) found that nurses working rotating shifts were twice as likely to make a medication error, and more likely to

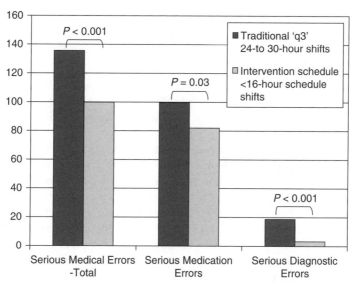

Fig. 17.2 Interns' rates of serious medical errors (total), serious medication errors, and serious diagnostic errors per 1,000 patient-days on traditional versus intervention schedule (Intern Sleep, and Patient Safety Study). On the traditional schedule, interns (first year postgraduate junior doctors) worked 30-hour shifts frequently, whereas on the intervention schedule, shifts were scheduled to a maximum of 16 consecutive hours. Interns' rates of serious errors (overall) were 36% higher on the traditional schedule than on the intervention schedule. Medication errors were 21% more common on the traditional schedule, and diagnostic errors were more than fivefold more common.
Source: Data from Landrigan, C.P., Rothschild, J.M., Cronin, J.W., et al. (2004). Effect of reducing interns' work hours on serious medical errors in intensive care units. *N Engl J Med*, **351**, 1838–1848.

suffer a motor vehicle crash than those working day or evening shifts. Rogers et al. (2004) reported that in the United States, 40% of all nursing shifts exceeded 12 hours, and that those working over 12.5 hours made three times as many errors as their peers working shorter shifts; Scott et al. (2006) reported a similar doubling in error risk among critical care nurses working >12 hours.

Consultant surgeons and obstetricians

A small body of literature has begun to emerge describing the consequences of sleep deprivation among senior physicians (attendings; consultants). In a retrospective study at the University of Virginia, Ellman et al. (2004) found no differences in the outcomes of coronary artery bypass graft surgeries performed by sleep deprived versus rested cardiac surgeons, or sleep deprived versus rested surgical residents (Ellman et al., 2005). The study had relatively low power to detect differences in mortality, as very few deaths occurred in the small sample of cases conducted by surgeons who were categorized as sleep deprived. Although better power existed to capture differences in complication rates, categorization of surgeons as 'sleep deprived' or 'not sleep deprived' was based on operating room logs, without validation of surgeons' actual work and sleep hours. In studying rates of surgical and obstetrical complications in a 10-year retrospective study at Brigham and Women's hospital, the Harvard Work Hours group similarly found no difference in overall rates of complications in surgeries performed after overnight duty versus those performed on other days, but we did find that in the subset of cases where surgeons or obstetricians had less than a 6-hour opportunity to sleep, compared with cases where they had more than a 6-hour sleep opportunity (based again on operating room logs), the odds of a complication occurring nearly doubled (Rothschild et al., 2009). A survey of neurosurgeons found that fatigue was identified by neurosurgeons as a leading factor contributing to wrong-site surgeries, though this impression was not substantiated by any objective data (Jhawar et al., 2007). Prospective studies carefully assessing the effects of sleep deprivation on consultants' alertness and performance are needed.

Improving safety

Systematically improving the safety of healthcare is a complex undertaking, and, as yet, efforts to do so both in the United Kingdom and the United States have only just begun. Although the past decade has seen the initiation of many efforts to implement safer systems of care, the safety of the healthcare system has not demonstrably improved (Altman et al., 2004; Vincent et al., 2008). Even the most promising interventions, such as computerized provider order entry (Bates et al., 1998; Potts et al., 2004), have been adopted by only a small fraction of medical centres (Cutler et al., 2005). Compliance with simple interventions such as use of maximal sterile barriers and hand washing remains poor (Pittet et al., 2004). The public reports dissatisfaction with the quality of care, and half report that it is unsafe (Altman et al., 2004; Kaiser Family Foundation, Agency for Healthcare Research and Quality, and Harvard School of Public Health, 2005). Although important questions about the effectiveness of many interventions remain, a critical element of the failure to make concrete improvements has been a failure to translate even well-proven interventions into common practice.

Work hour regulation: United States

Resident work hours

Despite the accumulation of the data outlined above, resident work hours in the United States continue at levels the evidence demonstrates are unsafe. The Accreditation Council for Graduate Medical Education (ACGME) continues to endorse 30-hour shifts and 80-hour workweeks, and in practice, even these permissive limits are frequently exceeded (Landrigan et al., 2006).

Reduction of work hours for physicians-in-training in the United States has proven difficult for many reasons. First, although recognition of the risks of extreme work hours has increased, it is not universal (ACGME, 2002; American Medical Association, 2005). Many physicians remain deeply committed to residents' traditional on-call schedules despite data about their risks, and others believe that implementation of the ACGME duty hour standards has effectively addressed the problem, despite data to the contrary. Concern about discontinuity of care (Petersen et al., 1994), particularly in hospitals where sign-out systems and tools (Petersen et al., 1998) have been inadequate, has slowed reduction of work hours. Justifiable concerns exist about how to effectively reschedule residents, how to train and hire more providers, and what effects these new personnel might have on the physician workforce. Consequently, inadequate resources have been invested in hiring needed personnel to allow for shorter hours. In addition, medical educators have expressed concern about how reduced residency hours might affect education, although, conversely, data have emerged demonstrating that sleep deprivation impairs consolidation of memory and learning as well as safety (Stickgold, 2005).

Nevertheless, the mounting data on the hazards of traditional extended shifts have prompted a critical re-examination of this issue and calls for policy change in the United States. In 2008, after conducting a comprehensive review of the topic and holding hearings over the course of a year, the IOM concluded that residents should not work for more than 16 hours in a row without sleep (Institute of Medicine, 2008) (Fig. 17.3).

To date, no action has been taken by the ACGME or other policy-makers on this recommendation, but active discussions are underway.

Nurse work hours

In a separate report, the IOM has also recommend that nurses' work be limited to no more than 12 hours per day (Institute of Medicine, 2006). Relatively few hospitals and health systems in the United States have implemented this recommendation, however, and nursing shifts continue to frequently exceed these limits (Rogers et al., 2004). A notable exception is the Veterans Affairs system for military veterans, which limits nurses in direct patient care to 12 consecutive hours of work and 60 hours of work per week (United States Department of Veteran Affairs, 2004). No regulatory agency, either professional or governmental, regulates nursing work hours in non-military hospitals.

Attending physician work hours

To date, no regulations have been implemented or formally called for regarding attending physician work hours in the United States.

Work hour regulation: United Kingdom

By contrast, the European Working Time Directive (EWTD) limits junior doctors, senior doctors, and nurses in Europe to work a maximum of 48 hours per week (see also Chapter 18). In the United Kingdom in particular, doctors' weekly work hours (averaged over a 6-month period) have been gradually reduced from a 72-hour weekly limit in 2004, to a 56-hour limit, to the current 48-hour limit, which was implemented in August 2009; shifts are limited to a maximum of 13 consecutive hours (British Medical Association, 2004). The full requirements of the EWTD, which have gradually been applied to doctors, are outlined in Fig. 17.4.

There has been ongoing controversy in the United Kingdom (as in the United States) about the appropriateness of these limits, with concerns about sleep deprivation being countered by concerns about care continuity and junior doctors training (Ahmed-Little, 2007; Murray et al., 2005;

Comparison of IOM Committee adjustments to current ACGME Duty Hour Limits		
	2003 ACGME Duty Hour Limits	**IOM Recommendation**
Maximum hours of work per week	80 hours, averaged over 4 weeks	No change
Maximum shift length	30 hours (admitting patients up to 24 hours then 6 additional hours for transitional and educational activities)	• 30 hours (admitting patients for up to 16 hours, plus 5-hour protected sleep period between 10:00 p.m. and 8:00 a.m. with the remaining hours for transitional and educational activities) • 16 hours with no protected sleep period
Maximum in-hospital on-call frequency	Every third night, on average	Every third night, no averaging
Minimum time off between scheduled shifts	10 hours after shift length	• 10 hours after day shift • 12 hours after night shift • 14 hours after any extended duty period of 30 hours and not return until 6:00 a.m. of next day
Maximum frequency of in-hospital night shifts	Not addressed	4 night maximum; 48 hours off after 3 or 4 nights of consecutive duty
Mandatory time off duty	• 4 days off per month • 1 day (24 hours) off per week, averaged over 4 weeks	• 5 days off per month • 1 day (24 hours) off per week, no averaging • One 48-hour period off per month
Moonlighting	Internal moonlighting is counted against 80-hour weekly limit	• Internal and external moonlighting is counted against 80-hour weekly limit • All other duty hour limits apply to moonlighting in combination with scheduled work
Limit on hours for exceptions	88 hours for select programs with a sound educational rationale	No change
Emergency room limits	12-hour shift limit, at least an equivalent period of time off between shifts; 60-hour workweek with additional 12 hours for education	No change

Fig. 17.3 A comparison of the 2009 IOM recommendations for resident-physician work hours in the United States with the 2003 ACGME regulations.
Source: Reproduced from Institute of Medicine (2008). *Resident Duty Hours: Enhancing Sleep, Supervision, and Safety*. Washington, DC: National Academies Press. Reproduced with permission from the National Academies Press, Copyright 2008, National Academy of Sciences.

Pounder, 2008). Relatively few data on the effects of these changes have emerged to date other than unsubstantiated survey studies, but one pilot study that collected objective data found that junior doctors working a 48-hour workweek, on a schedule built on principles of sleep and circadian medicine, made fewer errors than junior doctors on another clinical unit working a 56-hour week (Cappuccio et al., 2009) (see also Chapter 18).

Developing safer schedules

Regulation of work hours provides a foundation for safer care, but as suggested in reference to the United Kingdom study above, it is not sufficient to ensure safer care. Principles of sleep and circadian medicine must be incorporated into schedule design to translate absolute reductions in work hours into better performance and safety. For example, a 48-hour workweek built on a

European Working Time Directive requirements	
Maximum hours of work per week	48 hours
Maximum shift length	13 hours
Maximum work (per 24 hours) for night workers	8 hours
Minimum time off between scheduled shift	11 hours
Mandatory time off duty	1 day (24 hours) off in each 7-day period; One 48-hour period off in each 14-day period
Mandatory rest breaks	20 minutes for every 6 hours worked
Leave	4 weeks per year

Fig. 17.4 EWTD requirements: minimum requirements for work hours, rest, and leave*
*Over the past 5 years, these requirements have gradually been applied to junior doctors in the United Kingdom.
Source: Data from British Medical Association (2004). Time's up: a guide on the European Working Time Directive for junior doctors.

string of six 8-hour nights, followed by a string of six 8-hour days, followed by a string of six 8-hour nights is unlikely to be optimal—even though the total number of work hours is within EWTD standards—given the circadian misalignment and chronic sleep deprivation that such a schedule would induce. In addition, careful consideration of how to redesign infrastructure to minimize the risk of handover errors and to enhance medical education is needed as efforts to reduce work hours are implemented. Naps prior to night shifts should be encouraged, caffeine use and sleep hygiene education should be provided, and sleep disorders should be screened for and treated. In the absence of these efforts, and an effort to assure that reduction in work hours does not lead to systematic understaffing, efforts to reduce hours are unlikely to result in safer care, and will likely not be sustainable.

Conclusion

Healthcare provider sleep is critical to patient safety, as well as the safety of the providers themselves. Efforts are underway to safely reduce work hours in both the United Kingdom and the United States, but these efforts are still very early in their development. If such efforts are to succeed, a concerted effort must be made to ensure that principles of sleep and circadian medicine are incorporated into efforts to redesign work schedules. Concurrently, systematic efforts are needed to ensure the smooth transition from traditional systems of care to systems with reduced work hours, with an eye towards managing the workforce, handovers of care, and medical education.

Summary box

- This chapter reviews the epidemiology of medical error, and discusses fallible human cognitive processes as well as latent errors in the healthcare system that contribute to the genesis of error.
- It then proceeds to describe the manner in which sleep deprivation, circadian misalignment, and healthcare provider work schedules increase the propensity for cognitive errors to occur, leading both to medical errors and occupational injuries.
- It reviews the literature on sleep deprivation and extended work shifts among physicians and nurses, which includes studies in laboratory as well as in clinical settings.
- It concludes with a discussion of the policies regarding work schedules for physicians and nurses in the United Kingdom and the United States, and principles for advancing safer work scheduling practices.

References

ACGME (2002). Statement of justification/impact for the final approval of common standards related to resident duty hours. Accreditation Council for Graduate Medical Education.

Achermann, P., Werth, E., Dijk, D.J. & Borbély, A.A. (1995). Time course of sleep inertia after nighttime and daytime sleep episodes. *Arch Ital Biol*, **134**, 109–119.

Ahmed-Little, Y. (2007). Implications of shift work for junior doctors. *BMJ*, **334**, 777–778.

Åkerstedt, T., Fröberg, J.E., Friberg, Y. & Wetterberg, L. (1979). Melatonin excretion, body temperature and subjective arousal during 64 hours of sleep deprivation. *Psychoneuroendocrinology*, **4**, 219–225.

Åkerstedt, T., Torsvall, L. & Gillberg, M. (1983). Sleep-wake disturbances in shift work: implications of sleep loss and circadian rhythms. *Sleep Res*, **12**, 359.

Altman, D.E., Clancy, C. & Blendon, R.J. (2004). Improving patient safety—five years after the IOM report. *N Engl J Med*, **351**, 2041–2043.

American Medical Association (2005c). Medical Students and Residents Work-Hour Survey.

Angus, R.G., Heslegrave, R.J. & Myles, W.S. (1985). Effects of prolonged sleep deprivation, with and without chronic physical exercise, on mood and performance. *Psychophysiology*, **22**, 276–282.

Arnedt, J.T., Owens, J., Crouch, M., Stahl, J. & Carskadon, M.A. (2005). Neurobehavioral performance of residents after heavy night call vs after alcohol ingestion. *JAMA*, **294**, 1025–1033.

Aschoff, J., Giedke, H., Poppel, E. & Wever, R. (1972). The influence of sleep interruption and of sleep deprivation on circadian rhythms in human performance. In: Colquhoun, W.E. (ed.), *Aspects of Human Efficiency: Diurnal Rhythm and Loss of Sleep*. London: English University Press.

Ayas, N.T., Barger, L.K., Cade, B.E., et al. (2006). Extended work duration and the risk of self-reported percutaneous injuries in interns. *JAMA*, **296**, 1055–1062.

Babkoff, H., Caspy, T. & Mikulincer, M. (1991). Subjective sleepiness ratings: the effects of sleep deprivation, circadian rhythmicity and cognitive performance. *Sleep*, **14**, 534–539.

Barger, L.K., Cade, B.E., Ayas, N.T., et al. (2005). Extended work shifts and the risk of motor vehicle crashes among interns. *N Engl J Med*, **352**, 125–134.

Barger, L.K., Ayas, N.T., Cade, B.E., et al. (2006). Impact of extended-duration shifts on medical errors, adverse events, and attentional failures. *PLoS Med*, **3**, 1–9.

Bartle, E.J., Sun, J.H., Thompson, L., Light, A.I., McCool, C. & Heaton, S. (1988). The effects of acute sleep deprivation during residency training. *Surgery*, **104**, 311–316.

Bates, D.W., Leape, L.L., Cullen, D.J., et al. (1998). Effect of computerized physician order entry and a team intervention on prevention of serious medication errors. *JAMA*, **280**, 1311–1316.

Beatty, J., Ahern, S.K. & Katz, R. (1977). Sleep deprivation and the vigilance of anesthesiologists during simulated surgery. In: Mackie, R. (ed.), *Vigilance: Theory, Operational Performance, and Physiological Correlates*. New York, NY: Plenum Press, pp. 511–527.

Bertram, D.A. (1988). Characteristics of shifts and second-year resident performance in an emergency department. *N Y State J Med*, **88**, 10–14.

Blagrove, M., Alexander, C. & Horne, J.A. (1995). The effects of chronic sleep reduction on the performance of cognitive tasks sensitive to sleep deprivation. *Appl Cogn Psychol*, **9**, 21–40.

Bowser, B.A. (1996). Looking for Answers, Public Broadcasting Service, PBS Online Newshour.

British Medical Association (2004). Time's up: a guide on the European Working Time Directive for junior doctors.

Brunner, D.P., Dijk, D.J., Tobler, I. & Borbély, A.A. (1990). Effect of partial sleep deprivation on sleep stages and EEG power spectra: evidence for non-REM and REM sleep homeostasis. *Electroencephalogr Clin Neurophysiol*, **75**, 492–499.

Brunner, D.P., Dijk, D.J. & Borbély, A.A. (1993). Repeated partial sleep deprivation progressively changes the EEG during sleep and wakefulness. *Sleep*, **16**, 100–113.

Cappuccio, F.P., Bakewell, A., Taggart, F.M., et al. (2009). Implementing a 48 h EWTD-compliant rota for junior doctors in the UK does not compromise patients' safety: assessor-blind pilot comparison. *Q J Med*, **102**, 271–282.

Carskadon, M.A. & Dement, W.C. (1981). Cumulative effects of sleep restriction on daytime sleepiness. *Psychophysiology*, **18**, 107–113.

Carskadon, M.A. & Roth, T. (1991). Sleep restriction. In: Monk, T.H. (ed.), *Sleep, Sleepiness and Performance*. New York, NY: John Wiley and Sons, pp. 155–167.

Carskadon, M.A. & Dement, W.C. (1992). Multiple sleep latency tests during the constant routine. *Sleep*, **15**, 396–399.

Carskadon, M.A., Labyak, S.E., Acebo, C. & Seifer, R. (1999). Intrinsic circadian period of adolescent humans measured in conditions of forced desynchrony. *Neurosci Lett*, **260**, 129–132.

CBS News (2009). Quaid's Twins Given Accidental Overdose, CBS News.

Colquhoun, W.P., Hamilton, P. & Edwards, R.S. (1975). Effects of circadian rhythm, sleep deprivation, and fatigue on watchkeeping performance during the night hours. In: Colquhoun, W.P., Folkard, S., Knauth, P., et al. (eds.), *Experimental Studies of Shiftwork*. Opladen: Westdeutscher Verlag, pp. 20–28.

Cutler, D.M., Feldman, N.E. & Horwitz, J.R. (2005). U.S. adoption of computerized physician order entry systems. *Health Aff* (Millwood), **24**, 1654–1663.

Czeisler, C.A. (1978). Human circadian physiology: internal organization of temperature, sleep-wake, and neuroendocrine rhythms monitored in an environment free of time cues. Ph.D. Dissertation, Stanford University.

Czeisler, C.A., Weitzman, E.D., Moore-Ede, M.C., Zimmerman, J.C. & Knauer, R.S. (1980). Human sleep: its duration and organization depend on its circadian phase. *Science*, **210**, 1264–1267.

Czeisler, C.A., Dijk, D.J. & Duffy, J.F. (1994). Entrained phase of the circadian pacemaker serves to stabilize alertness and performance throughout the habitual waking day. In: Ogilvie, R.D. & Harsh, J.R. (eds.), *Sleep Onset: Normal and Abnormal Processes*. Washington, DC: American Psychological Association, pp. 89–110.

Deaconson, T.F., O'Hair, D.P., Levy, M.F., Lee, M.B.F., Schueneman, A.L. & Condon, R.E. (1988). Sleep deprivation and resident performance. *JAMA*, **260**, 1721–1727.

Deary, I.J. & Tait, R. (1987). Effects of sleep disruption on cognitive performance and mood in medical house officers. *BMJ*, **295**, 1513–1516.

Dement, W.C. (1972). Sleep deprivation and the organization of the behavioral states. In: Clemente, C.D., Purpura, D.P. & Mayer, F.E. (eds.), *Sleep and the Maturing Nervous System*. New York, NY: Academic Press, pp. 319–361.

Department of Transportation (2000). Washington, DC: National Archives and Records Administration, 65.

Dijk, D.J. & Czeisler, C.A. (1995). Contribution of the circadian pacemaker and the sleep homeostat to sleep propensity, sleep structure, electroencephalographic slow waves, and sleep spindle activity in humans. *J Neurosci*, **15**, 3526–3538.

Dijk, D.J., Duffy, J.F. & Czeisler, C.A. (1992). Circadian and sleep/wake dependent aspects of subjective alertness and cognitive performance. *J Sleep Res*, **1**, 112–117.

Dijk, D.J., Shanahan, T.L., Duffy, J.F., Ronda, J.M. & Czeisler, C.A. (1997). Variation of electroencephalographic activity during non-rapid eye movement and rapid eye movement sleep with phase of circadian melatonin rhythm in humans. *J Physiol (Lond)*, **505**, 851–858.

Dinges, D.F. (1989). The nature of sleepiness: causes, contexts, and consequences. In: Stunkard, A.J. & Baum, A. (eds.), *Perspectives in Behavioral Medicine: Eating, Sleeping, and Sex*. Hillsdale, NJ: Lawrence Erlbaum Associates, pp. 147–179.

Dinges, D.F. (1990). Are you awake? Cognitive performance and reverie during the hypnopompic state. In: Bootzin, R., Kihlstrom, J. & Schacter, D. (eds.), *Sleep and Cognition*. Washington, DC: American Psychological Association, pp. 159–175.

Dinges, D.F. (1993). Sleep inertia. In: Carskadon, M.A. (ed.), *Encyclopedia of Sleep and Dreaming*. New York, NY: Macmillan, pp. 553–554.

Dinges, D.F., Maislin, G., Kuo, A., et al. (1999). Chronic sleep restriction: neurobehavioral effects of 4 hr, 6 hr, and 8 hr TIB. *Sleep*, **22**(Suppl1), S115.

Eastridge, B.J., Hamilton, E.C., O'Keefe, G.E., et al. (2003). Effect of sleep deprivation on the performance of simulated laparoscopic surgical skill. *Am J Surg*, **186**, 169–174.

Ellman, P.I., Law, M.G., Tache-Leon, C., et al. (2004). Sleep deprivation does not affect operative results in cardiac surgery. *Ann Thorac Surg*, **78**, 906–911.

Ellman, P.I., Kron, I.L., Alvis, J.S., et al. (2005). Acute sleep deprivation in the thoracic surgical resident does not affect operative outcomes. *Ann Thorac Surg*, **80**, 60–64.

Folkard, S. & Åkerstedt, T. (1992). A three-process model of the regulation of alertness-sleepiness. In: Broughton, R.J. & Ogilvie, R.D. (eds.), *Sleep, Arousal, and Performance*. Boston, MA: Birkhäuser, pp. 11–26.

Friedman, R.C., Bigger, J.T. & Kornfield, D.S. (1971). The intern and sleep loss. *N Engl J Med*, **285**, 201–203.

Friedman, R.C., Kornfeld, D.S. & Bigger, T.J. (1973). Psychological problems associated with sleep deprivation in interns. *J Med Educ*, **48**, 436–441.

Fröberg, J.E., Karlsson, C.G., Levi, L. & Lidberg, L. (1975). Circadian rhythms of catecholamine excretion, shooting range performance and self-ratings of fatigue during sleep deprivation. *Biol Psychol*, **2**, 175–188.

Gillberg, M. & Åkerstedt, T. (1994). Sleep restriction and SWS-suppression: effects on daytime alertness and night-time recovery. *J Sleep Res*, **3**, 144–151.

Gold, D.R., Rogacz, S., Bock, N., et al. (1992). Rotating shift work, sleep, and accidents related to sleepiness in hospital nurses. *Am J Public Health*, **82**, 1011–1014.

Goldman, L.I., McDonough, M.T. & Rosemond, G.P. (1972). Stresses affecting surgical performance and learning I. Correlation of heart rate, electrocardiogram, and operation simultaneously recorded on videotapes. *J Surg Res*, **12**, 83–86.

Grantcharov, T.P., Bardram, L., Funch-Jensen, P. & Rosenberg, J. (2001). Laparoscopic performance after one night on call in a surgical department: prospective study. *BMJ*, **323**, 1222–1223.

Hart, R.P., Buchsbaum, D.G., Wade, J.B., Hamer, R.M. & Kwentus, J.A. (1987). Effect of sleep deprivation on first-year residents' response times, memory, and mood. *J Med Educ*, **62**, 940–942.

Hawkins, M.R., Vichick, D.A., Silsby, H.D., Kruzich, D.J. & Butler, R. (1985). Sleep and nutritional deprivation and performance of house officers. *J Med Educ*, **60**, 530–535.

Institute of Medicine (1999). *To Err is Human: Building a Safer Health System*. Washington, DC: National Academy Press.

Institute of Medicine (2006). *Keeping Patients Safe: Transforming the Work Environment of Nurses.* Washington, DC: National Academies Press.

Institute of Medicine (2008). *Resident Duty Hours: Enhancing Sleep, Supervision, and Safety.* Washington, DC: National Academies Press.

Jewett, M.E. (1997). Models of circadian and homeostatic regulation of human performance and alertness. Ph.D. Thesis, Harvard University.

Jewett, M.E. & Kronauer, R.E. (1999). Interactive mathematical models of subjective alertness and cognitive throughput in humans. *J Biol Rhythms*, **14**, 588–597.

Jhawar, B.S., Mitsis, D. & Duggal, N. (2007). Wrong-sided and wrong-level neurosurgery: a national survey. *J Neurosurg Spine*, **7**, 467–472.

Johnson, L.C. (1982). Sleep deprivation and performance. In: Webb, W.B. (ed.), *Biological Rhythms, Sleep, and Performance*. New York, NY: John Wiley and Sons, pp. 111–141.

Johnson, M.P., Duffy, J.F., Dijk, D.J., Ronda, J.M., Dyal, C.M. & Czeisler, C.A. (1992). Short-term memory, alertness and performance: a reappraisal of their relationship to body temperature. *J Sleep Res*, **1**, 24–29.

Kaiser Family Foundation, Agency for Healthcare Research and Quality & Harvard School of Public Health (2005). National Survey on Consumers' Experiences With Patient Safety and Quality Information.

Klein, D.C., Moore, R.Y. & Reppert, S.M. (1991). *Suprachiasmatic Nucleus: The Mind's Clock.* New York, NY: Oxford University Press.

Klose, K.J., Wallace-Barnhill, G.L. & Craythorne, N.W.B. (1985). Performance test results for anesthesia residents over a five day week including on-call duty. *Anesthesiology*, **63**, A485.

Kochanek, K.D., Murphy, S.L., Anderson, R.N. & Scott, C. (2004). Deaths: final data for 2002. *Natl Vital Stat Rep*, **53**, 1–115.

Koslowsky, M. & Babkoff, H. (1992). Meta-analysis of the relationship between total sleep deprivation and performance. *Chronobiol Int*, **9**, 132–136.

Lafrance, C., Dumont, M., Lesperance, P. & Lambert, C. (1998). Daytime vigilance after morning bright light exposure in volunteers subjected to sleep restriction. *Physiol Behav*, **63**, 803–810.

Landrigan, C.P. (2005). Sliding down the bell curve: effects of 24-hour work shifts on physicians' cognition and performance. *Sleep*, **28**, 1351–1353.

Landrigan, C.P., Rothschild, J.M., Cronin, J.W., et al. (2004). Effect of reducing interns' work hours on serious medical errors in intensive care units. *N Engl J Med*, **351**, 1838–1848.

Landrigan, C.P., Barger, L.K., Cade, B.E., Ayas, N.T. & Czeisler, C.A. (2006). Interns' compliance with accreditation council for graduate medical education work-hour limits. *JAMA*, **296**, 1063–1070.

Leape, L.L. (1994). Error in medicine. *JAMA*, **272**, 1851–1857.

Lewittes, L.R. & Marshall, V.W. (1989). Fatigue and concerns about quality of care among Ontario interns and residents. *CMAJ*, **140**, 21–24.

Lingenfelser, T., Kaschel, R., Weber, A., Zaiser-Kaschel, H., Jakober, B. & Kuper, J. (1994). Young hospital doctors after night duty: their task-specific cognitive status and emotional condition. *Med Educ*, **28**, 566–572.

Lockley, S.W., Cronin, J.W., Evans, E.E., et al. (2004). Effect of reducing interns' weekly work hours on sleep and attentional failures. *N Engl J Med*, **351**, 1829–1837.

Lorenzo, I., Ramos, J., Arce, C., Guevara, M.A. & Corsi-Cabrera, M. (1995). Effect of total sleep deprivation on reaction time and waking EEG activity in man. *Sleep*, **18**, 346–354.

Murray, A., Pounder, R., Mather, H. & Black, D.C. (2005). Junior doctors' shifts and sleep deprivation. *BMJ*, **330**, 1404.

Narang, V. & Laycock, J.R.D. (1986). Psychomotor testing of on-call anaesthetists. *Anaesthesia*, **41**, 868–869.

Orton, D.I. & Gruzelier, J.H. (1989). Adverse changes in mood and cognitive performance of house officers after night duty. *BMJ*, **298**, 21–23.

Petersen, L.A., Brennan, T.A., O'Neil, A.C., Cook, E.F. & Lee, T.H. (1994). Does housestaff discontinuity of care increase the risk for preventable adverse events? *Ann Intern Med*, **121**, 866–872.

Petersen, L.A., Orav, E.J., Teich, J.M. & O'Neil, A.C. (1998). Using a computerized sign-out program to improve continuity of inpatient care and prevent adverse events. *Jt Comm J Qual Improv*, **24**, 77–87.

Philibert, I. (2005). Sleep loss and performance in residents and non-physicians: a meta-analytic examination. *Sleep*, **28**, 1392–1402.

Pilcher, J.J. & Huffcutt, A.I. (1996). Effects of sleep deprivation on performance: a meta-analysis. *Sleep*, **19**, 318–326.

Pittet, D., Simon, A., Hugonnet, S., Pessoa-Silva, C.L., Sauvan, V. & Perneger, T.V. (2004). Hand hygiene among physicians: performance, beliefs, and perceptions. *Ann Intern Med*, **141**, 1–8.

Potts, A.L., Barr, F.E., Gregory, D.F., Wright, L. & Patel, N.R. (2004). Computerized physician order entry and medication errors in a pediatric critical care unit. *Pediatrics*, **113**, 59–63.

Pounder, R. (2008). Junior doctors' working hours: can 56 go into 48? *Clin Med*, **8**, 126–127.

Rasmussen, J. & Jensen, A. (1974). Mental procedures in real-life tasks: a case study of electronic trouble shooting. *Ergonomics*, **17**, 293–307.

Reason, J. (1990). *Human Error*. Cambridge: Cambridge University Press.

Reason, J. (2000). *Managing the Risks of Organizational Accidents*. Burlington, VT: Ashgate Publishing Company.

Reznick, R.K. & Folse, J.R. (1987). Effect of sleep deprivation on the performance of surgical residents. *Am J Surg*, **154**, 520–525.

Rogers, A.E., Hwang, W.T., Scott, L.D., Aiken, L.H. & Dinges, D.F. (2004). The working hours of hospital staff nurses and patient safety. *Health Aff* (Millwood), **23**, 202–212.

Rothschild, J.M., Keohane, C.A., Rogers, S., et al. (2009). Risks of complications by attending physicians after performing nighttime procedures. *JAMA*, **302**, 1565–1572.

Scott, L.D., Rogers, A.E., Hwang, W.T. & Zhang, Y. (2006). Effects of critical care nurses' work hours on vigilance and patients' safety. *Am J Crit Care*, **15**, 30–37.

Stickgold, R. (2005). Sleep-dependent memory consolidation. *Nature*, **437**, 1272–1278.

Strogatz, S.H., Kronauer, R.E. & Czeisler, C.A. (1986). Circadian regulation dominates homeostatic control of sleep length and prior wake length in humans. *Sleep*, **9**, 353–364.

Strogatz, S.H., Kronauer, R.E. & Czeisler, C.A. (1987). Circadian pacemaker interferes with sleep onset at specific times each day: role in insomnia. *Am J Physiol*, **253**, R172–R178.

Taffinder, N.J., McManus, I.C., Gul, Y., Russell, R.G. & Darzi, A. (1998). Effect of sleep deprivation on surgeons' dexterity on laparoscopy simulators. *Lancet*, **352**, 1191.

United States Department of Veteran Affairs (2004). Law Gives VA Flexible Pay for Physicians, Schedules for Nurses.

Vidacek, S., Kaliterna, L. & Vic-Vidacek, B.R. (1986). Productivity on a weekly rotating shift system: circadian adjustment and sleep deprivation effects? *Ergonomics*, **29**, 1583–1590.

Vincent, C., Neale, G. & Woloshynowych, M. (2001). Adverse events in British hospitals: preliminary retrospective record review. *BMJ*, **322**, 517–519.

Vincent, C., Aylin, P., Franklin, B.D., et al. (2008). Is health care getting safer? *BMJ*, **337**, a2426.

Wertz, A.T., Ronda, J.M., Czeisler, C.A. & Wright, K.P., Jr. (2006). Effects of sleep inertia on cognition. *JAMA*, **295**, 163–164.

Wikipedia (2009). TWA Flight 800. Wikipedia.

Wilkinson, R.T. (1969). Sleep deprivation: performance tests for partial and selective sleep deprivation. *Prog Clin Psychol*, **8**, 28–43.

Wilkinson, R.T. (1972). Effects of up to 60 hours' sleep deprivation on different types of work. *Ergonomics*, **7**, 175–186.

Chapter 18

European working time directive and medical errors

F.P. Cappuccio and M.A. Miller

Introduction

The modernization of the National Health Service (NHS) and medical careers have over the last 10 years or more brought growing pressures and demands for radical changes in the way we deliver safe and effective healthcare and train new doctors to fit these changes. At the same time, there has been an increasing awareness at European level that both patients and doctors are exposed to health risks due to excessive working hours of junior doctors. A legislative framework to reduce average working hours to no more than 48 hours per week was then introduced in Europe, which has added to the challenges and has sparked a much heated debate (see also Chapter 20). These proposals have met with support and criticisms from several camps, including doctors and their representative organizations, allied professions, NHS managers and, naturally, politicians. The debate has shifted emphasis continuously, neglecting a fundamental principle adopted in other areas of healthcare delivery (public health, medicine and surgery, health technology), that is, that our decisions should be supported by evidence.

European working time directive

The 1993 European Working Time Directive (EWTD) is intended to protect employees' health and safety and improve patient safety by limiting the maximum required working hours to 48 per week, averaged over up to 6 months, and was adopted into UK law through the Working Time Regulations 1998 (see also Chapter 20). The British government negotiated an extension of up to 12 years before full implementation in the United Kingdom was required, and changes affecting the medical profession have been phased in over a 5-year period, starting in August 2004, when junior doctors' 6-monthly average weekly working hours were reduced from 72 to 54 hours per week. This change took into account a European Court ruling specifying that resting and sleeping time, which occurred during periods of duty in hospital, should also be considered as working time (Jaeger v. Kiel, 2003) (see also Chapters 16 and 20). During the same timeframe the British Medical Association (BMA) conducted negotiations with the Department of Health to introduce a package of measures to improve the lives of junior doctors (the New Deal), a key feature of which was to reduce extended working hours and ensure that adequate rest time was built into rota systems (NHS Management Executive, 1991). Since August 2007, the average hours worked by junior doctors, which are still calculated over 6 months, have been further reduced to 56 hours per week with the intention of complying with the 48 hours required by the EWTD by August 2009 (British Medical Association, 2008). Under the political pressure of numerous professional bodies, the British government made a last attempt to block the implementation of the EWTD at European level, but it failed to stop it. The EWTD is now fully operational in the United Kingdom.

Working time and medical errors

Working at night is harder than working during the day, because this is the time when we are programmed to be asleep. Evidence from a range of industries where shift work is common shows that shift workers accumulate sleep debt, experience increased fatigue with negative effects on alertness, vigilance, performance, and cognitive reasoning. Therefore, working at night contributes to an increased risk of making errors (see also Chapter 16). The length of individual shifts and the number of shifts worked in succession are also very important (Folkard et al., 2005; Folkard and Tucker, 2003) (Fig. 18.1a), and the risk of an accident is always greater on the night shift than during the day (Fig. 18.1b).

Studies in the United States have shown that the rate of serious medical errors made by junior doctors is substantially higher when they work on a traditional on-call system involving

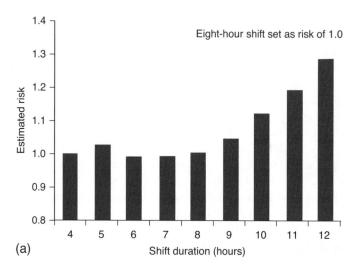

(a)

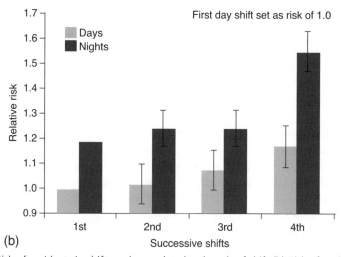

(b)

Fig. 18.1 (a) Risk of accidents in shift workers, related to length of shift (b) Risk of accidents in shift workers, related to the number of successive day or night-shifts.
Source: Based on figures from Folkard, S. & Tucker, P. (2003). Shift work, safety and productivity. *Occup Med (Lond)*, **53**(2), 95–101.

frequent periods of duty lasting for 24 hours or more (see also Chapter 17). The introduction of an intervention schedule, which limited scheduled continuous duty to 16 hours and reduced the total number of hours worked from ~85 to ~65 per week, resulted in more sleep, fewer attentional failures on duty, and fewer serious medical errors (Barger et al., 2005, 2006; Landrigan et al., 2004; Lockley et al., 2004). These results provided objective measurements of what had previously been mainly anecdotal reports about the effect on patient safety of doctors working for extended periods. Studies from industry have reported that the number of continuous hours worked increases the risk that safety incidents will occur, a risk that is compounded by night working and increases with each successive shift (Folkard et al., 2005; Folkard and Tucker, 2003) (see also Chapters 15 and 16). Similarly, US junior doctors were shown to have twice the risk of having a car crash driving home from an extended shift as compared to driving home after a non-extended shift (Barger et al., 2005) and are at increased risk of sharp injuries when working overnight and 'post-call' (Ayas et al., 2006).

Although junior doctors in the United Kingdom are not contracted to work such long hours on average as their American counterparts, their work hours can be similarly demanding and remain the subject of much discussion. The need to implement the requirements of EWTD competes with demands to maintain adequate medical cover at all times while ensuring that doctors are able to access the educational and training opportunities necessary to guarantee a safe and competent workforce in the future (Paice and Reid, 2004). Beyond issues of safety and effectiveness, concerns have been raised regarding the reduced time that is available for training junior doctors, the effect that this will have on clinical experience (including continuity of care), quality of care, and quality of life for doctors as a result of the new directive. Previous arrangements, in which on-call cover was provided during 'out of hours' periods, have given way to a wide variety of shift patterns, none of which have been evaluated objectively prior to implementation for their effect on patient safety and resident health.

Objections to the implementation of EWTD for junior doctors

There has been considerable controversy regarding the appropriateness of implementing the EWTD in the NHS. Concerns have been raised that the new directive would put doctors' and patients' lives at risk (Murray et al., 2005), would lead to reduced time available for training, and will have negative impacts on clinical experience and quality of care (Ahmed-Little, 2007; Benger, 2008; Pounder, 2008). These strong assertions are, without exception, based on opinions, anecdotes, or non-validated questionnaires and surveys (British Medical Association, 2008; Gander et al., 2007; Grover et al., 2008; Kara et al., 2008). For instance, the results of the Fourth National Survey of medical Specialist Registrars (SpRs) completed in December 2004 from the Royal College of Physicians (RCP) gave early indications that, contrary to expectations, 81% of the respondents suffered excess fatigue with 74% sleeping during night shifts with worsening of continuity and quality of patient care (Coward, 2005). Junior doctors' views about the impact of EWTD were generally of dissatisfaction with the changes in work pattern and concerns were raised about continuity of care, quality of care, and training, with deterioration in job satisfaction. The report concluded that dissatisfaction with the changes was 'almost unanimous' amongst medical SpRs. It is important to note that this survey was carried out by e-mail invitation of all SpRs on the Joint Committee on Higher Medical Training database. The overall response rate was 25% (i.e. one in four responded) with variations between specialities (22% in geriatric medicine and 30% in respiratory medicine). At around the same time, another e-mail-based survey of all acute hospitals in England and Wales, through the RCP college tutors (61% response rate), concluded that there was 'little overt evidence of dissatisfaction amongst junior staff' (Mather and Pounder, 2005). In March 2008, the BMA carried out a new postal survey of junior doctors' views on working hours and the EWTD; 3,000 members were written to and 470 (16%) replied (British Medical Association, 2008). Fewer that one in five respondents believed that a 48-hour working week would improve patient safety or the quality of patient care. Although they were reported to be most likely to believe that the new working week would have a negative impact on training, three in five reported that in their experience their ability to provide safe medical care to patients has been compromised by working excessive hours.

These surveys raise a number of questions: very low response rates introduce an important risk that the results may not be representative of the whole body of junior doctors and that they may be grossly biased. Indeed, the RCP surveys seem very inconsistent with each other and even within the BMA survey there are contradictions. These views, although informative of the degree of understanding, awareness, and personal acceptability of the changes in the rota systems amongst junior doctors, do not provide objective measures of effectiveness in terms of patients' and doctors' safety. Numerous opinions have been published opposing reductions in extended work hours due to concerns regarding continuity of patient care, reduced educational opportunities, and traditionally defined professionalism (Ahmed-Little, 2007; Benger, 2008; Fahrenkopf et al., 2008; Grover et al., 2008; Kara et al., 2008; Mann, 2009; Murray et al., 2005; Pounder, 2008; Waterman et al., 2009). However, there are remarkably few objective data in support of continuing to schedule medical trainees to work long shifts and long work weeks (Cappuccio et al., 2009b). There are currently no field data about the effect of implementing EWTD-compliant rotas in a medical setting, and previous surveys of doctors' subjective opinions on shift-working have not provided reliable objective data with which to evaluate its efficacy (Aitken and Paice, 2003). An evidence-based approach is needed to document the effect of work practices on junior doctors' health, access to education, on patient safety, and continuity of care (Lockley et al., 2006).

Recommendations from the Royal College of Physicians

In 2006, the UK Multidisciplinary Working Group of the RCP proposed a theoretically optimized schedule built around a 9-hour shift system which aimed to promote the design of a rota that would minimize the risk to doctors' health and patient safety particularly with regard to the length and frequency of night shifts (Horrocks and Pounder, 2006a).

The Working Group recommended:

i. that rotas involving seven consecutive 13-hour night shifts must be stopped due to their inherent high risk of fatigue and potential harm to patients and staff;
ii. that the number of night shifts in succession should not exceed four and the length of each night shift should be minimized;
iii. to encourage the use of three 9-hour shifts to cover 24 hours with the aim of improving patient health and safety, junior doctors' safety, teaching, supervision, and efficiency;
iv. to use evidence-based approaches in order to define optimal 48 hours rotas by 2009;
v. that a 'cell' of 10 junior doctors is necessary for any post that provides 24 hours cover.

In addition, the Working Group issued practical guidelines for the five 9-hour shift-work (Horrocks and Pounder, 2006b) and a guide for junior doctors on how to prepare for, survive, and recover from a night shift (Horrocks and Pounder, 2006c).

Inspired by the RCP recommendations, we proposed a study to test the feasibility of implementing a EWTD-compliant 48 hours a week schedule and to assess objectively its impact on patient safety. The intervention rota was based on the schedule that the RCP proposed as the most promising in its review in minimizing the risk to patient safety and doctors' health with particular regard to the length and frequency of night shifts (Horrocks and Pounder, 2006a).

EWTD-compliant rota in the United Kingdom and patients' safety

This study provides the first objective assessment of the impact of 2009 EWTD-compliant schedules on patient care, the primary concern of healthcare providers, and presents scientific evidence upon which to begin basing policy decisions. This study aims for the first time in Europe (Pounder, 2006) to address the lack of evidence on the effects of a 48-hour per week EWTD-compliant rota for junior doctors on patient care, as assessed objectively from medical error rates, in a large NHS Hospital Trust in England (Cappuccio et al., 2009a).

The study was carried out at the University Hospitals Coventry and Warwickshire NHS Trust, a 1,250-bed hospital in Coventry, over a 12-week period in 2007. During this period there were 1,707 admissions to the wards included in this study.

Rotas

The study was a single-blind between-groups clinical trial with an intervention group consisting of nine junior doctors covering in rotation the Clinical Decision Unit and the Endocrinology ward who were scheduled to a 2009 EWTD-compliant rota with an average of up to 48 hours per week (Fig. 18.2, right panel), and a group working on their traditional schedule, comprising 10 junior doctors covering in rotation the Care of the Elderly and the Respiratory ward, who were scheduled to a traditional rota of up to 54 hours per week on average (Fig. 18.2, left panel), for a duration of 12 weeks.

During the traditional rota, junior doctors were required to make an abrupt change from day shifts to night shifts, and were scheduled to work three or more consecutive 12.5-hour night shifts. During the intervention rota, the transition from day shifts to night shifts was made more gradually. Evening shifts were scheduled for the 2–3 days prior to starting the night shifts which were shorter and limited to a maximum three consecutive shifts, and usually only for two (61% of occasions). In the intervention group the sequence of shifts from day-evening-night was designed to facilitate sleep by permitting extended sleep before the evening shift. Doctors were also encouraged to take a nap in the afternoon before the night shift. This was a close approximation of the rota that the UK Multidisciplinary Working Group of the RCP had identified as the safer of possible rotas, the 'three 9-hour shifts for 24 hours', both New Deal and EWTD-compliant (Horrocks and Pounder, 2006a, b). The intervention rota was designed to allow doctors to have sequential shifts in optimal order for circadian adaptation 'early > evening > night', facilitating acclimatization to night-working. The night-shifts were shorter (maximum of 11 hours), reduced to blocks of two or less often three nights. The intervention group was given written advice on sleep hygiene and on the importance of naps. Doctors completed a work and sleep diary every day for the duration of the study.

Although the average weekly work hours differed by fewer than 10 hours per week between the traditional and intervention rotas (52.4 ± 11.2 vs. 43.2 ± 7.7 hours per week, respectively; $P < 0.001$), there was a remarkable difference in the range and distribution of weekly hours (Fig. 18.3a). Under the traditional rota, scheduled weekly work hours ranged from 30 to 77 hours per week, with 25% of work weeks lasting longer than 58 hours (Fig. 18.3a). In contrast, the intervention rota had a maximum of 60 hours per week (range 26–60) with only 2% of weeks with work ≥58 hours per week (Fig. 18.3a).

The intervention rota reduced the average duration of scheduled work shifts by nearly an hour as compared to the traditional rota (9.9 ± 1.7 hours [range 4.5–12.5; $n = 10$] vs. 9.0 ± 0.8 hours [3.0–11.0; $n = 9$]; $P < 0.001$) and abolished continuous duty shifts >12 hours, which were scheduled nearly 25% of the time on the traditional 56-hour rota (Fig. 18.3b). Shifts of 10 hours or more were scheduled only 7% of the time on the intervention rota, but were more than four times

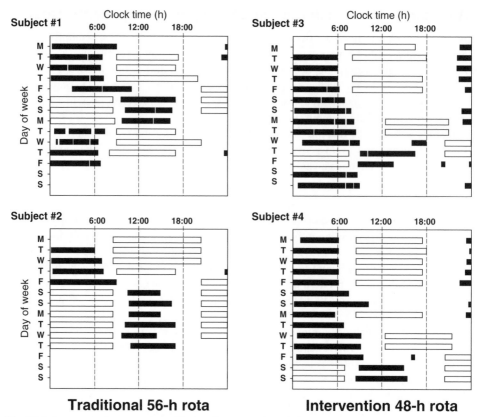

Fig. 18.2 Representative examples of junior doctor work and sleep patterns.

Self-reported sleep times (■) and work hours (□) are shown for four junior doctors while working on either a 56h schedule (Subjects 1 and 2, left panels) or a 48h schedule (Subjects 3 and 4, right panels). Clock time is plotted on the abscissa (0:00–0:00 h) with day of the week plotted on the ordinate over 14 consecutive days of the 12-week study. During the standard 56-hour schedule, junior doctors were required to make an abrupt change from day shifts to night shifts, and were scheduled to work 3 or more consecutive 12.5h night shifts (20:30–20:45 to 9:00–9:1 5h)(e.g., Fri-Sun, Subject 1; Fri-Wed, Subject 2). During the 48h intervention schedule, the transition from day shifts to night shifts was made more gradually. Evening shifts (8.5–9.0h; 12:30–21:00h or 1 5:00–00:00h) were scheduled for the 2–3 days prior to starting the night shifts (e.g. second Mon and Tue, Subject 3; second Wed and Thu, Subject 4), and shorter 8.75 to 11h night shifts (start range 20:30–23:00h, end range 7:30–9:00) were limited to a maximum three consecutive shifts, and usually only for two (61% of occasions). The sequence of shifts from day-evening-night also facilitated sleep by permitting extended sleep before the evening shift. Doctors were also encouraged to take a nap in the afternoon before the night shift.

Source: Reproduced from Cappuccio, F.P., Bakewell, A., Taggart, F.M., et al. (2009a). Implementing a 48 h EWTD-compliant rota for junior doctors in the UK does not compromise patients' safety: assessor-blind pilot comparison. *QJM*, **102**(4), 271–282, with permission.

more frequent (33%) during the traditional 56-hour rota (Fig. 18.3b). The average duration (9.9 ± 1.9 hours [3.0–13.0] vs. 9.2 ± 0.8 hours [5.5–11.5]; $P < 0.001$) and distribution of scheduled hours agreed closely with self-reported work hours from the subset of subjects with the most comprehensive diary data ($n = 9$) (Fig. 18.3c). Total sleep time/day tended to be longer during the intervention as compared to the traditional rota (7.26 ± 0.36 hours vs. 6.75 ± 0.40 hours,

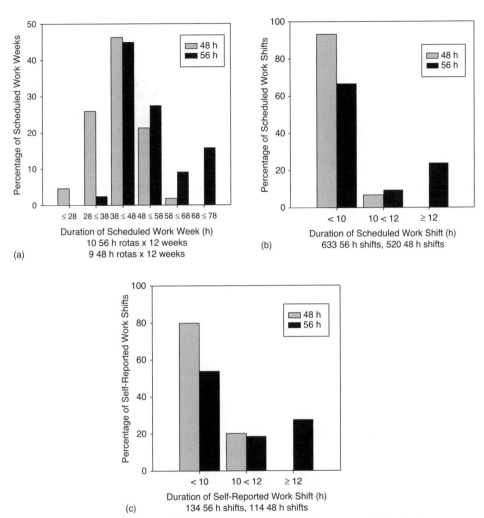

Fig. 18.3 (a) distribution of scheduled weekly work hours across the 12 weeks for the two groups. (b) distribution of scheduled work shift duration for all individuals (c) distribution of self-reported work shift duration in a subset of subjects working the 48-h (n = 4) or 56-h (n = 5) rotas.
Source: Reproduced from Cappuccio, F.P., Bakewell, A., Taggart, F.M., et al. (2009a). Implementing a 48 h EWTD-compliant rota for junior doctors in the UK does not compromise patients' safety: assessor-blind pilot comparison. *QJM*, **102**(4), 271–282, with permission.

respectively; $P = 0.095$) and as intended, the shift sequence during the intervention rota permitted a substantial recovery sleep of nearly 9 hours (8.68 ± 0.23 hours) after the evening shift, significantly more than after the day (6.93 ± 0.31 hours) or night (6.28 ± 1.41 hours) shift ($P < 0.05$; Fig. 18.4a). Sleep duration was shortest following the night shift on the traditional rota (5.69 ± 0.97 hours) (Fig. 18.4b).

Medical errors

Medical errors and adverse events were detected using retrospective case note review (Fahrenkopf et al., 2008; Landrigan et al., 2004). Direct observation identifies higher error rates than other techniques but its cost and organizational implications limit its use (Weingart et al., 2000).

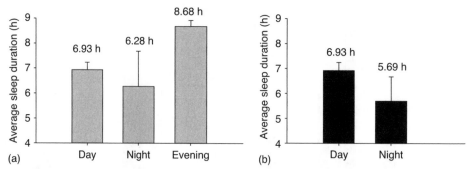

Fig. 18.4 Comparison of average duration of sleep after each shift type during the 48h a week intervention rota (a, n = 4) and the traditional 56h a week rota (b, n = 5) (mean and standard deviation. *Source*: Reproduced from Cappuccio, F.P., Bakewell, A., Taggart, F.M., et al. (2009a). Implementing a 48 h EWTD-compliant rota for junior doctors in the UK does not compromise patients' safety: assessor-blind pilot comparison. *QJM*, **102**(4), 271–282, with permission.

Retrospective case review is the most widely used clinical surveillance methodology for detecting medical errors and adverse events; rates of adverse events ranging from 2.9% to 16.6% have been reported from centres in North America and Australasia (Baker et al., 2004). A study in two acute hospital wards in the United Kingdom found an incidence rate of 11.7% (Vincent et al., 2001). Retrospective case note review, as used in this study, is less expensive and labour intensive than observation but nevertheless time-consuming and may not provide such a clear cut view of events especially since it is entirely dependent on the 'accuracy, completeness, and legibility' of medical records (Woloshynowych et al., 2003).

Out of a total of 1,707 admissions, 916 (54%) were randomly selected for review. Incidents with potential to cause harm were identified using an established methodology (Bates et al., 1995; Fahrenkopf et al., 2008; Walsh et al., 2006). An adverse event was defined as an incident in which medical management resulted in harm to the patient. In addition, any errors with potential to cause harm were documented, reviewed, and categorized. The rationale for this approach is based on the understanding that 'near-misses', represented by 'failures in process of care' (Griffin and Resar, 2007), afford 'free lessons' in the promotion of patient safety by highlighting error-prone areas of healthcare delivery (Reason, 2000). Blinded reviewers categorized each incident as an adverse event, non-intercepted potential adverse events, intercepted potential adverse events, or error with little potential for harm.

During a total of 4,782 patient-days involving 481 admissions, 32.7% fewer total medical errors occurred during the intervention than the traditional rota (27.6 vs. 41.0 per 1,000 patient-days, $P = 0.006$). The hazard ratio (HR) (95% confidence interval [CI]) was 0.62 (0.45–0.84), $P < 0.05$. There were 82.6% fewer intercepted potential adverse events (1.2 vs. 6.9 per 1,000 patient-days, $P = 0.002$) with HR 0.16 (95% CI: 0.05–0.57), $P < 0.05$ and 31.4% fewer non-intercepted potential adverse events (16.6 vs. 24.2 per 1,000 patient-days, $P = 0.067$) with a HR of 0.63 (95% CI: 0.42–0.94), $P < 0.05$ (Table 18.1). Preventable adverse events did not differ between groups.

Interviews

Doctors were asked a series of open-ended questions according to a semi-structured question-naire about the shift system, patient safety, their own rest and sleep, educational opportunities, and handover experiences. Interviews were recorded and transcribed and descriptive themes were extracted. Interviews were conducted in the last 3 weeks of the study for all but one doctor who was interviewed a week after the study period ended. All descriptive themes included for analysis were derived from comments made by doctors talking about their own experience of the shift

Table 18.1 Adverse events and error rates between intervention and traditional rotas

	Traditional	Intervention	Rate reduction % (95% CI)†	P value
Patients	2315	2467		
Preventable adverse events - *n* (rate*)	5 (2.2)	4 (1.6)	−27.3 (−85.1 to 24.9)	0.68
Intercepted potential adverse events - *n* (rate)	16 (6.9)	3 (1.2)	−82.6 (−97.7 to −38.5)	0.002
Non-intercepted potential adverse events - *n* (rate)	56 (24.2)	41 (16.6)	−31.4 (−55.2 to 4.6)	0.067
Minor errors - *n* (rate)	18 (7.8)	20 (8.1)	3.8 (−52.2 to 91.0)	0.90
Overall - *n* (rate)	95 (41.0)	68 (27.6)	−32.7 (−52.9 to −10.4)	0.006

*Rate is expressed as number (per 1,000 patient-days).

†Rate reduction = (rate of intervention − rate of traditional) × 100/rate of traditional.

system they were working. Descriptive themes were grouped into major themes according to broad category headings which corresponded to the four study objectives described above. Analysis was qualitative and performed according to principles of grounded theory (Strauss and Corbin, 1990) using a framework corresponding to the objectives of the study.

Workload issues and perception of patient safety

Comments were made about potential for delay in investigation when daytime junior staff levels were low. Another theme was lack of time for interaction with the rest of the team with less chance of feedback on their performance. In the general medical setting the perception of doctors in the intervention group was that because of frequent shift changes more time was needed to familiarize themselves with the new patients.

Learning opportunities

Most doctors in the intervention group felt that their educational opportunities were compromised. Doctors in the traditional group generally made positive comments about learning opportunities.

Rest and sleep

Comments on rest and sleep varied. Some of the intervention group doctors welcomed the shorter shifts because they were less tired and felt they were performing their duties better as a result, but others felt that they were performing worse because of the increased workload despite feeling less tired.

Quality of life (social life)

Both intervention and traditional groups reported that working in the evening or on night shifts and at weekends had a negative impact on social and family life.

Handovers

Thirty-four handover sessions were observed during the course of the study. Conversations between the participants were recorded using a portable sound recorder and notes taken by the observer regarding the identity of the speakers, who else attended, and how the handover was conducted. Doctors were almost unanimous in their description of procedures and selection of patients for handover. They usually compiled a list of patients and the jobs that needed to be done for each one either after clerking new patients or during a ward round. This list formed the basis of the handover. Patients would then be 'handed over' on a one-to-one basis, sometimes in person and sometimes over the phone. Doctors reported that patients would be selected for hand over according to the following criteria: (i) 'sick' or unstable patients whether or not specific tasks need doing so that the oncoming doctor is aware of the problem; (ii) patients who have investigations or results pending. Some also reported that they would hand over or be handed over jobs that had not been done because the outgoing doctor had not had time to do them. Few had concerns about the quality of handover but several spoke about the risk of omissions in care when patients were the subject of frequent handovers on the intervention rota.

Discussion

The study shows that 33% fewer medical errors occurred on an intervention rota up to 48 hours, as compared to a traditional 56 hours per week schedule. Although differences in clinical specialty may explain some differences in error rates between rotas, the study suggests that implementation of a 48-hour work week can be accomplished without an adverse effect on patient safety.

Considerations on rota design

The intervention rota had several important components that were based on well-established principles of sleep medicine and circadian biology (Horrocks and Pounder, 2006c; Lockley et al., 2006). First, it limited consecutive night shifts to three nights maximum and for the majority of weeks, only two, in order to reduce the build-up of chronic partial sleep deprivation due to the limited sleep between night shifts (Fig. 18.1b). Second, shift duration was limited to 12 hours maximum in order to minimize acute sleep deprivation, hence risk of fatigue (Fig. 18.1a), which represented a distinct difference from the current 56 hours a week rota which scheduled 25% of shifts >12 hours. Third, the sequence of shifts was designed to abolish 'slam shifts' in which doctors change from a day to a night shift immediately, which ensures complete circadian desynchrony (Czeisler et al., 1982), and instead gradually stagger the shifts from morning to evening to night in the direction to which the circadian system most easily adapts (Czeisler et al., 1999). This sequence also facilitates sleep and reduces performance decrements on the first night shift (Santhi et al., 2007) by providing an opportunity for a long recovery sleep after the evening shift prior to starting the first night shift. Finally, the intervention rota dramatically reduced the proportion of long work weeks, with an upper limit of 60 hours per week, again reducing chronic sleep deprivation, in stark contrast to the current 56-hour rota, during which 25% of the shifts were >58 hours per week and as long as 77 hours per week (see also Chapters 15 and 16).

These assumptions have recently been confirmed in an experimental comparison of the impact of schedule design feature on fatigue and well-being of 336 junior doctors working on different schedules throughout Wales (Tucker et al., 2009). Working seven consecutive nights was associated with greater accumulated risk and greater work-life interference, compared with working just three or four nights ($P < 0.01$ and < 0.05). Shift length and sleep duration were negatively correlated. Having only one rest day after working nights was associated with increased risk ($P < 0.01$) and work-life interference ($P < 0.05$). Napping before the first night shift reduced risk ($P < 0.05$). Working weekends increased work-life interference ($P < 0.01$) and psychological strain ($P < 0.01$). Working frequent on-calls increased work-life interference, as did longer on-calls. Inter-shift intervals of <10 hours were associated with shorter sleeps ($P < 0.01$) and increased risk ($P < 0.05$). Weekly hours were positively associated with work-life interference ($P < 0.01$) and with risk on night shifts ($P < 0.05$).

Considerations on medical error rates

Given that extended duration duty hours and long work weeks had previously been shown to be associated with increased risk to patient safety and resident health (Ayas et al., 2006; Baker et al., 2004; Barger et al., 2005; Cappuccio and Lockley, 2008; Landrigan et al., 2004), we hypothesized that medical errors rates would be reduced following introduction of the 2009 EWTD-compliant 48 hours a week rota as compared to the 56-hour rota currently in use. Indeed, we found that significantly fewer errors occurred on the 48-hour rota as compared to the 56-hour rota. This proportional benefit is comparable to that found in our previous study in medical and cardiac intensive care units in the United States (Landrigan et al., 2004) (see also Chapter 17) although it must be noted that the US study was carried out in units where the absolute rate of errors, given the intensity of work, was much higher than we found in medical wards. It also appears, on first impression, that much more substantive rota changes were introduced in the US study (continuous scheduled duty changed from 24–30 to 16 hours and scheduled work weeks changed from ~80 to ~63 hours per week) (Landrigan et al., 2004). On closer inspection, however, the fact that the 56-hour EWTD regulations allow averaging weekly work hours over 6 months permits work weeks in the United Kingdom that, during some weeks, are comparable to the US limit of 80 hours a week averaged over 4 weeks (Accreditation Council for Graduate Medical Education, 2008). It has been previously argued that such weekly limit terms are misleading (Lockley et al., 2006) given that, in both the United States and United Kingdom, weekly work hours can be much longer than the nominal 'limits' if they are balanced by shorter weeks elsewhere in the rota. In the English study, the reduction in error rates observed may have been due to the effect of the intervention on reducing the range of weekly work hours, rather than the average hours per week. The difference between 56 and 48 hours per week on average may appear small, but the difference may be much greater in any given week, as doctors still work nearly 80 hours a week for some weeks under the current regulations.

Considerations on hospital practices

For a full implementation of our rota in future iterations of the schedule, these changes should be synchronized with normal hospital practices (Ayas et al., 2006) and should include more doctors, recently argued to be between 12 and 13 per cell (Pounder, 2008), but at minimum 10. Nevertheless, the study in NHS-based medical wards was able to detect significant differences in work hours with important implications for patients' safety, despite doctors' perceptions that the new rota would worsen care and represent harm to patients.

Hospital at Night (H@N) is a Department of Health (England) driven programme being widely implemented across United Kingdom. It aims to redefine how medical cover is provided in hospitals during the out-of-hours period. It is a competency driven, patient focused, change programme that utilizes a multidisciplinary approach to delivering healthcare overnight, while retaining the ability to access specialist input as necessary. It employs a whole systems approach emphasizing patient safety while protecting doctor training in the face of the reduction of junior doctor hours, brought about by the EWTD. The ethos of H@N model is the provision of out-of-hours medical cover by a centralized multidisciplinary team, who have the full range of skills and competencies to meet the immediate needs of patients.

A recent study measured the impact of the implementation of H@N on both system and clinical outcomes (Beckett et al., 2009). The authors carried out an observational study during 14 consecutive nights before and 14 consecutive nights after the implementation of H@N within the Royal Infirmary of Edinburgh involving medical, surgical, and high-dependency wards. Following an overnight episode of concern, and using standardized methods, they gathered information on response time, seniority of reviewing staff, patient outcomes (including overnight transfers to critical care and cardiac arrests), and the use of Standardized Early Warning Score (SEWS). They compared the results before and after the implementation of H@N. Most importantly, the implementation of H@N was associated with a significant improvement in clinical outcomes in most circumstances. Cardiac arrests and transfers to critical care were significantly reduced in the Assessment Unit and in the wards from 17% to 6%, without compromising outcomes within the critical care settings. At the same time, significant inter-speciality differences were abolished (delays in reviewing patients and response time). Finally, patients were more likely to be seen by senior medical staff during H@N. The authors acknowledge the limitations of the study, noticeably that the action taken on patients triggering SEWS >4 did not improve during H@N.

Why is this study important? Acute care during out-of-hours in hospital can be sub-optimal and contribute to patient adverse outcomes. The research evidence indicating that H@N may improve numerous clinical outcomes is a significant step forward (Cappuccio, 2009). The study also indicates that a research approach can bring more objective information to guide policy changes within the NHS.

As in a previous study (Landrigan et al., 2004), the reduction in medical errors was achieved despite a modest increase in the number of handovers, which may be a source of error in its own right (Petersen et al., 1994). Regardless of shift length, the process of handing over care between shifts is error-prone, and should be a focus of future improvement efforts. Introduction of computerized handover tools (Petersen et al., 1998; Van Eaton et al., 2005) or standardized, consistent verbal handover procedures could further improve patient safety on these rotas.

Considerations on training opportunities

The English study was too short and not designed to assess the impact of the new 48-hour rota on educational opportunities. Educational issues are intertwined with both patient safety issues and doctors well-being in the context of a training post. Although the reduction of educational opportunities was raised as a concern, there are as yet no data testing the impact of shorter work hours on validated educational outcomes. Indeed, one could hypothesize that reducing work hours may enhance educational outcomes given the emerging importance of sleep in learning and memory consolidation (Stickgold, 2005; Stickgold and Walker, 2005) and the difficulty with learning while 'half asleep' on duty (Lockley et al., 2004). Additional controlled trials are needed to test these hypotheses.

Considerations on doctors' sleepiness

Although our intervention reduced the length of continuous duty and work week duration with the aim of reducing sleepiness and improving performance, most doctors did not consider that sleepiness was a major problem (see also Chapters 15–17). These comments are not surprising given that self-ratings of sleepiness when sleep deprived do not reflect objective measurements of poor performance. Similar to the misperception of one's own performance induced by alcohol, sleep-deprived individuals rate their alertness as better than their performance demonstrates (Arnedt et al., 2005; Van Dongen et al., 2003). This example illustrates a larger point, namely that policy decisions should not be made based on subjective opinions. Such unsubstantiated preconceptions are not valid when designing safe schedules. Decisions regarding work hour reform should be based on data derived from controlled clinical trials data, just as objective data form the basis of evidence-based medical decision (Horrocks and Pounder, 2006a). Current data represent the first step in this process and should be followed by additional hypothesis-driven studies.

Conclusion

Although concerns remain regarding continuity of patient care and reduced educational opportunities with the implementation of the EWTD, our objective data indicate that care can be safely provided on a 2009 EWTD-compliant rota. There is a need for a wider re-engineering of shift systems and hospital processes than was possible in this pilot study to ensure that the safety gains for patients cared for by less tired doctors are not compromised by delayed investigations and treatment, which can result from difficulties managing the routine daytime workload. Although our findings may not be directly applicable to all specialties, they do not indicate that a reduction in work hours inevitably leads to a reduction in the quality of patient care. Evidence-based policy decisions must be made for work hours in the same way as evidence-based medicine is used for clinical decisions (Muir Gray, 2004).

Summary box

- Working at night is harder than working during the day contributing to an increased risk of making errors.
- In the United States, longer working hours and longer night shifts amongst junior doctors cause reduced sleep, increased fatigue, more attentional failures on duty, more serious medical errors, and a greater risk of car accidents when returning home after a night shift.
- A legislative framework to reduce average working hours to no more than 48 hours per week has been implemented in European countries in 2009 (EWTD).
- A EWTD-compliant rota for junior doctors is associated with more sleep, less fatigue, and fewer medical errors.
- Care to patients can be safely provided on a 2009 EWTD-compliant rota.

References

Accreditation Council for Graduate Medical Education (2008). *Common Programme Requirements for Residents Duty Hours.*

Ahmed-Little, Y. (2007). Implications of shift work for junior doctors. *BMJ*, **334**(7597), 777–778.

Aitken, M. & Paice, E. (2003). Trainees' attitudes to shift work depend on grade and specialty. *BMJ*, **326**(7379), 48.

Arnedt, J.T., Owens, J., Crouch, M., Stahl, J. & Carskadon, M.A. (2005). Neurobehavioral performance of residents after heavy night call vs after alcohol ingestion. *JAMA*, **294**(9), 1025–1033.

Ayas, N.T., Barger, L.K., Cade, B.E., et al. (2006). Extended work duration and the risk of self-reported percutaneous injuries in interns. *JAMA*, **296**(9), 1055–1062.

Baker, G.R., Norton, P.G., Flintoft, V.,'et al. (2004). The Canadian Adverse Events Study: the incidence of adverse events among hospital patients in Canada. *CMAJ*, **170**(11), 1678–1686.

Barger, L.K., Cade, B.E., Ayas, N.T., et al. (2005). Extended work shifts and the risk of motor vehicle crashes among interns. *N Engl J Med*, **352**(2), 125–134.

Barger, L.K., Ayas, N.T., Cade, B.E., et al. (2006). Impact of extended-duration shifts on medical errors, adverse events, and attentional failures. *PLoS Med*, **3**(12), e487.

Bates, D.W., Cullen, D.J., Laird, N., et al. (1995). Incidence of adverse drug events and potential adverse drug events. Implications for prevention. ADE Prevention Study Group. *JAMA*, **274**(1), 29–34.

Beckett, D.J., Gordon, C.F., Paterson, R., et al. (2009). Improvement in out-of-hours outcomes following the implementation of Hospital at Night. *QJM*, **102**(8), 539–546.

Benger, J. (2008). Not just about working hours. *BMJ*, **336**, 345.

British Medical Association (2008). *BMA Survey of Junior Doctors' Views on Working Hours and the EWTD*, British Medical Association.

Cappuccio, F.P. (2009). 'Hospital at Night' improves outcomes: does the evidence support opinions? *QJM*, **102**(8), 583–584.

Cappuccio, F.P. & Lockley, S.W. (2008). Safety and the flying doctor. *BMJ*, **336**, 218.

Cappuccio, F.P., Bakewell, A., Taggart, F.M., et al. (2009a). Implementing a 48 h EWTD-compliant rota for junior doctors in the UK does not compromise patients' safety: assessor-blind pilot comparison. *QJM*, **102**(4), 271–282.

Cappuccio, F.P., Lockley, S.W. & Landrigan, C.P. (2009b). Cappuccio response to correspondence. *QJM*, **102**(5), 363–364.

Coward, R. (2005). *Medical SpRs and the European Working Time Directive*. London: Royal College of Physicians.

Czeisler, C.A., Moore-Ede, M.C. & Coleman, R.H. (1982). Rotating shift work schedules that disrupt sleep are improved by applying circadian principles. *Science*, **217**(4558), 460–463.

Czeisler, C.A., Duffy, J.F., Shanahan, T.L., et al. (1999). Stability, precision, and near-24-hour period of the human circadian pacemaker. *Science*, **284**(5423), 2177–2181.

Fahrenkopf, A.M., Sectish, T.C., Barger, L.K., et al. (2008). Rates of medication errors among depressed and burnt out residents: prospective cohort study. *BMJ*, **336**(7642), 488–491.

Folkard, S. & Tucker, P. (2003). Shift work, safety and productivity. *Occup Med (Lond)*, **53**(2), 95–101.

Folkard, S., Lombardi, D.A. & Tucker, P. (2005). Shiftwork: safety, sleepiness and sleep. *Ind Health*, **43**(1), 20–23.

Gander, P., Purnell, H., Garden, A. & Woodward, A. (2007). Work patterns and fatigue-related risk among junior doctors. *Occup Environ Med*, **64**(11), 733–738.

Griffin, F.A. & Resar, R.K. (2007). *IHI Global Trigger Tool for Measuring Adverse Events*. Cambridge, MA: Institute of Healthcare Improvement.

Grover, K., Gatt, M. & MacFie, J. (2008). The effect of the EWTD on surgical SpRs: a regional survey. *Ann R Coll Surg Engl*, **90**(Suppl), 68–70.

Horrocks, N. & Pounder, R. (2006a). *Designing Safer Rotas for Junior Doctors in the 48-Hour Week*. London: Royal College of Physicians.

Horrocks, N. & Pounder, R. (2006b). Who's for five nine-hour shifts a week? *Clin Med*, **6**(5), 440–442.

Horrocks, N. & Pounder, R. (2006c). Working the night shift: preparation, survival and recovery—a guide for junior doctors. *Clin Med*, **6**(1), 61–67.

Jaeger, N. v. Kiel, L. (2003). *Social policy—Concepts of Working Time and Rest Period—On-call Service Provided by Doctors in Hospitals*. European Commission, Council Directive 93/1 04/EC.

Kara, N., Patil, P.V. & Shimi, S.M. (2008). Changes in working patterns hit emergency general surgical training. *Ann R Coll Surg Engl*, **90**(Suppl), 60–63.

Landrigan, C.P., Rothschild, J.M., Cronin, J.W., et al. (2004). Effect of reducing interns' work hours on serious medical errors in intensive care units. *N Engl J Med*, **351**(18), 1838–1848.

Lockley, S.W., Cronin, J.W., Evans, E.E., et al. (2004). Effect of reducing interns' weekly work hours on sleep and attentional failures. *N Engl J Med*, **351**(18), 1829–1837.

Lockley, S.W., Landrigan, C.P., Barger, L.K. & Czeisler, C.A. (2006). When policy meets physiology: the challenge of reducing resident work hours. *Clin Orthop Relat Res*, **449**, 116–127.

Mann, C. (2009). Response to: implementing a 48 h EWTD-compliant rota for junior doctors in the UK does not compromise patients' safety: assessor-blind pilot comparison. *QJM*, **102**, 298.

Mather, H. & Pounder, R. (2005). *Coping with Problems in Acute Medicine in the Post-WTD Era—A December 2004 Survey of RCP College Tutors in December 2004*. London: Royal College of Physicians.

Muir Gray, J.A. (2004). Evidence based policy making. *BMJ*, **329**(7473), 988–989.

Murray, A., Pounder, R., Mather, H. & Black, D.C. (2005). Junior doctors' shifts and sleep deprivation. *BMJ*, **330**(7505). 1404.

NHS Management Executive (1991). *Hours of Work of Doctors in Training*. NHS Management Executive.

Paice, E. & Reid, W. (2004). Can training and service survive the European Working Time Directive? *Med Educ*, **38**(4), 336–338.

Petersen, L.A., Brennan, T.A., O'Neil, A.C., Cook, E.F. & Lee, T.H. (1994). Does housestaff discontinuity of care increase the risk for preventable adverse events? *Ann Intern Med*, **121**(11), 866–872.

Petersen, L.A., Orav, E.J., Teich, J.M., O'Neil, A.C. & Brennan, T.A. (1998). Using a computerized sign-out program to improve continuity of inpatient care and prevent adverse events. *Jt Comm J Qual Improv*, **24**(2), 77–87.

Pounder, R. (2006). European junior doctors who work at night. *Eurohealth*, **12**, 5–7.

Pounder, R. (2008). Junior doctors' working hours: can 56 go into 48? *Clin Med*, **8**(2), 126–127.

Reason, J. (2000). Human error: models and management. *BMJ*, **320**(7237), 768–770.

Santhi, N., Horowitz, T.S., Duffy, J.F. & Czeisler, C.A. (2007). Acute sleep deprivation and circadian misalignment associated with transition onto the first night of work impairs visual selective attention. *PLoS One*, **2**(11), e1233.

Stickgold, R. (2005). Sleep-dependent memory consolidation. *Nature*, **437**(7063), 1272–1278.

Stickgold, R. & Walker, M.P. (2005). Memory consolidation and reconsolidation: what is the role of sleep? *Trends Neurosci*, **28**(8), 408–415.

Strauss, A. & Corbin, J. (1990). *Basics of Qualitative Research: Grounded Theory Procedures and Techniques*. London: Sage.

Tucker, P., Osborne, M., Dahlgren, A., et al. (2009). *The Impact of Working Time Arrangements on Fatigue Among Junior Doctors in Wales*. Swansea: Swansea University, pp. 1–152.

Van Dongen, H.P., Maislin, G., Mullington, J.M. & Dinges, D.F. (2003). The cumulative cost of additional wakefulness: dose-response effects on neurobehavioral functions and sleep physiology from chronic sleep restriction and total sleep deprivation. *Sleep*, **26**(2), 117–126.

Van Eaton, E.G., Horvath, K.D., Lober, W.B., Rossini, A.J. & Pellegrini, C.A. (2005). A randomized, controlled trial evaluating the impact of a computerized rounding and sign-out system on continuity of care and resident work hours. *J Am Coll Surg*, **200**(4), 538–545.

Vincent, C., Neale, G. & Woloshynowych, M. (2001). Adverse events in British hospitals: preliminary retrospective record review. *BMJ*, **322**(7285), 517–519.

Walsh, K.E., Adams, W.G., Bauchner, H., et al. (2006). Medication errors related to computerized order entry for children. *Pediatrics*, **118**(5), 1872–1879.

Waterman, A.D., Hodgson, H.J.F., Cheshire, C.M. & Goddard, A. (2009). Cappuccio et al. paper. *QJM*, **102**, 298–299.

Weingart, S.N., Wilson, R.M., Gibberd, R.W. & Harrison, B. (2000). Epidemiology of medical error. *BMJ*, **320**(7237), 774–777.

Woloshynowych, M., Neale, G. & Vincent, C. (2003). Case record review of adverse events: a new approach. *Qual Saf Health Care*, **12**(6), 411–415.

Chapter 19

A commentary on sleep education

E. Peile

Sleep: an important focus for medical education?

Readers of this book will, I hope, have formed an understanding of the prevalence of sleep disorders, and translated this into a personal view of the health services needed to alleviate both the symptom burden and the social and economic impact. Factor in the demography of an ageing population (Ram et al., 2009), you are now ready to consider the implications for clinical training and medical education in sleep disorders.

Clinical training is not the same as medical education. We train for roles. 'To be trained is to have arrived; to be educated is to continue to travel' (Calman, 1994). Doctors, like all other health professionals, need training: training in the recognition of sleep disorders and in the skills of relevant procedures involved in diagnosis and treatment including prescribing. Most health professionals need some education on the physiology and pathophysiology of sleep, whatever their specialist discipline: care of children, adults, and elders benefits from a broad understanding of the concepts. For doctors, the educational need is clear. In the United Kingdom, there is, at last, consensus on the role of the doctor in healthcare (Medical Schools Council, 2008). Consider the implications of this statement for sleep education:

> Medical undergraduate education must provide a strong grounding in relevant science and in clinical practice as well as providing opportunities to develop an appreciation for research. Doctors must have the ability to assimilate new knowledge critically, have strong intellectual skills and grasp of scientific principles and be capable of dealing effectively with and of managing uncertainty, ambiguity and complexity. They must have the capacity to work out solutions from first principles when the pattern does not fit.
>
> (Medical Schools Council, 2008)

Having thus considered the educational need, now reflect on how this need has been met to date. In 1993, a national survey was conducted of 126 accredited medical schools in the United States to evaluate physician education in sleep and sleep disorders. Less than 2 hours of total teaching time was allocated to sleep and sleep disorders, on average, with 37 schools reporting no structured teaching time whatever in this area (Rosen et al., 1993). Little changed in the next 5 years and a survey of the two largest professional sleep societies in the United States revealed that, although the majority of respondent specialists were involved in teaching sleep to medical students or postgraduate trainees, the average amount of teaching time was only 2.1 hours for undergraduate and 4.8 hours for graduate education in sleep (Rosen et al., 1998). The most recent survey of the 4-year medical school curriculum reveals an average of less than 2 hours of formal education directed at sleep, even at Harvard Medical School, such that the average medical student graduates with little information on either the identification or the treatment of sleep disorders (Harvard Medical School, 2009, <<http://sleep.med.harvard.edu/what-we-do/medical-education>>).

The situation in the United Kingdom is, if anything, worse. In 1998, Stores and Crawford surveyed UK medical schools and found negligible amounts of teaching on sleep.

> The median total time given to sleep and its disorders in undergraduate teaching as a whole was five minutes, for preclinical teaching 15 minutes, and zero in clinical teaching. Teaching was particularly limited on the various types of sleep disorder common in clinical practice, and also on non-medication treatments

(Stores and Crawford, 1998)

Curriculum time is a rough guide: it is difficult to measure, as the boundaries around components of science teaching and clinical experience are intentionally fuzzy in integrated courses, but there is clearly an imbalance between educational need and provision at medical schools. It was this that stimulated us to design a Special Study Module on Sleep at Warwick Medical School in 2004.

The place of sleep in undergraduate education

There is, in my opinion, a particular rationale for learning based on 'sleep' in undergraduate medical education—one which is only rivalled by learning about 'pain' perhaps. These topics have important educational attributes. The subject comes within the compass of student experience—all students sleep; their experiences of sleep differ, yet most are acquainted with somebody for whom sleep is problematic. The subject also draws on many different strands of biomedical and social science learning. Finally, sleep, like pain, is relevant to almost all branches of clinical medicine.

As will be seen from Table 19.1, epidemiology is the foundation of our sleep teaching, and it is our experience that those students who select this course strengthen their applied understanding of epidemiological constructs. The course, which includes visits to clinical and research sleep centres, offers a wide variety of learning experiences including an opportunity to learn about counselling skills and apply them in sessions with simulated patients for whom sleep is a problem. Now versed in the elements of sleep hygiene, early phase students are able to practise for the first time, offering useful information to patients instead of just gathering information from them.

Curriculum coverage at other UK medical schools

In 2006, I was motivated to explore the websites of the other medical schools in the United Kingdom, looking for information about sleep. The majority of student support sites contained information on sleep and sleep hygiene, and many websites contained medical humanities material on sleep. Nearly all curricula made reference to covering the basic psychopharmacology of sleep. Sleep as a topic appeared from time to time across some, but by no means all, websites.

Table 19.1 Competencies predicated as learning outcomes for students on the original Warwick Sleep SSM

---

1. Relate recent biomedical research in circadian rhythms to a social perspective of sleep patterns in populations.
2. Interpret epidemiological data on sleeping habits in the light of reported individual variation in sleep patterns and sleep laboratory tests.
3. Engage with public health of sleep deprivation (e.g. accidents, shift-working, child health) and be able to discuss the relative merits of preventative strategies.
4. Counsel an individual patient about potential harm of sleep deprivation to psychological health and about healthy strategies.
5. Demonstrate causal links in the morbidity of obesity, diabetes, cardiovascular disease, and sleep disorder.
6. Discuss psychopharmacology of sleep.

Examples include reference in teaching Geriatric Medicine to 'Factors (diet, exercise, and sleep) affecting older people's life adjustments'; in paediatrics to a lecture on 'Sleep disorders in childhood'; and there was even a mention of sleep apnoea in a respiratory medicine clerkship. Sleep and mood disorders featured on two psychiatry curricula with one psychopharmacology course mentioning a lecture on sleep and waking. There was still scope for much more imaginative use of sleep for student learning at undergraduate level.

Resources are freely available for sleep teaching. For example, the American Academy of Sleep Medicine (AASM) maintains, reviews, and periodically updates the 'MEDSleep Educational Resources' which were designed to help medical schools increase the sleep-related knowledge and skills of students, staff, and community healthcare providers. These teaching tools were developed with funding from the US National Center for Sleep Disorders Research, which is a part of the National Heart, Lung, and Blood Institute (NHLBI). There are now nearly 80 presentations, case studies, and other resources (American Association of Sleep Medicine, 2009, http://www.aasmnet.org/ Education.aspx).

Postgraduate education and training

In the United Kingdom, there is, as yet, no recognition of sleep medicine as a specialist discipline. There is a varying emphasis on sleep in postgraduate curricula but it has not to date featured strongly on the core curricula for medicine.

In the United States, several American Board of Medical Specialties (ABMS) member boards began administering certification examinations in sleep medicine in 2007, coincident with the decision of the American Board of Sleep Medicine (ABSM) to cease offering their certification which had previously indicated substantial commitment to and expertise in sleep medicine. The ABSM had based the certification process on specific assumptions about sleep medicine (Table 19.2) (American Board of Sleep Medicine, 2009, http://www.absm.org/).

Unlike the United Kingdom, in the United States there are specific fellowships for training in sleep medicine, for example those offered at the Mayo Clinic (2009, http://www.mayo.edu/msgme/sleepmed-rch.html). Graduate education is supported by initiatives for specialists such as the excellent Harvard 'Sleep Grand Rounds' and Harvard continuing medical education online for the wider healthcare profession: 'Healthy Sleep: An Overview of the Processes Governing the Biology of Normal Sleep and the Consequences of Insufficient Sleep' (http://sleep.med.harvard.edu/what-we-do/medical-education). In the United States, the AASM lists opportunities for sleep specialists and other medical professionals to enhance their understanding of sleep and sleep disorders (American Association of Sleep Medicine, 2009), whereas to date the British Sleep Society

Table 19.2 The ABSM principles underlying certification

1. Sleep medicine is a clinical specialty with a focus on clinical problems that require accurate diagnosis and treatment.

2. The knowledge base of sleep medicine is derived from many disciplines including neuroanatomy, neurophysiology, respiratory physiology, pharmacology, psychology, psychiatry, neurology, general internal medicine, pulmonary medicine, paediatrics, as well as others.

3. Diagnosis of sleep disorders is based on clinical acumen, scientific knowledge, and appropriately applied laboratory studies.

4. Treatment of sleep disorders is based on accurate diagnosis.

5. Mastery of specific clinical skills and procedures is essential for the practice of sleep medicine.

has concentrated on the learning needs of a membership of clinicians, technicians, and scientists working in the field of sleep (British Sleep Society, 2009, http://www.sleeping.org.uk/).

A medical student attracted to the idea of a career in sleep medicine in the United Kingdom by working on the special studies module, has highlighted the difficulties of career progression without specific educational pathways (Currie et al., 2005).

Pedagogies for sleep

Much reference is made in medical education to the integrated curriculum, referring to vertical integration of topics as the learner progresses from novice to competent practitioner, and horizontal integration across domains taught at the same stage of the curriculum. The difficulty comes when faculty and students have different understandings of integration in the curriculum. The Sleep SSM at Warwick set out 'to demonstrate through learning linked to one broad topic how the scientific basis of medicine links into multiple clinical applications'. A further objective was to 'develop a process of clinical reasoning which integrates learning from different sources'. To this end, case presentations and tutoring on the interpretation of a polysomnograph were offered close to learning about counselling skills and clinical epidemiology.

Constructivist learning is predicated on learners creating their own meaning from their experience. Sleep teaching makes constant reference to the learner's own experience of sleep. Part of the value of studies in topics like pain or sleep is that learners can make their own connections across the domains of medicine and science. For this to happen effectively, it is important to avoid merely jumbling eclectic topics together because of a connection to sleep, and to invoke Biggs's concept of constructive alignment. Basically, constructive alignment means that for each course/theme there must be close interrelations between the defined learning outcomes, the selection of learning and teaching activities, and assessment of students' outcomes and grading of students' learning (Biggs and Tang, 2007).

Conclusion

Sleep offers unique opportunities in medical education, both at undergraduate and graduate level, for learners to connect interesting and rapidly advancing science with clinical presentations. This is fundamental to the development of sound clinical reasoning. Patients are underserved by the lack of understanding of sleep problems amongst clinicians. Medical educationalists and clinicians and scientists with a sleep interest should work to weave sleep topics into the curriculum, where they can have far-reaching benefits for learners and patients alike.

References

American Association of Sleep Medicine (2009). Avialable at: http://www.aasmnet.org/Education.aspx (accessed December 1, 2009).

American Board of Sleep Medicine (2009). Avialable at: http://www.absm.org/ (accessed December 1, 2009).

Biggs, J. & Tang, C. (2007). *Teaching for Quality Learning at University*. Maidenhead: McGraw-Hill.

British Sleep Society (2009). Avialable at: http://www.sleeping.org.uk/ (accessed December 1, 2009).

Calman, K. (1994). The profession of medicine. *BMJ*, **309**, 1140.

Currie, A., Peile, E. & Hanning, C. (2005). Dying for a kip student. *BMJ*, **13**, 89–132.

Medical Schools Council (2008). Consensus Statement on the Role of the Doctor. Available at: http://www.medschools.ac.uk/news.htm (accessed 1 December 2009).

Ram, S., Seirawan, H., Kumar, S.K. & Clark, G.T. (2010). Prevalence and impact of sleep disorders and sleep habits in the United States. *Sleep Breath,* **14**(1), 63–70.

Rosen, R.C., Rosekind, M., Rosevear, C., Cole, W.E. & Dement, W.C. (1993). Physician education in sleep and sleep disorders: a national survey of U.S. medical schools.*Sleep*, **16**(3), 249–254.

Rosen, R., Mahowald, M., Chesson, A., et al. (1998). The Taskforce 2000 survey on medical education in sleep and sleep disorders. *Sleep*, **21**(3), 235–238.

Stores, G. & Crawford, C. (1998). Medical student education in sleep and its disorders. *J R Coll Physicians Lond*, **32**, 149–153.

Mayo Clinic (2009). Available at: http://www.mayo.edu/msgme/sleepmed-rch.html (accessed December 1, 2009).

Harvard Medical School (2009). Available at: http://sleep.med.harvard.edu/what-we-do/medical-education (accessed 1 December, 2009).

Chapter 20

Sleep, law, and policy

C.B. Jones, C.J. Lee, and S.M.W. Rajaratnam

General introduction and scope

The detrimental effects of drowsiness on human performance have safety implications for drowsy persons and for anyone with whom they come into contact (Knauth, 2007). This is particularly so when the drowsy person is operating heavy machinery (e.g. driving a car) or has to make decisions that have potentially life-threatening consequences (e.g. a medical practitioner making a decision about a patient) (see also Chapters 15–18). Moreover, researchers are beginning to establish the long-term health implications of chronic sleep restriction (e.g. Sigurdson and Ayas, 2007) (see also Chapters 4 and 5).

The problems associated with drowsiness[1] have societal implications related to public and occupational health and safety which governments often seek to address as a matter of law and public policy (see also Chapter 21). This chapter focuses on the intersection between sleep, law, and policy, and briefly discusses the types of actions some governments around the world have taken in response to some of the societal problems and issues related to sleep.

Identification of high-risk groups

Sleep science has identified a number of critical factors that contribute to drowsiness, including the individual's sleep history and the phase or time of the internal circadian pacemaker that drives circadian rhythms (Lockley et al., 2006). As discussed elsewhere in this textbook, chronic sleep restriction will increase the sleep debt that a person carries, which is likely to adversely impact that person's cognitive performance (Bonnet and Arand, 1995). Based on this knowledge of the physiological determinants of drowsiness, it is possible to identify populations or occupational groups that are more likely to be affected by drowsiness, and for whom drowsiness may pose significant risks to personal and public health and safety. Examples of these groups include people who act or work:

+ extended hours;
+ shift-work schedules, including night work and rotating shifts;
+ early morning hours; and
+ in professions requiring safety-critical tasks to be performed immediately after waking.

------

[1] Lawmakers, policy-makers, and others use the terms 'sleepiness', 'fatigue', 'tiredness', and 'drowsiness' interchangeably at times and with specific meanings at others. In this chapter, 'drowsiness' is used to refer to the likelihood of falling asleep. This meaning does not extend to concepts associated with muscular exertion or to chronic fatigue syndrome. The reader should be aware that in some circumstances, including legislation or other sources of law or policy, other terms are used to describe drowsiness, and specific definitions for these terms may be provided that restrict or expand the definition used in this chapter. Whenever such alternative terms for drowsiness are used in a legislative, legal, or policy source discussed in this chapter, the alternative term also will be used in discussing the source.

Transport, medical and emergency services, manufacturing, mining, and defense are examples of industries that exhibit these characteristics and must therefore be considered to be at high risk of exposure to drowsiness and drowsiness-related incidents that may pose a threat to personal and public health and safety. Moreover, persons employed in these industries and others who attempt to drive in a drowsy state pose significant risks to their own safety and the safety of other drivers.

Role and reach of government

Governments have a legitimate interest in protecting public and occupational health and safety in their respective societies. It is therefore unsurprising that governments and other regulatory bodies have sought to address the drowsiness-related risks to public and occupational health and safety, particularly in the high-risk groups identified previously.

Government responses to the societal issues related to drowsiness have taken a number of forms, and in certain instances have involved the creation of schemes intended to address drowsiness directly as a matter of law and public policy. In countries that have adopted Britain's heritage of government and law, for example, work hours and shift structure arrangements historically have been addressed by industrial relations or labour law processes (Barnard et al., 2003). More recently, government interventions in this area have been justified on safety grounds (see also Chapters 17 and 18).

Some commentators argue that governments should take a multi-faceted approach to managing the societal risks posed by drowsiness (Fletcher et al., 2005; Heaton, 2005). This approach encourages governments to promote activities through official government channels, businesses, and individuals to address societal issues related to drowsiness, including:

◆ non-regulatory interventions, such as public awareness and education campaigns;

◆ the promotion of incorporating drowsiness management elements into workplace safety programs;

◆ assessments of shift structures to identify drowsiness risk;

◆ the adoption of corporate or professional codes of conduct or other means of corporate or industrial self-regulation; and

◆ official government regulation of certain private, public, and occupational activities through the legislative or regulatory process.

Regulatory and policy schemes to address drowsiness

Governments worldwide have established regulatory and policy schemes to address drowsiness in certain sectors of society (e.g. the high-risk groups identified previously), and the problems such drowsiness create for public and occupational health and safety. This part begins with a discussion of schemes applied in several countries[2] to three topical areas: (1) non-commercial road transport, (2) commercial road transport, and (3) resident physician training. In each of these areas, the schemes applied generally create legal duties or restrictions to address the public and occupational health and safety consequences of drowsiness. Following this discussion, the European Working Time Directive (EWTD) will be reviewed (see also Chapter 18). The EWTD represents a society-wide approach to addressing drowsiness in the workplace, requiring all

---

[2] Most of the schemes discussed in this part come from countries that have adopted the common law legal system (e.g. United States and Australia) rather than the civil law tradition (e.g. continental Europe).

European Union (EU) member states to enact provisions limiting working time throughout all sectors of their respective economies.[3]

Drowsy driving prevention in non-commercial transport in the United States

The issue of drowsy driving in the general population can be addressed as one concerning public health and safety to which the lessons learned from other successful public health and safety campaigns (e.g. those employed for combating and preventing drunk driving) may be applied. This is the approach taken by most drowsy driving prevention efforts in the United States, which are illustrative of drowsy driving prevention efforts in other countries.

National Sleep Foundation's efforts

As part of a US-wide public awareness campaign to reduce the number of drowsiness-related crashes among the nation's young drivers, the National Sleep Foundation (NSF) released its first *State of the States Report on Drowsy Driving* in November 2007.[4] In the report, NSF cites government statistics indicating that 100,000 police-reported crashes are the direct result of driver drowsiness each year in the United States, resulting in an estimated 1,550 deaths, 71,000 injuries, and $12.5 billion in monetary losses. NSF believes these statistics significantly underestimate the true magnitude of the problem of drowsy driving in the United States because:

- there is no test to determine drowsiness as there is for intoxication, for example, a 'breathalyzer';
- state reporting practices are inconsistent;
- there is little or no police training in identifying drowsiness as a crash factor;
- self-reporting is unreliable;
- drowsiness and fatigue may play a role in crashes attributed to other causes such as alcohol, and about one million such crashes annually are thought to be produced by driver inattention or lapses; and
- drowsy driving represents 10–30% of all crashes in countries with more consistent crash reporting procedures than in the United States (e.g. Australia, England, Finland, and other European nations).

In explaining its objectives in releasing the *State of the States* report, NSF comments:

> Like drugs and alcohol, fatigue needs to be addressed as a public health issue by dealing with the underlying causes of sleep deprivation such as lifestyles, work hours, shift work, or untreated sleep disorders, and as a public safety issue by employing traditional methods of traffic safety: education, enforcement, engineering and evaluation.

US federal efforts

The issue of drowsy driving prevention has attracted the attention of some US lawmakers at the federal level, and a proposed National Drowsy Driving Act was introduced in the US House of Representatives in February 2003 (Maggie's Law: National Drowsy Driving Act of 2003). Citing many of the statistics and findings that were later mentioned in the *State of the States* report, the bill was intended to provide incentives for US states to develop traffic safety programs to reduce

---

[3] The EWTD does not apply to transport workers, as specific Directives address the transport modalities.
[4] The NSF plans to update this report annually as part of each future Drowsy Driving Prevention Week.

crashes related to drowsy driving. The bill included provisions authorizing the granting of federal funds to state highway offices and other organizations for the purpose of:

- educating the public in all aspects of the dangers of drowsy driving, in recognizing the signs of drowsy driving, and in taking appropriate countermeasures to avoid fall-asleep crashes;
- educating law enforcement officials in all aspects of drowsy driving prevention, in identifying drowsiness among drivers and as a factor in car crashes, and in the sanctions available for drowsy driving accidents; and
- adopting 'formal codes on motor vehicle accident report forms to report fatigue-related or fall-asleep crashes' (Maggie's Law: National Drowsy Driving Act of 2003, § 3).

Although the National Drowsy Driving Act was not enacted into federal law, it has served as a model for subsequent drowsy driving bills introduced in various US states.

US state efforts

Lawmakers in several US states have introduced legislation concerning drowsy driving. These legislative proposals incorporate a variety of legal and policy approaches to combat and prevent drowsy driving and include changes to state driving laws and licensing processes, and the establishment of training requirements and new authorities for law enforcement officials. In some states without laws specifically addressing drowsy driving, courts have applied existing laws to situations involving drowsy driving.

Drowsy driving laws

Delaware and Virginia currently have laws that indirectly address drowsy driving in non-commercial drivers. The Delaware law considers the condition of the driver, targeting drivers who fail 'to give full time and attention to the operation of the vehicle' or 'to maintain a proper lookout while operating the vehicle' (DEL. CODE ANN. tit. 21, § 4176). The Virginia law considers the number of hours the driver has been behind the wheel, prohibiting a person from driving more than 13 hours in a 24-hour period (VA. CODE ANN. § 46.2-812).

In August 2003, New Jersey became the first US state to pass a law specifically addressing the issue of drowsy driving. Maggie's Law establishes driving while fatigued as recklessness under New Jersey's vehicular homicide statute[5]: under Maggie's Law, proof that a person 'fell asleep while driving or was driving after having been without sleep for a period in excess of 24 consecutive hours may give rise to an inference that the [person] was driving recklessly'. Proof of drowsy driving can therefore give rise to the same legal inference (i.e. driving recklessly) as proof of intoxicated or drunk driving (which 'shall give rise to an inference that the [person] was driving recklessly') under Maggie's Law (2003 N.J. Laws c. 143, § 1).

Since Maggie's Law was enacted in New Jersey, legislation pertaining to drowsy driving prevention has been proposed in several other states. Many of these bills feature similar proposals for substantive changes to the respective state's driving laws.

 i. **Definition and proof of drowsy or fatigued driving**

  All of the state bills proposing changes to driving laws as a means to prevent drowsy driving essentially provide the same meaning for the term 'drowsy' or 'fatigued': being without sleep for at least 24 consecutive hours. Bills in several states define drowsy or fatigued in this manner (S.B. 104 (Ill.) 2007; S.F. 2295 (Iowa) 2007; H.B. 150 (Ky.) 2007; H.B. 4332 (Mich.) 2007; H.B. 3021 (Or.) 2007).

---

[5] In the US legal system, 'statutes' are codified laws enacted by a state legislature (or Congress) with the approval of the Governor (or President) or over a gubernatorial (or Presidential) veto.

Several New York bills would create a rebuttable presumption that a person's ability to drive was impaired by drowsiness under a number of circumstances:

- proof that a person fell asleep while driving (A. 1234 (N.Y.) 2007; S. 1290 (N.Y.) 2007);
- proof that a person has been without sleep for at least 24 consecutive hours (A. 1234 (N.Y.) 2007; S. 1290 (N.Y.) 2007); or
- proof that a person is aware or should reasonably be expected to be aware that the person has been without sleep for at least 24 consecutive hours (A. 4143 (N.Y.) 2007; S. 2488 (N.Y.) 2007).

One Massachusetts bill provides that '[p]roof that the operator of a motor vehicle was awake for at least 22 of the 24 hours prior to said operation of a motor vehicle or at least 140 hours of the 168 hours prior to said operation of a motor vehicle shall constitute sufficient evidence to conclude that said motor vehicle operator was impaired by sleep deprivation' (S. 2124 (Mass.) 2005). This definition:

- addresses the potential argument that a driver was not legally impaired by sleep deprivation because the driver had obtained short bouts of sleep (e.g. 30–60 minutes) and therefore had not been awake for 24 consecutive hours prior to operating a motor vehicle; and
- accounts for impairment caused by chronic sleep restriction accumulated over the prior week.

ii. Drowsy or fatigued driving as a violation of law

Bills have been proposed in Massachusetts (S. 2124 (Mass.) 2005; S. 2072 (Mass.) 2008) and New York (A. 1234 (N.Y.) 2007; S. 1290 (N.Y.) 2007; A. 4143 (N.Y.) 2007; S. 2488 (N.Y.) 2007; A. 2332 (N.Y.) 2007) that would make driving while drowsy or fatigued a separate violation of law to be treated as a traffic infraction or a misdemeanour. The Massachusetts bills would establish the crime of:

- sleeping while driving (S. 2072 (Mass.) 2008); or
- falling asleep or being impaired by drowsiness or sleep deprivation while operating a motor vehicle, where the vehicle operator 'has fallen asleep while operating a motor vehicle, [or] was impaired by drowsiness of which the [operator] was aware or could reasonably be expected to be aware, or was impaired by sleep deprivation while operating a motor vehicle[]' (S. 2124 (Mass.) 2005).

Although most of the New York bills would establish the rebuttable presumptions regarding drowsiness mentioned previously, several of these specifically exempt emergency personnel engaged in the response to a catastrophic event affecting public safety or to certain other emergencies (A. 1234 (N.Y.) 2007; S. 1290 (N.Y.) 2007; A. 4143 (N.Y.) 2007; S. 2488 (N.Y.) 2007).

iii. Drowsy driving resulting in serious injury

Some of the New York bills concerning drowsy driving prevention provide criminal penalties for drowsy driving that cause serious injury to another person. Most of the bills would include driving while drowsy under the felony offense of vehicular assault in the second degree (A. 1234 (N.Y.) 2007; S. 1290 (N.Y.) 2007; A. 4143 (N.Y.) 2007; S. 2488 (N.Y.) 2007). One New York bill, however, provides that a person who causes serious physical injury to a person while committing the offense of driving while impaired by fatigue as defined under that bill also commits the misdemeanour offense of aggravated driving while ability impaired by fatigue (A. 2332 (N.Y.) 2007).[6]

---

[6] In the US legal system, the terms 'felony' and 'misdemeano[u]r' distinguish between serious and less serious crimes. The terms 'indictable' and 'summary' are used to make this distinction in many other common law jurisdictions.

iv. **Drowsy driving resulting in death**

Most state bills concerning drowsy driving prevention provide criminal penalties for drowsy driving that causes the death of another person. One Illinois bill exemplifies the most common approach—treating the act as reckless homicide rather than manslaughter—and further provides that:

- driving while the driver is aware that he or she is drowsy constitutes recklessness; and
- proof that the driver fell asleep while driving or was driving after having been without sleep for a period in excess of 24 consecutive hours may give rise to an inference that the driver was driving recklessly (S.B. 104 (Ill.) 2007).

In Tennessee, bills have been introduced that would allow triers of fact[7] to infer that if the driver of a motor vehicle fell asleep while driving or was driving after having been without sleep for a period in excess of 24 hours:

- such driver was driving in willful or wanton disregard for the safety of persons or property in violation of the Tennessee reckless driving statute; and
- where such conduct was the proximate cause of a fatal accident, such driver recklessly killed another in violation of the Tennessee reckless homicide statute (H.B. 117 (Tenn.) 2007; S.B. 71 (Tenn.) 2007).

Three different approaches to punishing drowsy driving resulting in death have been introduced in New York. One approach would treat the act as the existing felony offense of vehicular manslaughter in the second degree (A. 4143 (N.Y.) 2007; S. 2488 (N.Y.) 2007). Another approach would treat the act as the new felony offense of vehicular homicide caused by driving while ability impaired by drowsiness (A. 1234 (N.Y.) 2007; S. 1290 (N.Y.) 2007). The third approach would provide that a person who causes the death of a person while committing the new offense of driving while impaired by drowsiness also commits the new misdemeanour offense of aggravated driving while ability impaired by drowsiness (A. 2332 (N.Y.) 2007).

Procedural and administrative reforms in the state driver licensing process

Some recent Massachusetts bills relating to drowsy driving prevention include provisions for procedural and administrative reforms in the state's driver licensing process (S. 2124 (Mass.) 2005; S. 2072 (Mass.) 2008). These bills would require the licensing examination for non-commercial and school bus drivers in Massachusetts to include questions about the importance of obtaining adequate sleep and how to recognize the signs of reduced alertness and sleep disorders (S. 2124 (Mass.) 2005, §§ 2 and 3; S. 2072 (Mass.) 2008, §§ 2 and 3). By implication, making these topics part of the driving exams would require inclusion of information relating to these topics in the study materials for the exam (i.e. the Massachusetts Driver's Manual).

These bills would also add drowsy driving as a factor to consider in determining whether a person is a habitual traffic offender under Massachusetts law, thereby empowering the state's Registrar of Motor Vehicles to suspend or revoke the person's driving license (S. 2124 (Mass.) 2005, § 5; S. 2072 (Mass.) 2008, § 5). The bills would also require that at least one of the physicians appointed to the medical advisory board of the state's Registry of Motor Vehicles has expertise in sleep disorders or the effects of sleep deprivation (S. 2124 (Mass.) 2005, § 4; S. 2072 (Mass.) 2008, § 4).

---

[7] In the US legal system, the 'trier of fact' is the jury in jury trials, and the judge in bench trials.

Training law enforcement officials

The Massachusetts bills also include provisions for training and educating police and other law enforcement officials to recognize signs of drowsiness or reduced alertness associated with sleep deprivation or sleep disorders, requiring that:

- Massachusetts law enforcement officers learn about recognizing the symptoms of drowsy driving in their law enforcement and accident investigation training; and
- all Massachusetts court personnel be trained in recognizing the effects of sleep deprivation or sleep disorders (S. 2124 (Mass.) 2005, §§ 8 and 9; S. 2072 (Mass.) 2008, §§ 8 and 9).

Detention powers

Perhaps the boldest and most innovative proposal in the Massachusetts bills is a provision authorizing police officers to hold a drowsy driver in protective custody until the driver is rested. To determine whether or not a driver is impaired or incapacitated by reason of sleep deprivation or sleep disorder, the police officer would request the driver 'to submit to reasonable tests or other evidence' as established by regulation to determine if the driver was impaired or incapacitated by reason of sleep deprivation or disorder. Any driver who failed such test or who was unable to produce such evidence as required would be presumed impaired or incapacitated and would be placed in protective custody. Any person held in such protective custody would not be considered to have been arrested or charged with any crime (S. 2124 (Mass.) 2005, § 12; S. 2072 (Mass.) 2008, § 12).

Applying existing laws to drowsy driving situations

In some US states that have not enacted laws specifically aimed at combating and preventing drowsy driving, courts have applied existing vehicular homicide or reckless driving statutes to situations involving drowsy drivers. For example, a Maryland appellate court recently held that the following evidence was sufficient to show that a driver behaved in a grossly negligent manner so as to support a conviction for manslaughter by vehicle under Maryland law:

- that the driver recognized that he was extremely drowsy;
- that the driver was aware that he had repeatedly dozed off at the wheel; and
- that despite these premonitory symptoms of drowsiness, the driver made a deliberate decision to ignore the risk of falling asleep at the wheel and to continue driving.[8]

In a 1966 civil case involving the application of Michigan law, Maryland's highest court examined whether falling asleep at the wheel amounted to a *prima facie* case of gross negligence, which was defined under Michigan law as 'willful and wanton misconduct[.]' The Court held that the following evidence was sufficient for the issue of gross negligence to be submitted to a jury:

- that the driver had engaged in strenuous activities prior to a 500-mile car trip from Maryland to Michigan;
- that the driver had been warned numerous times of his sleepiness by passengers in his car, but had refused to relinquish the wheel to another passenger;
- that the driver had driven all except 2.5 hours of the trip from Maryland to Michigan;
- that the driver had driven off the road a fairly short time before the accident underlying the case at bar occurred, and had nearly driven into an overpass a short time later; and

---

8 Skidmore v. State, 887 A. 2d 92, 97 (Md. Ct. Spec. App. 2005). Under Maryland's manslaughter by vehicle statute, a person who causes the death of another as a result of driving, operating, or controlling a vehicle in a grossly negligent manner is guilty of the felony offense of manslaughter by vehicle (MD. CODE. ANN., CRIM. LAW § 2-209). 'Gross negligence' under Maryland law means 'a wanton or reckless disregard for human life or for the rights of others'. Johnson v. State, 132 A.2d 853, 855 (Md. 1957).

◆ that the accident underlying the case at bar had occurred on a limited access highway, which may have accentuated the driver's tendency to sleep.[9]

Given these court rulings, a person who has exhibited a pattern of behaviour that includes drowsy driving or falling asleep while driving may be found by a Maryland court to have acted in a grossly negligent manner; and a person who causes the death of another person as a result of driving, operating, or controlling a vehicle while drowsy may be criminally prosecuted for and convicted of manslaughter by vehicle under existing Maryland law.[10]

Commercial road transport

Given the significant risk posed by drowsiness in heavy or commercial vehicle drivers (e.g. National Transportation Safety Board, 1990), governments in most industrialized nations regulate the work hours of commercial drivers. Major reforms to these regulations have been implemented in the United States, Canada, and Australia over the last 5 years.

United States

Hours of Service (HOS) regulations have been in place for commercial vehicles in the United States since the middle of the twentieth century, with the most recent revision taking effect on 19 January 2009 (49 C.F.R. pt. 395). This revision has been the subject of considerable debate over the last decade, and the Federal Motor Carrier Safety Administration (FMCSA) has been required to revisit its proposed provisions several times (Hours of Service of Drivers, 2008). Although the FMCSA regulations only apply to inter-state travel, many US states have adopted identical (or near-identical) regulations for intra-state travel.

Under the HOS regulations, property-carrying commercial motor vehicle drivers may drive up to 11 hours in a 14-hour on-duty window after they come on-duty following 10 or more consecutive hours off-duty. The 14 hours on-duty includes non-driving activities such as re-fuelling, breaks, and meals. The regulations also place limits on cumulative driving hours over longer periods, prohibiting any driving after 60 hours on-duty in 7 consecutive days, or 70 hours in 8 consecutive days. In relation to the limits on the 7/8 day period, the regulations contain a 'restart' provision in which a driver may begin counting from zero hours towards the 7/8 day period limits after a driver has 34 consecutive hours off-duty.

The rules for passenger-carrying commercial motor vehicles are similar in form, although the specific limits on driving and working time are different. Drivers of passenger-carrying vehicles must not drive for more than 10 hours following 8 consecutive hours off-duty or for any period after having been on-duty 15 hours following 8 consecutive hours off-duty. The same 7/8 day limits applicable to property-carrying commercial motor vehicles are applicable to passenger-carrying commercial motor vehicles.

---

[9] White v. King, 223 A. 2d 763, 770-71 (Md. 1966).

[10] The mere fact that a person causes the death of another person as a result of drowsy driving will not sustain a conviction for manslaughter by vehicle under Maryland law; the drowsy driver must have demonstrated a pattern of conduct that reflected a wanton or reckless disregard for human life or for the rights of others. This concept was central to the recent decision of Maryland prosecutors not to criminally charge a driver who caused an accident on Maryland's Chesapeake Bay Bridge that resulted in the death of another motorist, even though the driver admitted to driving while drowsy and falling asleep at the wheel, because the facts of the case did not meet Maryland's 'gross negligence' standard for manslaughter (Williams, 2008; Weiss and Hohmann, 2008).

The regulations also address the use of sleeper berths, providing that if a driver cannot take the required 10 hours off-duty in a sleeper berth, a driver must take at least 8 consecutive hours in the sleeper berth plus 2 consecutive hours either in the sleeper berth, off-duty, or any combination of the two.

Canada

Canada has also comprehensively amended its regulations, the most recent of which became fully effective on 1 January 2007 (Commercial Vehicle Drivers Hours of Service Regulations, 2005). The Canadian regulations limit work hours and provide for minimum off-duty or rest periods. Based on the extreme climatic conditions in the far north of the country, however, a different set of more flexible limits are available to drivers who are above 60° N latitude. As with the United States, the federal Canadian regulations only apply to inter-provincial transport, whereas provincial regulations that largely mirror the federal regulations apply to intra-province transport.

The Commercial Vehicle Drivers Hours of Service Regulations impose limits on all commercial vehicle drivers of 13 hours of driving and 14 hours on-duty in a day. After the accumulation of 13 hours driving time or 14 hours on-duty time, the driver must take 8 consecutive hours off-duty. In addition, a motor carrier must ensure that a driver takes a minimum of 10 hours off-duty per day. This off-duty time must be taken in blocks of no less than 30 minutes. The regulations also prohibit any driving after 16 hours elapsed between two 8-hour off-duty periods, and provide for rules allowing the splitting or deferring of daily off-duty time.

Longer time period limits are also imposed, depending on which of two cycles a driver decides to follow: cycle 1 (7 days) or cycle 2 (14 days). Regardless of the cycle chosen, drivers must not drive unless they have at least one 24-hour period free from work in the preceding 14-day period. Drivers following cycle 1 must be on-duty for no more than 70 hours per 7 days, unless they 'reset'; drivers following cycle 2 must have no more than 120 hours of on-duty time per 14 days (including no more than 70 hours on-duty without 24 hours consecutively off-duty). The reset period is at least 36 consecutive off-duty hours for cycle 1, and at least 72 consecutive hours for cycle 2. Once the reset period is reached for the respective cycle, the driver begins a new cycle and the accumulated on-duty hours are reset to zero.

In addition to these duty hour restrictions, the federal regulations also impose a general duty on a range of parties (defined as 'motor carrier, shipper, consignee, or other person' as well as the driver) not to allow or require a driver to drive if that driver's faculties are impaired to the point that it would be unsafe for that driver to drive, or such that there would be a risk to the safety or health of the public, the driver, or the employees of the motor carrier. This 'catch-all' provision gives rise to the problem of determining how a duty holder could know that a driver was impaired. This is an important practical issue because any regulatory or policy scheme to address drowsiness that is not based on prescriptive work hour limitations would need to be accompanied by some method of assessing impairment or likely impairment.

Australia

A new framework for the regulation of heavy vehicle driver fatigue (HVDF) was introduced into four of the mainland Australian states in September 2008.[11] Unlike the United States and Canada, the constitutional power to regulate road transport in Australia is retained by the

---

[11] New South Wales, Queensland, South Australia, and Victoria. The Northern Territory and Tasmania will join this scheme at a later date, leaving Western Australia as the only major jurisdiction to remain outside of the national system and operating under its own regulatory framework.

states and territories.[12] The state regulations are based on the HVDF Model Legislation (National Transport Commission (Model Legislation—Heavy Vehicle Driver Fatigue) Regulations, 2007), but vary slightly from state to state.

The HVDF Model Legislation attempts to balance the challenges of allowing a flexible but safe set of rules for the operation of heavy vehicles[13] in Australia. The overall structure of the legislation incorporates three main features:

1. a general duty to manage fatigue;
2. a series of offences placing duties on an extended range of parties that require the parties not to cause anyone else to drive while fatigued; and
3. three options for work hours, of which two are linked to an accreditation system.[14]

The HVDF legislation therefore takes a multi-level approach to the management of drowsy driving beyond simply restricting working or driving hours.

The general duty to manage fatigue is a broad-based duty to not drive a regulated heavy vehicle on a road while a person is impaired by fatigue. This is in addition to any other existing legal duties that a driver may have. It is expressed similarly to state Occupational Health and Safety laws, although with a specific focus on drowsiness rather than general safety.

The second feature of the legislation is the 'chain of responsibility' (COR), which expands the parties upon whom duties are placed beyond those who are usually targeted (i.e. drivers and operators). The COR provisions place duties on parties who have influence over the operation of the logistic supply chain and whose demands and actions can lead to drivers driving when it may not be safe to do so. The COR is extended to nine parties that have been identified as having a role to play in commercial vehicle transport drowsiness, either directly (i.e. drivers, employers, schedulers, loaders, and unloaders) or indirectly through commercial arrangements (i.e. prime contractors, consignors and consignees, and loading managers). In addition to having the general duty not to do anything that would require a driver to drive while fatigued, some COR parties have certain specific duties (e.g. ensuring that loading and unloading occurs within a certain timeframe).

The third major component of the HVDF legislation is the operating hours limits. Two of these options (Standard Hours and Basic Fatigue Management) are drafted in a style similar to the regulations in the United States and Canada in that they prescribe minimum rest and maximum working times per period of time.[15] The third option (Advanced Fatigue Management) takes a different approach and allows a firm to submit a proposal indicating what steps it will take to manage drowsiness, and within which parameters and limits it proposes to operate. The Basic and Advanced Fatigue management options are also linked to an accreditation system whereby a firm must pass a third-party audit against a number of standards, including driver and scheduler fatigue management training.

---

[12] The combined effects of Section 51 and 107 of the Australian Constitution enumerate the powers of the Commonwealth Parliament, and preserve all others to the states. See Amalgamated Soc'y of Engineers v. Adelaide Steamship Co. Ltd. (1920) 28 C.L.R. 129.

[13] The definition for 'heavy vehicle' in the Model Legislation does not require the vehicle to be involved in commercial operations.

[14] Australia does not have a compulsory operator licensing system.

[15] See Sections 44 and 49 of the Model Legislation for the limits for solo drivers.

Resident work hours

The impact of long work hours and sleep deprivation on the performance of resident physicians has received much attention in recent years (see also Chapters 17 and 18).[16] Historically, residency has been a period in which the trainee is expected to gain exposure to a wide area of practical medical situations and to learn to take responsibility for patient care. It is also a period characterized by extremely long work hours.

The public in recent years has become increasingly concerned about medical errors committed by residents who are acutely and chronically sleep-deprived as a result of their long work hours (McCall, 1989; Sidney and Wolfe, 2001). A series of studies by the Harvard Work Hours, Health, and Safety Group has shown that half the residents surveyed worked more than an 80-hour week, including individual shifts of up to 30 hours, less than 5% of which were spent sleeping (2.6 ± 1.7 hours). This group also conducted an intervention study in which residents were assigned to a traditional shift pattern (in which they worked a ~30-hour shift every other shift) or an intervention pattern where no shift was longer than 16 hours. This study found twice as many attentional failures at night for residents on the traditional schedule; another study found that residents working extended duration on-call shifts made 35.9% more serious medical errors than residents working no more than a 16-hour shift (summarized in Czeisler, 2006).

Governments worldwide have attempted to address this issue as a matter of preserving public (i.e. patient) and occupational (i.e. physician) health and safety.[17] As in transport, a number of different approaches have been taken to regulate resident work hours around the world. Some countries have left the issue for the normal industrial relations mechanisms to address (e.g. Australia), while others have allowed collective agreements to address the issue within governmentally mandated limits (e.g. New Zealand). Some governments have stepped in directly to regulate resident work hours (e.g. France) (Institute of Medicine [IOM], 2008).

In recent years, there have been several attempts in the United Sates to regulate resident work hours at the federal (Patient and Physician Safety and Protection Act of 2001; Patient and Physician Safety and Protection Act of 2002) and state (American Medical Students Association, 2009) levels. No legal instrument is currently in effect at the federal level that directly addresses the working time arrangements of residents, and only New York (by regulation) (N.Y. COMP. CODES R. & REGS. tit. 10, § 405.4) and Puerto Rico (by legislation) (P.R. LAWS ANN., tit. 24, §§ 10005 to 10009) have taken action at the state level to regulate resident work hours as a matter of law.[18] Since July 2003, however, the Accreditation Council for Graduate Medical Education (ACGME) has had in place a set of accreditation standards that includes the following specific restrictions on resident work hours:

- ◆ an average maximum limit of 80 work hours per week for residents over a 4-week period;
- ◆ a maximum limit of 24 consecutive hours for on-call duty;

---

[16] Resident physicians are junior physicians who have completed their academic medical training at University and who are undergoing a period of intense practical training in a teaching hospital under the supervision of more experienced physicians. The 'residency' period varies between countries but typically lasts over a year, after which the resident may choose to enter a specialist training program or remain as generalists.

[17] Drowsy resident may also compromise public safety because of increased risk of getting into a motor vehicle crash while commuting from work. When one resident training in the United Kingdom was asked whether she experienced any events that could be attributed to drowsiness during non-working time, she responded: 'Definitely—trying to drive anywhere after a night shift is a bit of a disaster. I would often have to stop in a lay by and have a 10-minute power nap'.

[18] Although not a US state, Puerto Rico's government is similar to those of the 50 states.

- an average maximum for on-call frequency of every third night over a 4-week period;
- an average of 1 day off from work each week over a 4-week period; and
- a minimum period of 10 hours free from work in between duty periods (ACGME, 2002, 2003).

These ACGME guidelines represent an attempt by the US graduate medical education community to regulate itself on the issue of resident work hours, and at least one commentator has suggested that these guidelines were developed to avoid possible government intervention (Lee, 2006).

At the request of Congress and under a contract with the federal Agency for Healthcare Research and Quality, the IOM released a report in December 2008 that included:

- a synthesis of 'current evidence on medical resident schedules and healthcare safety';
- strategies to 'enable optimization of work schedules to improve safety in the healthcare work environment' that take into account 'the learning and experience residents must achieve during their training[]'; and
- recommendations 'structured to optimize both the quality of care and the educational objectives' (IOM, 2008, p. 5).

The IOM also assessed the effectiveness of the ACGME guidelines in its report and concluded:

- that 'greater attention should be focused on increasing the opportunities for sleep during resident training to prevent fatigue-related errors, rather than on simply reducing total duty hours[]';
- that only 'regulating resident duty hours and increasing adherence to them would be insufficient to improve conditions for resident and patient safety[]'; and
- that 'a number of additional interrelated changes are needed: more direct supervision of junior residents, adjustment of residents' workload, providing sufficient time for residents to reflect on their clinical experiences, and improved patient transfers[]' (IOM, 2008, pp. 3–4).

The IOM recommended that the ACGME guidelines be revised as summarized in Table 20.1. In looking to the future, the IOM remarked in its report:

> The past 5 years since the ACGME duty hour rules were implemented have been a period of change and adjustment for training programs in the United States. Many programs have replaced scheduling and staffing models adopted in the initial year, and they continue to refine them in their efforts to improve educational value, quality of patient care, and service coverage. Research studies tend to report institution-specific adaptations, and there are few national data or rigorous analyses of different scheduling models across institutions or specialties. However, based on the collective field experiences of programs, [IOM] concluded that some degree of flexibility in duty hour scheduling would have to be retained (IOM, 2008, p.7).

The IOM's remarks emphasize the importance of several questions that are often posed in response to efforts to reduce resident work hours, including:

- whether limiting the work hours of residents will limit their ability to gain hands-on experience treating patients;
- whether the sleep deprivation caused by extended duration shifts results in impaired learning in medical residents (Walker and Stickgold, 2004);
- whether more frequent handovers between residents 'changing shifts' will lead to increased errors; and
- whether the economic consequences of reducing the work hours of resident doctors in the public health system (e.g. the cost of training and hiring new doctors) may damage the viability of the healthcare system as it currently operates.

Table 20.1 Recommended adjustments to 2003 duty hour limits

	2003 ACGME duty hour limits	IOM recommendation
Maximum hours of work per week	80 hours, averaged over 4 weeks	No change
Maximum shift length	30 hours (admitting patients up to 24 hours then 6 additional hours for transitional and educational activities)	◆ 30 hours (admitting patients for up to 16 hours, plus 5-hour protected sleep period between 10:00 p.m. and 8:00 a.m. with the remaining hours for transition and educational activities) ◆ 16 hours with no protected sleep period
Maximum in-hospital on-call frequency	Every third night, on average	Every third night, no averaging
Minimum time off between scheduled shifts	10 hours after shift length	◆ 10 hours after day shift ◆ 12 hours after night shift ◆ 14 hours after any extended duty period of 30 hours and not return until 6:00 a.m. of next day
Maximum frequency of in-hospital night shifts	Not addressed	4 nights maximum; 48 hours off after 3 or 4 nights of consecutive duty
Mandatory time off duty	◆ 4 days off per month ◆ 1 day (24 hours) off per week, averaged over 4 weeks	◆ 5 days off per month ◆ 1 day (24 hours) off per week, no averaging ◆ One 48-hour period off per month
Moonlighting	Internal moonlighting is counted against 80-hour weekly limit	◆ Internal and external moonlighting is counted against 80-hour weekly limit ◆ All other duty hour limits apply to moonlighting in combination with scheduled work
Limit on hours for exceptions	88 hours for select programs with a sound educational rationale	No change
Emergency room limits	12-hour shift limit, at least an equivalent period of time off between shifts; 60-hour workweek with additional 12 hours for education	No change

Source: Reprinted with permission from the National Academies Press, Copyright 2009, National Academy of Sciences.

Notwithstanding these questions, based on accumulating evidence of the impact of extended duration shifts on the safety of residents, their patients, and the general public, urgent attention to the regulation of work hours in medical residents is warranted. Providing adequate opportunity for residents to sleep should be seen as a part of the hospital's duty to provide a safe working environment and to minimize potential harm to patients. Implementation of the 2008 IOM recommendations would be the first step in addressing these safety concerns.

The European Working Time Directive

The EWTD takes a different approach to the question of workplace drowsiness by imposing a society-wide limitation on working time arrangements (see also Chapter 18). This EU Directive explicitly addresses the social dimension of working time, as well as worker health and safety, and represents 'a practical contribution towards creating the social dimension of the internal market' (Council Directive 93/104/EC; Adnett and Hardy, 2001). The Directive also draws on international norms as expressed in International Labour Organization (ILO) Conventions on working time, which provide support for a number of the substantive limits contained in the Directive's Articles (Engelen-Kefer, 1990), and incorporates the World Health Organization's broad definition of health.[19]

The EWTD imposes the following limits:

- minimum daily rest: 11 hours per 24 (averaged over a 14-day reference period);
- short rest break after 6 hours continuous work;
- minimum weekly rest: 1 day per week;
- average work for a 7-day period is 48 hours (subject to averaging provisions);
- 4 weeks paid leave per year; and
- 8 hours night work per 24-hour period (subject to averaging provisions).

Although much literature has been published on the Directive's implementation, it has been argued that little empirical research has been published, other than in resident hours training (Cappuccio et al., 2009), and that there is a need for controlled studies to investigate the Directive's effects on health, well-being, and worker safety, particularly with regard to the implementation of flexible work hours arrangements (Costa et al., 2004).

Conclusion

It would be disingenuous to conclude that the regulatory and policy schemes discussed in this chapter have been completely successful in 'resolving' all the drowsiness-related issues affecting public and occupational health and safety that they were intended to address. Some of the challenges for designing and implementing such schemes include regulatory authority, jurisdictional limits, industry-specific demands, public awareness, and the fact that any given scheme may not take into account every effect and aspect of sleep and drowsiness (e.g. since sleep-wake history and circadian phase have a significant impact on drowsiness, regulatory schemes should at the very least account for these factors, where relevant). The last of these challenges may be the result of 'scientifically uninformed' decision-making.

Scientifically uninformed decisions are also apparent in judicial processes. A recent study found a notable difference between the way Finnish courts treated nine fatal car accident cases (Radun et al., 2009). When assessed by a multi-disciplinary team, all nine cases were assessed to have been most likely caused by the driver of the vehicle falling asleep. The courts only discussed fatigue or drowsiness in four of those cases, however, and in only one of the cases was the driver charged under the article of the Finnish Road Traffic Act covering drowsiness. This finding suggests that individuals or teams with expertise in the complex science underlying sleep medicine are invaluable resources in the judicial process and in the design of regulatory and policy schemes that:

- effectively address drowsiness-related issues affecting public and occupational health and safety; and

---

[19] 'A state of complete physical, mental, and social well-being and not merely the absence of disease or infirmity' (World Health Organization Const. pmbl.).

Although considerable progress has been made in identifying the determinants and effects of drowsiness, policy-makers and those who must implement drowsiness management strategies still face practical difficulties taking this information and turning it into workable solutions for their particular circumstance. Additional research could be fruitfully directed towards the following areas:

1. Determining a non-invasive method for assaying an individual's level of drowsiness at a given point in time.

2. Determining a widely-accepted metric for 'how tired is too tired' from a legal and public policy standpoint (cf. 0.05% or 0.08% blood alcohol concentration for alcohol).

3. Cost-benefit analysis of drowsiness interventions, to understand the economic implications of these interventions.

4. Systematic evaluation of the effectiveness of different systems of regulation (e.g. drowsiness or management system developed by employers vs. global limits on work hours).

5. Increased understanding of the causal relationship between irregular work hours and adverse health outcomes (e.g. gastrointestinal and cardiovascular disorders), and specific aspects of work schedules (e.g. night work) that increase the risk of these outcomes occurring, so that these risks may be minimized through regulation.

6. In the case of medical residents, assessment of the impact of sleep deprivation on training and learning, compared with the effect of reduced hours of exposure to training.

Fig. 20.1 Issues requiring further investigation.

- reflect the physiological and behavioural determinants and consequences of drowsiness and fatigue.

Such expertise can be used to assist policy-makers, lawmakers, and others in making scientifically informed decisions about drowsiness-related issues. Massachusetts policy-makers appear to have adopted this approach recently, creating a special commission that includes lawmakers, sleep experts, and law enforcement officials to consider whether to introduce state legislation to increase penalties for drowsy drivers who cause accidents and to educate the public about drowsy driving (2006 Mass. Acts c. 428, § 26). Other governments and entities interested in managing the risks associated with drowsiness as a matter of law or policy should consider taking this multi-disciplinary approach in the future (Fig. 20.1).

Summary box

- Drowsiness is now recognized as a hazard to public and occupational health and safety, and is of particular concern in certain occupational groups, such as transport and medicine (junior doctors and nurses), and in situations such as driving.

- Regulatory and policy schemes to address drowsiness vary widely and depend on the jurisdiction, the industry, and the perceived risks to health and safety.

- Efforts to address drowsy driving have proceeded in many jurisdictions, with approaches including amendments to traffic and criminal codes, education campaigns (of the motoring public and of enforcement agencies), and special conditions on junior drivers' licenses.

Summary box (continued)

♦ Commercial transport has received particular attention by regulators, and all major industrialized nations have schemes of varying complexity in place to address the risks posed by
drowsy operation.

♦ As an occupational group, junior doctors (residents) face drowsiness-related risks both in
terms of their own safety and that of their patients. In view of the well-documented safety
risks of extended duty shifts, the argument that such shifts are necessary to ensure that residents have adequate training is becoming increasingly untenable.

♦ The EWTD, which is society-wide in scope, may significantly impact the regulation of work-
related drowsiness, but empirical research remains to be carried out to assess its impact.

♦ A number of issues remain to be resolved from a policy standpoint, including establishing a
common definition of drowsiness as well as empirical questions, such as determining a non-
invasive method for assessing and establishing the threshold of unacceptable impairment.

References

Accreditation Council for Graduate Medical Education (ACGME) (2002). *Report of the ACGME Work
Group on Resident Duty Hours*. Available at: http://www.acgme.org (accessed March 3, 2009).

Accreditation Council for Graduate Medical Education (ACGME) (2003). *Common Program Requirements
for Resident Duty Hours* (Updated 2007). Available at: http://www.acgme.org (accessed March 3, 2009).

Adnett, N. & Hardy, S. (2001). Reviewing the Working Time Directive: rationale, implementation and case
law. *Ind Relat J*, 32(2), 114–125.

American Medical Students Association (2009). *The Resident Work Hour Issue: State Efforts*. Available at:
http://www.amsa.org/rwh/efforts.cfm (accessed March 3, 2009).

Barnard, C., Deakin, S. & Hobbs, R. (2003). Opting out of the 48 hour week: employer necessity or
individual choice? An empirical study of the Operation of Article 18(1)(b) of the Working Time
Directive in the UK. *Ind Law J*, 32(4), 223–252.

Bonnet, M.H. & Arand, D.L. (1995). We are chronically sleep deprived. *Sleep*, 18(10), 908–911.

Cappuccio, F.P., Bakewell, A., Taggart, F.M., et al. (2009). Implementing a 48h EWTD-compliant rota
for junior doctors in the UK does not compromise patients' safety: assessor blind pilot comparison.
Q J Med, 27 Jan 2009; Epub.

Costa, G., Åkerstedt, T., Nachreiner, F., et al. (2004). Flexible working hours, health, and well-being in
Europe: some considerations from a SALTSA project. *Chronobiol Int*, 21(6), 831–844.

Czeisler, C.A. (2006). Work hours, sleep and patient safety in residency training. *Trans Am Clin Climatol
Assoc*, 117, 159–187.

Engelen-Kefer, U. (1990). OPINION of the Economic and Social Committee on the Proposal for
a Council Directive concerning certain aspects of the organization of working time. COM(90) 317
final—SYN 295.

Fletcher, A., McCulloch, K., Baulk, S. & Dawson, D. (2005). Countermeasures to driver fatigue: a review of
public awareness campaigns and legal approaches. *Aust N Z J Public Health*, 29(5), 471–476.

Heaton, K. (2005). Truck driver hours of service regulations: the collision of policy and public health. *Policy
Polit Nurs Pract*, 6(4), 277–284.

Institute of Medicine (IOM) (2008). *Resident Duty Hours: Enhancing Sleep, Supervision, and Safety*.
Washington, DC: National Academies Press.

Knauth, P. (2007). Extended work periods. *Ind Health*, 45(1), 125–136.

Lee, C.J. (2006). Federal regulation of hospital resident work hours: enforcement with real teeth. *J Health Care Law Policy*, **9**, 162.

Lockley, S.W., Landrigan, C.P., Barger, L.K. & Czeisler, C.A. (2006). When policy meets physiology. The challenge of reducing resident work hours. *Clin Orthop Relat Res*, **449**, 116–127.

McCall, T.B. (1989). No turning back: a blueprint for residency reform. *JAMA*, **261**, 909.

National Transportation Safety Board (1990). *Fatigue, Alcohol, Other Drugs, and Medical Factors in Fatal-to-the-Driver Heavy Truck Crashes, Vol. 1*. Washington, DC: National Transportation Safety Board.

National Sleep Foundation (2007). *State of the States Report on Drowsy Driving*. Available at: http://www.drowsydriving.org (accessed March 2, 2009).

Radun, I., Ohisalo, J., Radun, J.E., Summala, H. & Tolvanen, M. (2009). Fell asleep and caused a fatal head-on crash? A case study of multidisciplinary in-depth analysis vs. the court. *Traffic Inj Prev*, **10**(1), 76–83.

Sidney, M. & Wolfe, D. (2001). *Public Citizen's Health Research Group, Petition to R. David Layne, Acting Ass. Sec'y for Occupational Safety & Health*, U.S. Dep't of Labor, 30 April.

Sigurdson, K. & Ayas, N. (2007). The public health and safety consequences of sleep disorders. *Can J Physiol Pharmacol*, **85**(1), 179–183.

Walker, M. & Stickgold, R. (2004). Sleep-dependent learning and memory consolidation. *Neuron*, **44**(1), 121–133.

Weiss, E.M. & Hohmann, J. (2008). Bay Bridge crash: 'It was Like a Bomb had Gone Off'. *Washington Post*, A01, 12 August.

Williams, C. (2008). No criminal charges in crash. *Washington Post*, B05, 19 December.

Bills, directives, regulations, and statutes

Australia

The Australian Constitution (The Commonwealth of Australia Constitution Act, 1900, 63 & 64 Vict., c. 12 (Eng.)), §§ 51 and 107.

National Transport Commission (Model Legislation—Heavy Vehicle Driver Fatigue) Regulations 2007, Fed. Reg. Legis. Instruments F2007L03869 (26 Sept. 2007).

Canada

Commercial Vehicle Drivers Hours of Service Regulations, SOR/2005-313.

European Union

Council Directive 93/104/EC (23 Nov. 1993), 1993 O.J. (L 307) 18, amended by Directive 2000/34/EC (22 June 2000), 2000 O.J. (L 195) 41.

United States of America

A. 1234, State Leg., 2007-2008 Reg. Sess. (N.Y. 2007).

A. 2332, State Leg., 2007-2008 Reg. Sess. (N.Y. 2007).

A. 4143, State Leg., 2007-2008 Reg. Sess. (N.Y. 2007).

Del. Code Ann. tit. 21, § 4176.

H.B. 117, 105th Gen. Assemb. (Tenn. 2007).

H.B. 150, Gen. Assemb., 2007 Reg. Sess. (Ky. 2007).

H.B. 3021, 74th Legis. Assemb., 2007 Reg. Sess. (Or. 2007).

H.B. 4332, Leg., 2007 Reg. Sess. (Mich. 2007).

Hours of Service of Drivers, 73 Fed. Reg. 69,567 (19 Nov. 2008).

Maggie's Law: National Drowsy Driving Act of 2003, H.R. 968, 108th Cong. (2003).

Md. Code Ann., Crim. Law § 2-209.
N.Y. Comp. Codes R. & Regs. tit. 10, § 405.4.
Patient and Physician Safety and Protection Act of 2001, H.R. 3236, 107th Cong. (2001).
Patient and Physician Safety and Protection Act of 2002, S. 2614, 107th Cong. (2002).
P.R. Laws Ann., tit. 24, §§ 10005 to 10009.
S. 1290, State Leg., 2007-2008 Reg. Sess. (N.Y. 2007).
S. 2072, 185th Gen. Ct., 2007-2008 Sess. (Mass. 2008).
S. 2124, 184th Gen. Ct., 2005-2006 Sess. (Mass. 2005).
S. 2488, State Leg., 2007-2008 Reg. Sess. (N.Y. 2007).
S.B. 71, 105th Gen. Assemb. (Tenn. 2007).
S.B. 104, 95th Gen. Assemb. (Ill. 2007).
S.F. 2295, 82nd Gen. Assemb., 2007-2008 Reg. Sess. (Iowa 2007).
Va. Code Ann. § 46.2-812.
2003 N.J. Laws c. 143, § 1 (codified as amended at N.J. Stat. Ann. § 2C:11-5(a)).
2006 Mass. Acts c. 428, § 26.
49 C.F.R. pt. 395.

World Health Organization

World Health Organization Const. pmbl.

Case Law

Australia

Amalgamated Soc'y of Engineers v. Adelaide Steamship Co. Ltd. (1920) 28 C.L.R. 129.

United States of America

Johnson v. State, 132 A.2d 853 (Md. 1957).
Skidmore v. State, 887 A.2d 92 (Md. Ct. Spec. App. 2005).
White v. King, 223 A.2d 763 (Md. 1966).

Chapter 21

Ethical considerations for the scheduling of work in continuous operations: physicians in training as a case study

C.A. Czeisler

Introduction

Thirty years ago, David A. Hamburg, who was then President of the Institute of Medicine (IOM) of the US National Academy of Sciences, challenged me to carve out a new area of occupational medicine related to the scheduling of work in round-the-clock operations. The overall concept was to begin applying in the workplace the results of laboratory and epidemiological research related to sleep and circadian rhythms. This led to some of the first successful translations of medical advances in sleep and circadian physiology to improvements in work-schedule design (Czeisler et al., 1982; Division of Sleep Medicine, Harvard Medical School, and WGBH Educational Foundation, 2010). Although considerable progress has since been made, in 2006 the IOM estimated that sleep deprivation and sleep disorders were under-recognized health problems that contributed substantially to occupational injuries and adversely affected health (Institute of Medicine, 2006). Extensive evidence indicates that long shift durations, particularly shifts that exceed 12 consecutive hours, are associated with increased risk of error and occupational injury. (Rogers et al., 2004; Landrigan et al., 2004; Ayas et al., 2006; Ayas et al., 2006) Yet, attempts to introduce regulations that would limit work hours in the United States, in the manner that the European Working Time Directive (EWTD) does for citizens of member states of the European Union, have met with little success. In fact, notwithstanding the increased unemployment rate caused by the economic tsunami of 2008, the trend in many occupations in the United States has been towards longer work hours for those who remain employed. Workers in many industries have moved from 8-hour work shifts to 10- or 12-hour work shifts. Some occupations, like firefighters, have even moved from 12-hour work shifts to 24-hour work shifts or even longer shifts.

One of the barriers that has repeatedly derailed attempts to address the issue of work-hour restrictions is the long hours worked by resident physicians during training. It is very difficult for specialists in occupational health, who champion workplace safety issues ranging from hearing protection to exposure to chemical carcinogens, to argue that 16-hour work shifts are hazardous when physicians routinely care for patients working 24-hour shifts. This inconsistency is not lost on regulatory agencies, employers, and labour unions, which routinely use the example of resident physician work hours in the United States as a precedent to justify perpetuation of extended duration work shifts and/or long work weeks. Thus, instead of the medical profession championing the elimination of a health and safety hazard decades ahead of a reluctant judiciary, as it did in the case of cigarette smoking (Cipollone v. Liggett Group, 1983; US Department of Health, Education, and Welfare, 1964), the judiciary has been decades ahead of the medical profession in recognizing the health and safety hazards associated with extended durations of work and night shift work (Faverty v. McDonald's Restaurants, 1995; Macdonald, 2009; Robertson v. LeMaster, 1983).

Thus, it was remarkable this past year when the blue-ribbon IOM Committee on Optimizing Graduate Medical Trainee (Resident) Hours and Work Schedules to Improve Patient Safety concluded, after conducting an exhaustive review of the medical and scientific literature, that it is unsafe for both physicians in training and their patients when physicians caring for patients work for more than 16 consecutive hours without sleep (Institute of Medicine, 2008). The IOM determined that the current practice of scheduling resident physicians to work for 30 consecutive hours without sleep promotes 'conditions for fatigue-related errors that pose risks to both patients and residents' (Institute of Medicine, 2008). This was the first time that the medical profession formally acknowledged the hazards of extended duration work shifts routinely worked by resident physicians. Moreover, based on the demonstration that the risk of a motor vehicle crash in resident physicians was more than doubled in residents driving home from an extended duration (>24 hours) shift than from a shift averaging about 12 hours in duration (Barger et al., 2005), the IOM recommended that hospitals immediately begin providing safe transportation home for residents impaired by fatigue (Institute of Medicine, 2008).

Regrettably, though it has been more than a year since those recommendations were made, there has been no change in the regulations governing resident physician work hours in the United States. Given that there are more than 100,000 resident physicians working extended duration shifts in the United States, and that this practice stands as an impediment to implementation of regulatory work-hour reform in other US industries, in this chapter I will use the work hours of physicians in training in the United States as a case study to address the issue of ethical considerations for the scheduling of work in continuous operations.

As shown in Tables 21.1 and 21.2, sleep deprivation degrades performance and safety and has adverse health effects.

Moreover, we have recently demonstrated that when an extended duration of wakefulness is preceded by chronic sleep curtailment, as occurs routinely among resident physicians, the impairments in performance are an order of magnitude more severe (Cohen et al., 2010) (Fig. 21.1).

Table 21.1 Some performance consequences of sleep deprivation

Slowed reaction times, comparably to blood alcohol concentration of 0.10 g/dL (Dawson and Reid, 1997)
Increased risk of attentional failures (Cohen et al., 2010; Van Dongen et al., 2003)
Enhanced distractibility (Anderson and Horne, 2006)
Impaired memory consolidation (Stickgold, 2005; Walker and Stickgold, 2004)
Increased mood lability (Dinges et al., 1997; Haack and Mullington, 2005; Yoo et al., 2007)
Impaired judgment (Killgore et al., 2006, 2007)
Increased risk of errors (fast and sloppy) (Horowitz et al., 2003)
Increased suggestibility (Blagrove, 1996)
Decreased vigilance (Cajochen et al., 1999; Durmer et al., 2005)
Degradation of general task performance to 15th percentile of rested performance (non-physicians) (Philibert, 2005)
Degradation of performance on clinical tasks to 7th percentile of rested performance (physicians) (Philibert, 2005)

Table 21.2 Some health consequences of chronic sleep curtailment

Increased blood pressure (Javaheri et al., 2008; Knutson et al., 2009)
Increased risk of calcification of coronary arteries (King et al., 2008)
Impairment of immune responses (Spiegel et al., 2002)
Altered glucose metabolism (Knutson et al., 2007; Spiegel et al., 1999)
Increased susceptlibility to infection (Cohen et al., 2009)
Increased carbohydrate craving (Spiegel et al., 2004a, b)
Increased risk of weight gain, obesity, and possibly diabetes (Knutson et al., 2008; Patel et al., 2008)
Decreased testosterone levels (men) (Åkerstedt et al., 1980)
Increased inflammatory markers (Patel et al., 2009)

Though a consolidated episode of 10 hours of sleep restores performance to baseline levels for a few hours, those with a history of chronic sleep loss deteriorate much more rapidly as the number of consecutive hours of wakefulness increases, particularly overnight. As shown in Table 21.3, in first-year resident physicians, extended duration work shifts in this setting more than double the risk of attentional failures at night, and significantly increase the risk of serious medical errors and fatigue-related preventable adverse events, including fatalities.

It was findings like these regarding the average impairment of performance associated with acute sleep loss that led the IOM to conclude that working for more than 16 consecutive hours without sleep posed an unacceptable safety risk for both patients and resident physicians themselves (Institute of Medicine, 2008). Yet, the publication of the IOM report on resident physician work hours has been met with great controversy (Association of Pediatric Program Directors, 2009; BBC News, 2008; Blanchard et al., 2009; Britt et al., 2009; Cappuccio et al., 2009a, b; Chen, 2008; Czeisler, 2009a, c; Higginson, 2009; Ingle, 2008; Jagannathan et al., 2009; Lopez and Katz, 2009; Moalem et al., 2009; Nasca, 2008, 2009; Reid and Coakley, 2008; Rybock, 2009;

Table 21.3 Some consequences of extended duration work shifts in first-year resident physicians

Double the risk of attentional failures while caring for ICU patients at night (Lockley et al., 2004)
Increased risk of making serious medical errors while caring for ICU patients (+35.9%) (Landrigan et al., 2004)
Increased risk of making serious medical errors that reaches the patient while caring for ICU patients (+56.6%) (Landrigan et al., 2004)
Increased risk of making serious diagnostic mistakes while caring for ICU patients (+464%) (Landrigan et al., 2004)
Increased risk of percutaneous injury while performing a procedure (odds ratio [OR]: 1.61; 95% confidence interval [CI]: 1.46–1.78) (Ayas et al., 2006)
Increased risk of motor vehicle crash on commute after extended duration work shift (OR: 2.3; 95% CI: 1.6–3.3) (Barger et al., 2005)
Increased risk of a fatigue-related preventable adverse event that injures a patient (OR: 7.0; 95% CI: 4.3–11) (Barger et al., 2006)
Increased risk of a fatigue-related fatal preventable adverse event (OR: 4.1; 95% CI: 1.4–12) (Barger et al., 2006)

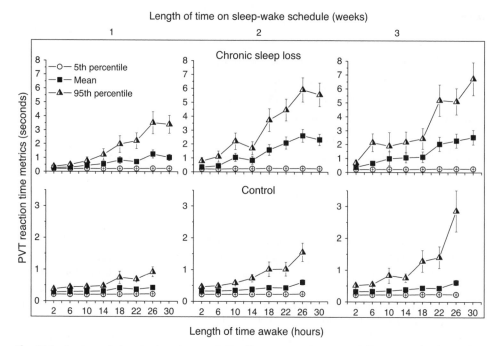

Fig. 21.1 Acute and chronic sleep homeostatic effects on psychomotor vigilance test (PVT) reaction time (RT) measures.

Effect of consecutive hours awake and weeks on the experimental schedule (averaged across all circadian phases) are shown for the 5th percentile, mean, and 95th percentile (mean and standard error of the mean) of reaction times. Data from the chronic sleep loss group (averaging 5.6h sleep opportunity per 24 hours) are shown in the top row and from the control group (averaging 8.0h sleep opportunity per 24 hours) are shown in the bottom row. Note that the protocols are shown on a different y-axis scales so that the relative deterioration with time awake is apparent in the control group. Apparent worsening across weeks in the control group, most evident in a sensitive measure such as 95th percentile, likely reflects some degree of chronic sleep loss that accumulated despite the 1:2 scheduled sleep-to-wake ratio. Unintentional sleep loss results from decreased sleep efficiency during sleep episodes scheduled during the circadian 'day', a potential factor leading to chronic sleep loss in shift-workers.

Source: Reproduced from Cohen, D.A., Wang, W., Wyatt, J.K., et al. (2010). Uncovering residual effects of chronic sleep loss on human performance. *Sci Transl Med*, **2**(14), 14ra3 supplementary online material, with permission.

The New York Times, 2008; USA Today, 2008; Warshaw, 2009; Willis, 2009). Moreover, four out of five resident physicians deny making a fatigue-related errors that cause patient injury during their internships. Could inter-individual differences in the vulnerability to the effects of sleep loss on performance account for this disparity? Although few are spared from the adverse effects of sleep loss on performance, there are considerable differences between people in the magnitude of the effect of sleep loss on performance (Chuah et al., 2006; Frey et al., 2004; Institute of Medicine, 2006; Leproult et al., 2003; Van Dongen, 2005, 2006; Van Dongen et al., 2004a, b, 2005). Based on our recent study of the synergistic interaction between chronic and acute sleep deprivation (Cohen et al., 2010), healthy well-rested sleepers are likely to be much more resistant to the effects of sleep loss than the 50–70 million Americans who suffer from chronic sleep deprivation or chronic disorders of sleep and wakefulness (Institute of Medicine, 2006). It is these inter-individual and intra-individual differences in the vulnerability to sleep loss that will serve as the premise that poses the ethical questions addressed in this chapter (Czeisler, 2009b).

Inter-individual differences in tolerance to sleep loss in healthy young adults

As shown in Table 21.4, there are many potential factors that could cause inter-individual differences in vulnerability to sleep deprivation, which are reviewed in detail elsewhere (Czeisler, 2009b).

From a survey of 3,283 randomly selected people from the Detroit area, Drake et al. (2004) identified and interviewed 162 night workers and 337 rotating shift workers, which represented 19.4% of the 2,449 working adults in that population sample. They found that 24.7% of night shift workers and 20.3% of rotating shift workers reported excessive sleepiness (i.e., an Epworth Sleepiness Scale [ESS] score > 13), as compared to 15.5% of day workers. The inter-individual differences in the severity of symptoms of shift-work disorder derived from workers participating in field studies are consistent with laboratory investigations that have revealed considerable differential vulnerability to the deterioration in neurobehavioural performance associated with sleep loss and night shift work (Van Dongen, 2004a, b, 2005, 2006). Based on these data, the prevalence of sleep disorders (Kryger et al., 2005), and the prevalence of each of the factors in Table 21.4 that are hypothesized to confer increased susceptibility to acute sleep loss, between 15% and 30% of resident physicians are likely to be differentially vulnerable to the effects of sleep loss on performance (Czeisler, 2009b).

Ethical considerations

To the extent that work hour policies limits for resident physicians in the U.S. have been evidence-based, the evidence upon which policy-makers have relied has been largely derived from laboratory studies of healthy subjects who have passed physical examinations and volunteered to participate in relatively brief sleep restriction or sleep deprivation studies. In continuing to

Table 21.4 Potential aetiology of inter-individual differences in vulnerability to acute sleep loss

History of chronic sleep curtailment (Belenky et al., 2003; Institute of Medicine, 2006; Van Dongen et al., 2003), as is common in residents working 80-hour weeks (Czeisler, 2004; Czeisler, 2009b)
Age (Duffy et al., 2009)
Biological trait, specific to task (Frey et al., 2004; Van Dongen et al., 2004)
Genetic variation (e.g., $PER3^{5/5}$ polymorphism, DEC2 or ADORA2A haplotype) (Bodenmann et al., 2007; Groeger et al., 2008; He et al., 2009; Viola et al., 2007) (Fig. 21.2)
Use of soporific agents (e.g., anti-histamines, hypnotics, alcohol, opiates) (Czeisler, 2009b; Frank et al., 2008; McBeth and Ankel, 2006; McLellan et al., 2008; Wang et al., 2008; Zgierska et al., 2007)
Stimulant use (e.g. caffeine, Adderall, cocaine) (Czeisler, 2009b; DeSantis et al., 2008; Wyatt et al., 2004)
Medical conditions (e.g., common cold, hepatitis, mononucleosis, nocturnal asthma) (Carter et al., 2003; Czeisler, 2009b)
Pregnancy (Czeisler, 2009b)

permit every other work shift to be 30 consecutive hours in duration throughout residency training, the Accreditation Council for Graduate Medical Education (ACGME) has implicitly assumed that the population of residents is entirely healthy, and highly resistant to the effects of sleep deprivation (Czeisler, 2009b). No one can become a licensed physician in the United States without running a gauntlet during residency training that tests their physical endurance to sleep loss; most, of course, want to prove that they are up to the challenge. Unlike military trainees who set out to prove their mettle in the very demanding but protected conditions of boot camp, resident physicians are often caring for critically ill patients, and it is these patients who often suffer the consequences whenever residents fail this sleep-loss endurance test. During residency training, it has been argued that the presence of nurses and the daily visits by attending physicians provide enough oversight to prevent most errors from reaching the patient. Although it is true that nurses catch most errors before they reach the patient (Rothschild et al., 2006), holes in the safety net leave patients at significantly greater risk of serious medical errors that cause injury or death when physicians work extended duration work shifts, despite supervisory oversight (Barger et al., 2006; Landrigan et al., 2004). This is why the IOM has concluded that scheduling residents to work for more than 16 hours without sleep is hazardous to both patients and to physicians themselves. Moreover, the schedule that physicians have been taught to work during training often carries over into their practices following training, with physicians in group practices taking 'call' on a rotating basis throughout their careers. In some practices, after taking care of their own patients all day on Friday, once a month physicians cover the patients of multiple other physicians from Friday afternoon until Monday morning, when they resume care for their own patients. Such physicians are thus working or are on call for 84 consecutive hours, and in many specialties, they may obtain very little sleep during this time.

Some physicians, and consequently the patients of those physicians, are much more vulnerable than others to the adverse effects on performance of sleep loss at an adverse circadian phase. After 17.5 hours of overnight call, the median error rate in a surgical simulator is more than *doubled* as compared to the rested condition, whereas the error rate for the 75th percentile is more than *tripled* and the highest error rate is *quadruple* that of the rested condition (Grantcharov et al., 2001). Yet, the work hours to which physicians in training and practising physicians are scheduled have not taken into account such inter-individual differences in the tolerance to sleep loss and circadian misalignment. That may be because under ordinary conditions, such differences are often not evident. For example, the internal medicine residency training program from the hospital where we performed our intervention studies (Landrigan et al., 2004; Lockley et al., 2004) has approximately 70 applicants for each internship slot, and prides itself on selecting a group of outstanding trainees every year. When rested, the sample we studied all performed remarkably well on managing medical problems on a sophisticated simulator of an ICU patient, comparable to physicians with many more years of experience. However, 10–15% of the same interns did so poorly in managing simulated ICU patients when the interns were post-call (Gordon et al., 2010), after having been awake all night in the ICU, that the Program in Medical Simulation at the Harvard Medical School expressed concern about their ability to care for patients after working all night.

Prompted by that concern, I began to focus on the issue of inter-individual differences. I wondered whether such differences could be affecting the debate about resident work hours. Notwithstanding considerable evidence demonstrating that 30-hour work shifts compromised both patient safety and physician safety, many key decision-makers continue to insist that 30-hour work shifts are essential. For example, despite our published findings demonstrating a significantly increased rate of serious medical errors in the ICU when interns were scheduled to work for 30 consecutive hours there as compared to when they were scheduled to work for

16 consecutive hours, once our intervention study was complete, interns in those same ICUs were once again scheduled to work 30 consecutive hours twice per week on ICU rotations. Could this be because the selective pressure resulting from working 30-hour work shifts twice per week for years during residency ensures that only those most genetically resistant to the adverse effects of sleep loss on performance become the decision-makers in clinical departments? Perhaps those medical practitioners who are now senior institutional leaders excelled in and benefited from the traditional schedule at a time before patient acuity was as high and length of stay was as short as it is today. It may be difficult for such decision-makers to appreciate the difficulties that others, whose genetic background or medical condition makes them vulnerable rather than resistant to the effects of sleep loss on performance, face on such a schedule. Pragmatic concerns regarding the staffing of academic medical centres to meet patient care needs must also affect the debate about resident work hours, notwithstanding effects on resident training or patient safety (Institute of Medicine, 2008).

Policy-makers who insist that physicians be pushed to the limits of their endurance during residency training should recognize that there are inter-individual differences in those limits and make appropriate accommodation for those differences. The fact that the adverse consequences of extended work hours are not uniformly spread across the population of physicians thus raises an ethical dilemma. Our data have revealed that fatigue-related mistakes account for tens of thousands of patient injuries and thousands of patient deaths annually (Barger, et al., 2006) (see also Chapter 17). Yet, a minority of residents report making the mistakes that caused these injuries and deaths. One out of five of the first-year residents we surveyed reported making a fatigue-related mistake during their internship that injured a patient, and one out of 20 reported making a fatigue-related mistake that resulted in the death of a patient (Barger et al., 2006). Since individuals differ in their vulnerability to sleep loss, it stands to reason that those whose performance is most adversely affected by sleep loss and circadian misalignment are responsible for a disproportionately large share of those fatigue-related injuries and deaths. In the interests of patient safety, every effort should therefore be made to identify those most susceptible to the adverse performance effects of sleep deprivation through programs to screen for sleep disorders and the use of sophisticated patient simulators that are validated against clinical performance to test the fitness of physicians to care for patients when sleep deprived. Once identified, appropriate treatments should be provided to those physicians who suffer from sleep disorders or other medical disorders that render them particularly susceptible to fatigue. In addition, given that the IOM has concluded that it is unsafe for the average physicians to work for more than 16 consecutive hours without sleep (Institute of Medicine, 2008), it would have to be considered negligent or reckless to require physicians who are most vulnerable to sleep deprivation and circadian misalignment—like an intern with narcolepsy or a resident with untreated sleep apnoea—to work 30-hour shifts twice per week. Given the magnitude and stability of inter-individual differences in the effect of sleep loss on performance, vulnerable individuals should be provided with a reasonable scheduling accommodation. Warning or educating particularly susceptible individuals, while necessary, would not be any more sufficient than a bartender warning an obviously intoxicated patron to be careful while driving home.

In the future, if and when the genetics of sleep loss vulnerability is well characterized, genetic screening could be used to quickly identify susceptible individuals. Employment of physicians identified as most vulnerable to the effects of sleep loss through genetic testing will be protected by the 2008 Genetic Information Nondiscrimination Act, which prohibits employers in the United States from using genetic information to make decisions about hiring, firing, or compensation, or from using such information to classify or segregate employees in such a way as to deprive them of employment opportunities. Hospitals in the United States will therefore not be allowed to screen out individuals from the intern match even if their genetic background were to indicate that scheduling them to work for 30 consecutive hours will subject hospital patients to an unreasonable risk of harm, nor would they be allowed to give preference to those whose genetic backgrounds suggest that they will be resistant to the effects of sleep deprivation. However, such information may prove to be a valuable aid to some individuals when making career choices, and also to hospitals in their scheduling practices.

Management of vulnerabilities secondary to sleep disorders

None of the potential oversight bodies or agencies (such as the ACGME, the Association of American Medical College, the Joint Commission, the Agency for Healthcare Research, and Quality or the Centers for Medicare and Medicaid Services [CMS]) provide any guidance or regulation to academic medical centres or residency review committees on how to ensure that patient safety is not compromised when residents suffering from a sleep disorder are scheduled to work for 30 consecutive hours twice per week. In fact, after a resident in a Boston graduate medical education program was diagnosed with narcolepsy, one of my colleagues was consulted about what strategies should be used to keep the intern awake all night so that he could work 30-hour shifts twice per week, caring for patients at this major tertiary referral hospital. Given that administration of FDA-Controlled Substance Class stimulants are required to maintain consolidated wakefulness for 16 hours in narcoleptic patients, it is patently unreasonable and unsafe for physicians with narcolepsy to be scheduled to care for gravely ill, hospitalized patients for 30 consecutive work hours without sleep. Yet, the ACGME has failed to provide guidance for the directors of graduate medical education programs on this issue, even after I posed the question to ACGME leadership at a national conference on resident work hours in 2009.

Similarly, no national guidance has been issued on the question as to whether academic medical centres have an obligation, under the Americans for Disabilities Act, to provide a reasonable scheduling accommodation to physician employees or other healthcare employees with sleep disorders. Some years ago, a Harvard Medical School student was being expelled for his failure to keep up with the extended duration work shift schedule required on clinical clerkships. The medical student successfully appealed for reinstatement when, after more than a year-long process involving multiple referrals, Harvard University Health Services ultimately diagnosed and effectively treated him for obstructive sleep apnoea/hypopnea syndrome. Once on nasal continuous positive airway pressure (CPAP), he successfully completed all of his required clinical clerkships, graduated from the Harvard Medical School, and eventually completed his postgraduate medical education training at another institution. If a resident physician were to be similarly diagnosed with obstructive sleep apnoea and experienced residual daytime sleepiness even after nasal CPAP treatment, it would not be safe to schedule an individual with this condition to work 30-hour shifts twice per week while caring for patients. By the same token, it would be unreasonable to terminate the employment of such a resident physician because a medical condition prevents her or him from working 30-hour shifts. It is evident that extended duration work shifts are not necessary for medical training, since graduate medical education programs in many other countries (Institute of Medicine, 2008) (Table 21.5) and at a number of academic medical centres in the United States have eliminated them.

Safer work schedules for all physicians

Some have argued that selecting those who are most resistant to the adverse effects of sleep deprivation on performance is one of the fundamental purposes of the gruelling work hours to which residents are scheduled. Dr. Richard Reiling, a Harvard-trained surgeon who was then

Table 21.5 Summary of work-hour regulations for various occupations in selected countries

Occupation	Limit
US airplane pilots (1–2 pilot airplanes): 1950s	<8 daily flight hours <16 daily work hours >8–12 hours rest required (since 1985) <34 hours flight time per week
US nuclear power plant operators: 1982; 2009	<16 consecutive work hours <72 work hours per week >34 consecutive hours off every 9 days
US railroad operators: 1907, modified 1969 and 1976	<12 work hours per day >8–10 hours rest required per day
US interstate truck and bus drivers: 1938; 1962; 2003; 2005; 2008	<11 driving hours within a 14-hour interval <14 consecutive hours from start to end of work >10 consecutive rest hours <60 work hours per 7 days; <70 work hours per 8 days >34 consecutive hours off between workweeks
EU all occupations (including resident physicians and practicing physicians): 2004; 2009	<13 consecutive work hours <56 work hours per week until 2009; 48 hours thereafter >11 hours rest time per day
New Zealand resident physicians: 1985	<16 consecutive work hours (labour agreement) <72 work hours per week
US resident physicians	Unlimited: no federal laws of regulations Self-regulation by profession (ACGME): all specialties since 2003 <30 consecutive work hours (two allowed per week) <80 work hours per week (averaged over 4 weeks) Monitoring by self-report (84% non-compliance)
El Salvador resident physicians	Unlimited Extended duration work shifts (36 hours) and long (>120 hours) workweeks common during internship

representing the American College of Surgeons at the American Medical Association, said as much in the following excerpt from a 2001 *Washington Post* interview:

> "Surgeons are built differently" and learn to become impervious to exhaustion. "That's part of the selection process in surgery", added Reiling, who dismisses complaints about fatigue as "whining".
>
> (Boodman, 2001)

Indeed, the gruelling work schedule of some residency programs may allow only those physicians who are resistant to the effects of sleep loss to 'survive' this *de facto* selection process. Perhaps those who complete such intensive training programs do differ in that they may, for example, have a lower proportion of individuals with the *PER3*[5/5] polymorphism, which may confer vulnerability to the effects of sleep loss on performance (Groeger et al., 2008; Viola et al., 2007) (Fig. 21.2), and a higher proportion of the haplotype of the adenosine A2A receptor gene (ADORA2A) that may confer resistance to the effects of sleep loss on performance (Bodenmann et al., 2007), or even a lower proportion of individuals who suffer from sleep disorders that confer vulnerability to sleep loss (Institute of Medicine, 2006).

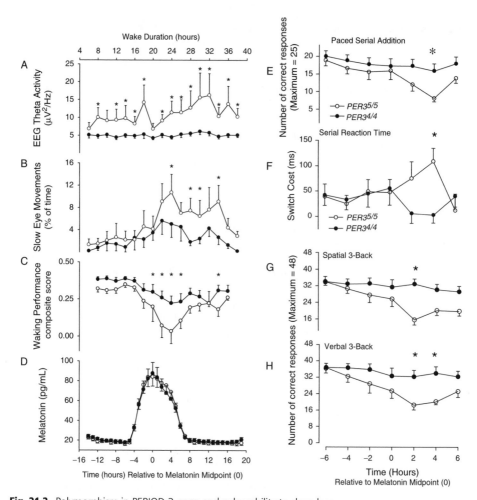

Fig. 21.2 Polymorphism in PERIOD 3 gene and vulnerability to sleep loss.
Left hand side: Deterioration of waking performance and increase of theta electroencephalography (EEG) activity and slow eye movements (SEMS) during sleep deprivation is greater in PER3^5/5 than in PER3^4/4 participants. Time course of central EEG theta (5–8 Hz) activity during wakefulness (Panel A), incidence of SEMs (percentage of 30 s epochs containing at least one SEM) (Panel B), and waking performance (composite performance score) (Panel C) are plotted relative to the timing of the plasma melatonin rhythm (Panel D) in 10 PER3^5/5 (open symbols) and 14 PER3^4/4 (filled symbols) homozygotes. EEG theta activity, SEMs, and waking performance data were averaged per 2-hour intervals, relative to the midpoint of the melatonin rhythm. (Asterisk [*] indicates a significant difference between genotypes, $P < 0.05$; upper abscissa indicates approximate wake duration.).
Right hand side: Overnight performance on the paced visual serial addition task in PER3^5/5 and PER3^4/4 participants. Mean numbers of correct responses are plotted relative to the midpoint of the melatonin rhythm (Panel E). Overnight performance on the serial reaction time task in PER3^5/5 and PER3^4/4 participants. Mean switch costs, that is, increase in time to respond to random rather than learned sequences of stimuli, are plotted relative to the melatonin midpoint. Higher values indicate poorer performance (Panel F). Overnight performance on spatial N-Back performance in relation to memory load in PER3^5/5 and PER3^4/4 participants. Mean numbers of correct responses are plotted separately for the 1-, 2-, and 3-back, relative to the melatonin midpoint (Panel G). Overnight performance on verbal N-Back performance in relation to memory load in PER3^5/5 and PER3^4/4 participants.

Fig. 21.2 (continued) Mean numbers of correct responses are plotted separately for the 1-, 2-, and 3-back, relative to the melatonin midpoint (Panel H). *P < 0.05, Bonferroni corrected. Error bars represent the standard error of the mean.
Sources: Figures and legends reprinted with permission from Viola, A.U., Archer, S.N., James, L.M., et al. (2007). PER3 polymorphism predicts sleep structure and waking performance. *Curr Biol*, **17**, 1–6 (left hand side) and Groeger, J.A., Viola, A.U., Lo, J.C.Y., von Shantz, M., Archer, S.N. & Dijk, D.J. (2008). Early morning executive functioning during sleep deprivation is compromised by a PERIOD3 polymorphism. *Sleep*, **31**(8), 1159–1167 (right hand side).

However, if screening for stamina were judged to be an important aim of the gruelling hours of residency (a premise with which I disagree), such screening could be better accomplished without risk to patients via overnight neurobehavioural performance testing designed to evaluate objectively the ability to sustain attention without stimulants while staying awake all day and all night. If this were done at the start of college, one overnight test under controlled laboratory conditions could also save vulnerable individuals the time and expense associated with 4 years of premedical course work, medical school entrance examinations, 4 years of medical school, three medical board certification examinations, and the first year or two of internship and residency training. It would also save the healthcare system from allocating limited resources towards training medical students and resident physicians who then elect not to practice medicine, and it would spare the patients who currently suffer the consequences of the errors made by residents susceptible to sleep loss. Moreover, it would ensure the identification of individuals who were indeed susceptible to sleep loss but who might manage to get through the rigours of residency training through reliance on stimulants, like high dose caffeine or attention-deficit hyperactivity disorder (ADHD) medications. The feasibility of such simple, objective testing debunks, the often-repeated notion that residency is a necessary mechanism to separate the wheat from the chaff.

Residency is a costly, labour-intensive, and unreliable method to screen for resistance to fatigue. It puts patients and the physicians themselves at an unacceptable risk of harm, which is not justified since such screening could be done more effectively without risk to patients. Even if one were to view residency as a way to separate those physicians who have the stamina to become surgeons versus those who, in Dr. Reiling's view, might be better suited to a less physically demanding medical specialty, then the task could be accomplished without risk to patients using patient simulator technology. Sophisticated patient simulators—much like the flight simulators that pilots use for flight training—would be a much safer alternative method than residency to screen for resistance to fatigue. Yet, concerns for patient safety have not been at the forefront in the design of the residency training system in the United States. As Dr. David Leach, former director of the ACGME once admitted:

> Residents live in the cracks of a broken health care system. They get things done. But what we badly need is a system that has many more elements of safety built into it.

(Boodman, 2001)

Selecting physicians resistant to the effects of fatigue rather than creating safer work schedules for all is a flawed and misguided approach that is doomed to failure. Even if hospitals were to select only those most resistant to the effects of sleep loss at the start of residency training, such selection would fail to protect patients from the hazards of extended duration work shifts, because the performance of even the most resistant to sleep loss is adversely affected by the acute and chronic sleep deprivation to which residents are currently exposed. Moreover, people and their situations often change. Some physicians may begin to use alcohol or other central nervous system depressants, which may increase their vulnerability (Czeisler, 2009b). Some physicians may gain weight or catch colds, both of which will put them at greater risk for sleep apnoea, which in turn will increase their vulnerability to sleep loss. Other physicians will have children, some of whom will have illnesses or sleep disorders, which will lead to acute or chronic sleep loss that increases vulnerability to sleep deprivation. Sometimes, physicians may be affected by a combination of factors, like the anaesthesia fellow who fell asleep at the wheel and crashed into a car carrying a driver and her 5-year-old child (Czeisler, 2006). Undiagnosed positional sleep apnoea (which has since been surgically corrected); behaviourally induced insufficient sleep syndrome; multiple interruptions of his limited sleep opportunities on prior nights caused by pages from the hospital ICU and by his young children; and a decision to avoid coffee before a 50-minute afternoon commute (so as not to disturb nocturnal sleep) likely all contributed to that crash (Czeisler, 2006). Just as redlining a car engine increases the risk of engine failure, pushing residents to the anticipated limit of their endurance is bound to precipitate human performance failures, often at the expense of patients. Scheduling physicians to be on call from home for weeks at a time is often justified on the presumption that calls will be infrequent. In such situations, contingencies should be in place to relieve the physician or surgeon from regularly scheduled daytime responsibilities whenever they have been required to handle emergency cases during the night that have deprived them of sleep.

There is an even more practical and compelling reason to implement safer work schedules that would accommodate a broader diversity in the tolerance to fatigue rather than selecting only those resistant to fatigue: the growing shortage of physicians and surgeons in the United States. The United States does not have enough physicians graduating from medical schools to implement a 'sleep resistance screening test' that would render at least one-quarter of medical school graduates ineligible to fulfill a residency requirement to work for 30 consecutive hours twice per week. How could the exclusion of one-quarter of physicians from residency, thereby denying them the opportunity to obtain a license to practice medicine, be justified on the basis of the argument that physician training requires 30-hour work shifts, given that New Zealand has limited the number of consecutive work hours to 16 hours for physicians in training there since 1985. How would the United States care for its sick if one-quarter of physicians graduating from medical schools were excluded from residency training? Interns and residents make up more than 10% of the workforce of physicians caring for patients in the United States. Given the extended duration hours that residents work caring for hospitalized patients, these physicians in training are likely providing an even greater share of the direct care for hospitalized patients. Therefore, instead of pushing all of the trainees to the limits of the endurance of those most resistant to sleep loss, a much safer and ethically justifiable strategy would be to implement work schedules that are safer for all trainees.

This is the purpose of the EWTD, which is intended to limit work hours for all employees— including physicians—in the European Union to a maximum of 13 hours per day and which provides for a minimum of 11 hours off per day. Recent evidence indicates that weekly work hour restrictions mandated by the directive have led to improvements in patient safety there (Cappuccio et al., 2009a, b) (see also Chapter 18).

Finally, an argument for the importance of developing safer schedules for all physicians can also be developed by applying common principles of bioethics to this discourse (University of Washington School of Medicine, 2009). The principle of *nonmaleficence* requires that the physician not create unnecessary harm or injury to the patient. Working for so many consecutive hours that our clinical performance *on average* declines to the 7th percentile of rested performance and the risk of making errors that harm patients rises by several hundred percent is clearly a violation of the principle of nonmaleficence. The fact that a substantial proportion of physicians, who could easily be identified, are at even greater risk of causing harm under such circumstances obligates us to do all that we can to remove this hazard. This is also why exhausted physicians who have worked for more than 16 consecutive hours without sleep should not be allowed to endanger themselves and others on roads and highways by driving motor vehicles (Czeisler, 2009b; Moore, 2009; Moore et al., 2009). The principle of *beneficence* indicates that it is a physician's duty to be of benefit to the patient, which requires physicians to take positive steps to prevent the patient from being harmed. As the IOM concluded based on an extensive, yearlong review of available evidence, working for more than 16 consecutive hours without sleep endangers patients and the physicians themselves. Now that this hazard has been identified, we are obligated as a profession to take appropriate steps to remove this harm. The principle of *autonomy* requires that physicians respect the right of the patient to make voluntary and informed healthcare decisions. It is for this reason that Boards of Directors of the Sleep Research Society and the National Sleep Foundation in 2005 endorsed model legislation that would establish 'a requirement for physicians who have been awake for more than 22 of the prior 24 hours to inform their patients of the extent and potential safety impact of their sleep deprivation and to obtain consent from such patients prior to providing clinical care or performing any medical or surgical procedures'. Given the extensive evidence that various aspects of neurobehavioural performance are degraded to a degree that is comparable to a blood alcohol concentration of 0.10 g/dL when a individual is awake for 24 hours (Dawson and Reid, 1997; Falleti et al., 2003; Lamond and Dawson, 1999; Powell et al., 2001; Williamson and Feyer, 2000), and that the average physician in training is impaired by an amount equivalent to a blood alcohol concentration of 0.05 g/dL when working frequent extended duration shifts (Arnedt et al., 2005), patients have a right to be informed that their physician is impaired by sleep loss and the right to decide whether to take the risk of receiving care from that provider.

The principle of *justice* in bioethics requires that both benefits and burdens be distributed fairly in our society. In connection with healthcare, this usually relates to distribution of scarce healthcare resources. Yet, there are many easily identifiable inter-individual differences in the vulnerability to the adverse effects of sleep loss that are based on genetic diversity and medical disorders. The IOM Resident Work-Hours Committee concluded that one of the greatest barriers to reducing resident work hours is the difficulty of finding other healthcare professionals who can provide the patient care services that are currently being provided by resident physicians (Institute of Medicine, 2008). Yet, more than double the full salaries of the ~100,000 resident physicians in the United States is being provided to academic medical centres by the US government through CMS at a cost of about $10 billion annually in order to defray the costs of educating these physicians. The costs of the patient care services being provided at those hospitals are billed separately to patients, the bulk of which are paid by private health insurance companies and by state and federal programs, such as those administered by CMS. To the extent that these young trainees are being scheduled to work extended duration shifts and long workweeks in order to provide patient care services that are being billed through other providers at academic medical centres, rather than for the sake of their training that is being subsidized by CMS, then it could be argued that the least powerful members of the academic medical hierarchy are being exploited by those who are in a more powerful position in order to have them work the least desirable and most dangerous hours. This is particularly significant given the evidence that working such extended duration shifts increases the risk of motor vehicle crashes and needle stick injuries of physicians in training (Ayas et al., 2006; Barger et al., 2005). It violates the principle of fairness to require this subset of vulnerable individuals to shoulder a disproportionately large burden (i.e. a higher rate of fatigue-related errors, accidents, and adverse health effects of sleep deprivation) (Institute of Medicine, 2006) than those who are resistant to the effects of sleep loss, for the convenience or financial benefit of teaching faculty or academic medical centres (Czeisler, 2009b). Such exploitation of junior doctors was most blatant when the EWTD limiting work hours to 56 hours per week was first implemented in the United Kingdom. By regulation, hospitals in England are only allowed to perform emergency surgeries at night, yet when the work hour restrictions were first implemented, the junior doctors training in surgery were scheduled to work all of their allotted weekly hours during 8-hour overnight shifts scheduled seven nights per week in order to provide patient coverage for the senior surgeons, despite the fact that the junior doctors could not observe or participate in any elective surgical cases at that time of night. It took further regulatory action to eliminate that practice. The very high rate of burnout among resident physicians, which is thought to be caused by occupational stress and sleep loss, suggests that it too may be a consequence of the exhaustion induced by these schedules in all but the most resistant individuals. Such adverse health and safety consequences are burdens that should be distributed fairly, but are instead disproportionately higher in those most vulnerable to sleep loss. Remarkably, when susceptible physicians whose performance is impaired by sleep loss inflict grievous harm—as occurred when first-year resident physician Dr. Sook Im Hong fell asleep at the wheel while driving home from a 36-hour work shift at the Rush Medical Center and rear-ended Heather Brewster's car, causing Ms. Brewster to suffer massive brain injuries (Gotbaum, 2005)—institutions often succeed in displacing the full criminal and/or financial burden of such incidents onto the resident physician instead of acknowledging the extent to which institutional work scheduling practices have contributed to the incident (Czeisler, 2006; Gotbaum, 2005), which violates the principle of justice.

The IOM discovered in its investigation that resident physicians routinely falsify the work-hour records they provide to the ACGME, as data from our research and others demonstrated (Carpenter et al., 2006; Cull et al., 2006; Institute of Medicine, 2008; Landrigan et al., 2006; Nasca, 2009a, b) and the ACGME has recently admitted after years of official denial. In an Open Letter to the GME Community, Thomas J. Nasca, MD, MACP, the new Chief Executive Officer of the ACGME, described the validity of the reporting to ACGME with a refreshing spirit of candor:

> I recently met with the 30 residents who are members of the various Residency Review Committees of the ACGME. These are committed young individuals who bring much to our discussions and deliberations. I asked them a pointed question, whether they "systematically under represent" their hours worked, specifically in relation to the 24/6 standard. To a person, without question, they answered that most residents do systematically under represent the number of times they violate this standard. They give the following three reasons why a resident would misrepresent their actions. First, and foremost, one of their patients needed them. Second, it is the culture of their program that all work be done and not signed out prior to leaving. Third, (and this occurs rarely) their program director or faculty compel them to answer in that fashion.

> (Nasca, 2009a, b)

Such systematic falsification of work-hour records, at least sometimes with the tacit approval, awareness, or expectation of their program directors, violates the principle of *truthfulness and honesty* and sets a regrettable precedent for the trainees of a profession that fundamentally depends on integrity. There are many reasons that may underlie such falsification (Landrigan et al., 2006), including fear of reprisal or loss of program accreditation, as reportedly occurred to Dr. Troy Madsen, a resident who reported resident work-hour violations at Johns Hopkins to the ACGME. Dr. Madsen felt compelled to transfer to Ohio State University Medical Center in order to complete his residency after his report led the ACGME to put the accreditation of the Johns Hopkins internal medicine residency program in which he was enrolled on probation (Madsen, 2004). Our survey data from 4,015 interns revealed that 83.6% of interns reported work hours that were not in compliance with ACGME work-hour limits, which represented 85.4% of the programs in 90.8% of the hospitals. These were not occasional violations, but were systematic, as Dr. Nasca suggests, occurring in 61.5% of inpatient intern-months. The data from our surveys, in which respondent confidentiality was protected by federal statute, was in stark contrast with the data reported by the ACGME. For the same period, the ACGME reported that only 3.3% of residents were non-compliant with the 80-hour rule, based on its national survey; only 2.6% of residency programs were cited by the

ACGME for non-compliance with the 80-hour rule, 1.3% of programs for non-compliance with the 30-hour rule, and 1.4% of programs for non-compliance with the 7-day rule (Landrigan et al., 2006). In other safety-sensitive industries, such falsification of work-hour records have led to felony convictions, hefty fines, and imprisonment, not only for those who falsified the reports but also for company owners and supervisors who were complicit in the falsifications of work-hour records. [See rulings in: (Office of Inspector General, U.S. Department of Transportation, 1999; 2002; 2003; 2005; 2006a, b, c, d; 2007; 2008; 2009) and (Czeisler, 2009b)]. Such work-hour records can have important legal ramifications, as the United States Supreme Court has ruled that, as a matter of law, a railroad operator is considered to be impaired by fatigue after 12 hours of work. Furthermore, how can faculty members instill in trainees the importance of honesty and integrity in clinical and research recordkeeping if they turn a blind eye to the systematic falsification of resident work-hour records? The IOM has therefore recommended that the CMS, which spends nearly $10 billion annually to support the salaries and associated teaching costs of more than 100,000 interns and residents in the United States, together with the Joint Commission, oversee the monitoring of and compliance with its recommended resident physician work-hour restrictions (Institute of Medicine, 2008).

For all these reasons, at its heart, the issue of resident work-hour reform relates to the principle of *human dignity*, both for the patient and for the physician (Czeisler, 2009b). Burdening a physician with a workload that s/he cannot carry creates an ethical dilemma with no good solution. On the one hand, the more hours that the physician works, the greater is the risk to both the patient and to the physician, whereas on the other hand the physician cannot ethically stop working and abandon a patient in need of medical care (Czeisler, 2009b). Thus, a high proportion of dedicated physicians in training, who are attempting to do their best, report making fatigue-related mistakes that injure or result in the death of patients (Barger et al., 2006). In addition to the harm this causes to patients, the guilt over such mistakes causes considerable psychological distress in the physicians themselves (West et al., 2006). Sleep deprivation should not be seen as a proxy for dedication. Instead, working when deprived of sleep should be regarded as working in an impaired state, comparable to being under the influence of alcohol (Czeisler, 2009b). Ensuring that an individual is fit for duty is a shared responsibility between the employer and the employee. Optimizing the work schedule alone is not sufficient. It is the responsibility of the physician to obtain the sleep that s/he needs during off-duty hours. As the IOM recommended in their report on sleep deprivation and sleep disorders in 2006, education about the impact of sleep deprivation and sleep disorders on performance, health, and safety should therefore be provided to medical students, physicians in training, and physicians in practice, so that these healthcare providers understand the importance of that responsibility and so that they recognize the signs and symptoms of sleep disorders (Institute of Medicine, 2006). Towards this end, the Harvard Medical School Division of Sleep Medicine has worked with WGBH, a Boston-based public broadcasting station, to produce a series of web-based educational documentaries on healthy sleep, sleep deprivation, and sleep disorders, which can be accessed at: http://understandingsleep.org.

Education alone is not enough to ensure that physicians are able to minimize impairment by sleep deprivation. The work schedule must be designed to afford the individual a reasonable opportunity for sleep, and to accommodate inter-individual differences in the tolerance to sleep loss and circadian misalignment. As in other safety-sensitive industries in the United States and in residency training in many other countries, work-hour limits for physicians in training should be based on work hours that are safe for most of the population, not a select few (Table 21.5) (Czeisler, 2009b).

Prior to the threat of federal legislation (Nasca, 2009a, b), some medical and surgical training programs in the United States routinely required resident physicians to work 120–140 hours per week (Barger et al., 2005; Czeisler, 2006), just as they currently do in El Salvador (Czeisler, 2009b; Fernández-Taylor, 2007), which still lacks any regulation of resident physician work hours (Table 21.5). At the time, resident physicians nationwide together worked more than an estimated thousand shifts per year that exceeded 70 consecutive hours in duration (Barger et al., 2005). When the fear of legislative intervention finally motivated the ACGME to curtail these egregiously unsafe practices, some decried the limits. Dr. Josef Fischer, then Chair of the Department of Surgery at the Beth Israel Deaconess Medical Center and Harvard Medical School, solemnly declared that the '… total destruction of medicine, and more specifically general surgery, is upon us as a profession…' and that the 80-hour work week limit '… is the antithesis of a profession…' Given the inability of the American medical profession to establish or enforce meaningful comprehensive resident physician work-hour reform in the 25 years since the tragic death of Libby Zion rushed the issue onto the national stage (Lerner, 2009), the time has come for the establishment of reasonable work-hour limits that are enforced by law or regulation (Czeisler, 2006; Czeisler, 2009a; Moore, 2008), an approach that has been endorsed by the boards of directors of the Sleep Research Society and the National Sleep Foundation (Rajah et al., 2009). The fact that a substantial fraction of physicians believe that they are able to exceed proposed limits safely is reminiscent of the position of those opposing drunk driving legislation a half century ago (Fischer, 2005), who argued vehemently that it was not fair to restrict everyone from drinking and driving just because some people could not 'hold their liquor'. Notwithstanding considerable inter-individual differences in the extent to which alcohol impairs cognitive and psychomotor performance, society has resoundingly rejected this line of reasoning and all 50 states have established blood alcohol concentrations above which drivers are judged to be impaired. As the IOM has recently concluded, now is the time for meaningful resident physician work-hour limits as well (Institute of Medicine, 2008), which the federal government has the authority to implement (Czeisler, 2009a; Lee, 2006). This should include a provision to require disclosure to patients if a physician has been awake for more than 22 of the prior 24 hours, or more than 140 of the prior 168 hours, so that the patient can make a decision as to whether s/he wishes to receive medical care from a physician who may be considerably impaired by the effects of acute or chronic sleep deprivation. Once physician work-hour reform has been implemented successfully in the United States, it will serve as the foundation for implementation of safer work schedules in a wide variety of industries.

References

Åkerstedt, T., Palmblad, J., de la Torre, B., Marana, R. & Gillberg, M. (1980). Adrenocortical and gonadal steriods during sleep deprivation. *Sleep*, **3**(1), 23–30.

Anderson, C. & Horne, J.A. (2006). Sleepiness enhances distraction during a monotonous task. *Sleep*, **29**(4), 573–576.

Arnedt, J.T., Owens, J., Crouch, M., Stahl, J. & Carskadon, M.A. (2005). Neurobehavioral performance of residents after heavy night call vs after alcohol ingestion. *JAMA*, **294**(9), 1025–1033.

Association of Pediatric Program Directors (2009). Association of Pediatric Program Directors (APPD) Position Statement in Response to the IOM Recommendations on Resident Duty Hours.

Ayas, N.T., Barger, L.K., Cade, B.E., et al. (2006). Extended work duration and the risk of self-reported percutaneous injuries in interns. *J Am Med Assoc*, **296**(9), 1055–1062.

Barger, L.K., Cade, B.E., Ayas, N.T., et al. (2005). Extended work shifts and the risk of motor vehicle crashes among interns. *N Engl J Med*, **352**, 125–134.

Barger, L.K., Ayas, N.T., Cade, B.E., et al. (2006). Impact of extended-duration shifts on medical errors, adverse events, and attentional failures. *PLoS Med*, **3**(12), e487.

BBC News (2008). Doctor hour cuts 'will harm care'. BBC News.

Belenky, G., Wesensten, N.J., Thorne, D.R., et al. (2003). Patterns of performance degradation and restoration during sleep restriction and subsequent recovery: a sleep dose-response study. *J Sleep Res*, **12**, 1–12.

Blagrove, M. (1996). Effects of length of sleep deprivation on interrogative suggestibility. *J Exp Psychol*, **2**, 48–59.

Blanchard, M.S., Meltzer, D. & Polonsky, K.S. (2009). To nap or not to nap? Residents' work hours revisited. *N Engl J Med*, **360**(21), 2242–2244.

Bodenmann, S., Hohoff, C., Grietag, C., Deckert, J., Retey, J. & Landolt, H.-P. (2007). Genetic variation in the adenosine A2A receptor gene modulates performance on the psychomotor vigilance task. *Sleep Biol Rhythms*, **5**, A47.

Boodman, S.G. (2001). Low experience, high expectations. *Washington Post*. Health Section, T_{12}

Britt, L.D., Sachdeva, A.K., Healy, G.B., Whalen, T.V. & Blair, P.G. (2009). Resident duty hours in surgery for ensuring patient safety, providing optimum resident education and training, and promoting resident well-being: a response from the American College of Surgeons to the Report of the Institute of Medicine, 'Resident Duty Hours: Enhancing Sleep, Supervision, and Safety'. *Surgery*, **146**(3), 398–409.

Cajochen, C., Khalsa, S.B.S., Wyatt, J.K., Czeisler, C.A. & Dijk, D.J. (1999). EEG and ocular correlates of circadian melatonin phase and human performance decrements during sleep loss. *Am J Physiol*, **277**, R640–R649.

Cappuccio, F.P., Bakewell, A., Taggart, F.M., et al. (2009a). Implementing a 48 h EWTD-compliant rota for junior doctors in the UK does not compromise patients' safety: assessor-blind pilot comparison. *Q J Med*, **102**, 271–282.

Cappuccio, F.P., Lockley, S.W. & Landrigan, C.P. (2009b). Cappuccio response to correspondence. *QJM*, **102**(5), 363–364.

Carpenter, R.O., Austin, M.T., Tarpley, J.L., Griffin, M.R. & Lomis, K.D. (2006). Work-hour restrictions as an ethical dilemma for residents. *Am J Surg*, **191**(4), 527–532.

Carter, N., Ulfberg, J., Nystrom, B. & Edling, C. (2003). Sleep debt, sleepiness and accidents among males in the general population and male professional drivers. *Accid Anal Prev*, **35**(4), 613–617.

Chen, P.W. (2008). Does more sleep make for better doctors? *NY Times*. Health section

Chuah, Y.M., Venkatraman, V., Dinges, D.F. & Chee, M.W. (2006). The neural basis of interindividual variability in inhibitory efficiency after sleep deprivation. *J Neurosci*, **26**(27), 7156–7162.

Cipollone v. Liggett Group (1983). 693 F. Supp. 208 (D.N.J. 1988) aff'd in part, rev'd in part, 893 F. 2d 541 (3rd Cir. 1990), aff'd in part, rev'd in part 505 U.S. 504 (1992).

Cohen, S., Doyle, W.J., Alper, C.M., Janicki-Deverts, D., & Turner, R.B. (2009). Sleep habits and susceptibility to the common cold. *Arch Intern Med*, **169**(1), 62–67.

Cohen, D.A., Wang, W., Wyatt, J.K., et al. (2010). Uncovering residual effects of chronic sleep loss on human performance. *Sci Transl Med*, **2**(14), 14ra3.

Cull, W.L., Mulvey, H.J., Jewett, E.A., et al. (2006). Pediatric residency duty hours before and after limitations. *Pediatrics*, **118**(6), e1805–e1811.

Czeisler, C.A. (2004). Work hours and sleep in residency training. *Sleep*, **27**(3), 371–372.

Czeisler, C.A. (2006). The Gordon Wilson Lecture: work hours, sleep and patient safety in residency training. *Trans Am Clin Climatol Assoc*, **117**, 159–189.

Czeisler, C.A. (2009a). It's time to reform work hours for resident physicians. *Sci News*, **176**(9), 36.

Czeisler, C.A. (2009b). Medical and genetic differences in the adverse impact of sleep loss on performance: ethical considerations for the medical profession. *Trans Am Clin Climatol Assoc*, **120**, 249–285.

Czeisler, C.A. (2009c). Operating over the limit. *Boston Globe*, A17.

Czeisler, C.A., Moore-Ede, M.C. & Coleman, R.M. (1982). Rotating shift work schedules that disrupt sleep are improved by applying circadian principles. *Science*, **217**, 460–463.

Dawson, D. and Reid, K. (1997). Fatigue, alcohol and performance impairment. *Nature*, **388**, 235.

DeSantis, A.D., Webb, E.M. & Noar, S.M. (2008). Illicit use of prescription ADHD medications on a college campus: a multimethodological approach. *J Am Coll Health*, **57**(3), 315–324.

Dinges, D.F., Pack, F., Williams, K., et al. (1997). Cumulative sleepiness, mood disturbance, and psychomotor vigilance performance decrements during a week of sleep restricted to 4-5 hours per night. *Sleep*, **20**(4), 267–277.

Division of Sleep Medicine, Harvard Medical School, and WGBH Educational Foundation (2010). Lou's Killer Shift. Available at: http://healthysleep.med.harvard.edu/need-sleep/success-stories/lou-killer-shift. Accessed 1 February 2010.

Drake, C.L., Roehrs, T., Richardson, G., Walsh, J.K. & Roth, T. (2004). Shift work sleep disorder: prevalence and consequences beyond that of symptomatic day workers. *Sleep*, **27**(8), 1453–1462.

Duffy, J.F., Willson, H.J., Wang, W. & Czeisler, C.A. (2009). Healthy older adults better tolerate sleep deprivation than young adults. *J Am Geriatr Soc*, **57**(7), 1245–1251.

Durmer, J.S. & Dinges, D.F. (2005). Neurocognitive consequences of sleep deprivation. *Semin Neurol*, **25**(1), 117–129.

Ekstedt, M., Soderstrom, M., Åkerstedt, T., Nilsson, J., Sondergaard, H.P. & Aleksander, P. (2006). Disturbed sleep and fatigue in occupational burnout. *Scand J Work Environ Health*, **32**(2), 121–131.

Falleti, M.G., Maruff, P., Collie, A., Darby, D.G. & McStephen, M. (2003). Qualitative similarities in cognitive impairment associated with 24 h of sustained wakefulness and a blood alcohol concentration of 0.05%. *J Sleep Res*, **12**(4), 265–274.

Faverty v. McDonald's Restaurants (1995). 892 P. 2d 703 (Or. Ct. App. 1995) appeal dismissed, petition for review dismissed, 971 P. 2d 407 (Or. 1998).

Fernández-Taylor, K.R. (2007). Excessive work hours of physicians in training in El Salvador: putting patients at risk. *PLoS Med*, **4**(7), e205.

Fischer, J.E. (2005). Surgeons: Employees o professionals? *Am J Surg*, **190**, 1–3.

Four truck drivers sentenced in logbook falsification case. (2009). U.S. District Court, Fresno, CA. Available at: http://www.oig.dot.gov/library-item/3435. Accessed 25 May 2010.

Frank, E., Elon, L., Naimi, T. & Brewer, R. (2008). Alcohol consumption and alcohol counselling behaviour among US medical students: cohort study. *BMJ*, **337**, a2155.

Frey, D.J., Badia, P. & Wright, K.P., Jr. (2004). Inter- and intra-individual variability in performance near the circadian nadir during sleep deprivation. *J Sleep Res*, **13**(4), 305–315.

Gordon, J.A., Alexander, E.K., Lockley, S.W., et al. (2010). Does simulator-based clinical performance correlate with actual hospital behavior? The effect of extended work hours on patient care provided by medical interns. *Acad Med*, in press

Gotbaum, R. (2005). *Safety of Medical Residents' Long Hours Questioned*. Washington, DC: National Public Radio.

Grantcharov, T.P., Bardram, L., Funch-Jensen, P. & Rosenberg, J. (2001). Laparoscopic performance after one night on call in a surgical department: prospective study. *BMJ*, **323**, 1222–1223.

Groeger, J.A., Viola, A.U., Lo, J.C.Y., von Shantz, M., Archer, S.N. & Dijk, D.J. (2008). Early morning executive functioning during sleep deprivation is compromised by a *PERIOD3* polymorphism. *Sleep*, **31**(8), 1159–1167.

Haack, M. & Mullington, J.M. (2005). Sustained sleep restriction reduces emotional and physical well-being. *Pain*, **119**(1–3), 56–64.

He, Y., Jones, C.R., Fujiki, N., et al. (2009). The transcriptional repressor DEC2 regulates sleep length in mammals. *Science*, **325**(5942), 866–870.

Higginson, J.D. (2009). Limiting resident work hours is a moral concern. *Acad Med*, **84**(3), 310–314.

Horowitz, T.S., Cade, B.E., Wolfe, J.M. & Czeisler, C.A. (2003). Searching night and day: a dissociation of effects of circadian phase and time awake on visual selective attention and vigilance. *Psychol Sci*, **14**(6), 549–557.

Ingle, J. (2008). Resident work hours: standing up for patient safety is not 'whining'. *Huffington Post*.

Institute of Medicine (2006). In: Colten, H.R. & Alteveogt, B.M. (eds.), *Sleep Disorders and Sleep Deprivation: An Unmet Public Health Problem*. Washington, DC: National Academies Press, pp. 1–500; ISBN: 0-309-66012-2.

Institute of Medicine (2008). In: Ulmer, C., Wolman, D.M. & Johns, M.M.E. (eds.), *Resident Duty Hours: Enhancing Sleep, Supervision, and Safety*. Washington, DC: National Academies Press, pp. 1–322.

Jagannathan, J., Vates, G.E., Pouratian, N., et al. (2009). Impact of the Accreditation Council for Graduate Medical Education work-hour regulations on neurosurgical resident education and productivity. *J Neurosurg*, **110**(5), 820–827.

Javaheri, S., Storfer-Isser, A., Rosen, C.L. & Redline, S. (2008). Sleep quality and elevated blood pressure in adolescents. *Circulation*, **118**(10), 1034–1040.

Killgore, W.D., Balkin, T.J. & Wesensten, N.J. (2006). Impaired decision making following 49 h of sleep deprivation. *J Sleep Res*, **15**(1), 7–13.

Killgore, W.D., Killgore, D.B., Day, L.M., Li, C., Kamimori, G.H. & Balkin, T.J. (2007). The effects of 53 hours of sleep deprivation on moral judgment. *Sleep*, **30**(3), 345–352.

King, C.R., Knutson, K.L., Rathouz, P.J., Sidney, S., Liu, K. & Lauderdale, D.S. (2008). Short sleep duration and incident coronary artery calcification. *J Am Med Assoc*, **300**(24), 2859–2866.

Knutson, K.L., Spiegel, K., Penev, P. & Van Cauter, E. (2007). The metabolic consequences of sleep deprivation. *Sleep Med Rev*, **11**(3), 163–178.

Knutson, K.L. & Van Cauter, E. (2008). Associations between sleep loss and increased risk of obesity and diabetes. *Ann N Y Acad Sci*, **1129**, 287–304.

Knutson, K.L., Van Cauter, E., Rathouz, P.J., et al. (2009). Association between sleep and blood pressure in midlife: the CARDIA sleep study. *Arch Intern Med*, **169**(11), 1055–1061.

Kryger, M.H., Roth, T. & Dement, W.C. (eds.) (2005). *Principles and Practice of Sleep Medicine*. Fourth edition. Philadelphia, PA: W.B. Saunders.

Lamond, N. & Dawson, D. (1999). Quantifying the performance impairment associated with fatigue. *J Sleep Res*, **8**(4), 255–262.

Landrigan, C.P., Rothschild, J.M., Cronin, J.W., et al. (2004). Effect of reducing interns' work hours on serious medical errors in intensive care units. *N Engl J Med*, **351**(18), 1838–1848.

Landrigan, C.P., Barger, L.K., Cade, B.E., Ayas, N.T. & Czeisler, C.A. (2006). Interns' compliance with accreditation council for graduate medical education work-hour limits. *J Am Med Assoc*, **296**(9), 1063–1070.

Lee, C.J. (2006). Federal regulation of hospital resident work hours: enforcement with real teeth. *J Health Care Law Policy*, **9**(1), 1–55.

Leproult, R., Colecchia, E.F., Berardi, A.M., Stickgold, R., Kosslyn, S.M. & Van Cauter, E. (2003). Individual differences in subjective and objective alertness during sleep deprivation are stable and unrelated. *Am J Physiol Regul Integr Comp Physiol*, **284**, R280–R290.

Lerner, B.H. (2009). A life-changing case for doctors in training. *NY Times*.

Lockley, S.W., Cronin, J.W., Evans, E.E., et al. (2004). Effect of reducing interns' weekly work hours on sleep and attentional failures. *N Engl J Med*, **351**(18), 1829–1837.

Lopez, L. & Katz, J.T. (2009). Creating an ethical workplace: reverberations of resident work hours reform. *Acad Med*, **84**(3), 315–319.

Macdonald, K. (2009). Night shifts spark cancer pay-out. BBC News.

Madsen, T.A. (2004). Whistleblower's story: reflections on making that report. *New Physician*.

McBeth, B.D. & Ankel, F.K. (2006). Don't ask, don't tell: substance use by resident physicians. *Acad Emerg Med*, **13**(8), 893–895.

McLellan, A.T., Skipper, G.S., Campbell, M. & DuPont, R.L. (2008). Five year outcomes in a cohort study of physicians treated for substance use disorders in the United States. *BMJ*, **337**, a2038.

Moalem, J., Salzman, P., Ruan, D.T., et al. (2009). Should all duty hours be the same? Results of a national survey of surgical trainees. *J Am Coll Surg*, **209**(1), 47–54.

Moore, R.T. (2008). An act relative to safe work hours for physicians in training and protection of patients. Commonwealth of Massachusetts Senate Docket No. 1178.

Moore, R.T. (2009). An act relative to health care provider transportation. Commonwealth of Massachusetts Senate Docket No. 1901.

Moore, R.T., Kaprielian, R. & Auerbach, J. (2009). Asleep at the wheel. Report of the Massachusetts commission on drowsy driving. http://www.boston.com/news/local/breaking_news/Drowsy%20 Driving%20Commission%20Report.pdf

Nasca, T.J. (2008). Opposing view: teaching hospitals excel. *USA Today*.

Nasca, T.J. (2009a). Resident issues need close examination. AAMC Reporter. http://www.boston.com/ news/local/breaking_news/Drowsy%20Driving%20Commission%20Report.pdf

Nasca, T.J. (2009b). Open letter to the GME community. Office of Inspector General, U.S. Department of Transportation (2007).

Office of Inspector General, U.S. Department of Transportation (1999). Trucking company, owner sentenced in driver log-fraud case. 1-22-1999. Federal Court, MN. Available at: http://www.oig.dot.gov/library-item/5041; accessed on 24 May 2010.

Office of Inspector General, U.S. Department of Transportation (2002). Trucking firm and president sentenced in hours-of-service violations. 7-24-2002. U.S. District Court, Bangor, ME. Available at: http://www.oig.dot.gov/library-item/3006; accessed on 24 May 2010.

Office of Inspector General, U.S. Department of Transportation (2003). Truck driver imprisoned for falsifying his driver's log. 12-16-2003. U.S. District Court, Philadelphia, PA. Available at: http://www.oig.dot.gov/library-item/3176; accessed on 24 May 2010.

Office of Inspector General, U.S. Department of Transportation (2005). South Dakota trucking firm and president ordered to pay over $325,000 in driver logbook falsification case. 9-22-2005. U.S. District Court, Sioux Falls, SD. Former executive, dispatcher, and two drivers of Virginia trucking company sentenced for their roles in falsifying drivers' logbooks. 1-18-2006a. U.S. District Court, Lynchburg, VA. Ref Type: Case. Available at: http://www.oig.dot.gov/library-item/3389; accessed on 24 May 2010.

Office of Inspector General, U.S. Department of Transportation (2006). Former owner and dispatcher for Pennsylvania trucking company sentenced in logbook falsification case. 3-14-2006b. U.S. District Court, Williamsport, PA.

Office of Inspector General, U.S. Department of Transportation (2006). Virginia truck driver gets jail time for falsifying logbooks. 8-11-2006c. U.S. District Court, Brunswick, GA.

Office of Inspector General, U.S. Department of Transportation (2008). California trucking company safety director and four drivers sentenced for their role in a false driver's logbook scheme. 7-21-2008. U.S. District Court, Fresno, CA. Available at: http://www.oig.dot.gov/library-item/3644; accessed 24 May 2010.

Patel, S.R. & Hu, F.B. (2008). Short sleep duration and weight gain: a systematic review. *Obesity (Silver Spring)*, **16**(3), 643–653.

Patel, S.R., Zhu, X., Storfer-Isser, A., et al. (2009). Sleep duration and biomarkers of inflammation. *Sleep*, **32**(2), 200–204.

Pennsylvania truck driver sentenced to 2 years in prison for vehicular homicide relating to hours-of-service violations. 3-7-2007. State Court, Easton, PA. Available at: http://www.oig.dot.gov/library-item/3554. Accessed on 24 May 2010.

Philibert, I. (2005). Sleep loss and performance in residents and nonphysicians: a meta-analytic examination. *Sleep*, **28**(11), 1392–1402.

Powell, N.B., Schechtman, K.B., Riley, R.W., Li, K., Troell, R. & Guilleminault, C. (2001). The road to danger: the comparative risks of driving while sleepy. *Laryngoscope*, **111**(5), 887–893.

Rajah, M.N., Bastianetto, S., Bromley-Brits, K., et al. (2009). Biological changes associated with healthy versus pathological aging: a symposium review. *Ageing Res Rev*, **8**(2), 140–146.

Reid, W. & Coakley, J. (2008). Junior doctors' working hours: 48 hours in 2009. Meeting the challenge. *Clin Med*, **8**(3), 346–347.

Robertson v. LeMaster (1983). 301 SE. 2d 563 (W. Va. 1983).

Rogers, A.E., Hwang, W.T., Scott, L.D., Aiken, L.H., & Dinges, D.F. The working hours of hospital staff nurses and patient safety. *Health Aff. (Millwood.)*, **23**(4), 202–212.

Rothschild, J.M., Hurley, A.C., Landrigan, C.P., et al. (2006). Recovery from medical errors: the critical care nursing safety net. *Jt Comm J Qual Patient Saf*, **32**(2), 63–72.

Rybock, J.D. (2009). Residents' duty hours and professionalism. *N Engl J Med*, **361**(9), 930–931.

Spiegel, K., Leproult, R. & Van Cauter, E. (1999). Impact of sleep debt on metabolic and endocrine function. *Lancet*, **354**, 1435–1439.

Spiegel, K., Sheridan, J.F. & Van Cauter, E. (2002). Effect of sleep deprivation on response to immunization. *J Am Med Assoc*, **288**(12), 1471–1472.

Spiegel, K., Leproult, R., Tasali, E., Penev, P. & Van Cauter, E. (2004a). Sleep curtailment results in decreased leptin levels, elevated ghrelin levels and increased hunger and appetite. *Ann Intern Med*, **141**, 846–850.

Spiegel, K., Tasali, E., Penev, P. & Van Cauter, E. (2004b). Brief communication: sleep curtailment in healthy young men is associated with decreased leptin levels, elevated ghrelin levels, and increased hunger and appetite. *Ann Intern Med*, **141**(11), 846–850.

Stickgold, R. (2005). Sleep-dependent memory consolidation. *Nature*, **437**(7063), 1272–1278.

The New York Times (2008). Napping during hospital shifts.U.S. Department of Health, Education, and Welfare (1964). *Smoking and Health: Report of the Advisory Committee to the Surgeon General of the Public Health Service*. Washington, DC: U.S. Department of Health, Education, and Welfare. PHS Publication No. 1103.

University of Washington School of Medicine (2009). *Ethics in Medicine*. Available at: http://depts. washington.edu/bioethx/tools/princpl.html.

USA Today (2008). Our view on medical care: sleep-deprived residents still pose risk for patients.

Van Dongen, H.P.A. (2005). Brain activation patterns and individual differences in working memory impairment during sleep deprivation. *Sleep*, **28**(4), 386–388.

Van Dongen, H.P.A. (2006). Shift work and inter-individual differences in sleep and sleepiness. *Chronobiol Int*, **23**(6), 1139–1147.

Van Dongen, H.P.A., Maislin, G., Mullington, J.M. & Dinges, D.F. (2003). The cumulative cost of additional wakefulness: dose-response effects on neurobehavioral functions and sleep physiology from chronic sleep restriction and total sleep deprivation. *Sleep*, **26**(2), 117–126.

Van Dongen, H.P.A., Baynard, M.D., Maislin, G. & Dinges, D.F. (2004a). Systematic interindividual differences in neurobehavioral impairment from sleep loss: evidence of trait-like differential vulnerability. *Sleep*, **27**, 423–433.

Van Dongen, H.P.A., Maislin, G. & Dinges, D.F. (2004b). Dealing with inter-individual differences in the temporal dynamics of fatigue and performance: importance and techniques. *Aviat Space Environ Med*, **75**(Suppl 3), A147–A154.

Van Dongen, H.P.A., Vitellaro, K.M. & Dinges, D.F. (2005). Individual differences in adult human sleep and wakefulness: leitmotif for a research agenda. *Sleep*, **28**(4), 479–496.

Van Dongen, H.P.A., Caldwell, J.A., Jr. & Caldwell, J.L. (2006). Investigating systematic individual differences in sleep-deprived performance on a high-fidelity flight simulator. *Behav Res Methods*, **38**(2), 333–343.

Viola, A.U., Archer, S.N., James, L.M., et al. (2007). *PER3* polymorphism predicts sleep structure and waking performance. *Curr Biol*, **17**, 1–6.

Walker, M.P. & Stickgold, R. (2004). Sleep-dependent learning and memory consolidation. *Neuron*, **44**(1), 121–133.

Wang, D., Teichtahl, H., Goodman, C., Drummer, O., Grunstein, R.R. & Kronborg, I. (2008). Subjective daytime sleepiness and daytime function in patients on stable methadone maintenance treatment: possible mechanisms. *J Clin Sleep Med*, **4**(6), 557–562.

Warshaw, A.L. (2009). Walking a tightrope on MGH's training hours. *Boston Globe*.

West, C.P., Huschka, M.M., Novotny, P.J., et al. (2006). Association of perceived medical errors with resident distress and empathy: a prospective longitudinal study. *JAMA*, **296**(9), 1071–1078.

Williamson, A.M. & Feyer, A.M. (2000). Moderate sleep deprivation produces impairments in cognitive and motor performance equivalent to legally prescribed levels of alcohol intoxication. *Occup Environ Med*, **57**, 649–655.

Willis, R.E. (2009). Views of surgery Program Directors on the current ACGMA and proposed IOM duty-hour standards. *J Surg Educ*, **66**(4), 216–221.

Wyatt, J.K., Cajochen, C., Ritz-De Cecco, A., Czeisler, C.A. & Dijk, D.J. (2004). Low-dose repeated caffeine administration for circadian-phase-dependent performance degradation during extended wakefulness. *Sleep*, **27**(3), 374–381.

Yoo, S.S., Gujar, N., Hu, P., Jolesz, F.A., Walker, M.P. The human emotional brain without sleep - a prefrontal amygdala disconnect. *Curr Biol*, **17**(20), R877–R878.

Zgierska, A., Brown, R.T., Zuelsdorff, M., Brown, D., Zhang, Z. & Fleming, M.F. (2007). Sleep and daytime sleepiness problems among patients with chronic noncancerous pain receiving long-term opioid therapy: a cross-sectional study. *J Opioid Manag*, **3**(6), 317–327.

Index